AF548594

PATHOLOGY OF LYMPH NODES

CONTEMPORARY ISSUES IN SURGICAL PATHOLOGY VOLUME 21

SERIES EDITOR

Lawrence M. Roth, M.D.

Professor of Pathology
Director, Division of Surgical Pathology
Indiana University School of Medicine
Indianapolis, Indiana

Previously published

Vol. 6 Tumors and Tumorlike Conditions of the Ovary
Lawrence M. Roth, M.D., and Bernard Czernobilsky, M.D.

Vol. 7 Pathology of the Testis and Its Adnexa
Aleksander Talerman, M.D., and Lawrence M. Roth, M.D

Vol. 9 Pathology of the Vulva and Vagina
Edward J. Wilkinson, M.D.

Vol. 12 Pathology of the Heart and Great Vessels
Bruce F. Waller, M.D.

Vol. 13 Pathology of the Urinary Bladder
Robert H. Young, M.D.

Vol. 15 Pathology of the Prostate
David G. Bostwick, M.D.

Vol. 16 Tumors and Tumor-like Conditions of the Kidneys and Ureters
John N. Eble, M.D.

Vol. 17 Pathology of the Colon, Small Intestine, and Anus, 2nd Ed.
H. Thomas Norris, M.D.

Vol. 18 Tumors and Tumorlike Lesions of Soft Tissue
Vito Ninfo, M.D., E.B. Chung, M.D., M.Sc., Ph.D., and
Andrea O. Cavazzana, M.D.

Vol. 19 Tumors and Tumorlike Lesions of the Uterine Corpus and Cervix
Philip B. Clement, M.D., and Robert H. Young, M.D., M.R.C. Path.

Vol. 20 Gastrointestinal Mucosal Biopsy
Harvey Goldman, M.D.

PATHOLOGY OF LYMPH NODES

Edited by

Lawrence M. Weiss, M.D.
Director of Surgical Pathology
Division of Pathology
City of Hope National Medical Center
Duarte, California

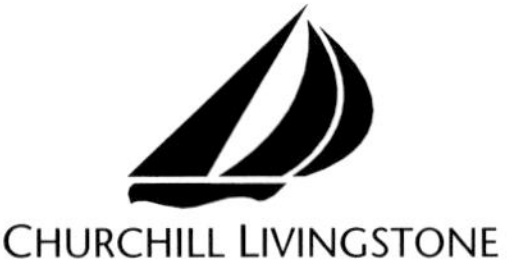

CHURCHILL LIVINGSTONE

New York, Edinburgh, London, Madrid, Melbourne, San Francisco, Tokyo

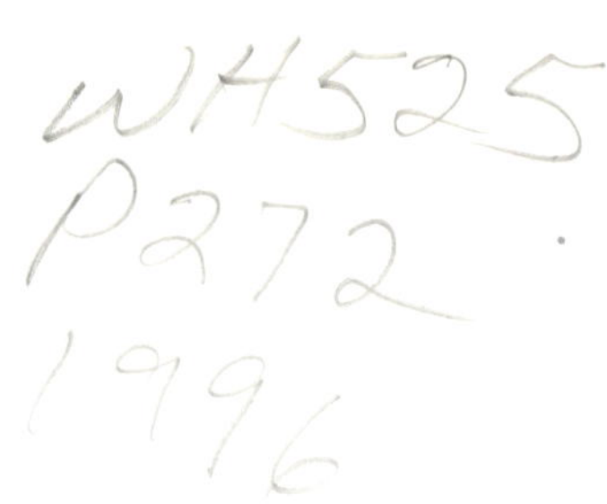

Library of Congress Cataloging-in-Publication Data

Pathology of lymph nodes / edited by Lawrence M. Weiss.
p. cm. — (Contemporary issues in surgical pathology ; vol. 21)
Includes bibliographical references and index.
ISBN 0-443-07620-0
1. Lymph nodes — Biopsy. 2. Lymph nodes— Diseases— Cytodiagnosis. 3. Pathology, Surgical. I. Weiss, Lawrence M. II. Series.
[DNLM: 1. Lymphoma— pathology. 2. Lymphatic Diseases— pathology. W1 CO769MS v.21 1996 / WH 525 P297 1996]
RC646.P38 1996
616.4′207—dc20
DNLM/DLC
for Library of Congress 96-19840
CIP

Distributed in the United Kingdom by Churchill Livingstone, Robert Stevenson House, 1–3 Baxter's Place, Leith Walk, Edinburgh EH1 3AF, and by associated companies, branches, and representatives throughout the world.

Accurate indications, adverse reactions, and dosage schedules for drugs are provided in this book, but it is possible that they may change. The reader is urged to review the package information data of the manufacturers of the medications mentioned.

The Publishers have made every effort to trace the copyright holders for borrowed material. If they have inadvertently overlooked any, they will be pleased to make the necessary arrangements at the first opportunity.

Assistant Editor: *Marc Strauss*
Production Editor: *David Terry*
Production Supervisor: *Laura Mosberg Cohen*

Printed in the United States of America

First published in 1996 7 6 5 4 3 2 1

Contributors

Bjarni A. Agnarsson, M.D.
Associate Professor, Department of Pathology, University of Iceland Faculty of Medicine, Reykjavík, Iceland

Lawrence J. Burgart, M.D.
Assistant Professor, Department of Pathology, Mayo Medical School; Senior Associate Consultant, Department of Pathology, Mayo Clinic, Rochester, Minnesota

John K. C. Chan, M.B.B.S., M.R.C.Path., F.R.C.P.A.
Consultant, Department of Pathology, Queen Elizabeth Hospital, Kowloon, Hong Kong

Karen L. Chang, M.D.
Staff Pathologist, Division of Pathology, City of Hope National Medical Center, Duarte, California

Glauco Frizzera, M.D.
Professor, Department of Pathology, New York University School of Medicine; Director, Division of Hematopathology, Department of Pathology, New York University Medical Center, New York, New York

Thomas M. Grogan, M.D.
Professor, Department of Pathology, University of Arizona College of Medicine, Tucson, Arizona

Nancy Lee Harris, M.D.
Professor, Department of Pathology, Harvard Medical School; Director, Section of Anatomic Pathology, Department of Pathology, Massachusetts General Hospital, Boston, Massachusetts

Marshall E. Kadin, M.D.
Professor, Department of Pathology, Harvard Medical School; Director, Division of Hematopathology, Department of Pathology, Beth Israel Hospital, Boston, Massachusetts

William F. Kern, M.D.
Assistant Professor, Department of Pathology, University of Oklahoma College of Medicine; Attending Physician, Department of Pathology, University of Oklahoma Health Sciences Center, Oklahoma City, Oklahoma

Catherine P. Leith, M.D.
Assistant Professor, Department of Pathology, University of New Mexico School of Medicine; Director, Clinical Flow Cytometry Laboratory, University Hospital, Albuquerque, New Mexico

L. Jeffrey Medeiros, M.D.
Director of Hematopathology, Division of Pathology, City of Hope National Medical Center, Duarte, California

Michael A. Nalesnik, M.D.
Associate Professor, Division of Transplantation Pathology, Department of Pathology, University of Pittsburgh School of Medicine, Pittsburgh, Pennsylvania

Bharat N. Nathwani, M.D.
Professor, Department of Pathology, University of Southern California School of Medicine; Chief, Division of Hematopathology, Department of Pathology, Los Angeles County-University of Southern California Medical Center, Los Angeles, California

Sibrand Poppema, M.D., Ph.D.
Chairman, Department of Pathology, University of Groningen Faculty of Medicine; Head, Department of Pathology, Academic Hospital, Groningen, the Netherlands

John G. Strickler, M.D.
Associate Professor, Department of Pathology, Mayo Medical School; Consultant, Department of Pathology, Mayo Clinic, Rochester, Minnesota

William Y. W. Tsang, M.B.B.S., F.R.C.P.A.
Senior Pathologist, Department of Pathology, Queen Elizabeth Hospital, Kowloon, Hong Kong

Lawrence M. Weiss, M.D.
Director of Surgical Pathology, Division of Pathology, City of Hope National Medical Center, Duarte, California

Preface

This volume of *Contemporary Issues in Surgical Pathology* provides up-to-date discussion of several important topics in lymph node pathology by some of the foremost experts in the field. It is not intended to cover the complete gamut of hematopathology; for this, the reader is referred to several excellent texts. Rather, this book focuses on important topics in a timely fashion, providing in-depth coverage not generally possible in textbooks that cover the entire field. For example, the chapter on molecular hematopathology by Medeiros provides an introduction to molecular analysis as well as a comprehensive and up-to-date review of molecular genetic findings in specific lymphoma types. The chapter on reactive lymphadenopathies by Chan and Tsang gives a general approach to benign lymphadenopathies, with extensive description and illustration of newly recognized entities. With established entities, relevant new information is highlighted. The chapter on posttransplant lymphoproliferative disorders by Nalesnik and Frizzera discusses a very difficult and controversial area within hematopathology, offering a coherent account of this disorder from the anatomic pathologist's standpoint and a practical framework with which to evaluate cases.

One highlight of this book is extensive discussion of the recently proposed Revised European-American Classification of Lymphomas (REAL classification). The chapter on lymphoma classification provides a historical review, with critical analysis and comparison of the Working Formulation with the REAL classification. The chapter on low grade B-cell lymphomas by Harris and the chapter on peripheral T-cell lymphomas by Leith, Kern, and Grogan provide in-depth discussion of some of the more recently described entities in the REAL classification, with precise criteria for their identification and discussion of differential diagnosis. The chapter on aggressive non-Hodgkin's lymphoma by Weiss and Nathwani gives an overview of these lymphomas, with coverage of the difficult areas of T-cell-rich and B-cell lymphoma, mediastinal large B-cell lymphoma, and angiotropic lymphoma, as well as coverage of HIV-associated lymphoma, a lymphoma of increasing importance throughout the world. The chapter on anaplastic large cell lymphoma by Agnarsson and Kadin describes the histology and immunohistochemistry of this controversial lymphoma, with special emphasis on its differential diagnosis from other disorders with which it may be confused.

This book also provides extensive coverage of Hodgkin's disease. Our current knowledge of Hodgkin's disease suggests that nodular lymphocyte predominance Hodgkin's disease should be separated from the other types as a discrete disease entity. Therefore, we have chosen to discuss these topics in separate chapters. The chapter by Strickler, Burgart, and Weiss reviews classical Hodgkin's disease, emphasizing recent histologic, immunologic, molecular, cytogenetic, viral, and clinical studies. Following this, a chapter by Poppema reviews nodular lymphocyte predominance Hodgkin's disease, with discussion of diffuse variants and transformation to large cell lymphoma. Finally, the chapter on histiocytic and dendritic disorders by Chang and Weiss discusses recent findings in this area, particularly within the controversial area of true histiocytic neoplasms.

I wish to give special thanks to my colleague Dr. Karen L. Chang, not only for her contribution to Chapter 11, but also for her suggestions and help with editing this book and many of my other publications.

Lawrence M. Weiss, M.D.

Contents

1

Molecular Hematopathology

L. Jeffrey Medeiros

ROLE OF MOLECULAR GENETIC STUDIES IN THE WORK-UP OF LYMPHOID NEOPLASMS

The histologic findings of malignant lymphomas and leukemias, although essential, may be insufficient for complete diagnosis. Immunophenotypic and molecular genetic findings have contributed greatly to our ability to diagnose and subclassify these tumors. Usually, immunophenotypic studies using either flow cytometry or immunohistochemistry represent the first step in the work-up of lymphomas and leukemias.[1,2] The clonality of B-cell neoplasms may be determined by analysis of Igκ and Igλ light chain expression. Monoclonal B cells often express either one or the other Ig light chain, whereas polyclonal B cells express a mixture of Ig light chains. The expression of various lineage-specific antigens such as CD19 or CD3 by lymphoid cells is also useful. However, there are drawbacks to immunophenotypic analysis. There are no clonal markers analogous to the Ig light chains that are expressed by neoplastic T cells.[1,2] Furthermore, immunophenotyping is based on gene expression; in other words, protein must be produced by the cells in a quantity sufficient to be detected by immunophenotypic methods.[1,2]

Molecular genetic techniques are a second step, usually performed after immunophenotyping is completed, and are complementary studies that provide additional information. Molecular methods are generally more sensitive than immunophenotyping, particularly when the assays use the polymerase chain reaction (PCR) technique. Molecular analyses do not require gene expression; instead, they assess the genes directly. Also, molecular studies are essential for the assessment of clonality in T-cell lesions.[1,2]

Molecular genetic analyses are best performed on either fresh or viably frozen tissue. Thus, if a lymphoproliferative process is a possible diagnosis, a portion of the fresh tissue should be preserved in a frozen state (less than $-70°C$) and stored, at least until the diagnosis is confirmed. If the quantity of tissue is adequate, a cell suspension should be prepared and rapidly frozen for possible flow cytometric studies. When it is not possible to prepare a cell suspension, tissue frozen in cryostat section-embedding medium can be used for immunohistochemical studies and is also suitable for DNA extraction and molecular genetic analysis, if necessary. Commonly, molecular studies will not be needed to establish the diagnosis. However, the stored tissue sample can be used for additional purposes. For example, antigen receptor gene rearrangements or specific chromosomal translocations are unique tumor markers and thus can be used subsequently for monitoring the presence or absence of disease during or following therapy.[1–3]

With the advent of PCR-based assays, it is not always essential to have fresh or frozen tissue. Assays using PCR do not require the presence of high molecular weight DNA, and therefore analysis can be performed on formalin-fixed, paraffin-embedded tissue, and/or histologic sections.[1]

MOLECULAR GENETIC BASIS OF ANTIGEN RECEPTOR GENE REARRANGEMENT

Non-Hodgkin's lymphomas are neoplasms of lymphoid cells of B-cell or T-cell lineage. The immunoglobulin (Ig) molecule, the antigen receptor of B lymphocytes, is a multidimeric protein composed of two heavy and two light (either κ or λ) polypeptide chains.[4,5] The T-cell receptor (TCR), the antigen receptor of T lymphocytes, is a heterodimeric protein analogous in structure to the Ig molecule. There are two types of TCRs: α/β and γ/δ. Approximately 95 percent of mature T cells express the α/β TCR, which is composed of α and β polypeptide chains. Approximately 5 percent of mature T cells express the γ/δ TCR, composed of γ and δ polypeptide chains.[1,2]

Early in normal lymphocyte differentiation the antigen receptor genes rearrange, resulting in the synthesis of Igs in B cells and TCRs in T cells. In the germline configuration, the antigen receptor genes are encoded by discontinuous regions of DNA: variable (V), diversity (D), joining (J), and constant (C) regions. All of the antigen receptor genes contain V, J, and C regions. The D regions are components of only the Ig heavy and the TCRβ and TCRδ chain genes.[1,2,4,6] The genomic configuration of the antigen receptor genes is shown in Figs. 1-1 and 1-2.

For those genes without D regions, such as the Igκ light chain gene, one of many Vκ segments is directly joined with a Jκ segment. This step alone generates many different DNA sequences that code for slightly different Igκ light chain proteins. For other genes with D regions, such as the Ig heavy chain (H) gene, rearrangement begins with D–J joining, followed by V–DJ joining (Fig. 1-3). Because there are numerous V, D, and J segments in the Ig heavy chain gene, many more combinations are possible than for the Igκ light chain gene. Each combination of segments results in slightly different DNA sequences being used to form an antigen receptor gene and corresponding protein with unique specificity.[1,3] No rearrangement occurs between the fused VJ or VDJ segments and the C regions (Fig. 1-3). The message encoded by the C region is incorporated into the Ig or TCR molecules at the time of transcription into VDJC mRNA and then translated into protein.

The process of gene rearrangement is made possible by heptamer-nonamer sequences of DNA (Fig. 1-4), 3′ to V regions, flanking D regions, and 5′ to J regions.[1,3] These sequences are composed of an identical 7 basepair (bp) sequence, either a 12 or 23 bp random spacer sequence, and an identical 9 bp sequence. Rearrangement occurs between a region with a 12 bp spacer and a region with a 23 bp spacer. Rearrangement is mediated with high efficiency by two recombinase enzymes, RAG-1 and RAG-2, encoded by two closely linked genes.[7] The recombinase enzymes are identical in B cells and T cells.

Using the gene rearrangement process, a relatively limited amount of genetic information inherited in the germline is translated into a wide array of possible gene sequences that encode the antigen-binding sites of either Ig or TCR molecules. The actual shuffling and joining of these discontinuous segments, in large part, explains at a statistical level the vast diversity of antigen receptors that can be generated by the immune system of humans.[1,2,4,6] In addition, other factors raise the possible number of DNA sequences that encode for unique antigen receptor specificities. These factors include flexibility at the joining sites between the V–J, D–J, and V–D segments and the addition of nontemplated nucleotides, so-called N insertions, at the joining sites.[4] Both of these mechanisms may alter the open reading frame of the sequence. Another factor that adds to the number of possible DNA sequences is a high rate of point mutations, particularly within the Ig complementarity-determining regions, the regions that appear to be responsible for encoding antigen receptor specificity.[4,5]

In addition, the IgH, Igλ, and TCRβ genes have more than one C region, which further increases the number of Ig molecules with different specificity.[1,4] The IgH gene has the greatest number of C regions that also may rearrange temporally subsequent to VDJ join-

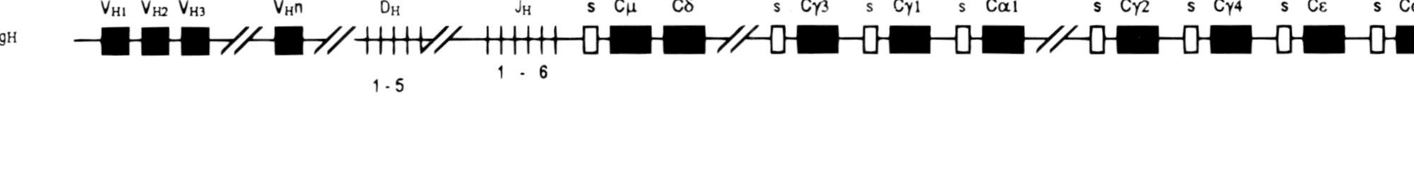

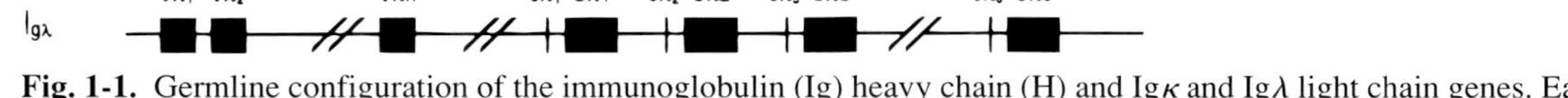

Fig. 1-1. Germline configuration of the immunoglobulin (Ig) heavy chain (H) and Igκ and Igλ light chain genes. Each gene is composed of variable (V), joining (J), and constant (C) regions. The IgH gene also contains diversity (D) regions.

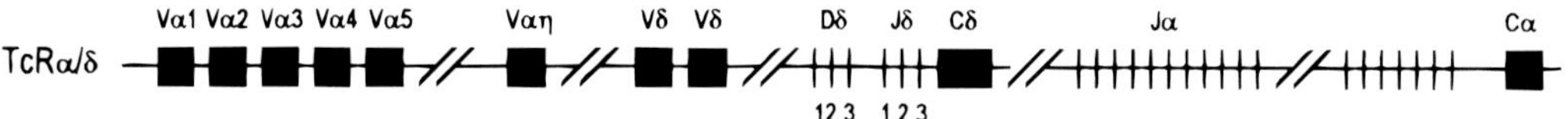

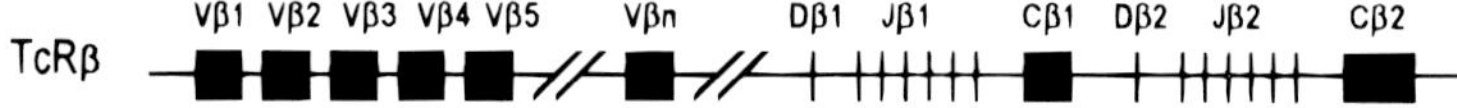

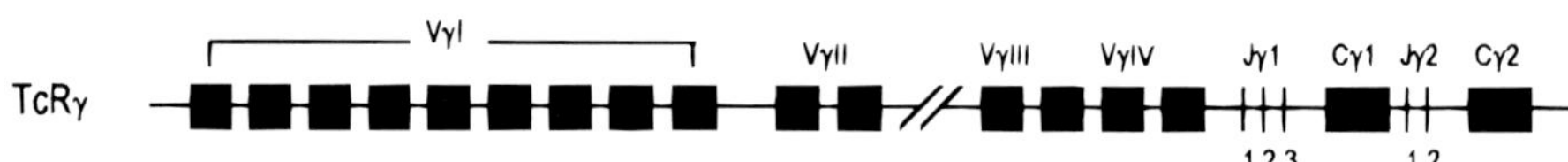

Fig. 1-2. Germline configuration of the T-cell receptor (TCR) α/δ, β, and γ chain genes. Each gene is composed of variable (V), joining (J), and constant (C) regions. The TCRδ and TCRβ chain genes also contain diversity (D) regions.

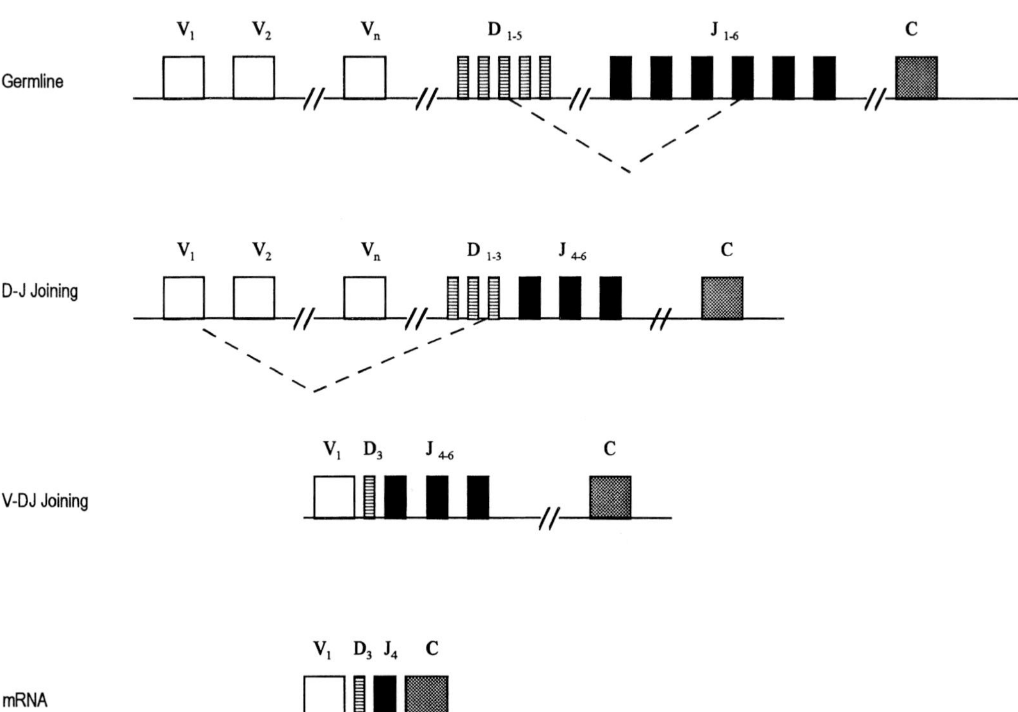

Fig. 1-3. Schematic representation of immunoglobulin heavy chain gene (IgH) rearrangement. Initially, D–J joining occurs followed by V–DJ joining. After transcription and mRNA splicing take place, one of each V, D, and J region are joined to a C region.

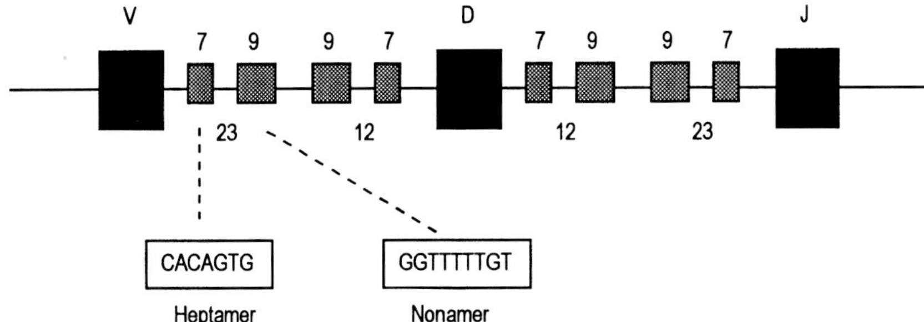

Fig. 1-4. The *IgH* gene. Heptamer-nonamer sequences, present in all antigen receptor genes, are thought to mediate V–(D)–J rearrangement. In all genes these sequences are found 3′ to the variable (V) and 5′ to the joining (J) regions. In genes with diversity (D) regions, heptamer-nonamer sequences are also found 5′ and 3′ to the D regions. The sequences illustrated are consensus sequences that may vary in different genes. (Modified from Kirsch and Kuehl,[3] with permission.)

ing through a mechanism that allows an antigen receptor encoded by a single VDJ rearrangement to become contiguous with any of the C regions.[1,4] In other words, the identical antigen receptor can be combined with IgM, IgG, IgA, IgD, or IgE. This phenomenon is known as *IgH switching*.

Switching is possible because there is a DNA sequence 5′ to all the different C regions except IgD. When the switch occurs, the $C\mu$ region is deleted, and one of several C regions (e.g., $C\alpha$) is brought into continuity with the VDJ rearrangement.[4] Transcription and translation into an Ig molecule of the heavy chain class encoded by the rearranged C segment follows. The combination of the Ig light and heavy chains further adds to the possible number of different Ig antigen receptors. It is estimated that the mechanisms of gene rearrangement can generate more than 10^8 different Igs and TCRs, more than enough to react specifically with the large number of foreign antigens that the mammalian organism may encounter.[6]

It needs to be emphasized that the gene rearrangement process is *not* involved in mechanisms that lead lymphoid cells to become malignant. Instead, the gene rearrangement process is normal and usually occurs *prior* to neoplastic transformation. Thus, all of the neoplastic cells will carry an identical Ig of TCR gene rearrangement, distinct from reactive, polyclonal lesions within which each cell carries its own, unique gene rearrangement.[1–4]

GERMLINE CONFIGURATION OF THE ANTIGEN RECEPTOR GENES

Immunoglobulin Heavy Chain Gene

The IgH gene (Fig. 1-1), located on chromosome 14q32, is complex and is composed of up to 100 V_H segments, approximately 30 D_H segments, six J_H segments, and numerous C regions: α, γ, μ, δ, and ϵ, including genes encoding Ig heavy chain subclasses (e.g., γ_1, γ_2, γ_3, γ_4).[4,5] D–J and V–DJ joining occur at the time of commitment to B-cell lineage, in the bone marrow, whereas IgH switching occurs later, with antigen exposure (e.g., in the follicle germinal center of a lymph node).

The numerous V_H segments of the IgH gene can be grouped into seven families.[5] In each family there are DNA sequences that are relatively conserved and similar in each family, such as sequences within the framework complementarity-determining region III (CDR III), framework CDR I, framework CDR II, and leader sequence. The six J_H segments are homologous at their 5′ ends.[4] These similarities in DNA sequence between V_H or J_H segments allow the construction of consensus primers that can be used in PCR-based assays to detect IgH gene rearrangements (discussed subsequently).

Immunoglobulin κ Light Chain Gene

The Igκ light chain gene (Fig. 1-1), located on chromosome 2p11 (reported as p11–13 in some studies),[4] is composed of many (perhaps up to 100) distinct Vκ regions, five Jκ segments, and a single Cκ region.[1,4] Also, 3′ to the Cκ region, a κ-deleting element is present. In Igλ-positive B cells in which the Igκ genes are nonproductively rearranged, the κ-deleting element rearranges specifically and deletes the Cκ loci.[1,4] In addition, the Jκ regions may be also deleted in approximately 25 percent of Igλ-positive cells.

Immunoglobulin λ Light Chain Gene

The Igλ gene (Fig. 1-1), situated on chromosome region 22q11, is organized quite differently from the Igκ light chain gene. The Igλ gene is composed of a series of Vλ segments followed by tandemly arranged Jλ and Cλ segments.[1,4] The number of Cλ regions is polymorphic in the human population because a 5 kilobase (kb) segment of DNA containing a Cλ gene is carried as one copy per allele in the germline of some individuals, whereas this segment is present in many copies per allele in other individuals.[1,4] Thus, the number of Cλ regions in each allele of the Igλ gene may vary from six to nine.

T-Cell Receptor δ Chain Gene

The TCRδ gene (Fig. 1-2), located at chromosome 14q11, contains very few (six or less) Vδ elements, two or three Dδ regions, and three Jδ segments.[1,2] The TCRδ gene is situated within the TCRα chain gene, immediately 5′ to the Jα segments and 3′ to the Vα genes.[8] This position is critical, since rearrangement of the TCRδ gene plays a role in the decision of a developing T cell to differentiate into an α/β or γ/δ T cell. If TCRδ gene rearrangement is productive, the cell goes on to express the γ/δ TCR. If TCRδ gene rearrangement is nonproductive, the TCRδ gene is deleted by a specific mechanism involving DNA sequences that flank the TCRδ locus and mediate deletion.

T-Cell Receptor α Chain Gene

The TCRα gene (Fig. 1-2), also located on chromosome 14q11, flanks the TCRδ gene.[2,4] The TCRα gene is very complex and is composed of numerous Vα segments, a large Jα region that spans over approximately 80 kb and contains up to 50 Jα segments, and one Cα locus.[1,2,4] Following nonproductive TCRδ gene rearrangement and deletion, a Vα segment may then directly join one of the Jα genes to form a productively rearranged TCRα gene, and the cell may eventually express the α/β TCR. Thus, T cells expressing the α/β TCR, in most cases, have deleted the TCRδ locus from both chromosomes.

T-Cell Receptor β Chain Gene

The TCRβ gene (Fig. 1-2), located on chromosome 7q34, has approximately 75 to 100 Vβ gene segments followed by two distinct Dβ, Jβ, and Cβ regions.[1,2] Each of these regions is composed of one Dβ segment, six or seven Jβ segments, and one Cβ segment. The $C\beta_1$ and $C\beta_2$ segments have almost identical nucleotide sequences. The Vβ segments may rearrange with either the $D\beta_1J\beta_1$ or the $D\beta_2J\beta_2$ regions.[2,4]

T-Cell Receptor γ Chain Gene

The TCRγ gene (Fig. 1-2), located on chromosome 7q15, is composed of only a few Vγ elements (up to 11 or 12) that may rearrange to either one of two Jγ regions.[1,9] Each Jγ region precedes nearly identical Cγ regions on the chromosome.

The relative simplicity of this gene, relative to the other TCR genes, has led many investigators to use the TCRγ gene for PCR-based assays to detect TCR gene rearrangement. The 11 Vγ gene segments can be divided into four groups: Vγ1–8, Vγ9, Vγ10, and Vγ11. The two Jγ regions contain five Jγ genes: Jγ1, Jγ2, Jγp, Jγp1, Jγp2. Thus, PCRs with a limited number of primers can be used to detect TCRγ gene rearrangements (discussed subsequently).

DEVELOPMENTAL HIERARCHY OF ANTIGEN RECEPTOR GENE REARRANGEMENTS

The study of acute lymphoblastic leukemias led investigators to understand that there appears to be a normal developmental hierarchy of antigen receptor gene rearrangement, which is more clearly established in B cells than in T cells.[10]

In neoplastic B cells and (by inference) normal lymphocytes, the Ig genes rearrange sequentially. At the earliest stage of B-cell differentiation, the IgH chain gene rearranges, subsequently followed by Igκ gene rearrangement. If neither Igκ allele is rearranged functionally, then the Igλ gene undergoes rearrangement.[10] In other words, Igλ gene rearrangements do not occur unless both alleles of the Igκ gene are either rearranged or deleted. This molecular mechanism allows an individual mature B cell to express only one Ig light chain, known as the principle of allelic exclusion. However, exceptions to this principle can occur.[11]

Studies of T-cell acute lymphoblastic leukemias have led to an understanding of a similar developmental hierarchy in neoplastic and (by inference) normal T cells. The TCRδ gene appears to be the first TCR gene to rearrange, followed by rearrangements of the TCRγ and TCRβ genes. The TCRα gene appears to be the last TCR gene to rearrange.[12]

The mechanisms that regulate the timing of antigen receptor gene rearrangements are poorly understood.

LINEAGE INFIDELITY

The occurrence of TCR gene rearrangements in B-cell neoplasms and Ig gene rearrangements in T-cell tumors is known by a variety of names, including *lineage infidelity, lineage promiscuity,* and *lineage crossover.* Lineage infidelity is common in lymphoid neoplasms arising from immature precursor B cells and T cells and is much less common in tumors arising from mature lymphoid cells.[1,2,13] The mechanism of lineage infidelity is unknown, but may be explained by the common use of heptamer-nonamer germline DNA sequences as recognition sites for rearrangement by both the Ig and TCR genes, as well as the recombinase enzymes RAG-1 and RAG-2.[7]

Since the mechanisms of Ig and TCR gene rearrangement are similar, it is perhaps not a surprise that lineage-inappropriate gene rearrangements occur. Why lineage infidelity is more common in neoplasms derived from precursor rather than from mature lymphoid cells is unknown, as are the exact mechanisms that restrict Ig gene rearrangement to B cells and TCR gene rearrangement to T cells. Importantly, Ig light chain gene rearrangement in T-cell tumors is rare. Therefore, the presence of both IgH and Ig light chain gene rearrangements occurs almost exclusively in B-cell neoplasms.[1,3,4,14]

CLONAL EVOLUTION

The restriction fragment profile of an individual lymphoid neoplasm is unique to the tumor. This "fingerprint" is a consequence of the extraordinarily large number of possible gene rearrangements and the randomness of the rearrangement process.[1–3] Thus, each B-cell or T-cell neoplasm carries its own particular gene rearrangement profile. This profile can be used as a tumor marker to monitor the course of disease, assess minimal residual disease after therapy, and assess tumor recurrence.

Although the above statements are true, the Ig gene locus is highly labile, especially in certain B-cell neoplasms such as follicular lymphoma, and a high rate of secondary gene rearrangements and somatic mutations occur.[4,5] For example, when sequential follicular lymphoma biopsy specimens from the same patient are analyzed, secondary changes in the Ig gene loci are detected in up to 40 percent of cases.[15] These changes include IgH constant region gene switching (e.g., from $C\mu$ to $C\alpha$), replacement of one V region with another, or mutations, some of which may alter restriction enzyme sites. However, despite these changes, usually one Ig gene allele remains unchanged or cytogenetic abnormalities remain constant, allowing recognition of these changes as clonal evolution and not as the emergence of a second neoplasm.

Unlike the Ig genes, the TCR genes rarely undergo somatic mutation. Thus, TCR gene rearrangements are much more stable tumor markers.

CLONALITY AND THE DIAGNOSIS OF MALIGNANCY

Virtually all non-Hodgkin's lymphomas and lymphocytic leukemias contain rearranged antigen receptor genes. However, an important question remains: Are the results of gene rearrangement analysis useful for distinguishing clinically benign from malignant lymphoproliferative processes?

In general, the answer is yes for biopsy specimens obtained from patients with intact immune systems and analyzed by Southern blot hybridization. Monoclonal or oligoclonal populations of cells are very rarely detected in lymphoid lesions obtained from patients with intact immune systems. However, in patients with abnormal immune systems monoclonal or oligoclonal Ig or TCR gene rearrangements may be detected in clinically and histologically benign lymphoproliferative processes. Diseases associated with immune system abnormalities, in which gene rearrangements may be detected in the absence of overt neoplasia, include angioimmunoblastic lymphadenopathy with dysproteinemia,[16] congenital immunodeficiency syndromes,[17] the plasma cell variant of Castleman's disease,[18,19] autoimmune diseases (e.g., Sjögren syndrome),[20] iatrogenic immunosuppression following organ transplant,[21] lymphoproliferations occurring in patients with rheumatoid arthritis or dermatomyositis treated with methotrexate, and the acquired immunodeficiency syndrome (AIDS).[22] In each of these conditions, the detection of monoclonal populations in biopsy specimens cannot be equated with malignancy without histologic evidence of malignant lymphoma. In fact, Lipford and colleagues[16] have demonstrated Ig and TCR gene rearrangements that arose and spontaneously disappeared in patients with angioimmunoblastic lymphadenopathy with dysproteinemia who did not develop lymphoma, even after long follow-up. Furthermore, marked lymphadenopathy resembling lymphoma that occurs in patients following organ transplantation or in patients with connective tissue diseases treated with methotrexate may resolve, in some cases, by withdrawing or reducing immunosuppression.[21,23]

It is important to note that in each of these clinical settings the patients are at a markedly heightened risk of developing lymphoma, usually diffuse, aggressive non-Hodgkin's lymphomas. The mechanism underlying the phenomenon of "benign" oligoclonal lymphoproliferative processes and the subsequent increased risk of lymphoma appears to be a consequence of reduced immunoregulation, which permits antigenically stimulated cells (usually B cells) to divide and expand beyond their usual limits in the immunologically intact host. Epstein-Barr virus is likely to be one of the antigens expanding the B-cell pool. An expanded pool of dividing B cells is thus at risk for secondary genetic events, such as chromosomal translocation, which by imparting genetic damage may transform these cells into malignant lymphoma. In fact, examples of this hypothesis have been directly demonstrated in patients with AIDS. Pelicci and colleagues[22] have shown that early lymphoproliferative processes in patients with human immunodeficiency virus (HIV) infection are often monoclonal or oligoclonal, as demonstrated by Ig gene rearrangement analysis. However, lymphomas arising in this setting also carry rearrangements of the c-*myc* oncogene.[22] Thus, at least one secondary genetic event has occurred in these cells; presumably, this event is responsible for transforming the cells into an aggressive non-Hodgkin's lymphoma. The presence of secondary genetic alterations, such as a chromosomal translocation, may also provide a diagnostic marker to assist in the differential diagnosis between a limited lymphoproliferation and an aggressive malignant lymphoma.

However, the general statements above may not apply to gene rearrangement data obtained by PCR. The increased sensitivity of PCR, particularly modified PCR assays to maximize sensitivity, compared with Southern blot analysis for detecting Ig and TCR gene rearrangements is likely to detect gene rearrangements in histologically benign lymphoid lesions with a higher frequency and probably in patients with intact immune systems. Examples of this phenomenon have been recently reported. Elenitoba-Johnson and colleagues[24] reported a case of low grade B-cell lymphoma of the lung mucosa-associated lymphoid tissue (MALT) associated with multiple microscopic aggregates of histologically benign lymphoid tissue. The lymphoma and the benign aggregates were studied separately using PCR to analyze IgH. IgH gene rearrangements of identical size were detected in the lymphoma and in the majority of the histologically benign lymphoid aggregates. A second example has been reported in abstract form by Hsi and colleagues.[25] They have reported IgH gene rearrangements, detected by PCR, in patients with *Helicobacter pylori*-induced chronic active gastritis, without clinical or histologic evidence of malignant lymphoma. Furthermore, using very sensitive microdissection or semi-nested PCR methods (discussed later), small populations of B cells with the t(14;18) have been detected in hyperplastic tonsils and lymph nodes from healthy individuals.[26,27]

Thus, detection of monoclonal populations of cells is likely to become even more common in patients with both compromised and intact immune systems, particularly when PCR-based methods for antigen receptor gene rearrangement analysis are used.

CHROMOSOMAL TRANSLOCATIONS

Chromosomal translocations are another form of gene rearrangement, but, unlike the antigen receptor genes, translocations generally do not occur in normal cells.[28] In chromosomal translocations, a portion of one chromosome becomes separated and attached to a different chromosome. Commonly, the translocations are also reciprocal; in other words, segments from two chromosomes exchange places. For example, in the t(11;14) the detached portion of chromosome 11 becomes joined to chromosome 14 and the detached portion of chromosome 14 becomes joined to chromosome 11. Reciprocal translocations may be further characterized as balanced or unbalanced. In balanced translocations there is no net loss of DNA.

Many different chromosomal translocations have been identified. In a recent review, Rabbitts[28] listed 55 distinct chromosomal translocations in hematopoietic neoplasms, the majority identified in lymphomas and lymphoid leukemias. In general, these translocations can be divided into two groups. In one group, the chromosomal translocations result in an oncogene being brought into continuity with an antigen receptor gene locus. This causes the oncogene to become deregulated, with increased expression of oncoprotein driving cell proliferation. Examples of this type of translocation are common in B-cell lymphomas and include the t(8;14), t(2;8), and t(8;22) in Burkitt's lymphoma; the t(11;14) in mantle cell lymphoma; and the t(14;18) in follicular lymphoma.[28]

In the second group, chromosomal translocations result in two nonantigen receptor gene loci being made contiguous to form a fusion gene.[28] Transcription results in the formation of chimeric transcripts that are translated into novel proteins. The most well-known example of this type of translocation is the t(9;22) that occurs in chronic myeloid leukemia and a subset of B-cell acute lymphoblastic leukemias.[28] The corresponding proteins, either p210 or p190, respectively, result in increased tyrosine kinase activity that is thought to drive cell proliferation. In general, the majority of chromosomal translocations that are recognized in either B-cell or T-cell acute lymphoblastic leukemias result in the formation of fusion genes and novel proteins.[28]

The mechanisms involved in chromosomal translocations are poorly understood. However, the evidence suggests that normal cell gene rearrangement mechanisms, such as IgH gene switching and V(D)J recombination, are involved in some chromosomal translocations. For example, in some chromosomal translocations an oncogene is brought into continuity with a C region of the IgH gene. This finding suggests that the IgH gene switch mechanism may be involved in the translocation. The t(8;14) in some cases of Burkitt's lymphoma is one example of this type of translocation. Alternatively, in other translocations the oncogene is juxtaposed with D or J segments and extraneous nucleotides (N insertions, typically added by terminal deoxynucleotidyl transferase) may be present between the spliced chromosomes. These findings suggest that the translocations occurred as an error in V(D)J joining mediated by the recombinase enzymes. As mentioned earlier, heptamer-nonamer recognition sequences flank the 3′ ends of the V genes, the 5′ and 3′ ends of D genes, and the 5′ ends of J genes. DNA sequences that flank or are located within some oncogenes may share homology with these heptamer-nonamer sequences. The cell V(D)J rearrangement mechanism may mistakenly recognize these homologous sequences during the process of recombination. An example of this mechanism is the t(1;14), which occurs in 30 percent of T-cell acute lymphoblastic leukemias, and results in two nonantigen receptor genes being brought into continuity. In the t(1;14), the recombinase enzymes recognize DNA sequences that mimic heptamer-nonamer sequences.[29]

Other types of DNA sequences may facilitate V(D)J or other types of DNA rearrangement. For example, χ-like sequences have been identified in human DNA. χ is a procaryotic recombination signal. In follicular lymphomas, Wyatt and colleagues[30] recognized χ-like sequences within the major breakpoint region of the *bcl*-2 gene and suggested that these sequences are responsible for the t(14;18). Others have suggested that alternating stretches of purines and pyrimidines may form "Z" DNA configurations that may promote translocation.[31]

Since all of the antigen receptor genes have heptamer-nonamer recognition sequences, one might surmise that different antigen receptor genes can recombine with each other. This does occur, uncommonly in normal cells, with the resulting genes being known as hybrid immune receptor genes. An IgH variable region–TCRα constant region hybrid gene is most common and can be detected in up to 0.1 percent of normal peripheral blood T cells.[32] Hybrid genes can also be transcribed and translated. The significance of hybrid genes is currently unknown, and perhaps it is surprising that hybrid immune receptor genes are not more commonly detected in normal cells. Hybrid immune receptor genes are known to be more common in certain diseases. For example, in patients with the congenital immunodeficiency syndrome ataxia-telangiectasia, hybrid immune receptor genes are detected in peripheral blood T cells 100 times more commonly than in normal patients.[32]

ONCOGENES AND TUMOR SUPPRESSOR GENES

Many of the oncogenes and tumor suppressor genes known to be involved in lymphoid neoplasia are listed in Tables 1-1 and 1-2.

Proto-oncogenes can be defined as normal cellular genes, usually actively transcribed in embryogenesis or early development, that are usually turned off in mature cells.[33,34] Proto-oncogenes typically encode for proteins that are involved in the control of cell proliferation or differentiation. The majority of known oncoproteins can be subdivided into four groups: growth factors, growth factor receptors, intracellular signal transducers (e.g., c-*abl*, H-*ras*), and nuclear transcription factors (e.g., c-*myc*).[33] There are also proto-oncogenes that do not fit these categories, such as *bcl*-1, which encodes for a cyclin that acts to drive the cell cycle, and *bcl*-2, which encodes a protein that inhibits apoptosis.[33] Historically, proto-oncogenes were recognized as cellular homologs of retroviral oncogenes. In retroviruses, oncogenes encode proteins that activate host cell replication and drive cell proliferation, allowing the virus to reproduce itself and survive. Thus, these viral proteins

Table 1-1. Oncogenes and Candidate Oncogenes Involved in Lymphoid Neoplasms

Oncogenes	Chromosome Location
c-*abl*	9q34
bcr	22q11
*Pbx*1	1q23
E2A	19q13
MLL/ALL1/HRX	11q23
AF-4/*FEL*	4q21
AF-9	9p22
ENL	19p13
tcl-1	14q32
tal-1/*Scl*/*tcl*-5	1p32
SIL	14q11
tcl-3/*HOX11*	10q24
bcl-1/*PRAD*-1/*CCND*1	11q13
bcl-2	18q21
bcl-3	19p13
bcl-6/*LAZ3*	3p27
c-*myc*	8p24
N-*ras*	1p11-13
K-*ras*	12p11-12
H-*ras*	11p15
c-*rel*	2p11-14
lyt-10	10q24
ttg-1	11p15
ttg-2	11p13
lyl-1	19p13
tan-1	9q34

function as oncoproteins in host cells. Similarly, activation of cellular proto-oncogenes invariably results in the potentiation of function.[33,34]

Proto-oncogenes may be activated by a variety of mechanisms including chromosomal translocation, point mutation, DNA amplification, and viral insertion into oncogene DNA.[33,35] These molecular abnormalities result in the translation of cellular oncoproteins that are qualitatively normal but overexpressed or are mutant with novel or increased activity. In general, the effect of an inappropriately expressed oncogene is dominant.[34,36] In other words, if an oncogene on one allele is activated, the corresponding oncoprotein drives cell proliferation.

Table 1-2. Tumor Suppressor Genes Involved in Lymphoid Neoplasms

Tumor Suppressor Genes	Chromosome Location
p53	17q13
Rb-1	13q14
p15/*MTS*-2	9p21
p16/*MTS*-1/*CDK4I*	9p21
TEL	12p13
KIP1	12p13

Historically, tumor suppressor genes (also known as anti-oncogenes) were discovered after oncogenes and are the antithesis of oncogenes. Tumor suppressor genes are genes that encode for proteins that are involved in controlling cell growth, and many of these proteins block cell proliferation at the level of the cell cycle.[35,36]

A variety of mechanisms may inactivate tumor suppressor genes, such as chromosomal translocations involving the gene locus, point mutations, and deletions. When a tumor suppressor gene is inactivated, the corresponding protein encoded by this gene is no longer translated, or a mutant and dysfunctional protein is translated that can no longer check cell growth. In general, the effect of a tumor suppressor gene is recessive.[35,36] In other words, the tumor suppressor genes of both alleles must be inactivated before the cell inappropriately proliferates. Both tumor suppressor genes may be inactivated as acquired abnormalities. However, in familial cancer syndromes one defective allele is inherited, greatly increasing the statistical chance of cancers developing in the target tissues where only one allele needs to be inactivated by somatic mutation for neoplasms to arise.

The first tumor suppressor gene to be discovered was the retinoblastoma (*Rb*) gene, situated on chromosome 13q14.[35,37] The *Rb* gene encodes for a 110 kilodalton (kd) protein that is involved in controlling the cell cycle and is regulated by phosphorylation. For sporadic or familial retinoblastomas to develop in the retina, both *Rb* alleles need to be inactive. In sporadic tumors, both *Rb* alleles are inactivated via acquired mutations.[35,37] In patients with familial tumors, which represent approximately 40 percent of cases, all cells contain one inherited inactive *Rb* allele. A second sporadic mutation in the retina results in two mutated *Rb* alleles and the development of retinoblastoma. Approximately 80 percent of all patients who inherit one defective *Rb* allele will develop retinoblastoma. Patients who inherit one inactive *Rb* allele are also at increased risk of other tumors at a variety of anatomic sites such as osteosarcoma, breast, lung, and prostate carcinomas and lymphoid neoplasms.[35]

The *p53* gene is another tumor suppressor gene, situated on chromosome 17q13.[38] Mutations of the *p53* gene are common and are found in a variety of neoplasms, including lymphoid neoplasms. The *p53* gene encodes a protein that is involved in controlling the cell cycle, particularly in the transition of the cell from G1 to S phase. The p53 protein is thought to delay this transition when DNA damage is present, allowing the cell to repair DNA before replication. The p53 protein also can induce apoptosis. The *p53* gene mutations most often occur as acquired abnormalities. However, a subset of patients with the Li-Fraumeni syndrome are known to inherit one defective *p53* allele, perhaps explaining the susceptibility of these patients to the variety of neoplasms involving many anatomic sites that characterize this syndrome.[38,39]

Most investigators now agree that cancer appears to result from the stepwise accumulation over time of a variety of independently acquired genetic defects.[34] A single mutation or ''hit'' involving an oncogene or tumor suppressor gene is usually inadequate for neoplastic transformation, although a preneoplastic state may result. Two or more mutations involving different genes are required for neoplastic transformation to occur.

INTRODUCTION TO METHODS USED IN MOLECULAR DIAGNOSIS

Conventional Cytogenetics

These conventional methods are usually the first step in the molecular characterization of neoplasms.

Karyotyping of a lymphoid neoplasm allows the recognition of gross alterations in chromosome content or structure. As an example of altered chromosome content, trisomy 12 has been detected in 20 to 40 percent of cases of B-cell chronic lymphocytic leukemia (discussed subsequently). With this information one suspects that there is genetic abnormality in B-cell chronic lymphocytic leukemia located somewhere on chromosome 12, although the exact site of this lesion is unknown. Since the total copy number of chromosome 12 is increased, one may suspect that amplification of a gene or genes on chromosome 12 may be involved in the pathogenesis of B-cell chronic lymphocytic leukemia. Much less commonly, lymphoid neoplasms may be characterized by complete loss of a chromosome. Instead, small deletions of chromosomes occur. In this scenario, one suspects that loss of a gene or genes is involved in lymphomagenesis, as is the case for a variety of tumor suppressor genes.

Chromosomal translocations are commonly identified in a variety of lymphoid neoplasms.[28] When found, the chromosomal bands involved in the translocation, in other words, the sites of the breakpoints, are likely sites of one or more genes that are involved in the pathogenesis of the neoplasm. Most commonly these loci are the sites of oncogenes. As an example of the former, one of the first lymphomas known to have a characteristic translocation was Burkitt's lymphoma.[4] Approximately 75 percent of these neoplasms carry the t(8;14)(q24;q32). This cytogenetic result led molecular biologists to clone, map, and sequence the sites of the breakpoints, 8q24 and 14q32, leading to the recognition of the c-*myc* and the IgH genes, respectively. As will be discussed subsequently, the t(8;14) translocation results in the juxtaposition of the c-*myc* oncogene, derived from chromosome 8q24, with the IgH locus on chromosome 14q32. It is thought that the active enhancer of the IgH gene is juxtaposed with the c-*myc* oncogene, resulting in constitutive activation of c-*myc*, which encodes a protein involved in mitogenesis.[4] Other mechanisms are also involved in the increased expression of c-myc protein.

Since each chromosome band is relatively

large, containing 1 to 4 $\times$ 10^7 bp of DNA and therefore many genes, translocations may involve the same chromosome band, and yet different genes are affected in different lymphoid neoplasms. For example, the 10q24 locus is involved in at least two known translocations, the t(10;14)(q24;q32) and the t(10;14)(q24;q11). In the former translocation, the *lyt*-10 gene at 10q24 is involved in B-cell lymphomas. In the latter translocation, the *HOX11* gene at 10q24 is involved in T-cell ALL.

Chromosomal translocation can also be a mechanism of tumor suppressor gene inactivation, and thus the sites of breakpoints can identify a chromosome locus that contains one or more of these genes. For example, such translocations played a role in establishing the location of the *Rb* tumor suppressor gene at chromosome 13q14.

In summary, conventional cytogenetics studies have been essential to the identification of genetic abnormalities in cancer. These studies usually represent the first step, often localizing the abnormality to a relatively small chromosome locus, where research efforts can be focused to identify the exact genes involved. Once the genes are recognized, in many instances molecular genetic testing is superior to conventional cytogenetics methods for assessing the presence of the abnormality. However, in many other instances molecular testing is far behind conventional cytogenetics for assessing the presence of a molecular lesion, and in other diseases conventional cytogenetics and molecular testing have become complementary.

Southern Blot Hybridization

Method

To perform Southern blot hybridization, DNA must first be extracted from fresh or frozen cells or tissues using standard methods. The most commonly used DNA extraction protocols are conventional chemical methods that use cold ethanol and salt to precipitate high molecular weight, genomic DNA and phenol/chloroform to remove cell lipids, further purifying the DNA.

The second step is to cut the DNA into relatively small fragments in order that the DNA may be analyzed by electrophoresis.[1,3] The upper size limit of standard electrophoresis is 25 kb. Restriction enzymes, bacterial enzymes that cut specific or ''restricted'' sequences of bases, are known that are four, six, or eight base cutters. Six base cutters are most convenient because they digest DNA into fragments that statistically should average 4,096 (4^6) bp, since any one of four bases may occur at any of the six positions. Four base and eight base cutters statistically cut DNA into fragments that are too small or too large for standard electrophoresis. Typically, the restriction fragment sizes generated by digestion with a six base cutter represent a range of sizes, from several hundred bases to more than 20 kb. The restriction enzymes used are selected on the basis of the known structure of the DNA. For the analysis of the antigen receptor genes, the *Eco*RI, *Hin*dIII, and *Bam*HI restriction enzymes, all six base cutters, are most commonly used. The cut DNA is then electrophoresed in a gel. Agarose gels are often used because they allow adequate separation of the DNA restriction fragments and agarose is relatively inexpensive. Following separation, a solid matrix such as a nylon membrane is overlaid on the gel, and the DNA fragments are transferred onto the solid matrix or blot. One of the simplest methods to accomplish transfer is to place the gel between filter paper below and blotting paper above. The filter paper has long wicks immersed in buffer, and the blotting paper is stacked in the form of a tower. Capillary pressure results in buffer migrating up the filter paper wicks, through the gel, and into the tower carrying the DNA fragments onto the nylon membrane. After transfer, the blot contains an exact imprint of the fragments separated on the electrophoretic gel.

The location of the restriction fragment carrying the gene of interest is then detected by hybridizing the blot in a liquid solution containing a labeled probe. Both the DNA fixed to the blot and the probe DNA need to be denatured (i.e., made single stranded) to allow hybridization.

The probe will seek out complementary single strands of DNA on the blot and hybridize with them. Unbound probe is then washed away under precise conditions of temperature and salt concentration so that only specifically hybridized probe remains on the blot. If the probe is radioactive, the blot is then exposed to x-ray film, and the resulting autoradiograph is developed to reveal the position of the restriction fragment containing the gene sequence recognized by the probe. Multiple probes are available commercially, and systems that use nonradioactively labeled probes and colorimetric or chemiluminescent detection methods are also now available.

The gene rearrangement process is suited to detection by Southern blotting because DNA rearrangement deletes intervening DNA sequences including restriction enzyme sites, resulting in a change in size from the germline (embryonic) restriction fragment size.[3,4] Thus, to interpret Southern blot results one must know the germline configuration of the gene being analyzed, including the location of relevant restriction enzyme sites.

In the schematic example of the Igκ gene (Fig. 1-5), a sequence of six bases recognized by the *Eco*RI restriction enzyme site within the deleted segment is lost from the cell, and another 5′ *Eco*RI site is brought in with Vκ, which is now joined to Jκ. The downstream *Eco*RI site immediately 3′ to the Jκ gene remains unchanged. Thus, the two *Eco*RI sites are approximately 9,400 bp (or 9.4 kb) apart in the germline configuration of Igκ. By contrast, the rearranged Igκ allele shown has two *Eco*RI sites 6.5 kb apart, resulting in a 6.5 kb restriction fragment (Fig. 1-5).

An example of an actual tumor with Igκ gene rearrangement is shown in Fig. 1-6. The unrearranged or germline configuration of the Igκ gene (dashes) has a restriction fragment size of 5.5 kb in a *Hin*dIII digest of genomic DNA, whereas its size in a *Bam*HI digest is 12 kb. Only the germline fragments are present in the negative control (placenta; P). However, the follicular lymphoma (L) contains one fragment or band (dash) equal in size to the germline band of the negative control and two additional bands (arrows) indicating bi-allelic rearrangement of the Igκ gene. This result indicates that the lymphoma is monoclonal, since two uniformly sized restriction fragments (both alleles) are detected. A polyclonal population of B cells, in contrast,

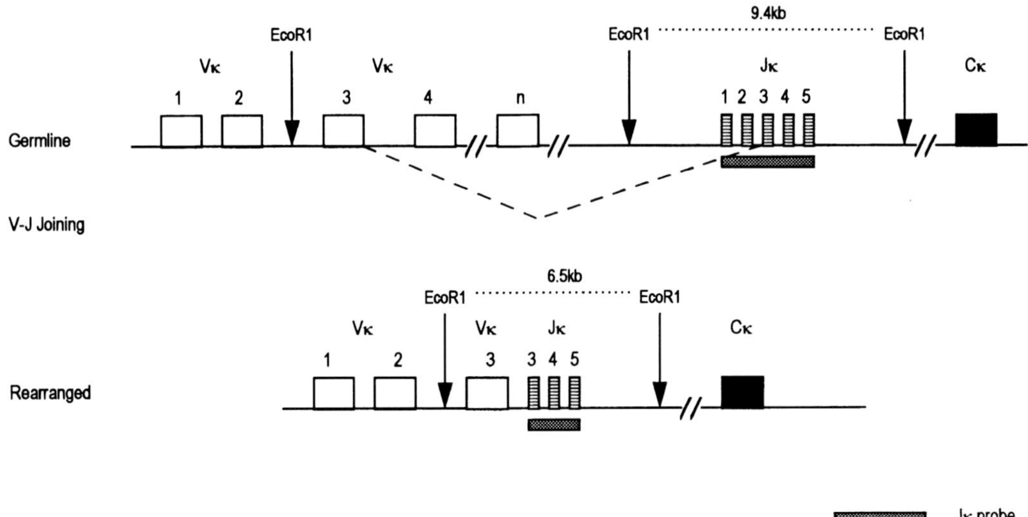

Fig. 1-5. Hypothetical example of Igκ light chain gene rearrangement. The rearrangement results in deletion of an *Eco*RI restriction enzyme site, changing the size of the fragment detected by an Igκ joining region probe (Jκ) using *Eco*RI-digested genomic DNA.

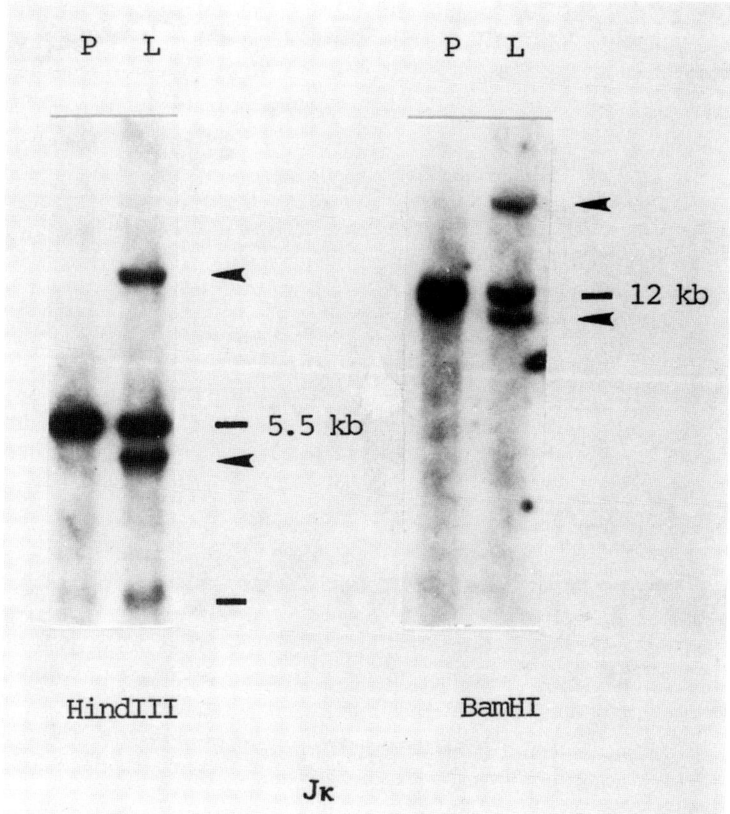

Fig. 1-6. B-cell lymphoma (L) and control placenta (P) DNA. Two extra bands are detected in the lymphoma, consistent with bi-allelic gene rearrangement. Southern blot hybridization analysis using *Hin*dIII and *Bam*HI digested genomic DNA and a ^{32}P-labeled genomic probe specific for the Igκ gene joining region (Jκ). (*Dashes,* germline fragments; *arrows,* rearranged fragments.)

would generate a smear of differently sized fragments that are usually not detected by this method.

Sensitivity

The distinction between a monoclonal and a polyclonal process, as determined by Southern blot hybridization, relies on the sensitivity of the assay. A polyclonal B-cell lesion contains cells that have rearranged their immunoglobulin genes. However, these rearrangements are not sufficiently abundant to be detected as a single band by this technique. To be detected, cells containing a single rearrangement must represent at least 1 to 5 percent of the total cell population, making this technique sensitive for the detection of a clone down to the 1 to 5 percent level.[1,2,17,41] This sensitivity has been demonstrated through the use of mixing experiments in which monoclonal B cells are added in varying amounts to a polyclonal cell population. Thus, polyclonal lymphoid cells that also rearrange their antigen receptor genes will not be detected because these cells will not represent more than 1 percent of the total cell population analyzed.

Southern blotting is approximately 5 to 10 times more sensitive than conventional immunophenotypic analysis for detecting clonality.[1] However, even with restriction fragment analysis and Southern blot hybridization, low numbers of clonal malignant cells may be missed. Thus, the PCR technique with its much greater sensitivity is better suited than Southern blot analysis for the detection of minimal residual disease.

Choice of Probes

For the detection of antigen receptor gene rearrangements, probes of the J regions are the most practical. The J regions are involved in most gene rearrangements, and, for the majority of the antigen receptor genes, the J segments are limited in number. Thus, J region probes can detect most gene rearrangements.[1,2]

IgH Gene. A genomic DNA fragment containing the JH region will detect rearrangements in virtually any B-cell neoplasm. Since the IgH gene is the first to rearrange in B-cell development, and is rearranged in even the most immature B-cell neoplasm, this single probe can detect rearrangements in all B-cell neoplasms. In contrast, Cμ probes were used in early studies before J region probes were generally available. The Cμ region may be deleted in B cells that have undergone Ig heavy chain switching.[4] Thus, using a Cμ probe, an IgH gene rearrangement may be missed.[1,4]

Igκ Gene. During B-cell differentiation, the Igκ genes rearrange prior to the Igλ gene rearrangement.[1,4] If the Igκ genes rearrange productively, the Igλ genes remain in the germline configuration. If, instead, the Igκ genes rearrange nonproductively, then the Igλ gene rearranges. Therefore, Igλ-expressing B cells and B-cell neoplasms have rearranged Igκ genes that also may be subsequently deleted. Because most normal B cells (approximately two-thirds) and B-cell neoplasms express Igκ, the Igλ light chain gene is germline in most instances. For practical purposes, then, testing for Igκ gene rearrangement is generally more informative than analyzing the Igλ gene.[1,3]

Igκ gene rearrangements are best detected with a Jκ probe, which will identify virtually any Vκ–Jκ joining. Historically, Cκ probes were first cloned and used to analyze B-cell lymphomas. However, among the B-cell neoplasms that express Igλ light chain (approximately 20 to 35 percent of mature B-cell neoplasms), the majority of cases will have deleted both Cκ loci.[1,4] In contrast, in the same cases the Jκ loci will be similarly deleted in approximately 25 percent of cases. Thus, Jκ probes are more useful than Cκ probes for detecting Igκ gene rearrangements in Igλ-expressing B-cell neoplasms. In those cases in which the Jκ segments have been deleted, probes specific for the κ-deleting element show rearrangement. Such cases would be expected to represent fewer than 10 percent of all B-cell neoplasms.[1]

Igλ Gene. The Cλ region has been cloned and can be used as a probe for rearrangement. However, the Igλ gene is polymorphic, and there may be multiple germline Cλ regions per allele, resulting in many germline bands that may be difficult to differentiate from a gene rearrangement.[1,3] Thus, the Igλ gene is not routinely assessed in the work-up of B-cell lymphoproliferative processes.

TCRβ Chain Gene. Of the TCR genes, the TCRβ chain locus provides the most information for the diagnosis of clonality. The TCRβ gene is rearranged in 90 to 95 percent of all mature T-cell neoplasms[1,2] as well as immature T-cell acute lymphoblastic leukemias and lymphoblastic lymphomas.[42] Generally, most studies have reported the use of constant region probes (Cβ), since the Cβ1 and Cβ2 regions are nearly identical in sequence and a single probe can detect rearrangements in either locus. However, the germline configuration of the TCRβ gene has an *Eco*RI restriction enzyme site between the Jβ2 and Cβ2 regions and a *Hin*dIII restriction enzyme site between the Jβ1 and Cβ1 loci. Thus, using a Cβ probe and *Eco*RI-digested DNA, rearrangements involving the Jβ2 allele cannot be detected, nor can rearrangements involving the Jβ1 allele be observed using *Hin*dIII-digested DNA. J region probes are more informative, and the cloning of the two Jβ1 and Jβ2 segments has permitted more thorough analysis of the TCRβ gene using these probes.[1,2]

The Cβ probe has two advantages over Jβ region probes, however. First, an estimate of the percentage of polyclonal T cells in a patient sample may be made because of the location of the *Eco*RI and *Hin*dIII sites in the TCRβ gene germline configuration.[2] For example, using *Eco*RI-digested DNA, the Cβ probe hybridizes with two germline restriction fragments that contain the Cβ1 and Cβ2 loci. Polyclonal T cells that use the Cβ1 allele in TCRβ chain gene rearrangement will have Cβ1 restriction fragments that differ from those of the germline configuration, reducing the overall intensity of the Cβ1 germline band. In contrast, the presence of an *Eco*RI site 5′ to the Cβ2 allele results in the DNA of polyclonal T cells that used the Cβ2 allele in gene rearrangement being seen by the Cβ probe as a part of the Cβ2 germline band, with no decrease in band intensity. Thus, in an *Eco*RI digest the reduction of the Cβ1 germline fragment, compared with the Cβ2 germline fragment, is proportional to the percentage of polyclonal T cells present.[2] Furthermore, in contrast with the Cβ probe, the Jβ1 and Jβ2 regions are not sufficiently homologous to allow a probe from one region to cross-hybridize with the other region. Both probes are necessary for analysis, although in practice both the Jβ1 and Jβ2 probes can be added to the same hybridization mixture, allowing detection of rearrangements involving either J region simultaneously.

TCRα Chain Gene. The TCRα chain gene is composed of an enormous J region, approximately 80 kb long, within which approximately 50 Jα segments are dispersed.[1,2] The size of the J region precludes analysis using one or two J region probes and standard electrophoresis. Thus, analysis of the TCRα chain gene is impractical for routine diagnostic testing. This gene, however, can be assessed by other methods that are capable of studying large fragments of DNA, such as pulsed field gel electrophoresis.

TCRδ Chain Gene. The TCRδ locus lies within the TCRα gene, immediately upstream (5′) of the Jα region. Rearrangements of the TCRδ chain gene are best detected with Jδ probes. The Jδ1 probe is most helpful since the Jδ1 segment is usually involved in TCRδ gene rearrangements.[12] TCRδ gene rearrangements are of interest because many of these are the result of chromosomal translocations involving chromosome region 14q11, the site of the TCRδ and TCRα genes.

The majority of T-cell neoplasms express the α/β TCR and have deleted both copies of their TCRδ genes. However, TCRδ gene rearrangement does not preclude TCRβ gene rearrangement, and T-cell neoplasms with TCRδ rearrangements often also have TCRβ rearrangements.[12]

TCRγ Chain Gene. The TCRγ gene is rearranged in most immature as well as mature T-cell neoplasms, even if the neoplastic cells express the α/β TCR rather than the γ/δ TCR. Jγ probes have been cloned, allowing detection of TCRγ rearrangements that can serve as clonal markers in T-cell neoplasms.[1,2] However, the TCRγ gene has a limited number of Vγ genes, up to 11.[9] As a consequence, there is a restricted number of productive Vγ–Jγ joinings with a corresponding limited number of restriction fragments generated by an enzyme such as *Eco*RI or *Hin*dIII. Because there is a low number of Vγ–Jγ joinings, Southern blotting can detect TCRγ gene rearrangements in polyclonal T cells, since each different rearrangement will be found in approximately 10 percent of the T cells, above the sensitivity of the technique. Thus, when polyclonal T cells are admixed with the neoplastic cells, the TCRγ gene rearrangements in the polyclonal T cells confound the interpretation of Southern blot results. These bands can be detected when polyclonal T cells represent approximately 10 percent of the cell sample and can obscure a neoplastic clone when as few as 25 percent of cells in the sample are normal polyclonal T cells.[43] Thus, when analyzing the TCRγ gene, one must ensure that bands attributable to the germline patterns of polyclonal T cells not be misconstrued as a neoplastic T-cell clone.[43]

Detection of Chromosome Translocations

Southern blot hybridization can be used to detect chromosome translocations. Similar to antigen receptor gene rearrangement, the translocation alters the germline configuration and corresponding restriction enzyme sites.[1,3] The change in size of restriction fragments implies the presence of the translocation.

For example, the t(14;18) in follicular lymphoma juxtaposes the IgH gene on chromosome 14q32 with the *bcl*-2 oncogene on chromosome 18q21. The restriction enzyme sites surrounding these genes in the germline configuration are known. The translocation is balanced, resulting in the formation of two different fused segments of 14;18 DNA. Analysis with either an IgH joining region probe (J_H) or a *bcl*-2 probe will demonstrate a change in the restriction fragment sizes of chromosomes 14 and 18, implying that the translocation has occurred (Fig. 1-7). Furthermore, in many cases the same restriction fragment can be shown to hybridize with both the J_H and *bcl*-2 probes, a phenomenon referred to as comigration (Fig. 1-7), proving the presence of both chromosomes within the same fragment and unequivocally demonstrating the t(14; 18).[1,3]

Polymerase Chain Reaction

The PCR technique allows the synthesis and amplification of double-stranded DNA in vitro.[44,45] This technique accommodates the unique characteristics of DNA polymerase, which proceeds only in the 5′ to 3′ direction, and can extend DNA only at the 3′ end of one strand that is annealed to a DNA template (a second complete strand of DNA).

Method

The simplest of PCR protocols usually is as follows.[44,45] To begin, all of the components of DNA must be added to a test tube: the four nucleotides in an appropriate buffer containing an optimum concentration of magnesium. Primers are also needed. Typically, primers are synthesized oligonucleotides, 20 to 25 bases long, that are complementary to the template DNA. The primers serve two functions. One, they provide a 3′ end of DNA that can be extended by the DNA polymerase. Two, the primers provide the specificity of the reaction and are designed to anneal with the 5′ end of each template strand of DNA, flanking the target DNA sequence to be amplified. To design these primers, the sequence of the target DNA and particularly the sequences flanking the target DNA must be known. The last ingredient to be added is DNA polymerase.

The PCR itself is based on repetitive cycles of three reactions, each differing only in temperature and time of incubation. In the first reaction, high temperature (e.g., 90° to 95°C) is used to denature DNA template double stranded DNA into single stranded DNA. This maximizes the opportunity for the primers to anneal with complementary sequences located at the 5′ ends of both single strands of template DNA flanking the target region, a reaction that best occurs at 50° to 60°C. In the last reaction, an intermediate temperature (e.g., 72°C) is used to optimize the activity of a heat stable DNA polymerase, with DNA synthesis then occurring at the 3′ ends of the annealed primers. Following one such cycle, the target region of DNA template strand is exactly duplicated.

An important feature of PCR is that all synthesized DNA sequences can then serve as templates for additional DNA synthesis in subsequent cycles. Theoretically, after the third cycle, DNA amplification becomes geometric. In other words, the target DNA sequence is exponentially amplified 2^n, with n representing the number of cycles.

A great advance in the development of PCR was the isolation and commercial availability of *Taq* polymerase, isolated from the bacterium *Thermus aquaticus,* a thermophilic species originally isolated from the water of hot springs. *Taq* polymerase is heat stable, and its use allows PCR to be done as a closed system that is fully automated in a thermal cycler. Prior to the use of *Taq* polymerase, heat would denature other DNA polymerases, and thus enzyme needed to be added (usually manually) after each cycle.

Commonly, 30 to 40 cycles are done to amplify DNA by PCR. Thus, initially primers and

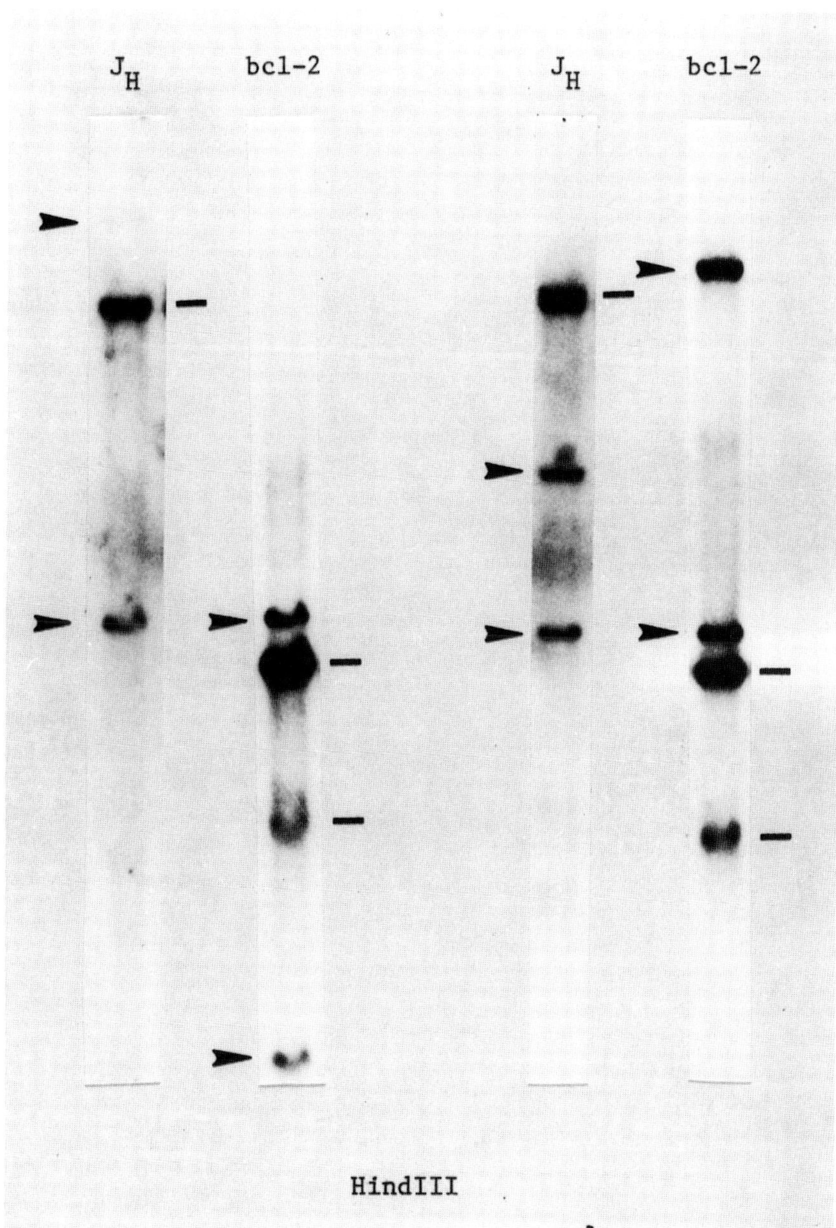

Fig. 1-7. Two follicular lymphomas. In both tumors two extra bands are detected, indicating the presence of bi-allelic rearrangement of both the IgH and *bcl*-2 genes. In both tumors there is also comigration of IgH and *bcl*-2 rearranged bands, demonstrating the presence of the t(14;18). Southern blot hybridization analysis using *Hin*dIII-digested genomic DNA and ^{32}P-labeled genomic probes specific for the IgH gene joining region (JH) and the *bcl*-2 gene. (In the left lane, the larger IgH gene rearrangement is very faint secondary to incomplete transfer).

nucleotides need to be added to the reaction in great excess compared with template DNA. With an adequate amount of *Taq* polymerase, the test tube(s) are placed in the thermal cycler, the conditions for the three reactions are programmed, and PCR takes place in only a few hours, often done overnight for convenience.

Product Visualization

Once the PCR is complete, the amplified product is usually analyzed by gel electrophoresis.[44,45] After electrophoresis the product amplified can be visualized by staining the gel with ethidium bromide. Furthermore, these products can be transferred to a nylon membrane by Southern blotting, and the membrane can be hybridized with a labeled probe specific for the target sequence amplified and internal to the primers. A successful PCR will yield a discrete band that corresponds to the expected size of the product, as predicted from the sites of the primers selected.

Both agarose and polyacrylamide gels may be used, depending on the PCR application. Agarose gels are inexpensive and easy to prepare, and amplified products are easily transferred to a solid membrane that can be hybridized with a specific internal probe. Although often not necessary for many applications, Southern blotting and hybridization with an internal labeled probe is the most sensitive and specific method for detecting PCR amplified products. However, the separation of PCR products with very small differences in size is suboptimal in agarose gels. Polyacrylamide gels are far superior for this purpose. Furthermore, denaturing chemicals such as urea or formamide can be added to polyacrylamide to create denaturing gradient gels. In addition to size, the concentration of urea or formamide required for denaturation of double stranded DNA into single strands depends on the nucleotide sequence and can be used to separate DNA molecules. Single stranded DNA migrates through the gel much more slowly than double stranded DNA. Using denaturing gradient polyacrylamide gels, DNA molecules that differ only by a single base change may be separated. Polyacrylamide also has disadvantages compared with agarose. Polyacrylamide gels are more expensive and difficult to prepare, and Southern blot transfer of DNA from polyacrylamide to solid membranes is inefficient.

Sensitivity

The sensitivity of PCR depends, in large part, on its application. For example, for the detection of a chromosomal translocation such as the t(14; 18), which does not occur in normal cells, PCR can detect one cell with the translocation in up to 10^5 to 10^6 cells.[46]

The sensitivity of PCR to detect antigen receptor gene rearrangements is substantially less. Since these gene rearrangements occur normally in all lymphoid cells, PCR is being used to detect a monoclonal population of cells, each with a similarly sized amplifiable product, from a background of differently sized gene rearrangements found in polyclonal cells. This polyclonal background explains the reduced sensitivity. In most studies, PCR has been reported to detect one monoclonal cell in a population of 10^2 or 10^3 polyclonal cells, although this sensitivity can be increased by modifying standard protocols.[26,27]

Applications

Chromosome Translocations. Chromosomal translocations in which the precise breakpoints and their flanking sequences are known can be readily detected by PCR.[46,47] For example, in the t(14;18) there are a variety of breakpoints within the *bcl*-2 gene on chromosome 18. Approximately 50 to 60 percent of these translocations occur within 150 bp, the major breakpoint cluster region. An additional 20 to 30 percent of cases are clustered further 3′ in the minor breakpoint cluster region, and a small subset of cases involve other breakpoints. The breakpoints on chromosome 14 occur within the J_{H5} and J_{H6} segments of the IgH gene J region. The sequences flanking these breakpoints are known, allowing the design of primers that flank the site of 14;18 fusion.

Simultaneous screening for several breakpoint cluster regions of *bcl*-2 can be done, known as multiplex PCR, using a mixture of different primers each flanking a different breakpoint site in a single reaction.[48] The mixture of primers must be selected in order that all primers may anneal sufficiently with template DNA. This approach obviously simplifies the screening process.

Chromosomal translocations that have widely dispersed breakpoint sites are less amenable to PCR-based assays for detection. For example, in Burkitt's lymphoma the t(8;14), t(2;8), or t(8; 22) translocations may be identified. Furthermore, in the t(8;14) the breakpoint sites on both chromosomes 8 and 14 are variable. Thus, although the flanking sequences for a variety of these breakpoints are known, PCR-based detection of these translocations is more complicated and requires the use of multiple primer sets.

Antigen Receptor Gene Rearrangements. PCR-based assays for detecting antigen receptor gene rearrangements are currently an area of great interest. Although Southern blot hybridization remains the "gold standard" for this purpose, an equally effective PCR-based method is faster, less expensive, and can be done using small amounts of low quality DNA such as that obtained from fixed, paraffin-embedded tissue. To date, most efforts using PCR have been directed toward the analysis of the Ig heavy and light chain genes and the TCRγ chain genes.[49–62]

Unlike a chromosome translocation, in which there may be only one or a limited number of breakpoint sites, any of the variable (V) and joining (J) segments of an antigen receptor gene may be used in the process of gene rearrangement. For example, the Ig heavy chain gene has up to 100 V and 6 J segments. Using a different set of primers for each possible combination is impractical. Thus, investigators have searched for consensus sequences, shared by all of the V or J segments, that can be used to detect all combinations. For the V segments, a number of consensus sequences may be used as 5′ primers, with perhaps the best primer being a sequence 5′ to the framework of the CDR III. A consensus sequence from the 5′ end of the J segments also has been identified for use as a 3′ primer.

Investigators have focused on the TCRγ chain gene for PCR-based assays to detect TCR gene rearrangements because the TCRγ gene is relatively simple.[57,60,61] There are four families (11 segments) of V genes and five J genes (two highly homologous) that can be assayed with only four sets of V and J primers.[61]

The theory behind a PCR-based assay for detecting antigen receptor gene rearrangements is as follows. In the germline configuration the V and J segments are widely separated, and thus PCR amplification of intervening DNA cannot occur. In contrast, VJ or VDJ gene rearrangement brings the flanking V and J primers into close proximity, allowing successful amplification of intervening DNA. Monoclonal cells contain one or two rearranged alleles, and thus PCR will amplify one (or two) predominant band(s). In contrast, polyclonal cells each carry a distinctive gene rearrangement that PCR will amplify as a smear of bands of slightly different size.[54–56]

The major problem for PCR-based assays is the relatively high false negative rate, from less than 10 percent to 40 percent in prior studies, compared with Southern blot hybridization.[49–62] There may be a variety of explanations for false negative results. PCR, unlike Southern blotting, will not detect antigen receptor gene rearrangements that result from chromosomal translocation or partial DJ rearrangements. In these circumstances the V and J segments are not brought into proximity, and intervening DNA cannot be amplified. Somatic mutations occurring in the V region genes are also a major problem, particularly involving the IgH gene in tumors with a high somatic mutation rate, such as follicular center cell lymphomas.[62] The mutations in the V genes of the template DNA probably prevent the oligonucleotide primers from annealing. Another problem is the great diversity of the V segments of the Ig heavy chain gene, making it almost impossible to select a consensus V region sequence that will anneal with all of the V segments.[62]

Some of the above problems can be overcome with the use of multiple primer sets, which can be chosen to optimize the yield for certain types of lymphoid tumors that may be suspected a priori.[62] Currently, however, PCR-based detection of antigen receptor gene rearrangements is best used as a screening method in daily practice. A negative result should not be considered negative unless confirmed by Southern blotting.[54–56,61,62]

Monitoring Residual Disease. A variety of approaches have been taken for monitoring residual disease. For example, one may monitor a chromosomal translocation, an antigen receptor gene rearrangement, or a tumor-specific DNA sequence. Of these, the latter approaches are the most specific and sensitive but also require the most effort, usually in the form of sequencing tumor cell DNA at the time of initial diagnosis.

Chromosome translocations are useful for monitoring residual disease. Because most translocations are restricted to neoplastic cells, the sensitivity of PCR is high, and one tumor cell with the translocation can be detected in 10^5 or 10^6 normal cells.[46]

The use of antigen receptor gene rearrangements is inherently less specific, since normal B cells and T cells rearrange their antigen receptor genes and tumor gene rearrangements must be distinguished from reactive cell gene rearrangements. PCR for this purpose can detect one tumor cell in at least 10^2 or 10^3. Another problem complicating the analysis of antigen receptor genes is that additional rearrangements, deletions, and somatic mutations may occur that can result in the disappearance of a previous amplifiable signal (i.e., a false negative).

A more specific approach is the isolation and sequencing of an antigen receptor gene rearrangement at the time of initial diagnosis, which then allows the design of tumor-specific probes that can then be used to monitor residual disease. A number of different methods to accomplish this goal have been developed.[63,64] A disadvantage to this approach is that initial tumor sample may not be available for molecular analysis, which in our experience is not uncommon when a patient is referred to a tertiary care institution for definitive therapy.

Regardless of the method used to assess minimal residual disease, the clinical significance of residual tumor when detected is not completely established in a variety of clinical settings. For example, PCR-based detection of the t(14;18) may be valuable for detecting minimal residual t(14;18)-positive B-cell lymphomas following induction or salvage chemotherapy.[65] However, Price and colleagues[66] studied 15 patients with follicular lymphomas in continuous clinical remission for at least 10 years and detected the t(14;18) in six patients (40 percent). The latter patients did not develop lymphoma after 1 year follow-up. Acute lymphoblastic leukemia is another disease in which PCR studies have yielded conflicting data. In some studies, negative and positive PCR results have correlated with sustained clinical remission and relapse, respectively.[67,68] However, in other studies patients with acute lymphoblastic leukemia in complete clinical remission have had persistent residual disease as shown by PCR for months after treatment, without subsequent relapse.[67] Quantitative PCR assays may be helpful in distinguishing patients at high risk of relapse from those likely to be cured.

Reverse Transcriptase PCR. Reverse transcriptase PCR is of particular value when a gene involved in a chromosome translocation contains relatively large introns. These introns can result in the sites of the flanking primers being widely separated, precluding amplification by standard PCR. However, the mRNA transcripts of the translocation can be isolated, cDNA can be synthesized with reverse transcriptase, and then standard PCR methods to amplify cDNA can be done. The reverse transcriptase PCR method is of great utility in the study of certain neoplasms, such as the t(9;22) in chronic myelocytic lymphoma and acute lymphoblastic leukemia.[69] Manufacturers also have simplified reverse transcriptase PCR methods by providing kits that are easy to use, some of which utilize an enzyme that has both reverse transcriptase and DNA polymerase activity.

Single Cell PCR. The great advantage of single cell PCR is that it allows the amplification of DNA from a single cell.[70] This method is of great value when the cells of interest represent only a minor fraction of the cell population, for example, in Hodgkin's disease. Prior molecular studies of Hodgkin's disease have been limited by the inability to distinguish the DNA of the Reed-Sternberg and Hodgkin cells from the reactive cells.

Compared with standard PCR, in single cell PCR the cell(s) of interest are initially isolated from other cells, usually using micromanipulation or flow cytometry. Then PCR primers and methods are designed for maximum sensitivity, allowing the amplification of DNA from a single cell. For example, two sets of nested primers can be used, the first set external to the second set, with sequential PCR amplifications.

Assessing Gene Mutations. Standard PCR methods play an essential role in studies to search for possible gene mutations in malignant tissues. PCR is the first step used to amplify tumor cell DNA prior to screening for gene mutations with other methods, for example, single stranded conformational polymorphism analysis.

Advantages and Disadvantages of PCR

PCR offers many technical advantages. First, the power of PCR amplification allows studies to be done on very small amounts of DNA. As a corollary to this, PCR is extremely sensitive, far superior to flow cytometry or Southern blotting. Second, DNA can be amplified from poorly preserved mixtures of DNA such as those obtained from fixed, paraffin-embedded tissue blocks and scrapings from routinely stained, archival glass slides.[71] Although formalin fixation and paraffin embedding of tissue denature DNA and preclude the analysis of large fragments, statistically there are usually a few small DNA fragments that remain intact and can therefore be amplified by PCR. However, it needs to be emphasized that certain fixatives, such as B5, Zenker's, and Bouin's, particularly degrade DNA, significantly compromising PCR amplification.[72] Third, PCR studies can be done very quickly, often in 2 days. Fourth, the oligonucleotide primers direct amplification, providing great specificity, and a small DNA sequence can be specifically amplified from an impure mixture of DNA. Lastly, the results of PCR studies for antigen receptor gene rearrangements are easier to interpret than those generated by Southern blot hybridization. With PCR, antigen receptor gene rearrangements cannot be confused with germline bands, which are not amplified. Furthermore, the problems of incomplete transfer and the poor resolution of large DNA fragments are avoided.

The major disadvantage of PCR also is a consequence of its extraordinary sensitivity. Even the slightest contamination from a positive sample can result in false positive results. Thus, rigorous attention to quality control is needed to prevent contamination. Other disadvantages to PCR are minor. In some instances, PCR may nonspecifically amplify DNA sequences. Usually the size of these products is sufficiently different from the desired product, and this artifact can be recognized. Hybridization with an internal probe will also detect only the specific product. Also, as mentioned above, PCR studies for antigen receptor gene rearrangements currently result in a significant false negative rate.

In Situ Hybridization

A major disadvantage of both the Southern blot and PCR methods is that the cellular location of a gene or virus cannot be determined. The great utility of in situ hybridization (ISH) is that it allows for direct observation of target DNA or RNA within tissue sections, single cells, or chromosomal preparations.[73]

Method

In situ hybridization begins with the selection of an appropriate DNA, RNA, or synthetic oligonucleotide probe. This probe may be radioactively or colorimetrically labeled. If fixed, paraffin-embedded sections are to be analyzed, ISH generally comprises the following steps.[73] The sections are first de-paraffinized in xylene and dehydrated in ethanol. Next, if DNA is to be analyzed, the DNA in the sections needs to be denatured in order that hybridization may occur. The probe is then overlaid on the sections to allow hybridization, followed by washing steps of appropriate stringency. If the probe is radioactive, autoradiography follows. If the probe is linked to a molecule such as biotin, substrate needs to be placed on the sections to produce a colored product at the sites of probe binding. In many ways the procedure resembles immunohistochemistry, although the binding of probe to tissue is via hydrogen bonds between complementary bases and not antigen-antibody binding.

Fluorescence In Situ Hybridization

Fluorescence in situ hybridization (FISH), also known as interphase cytogenetics, combines the techniques of ISH and cytogenetics.[74] In conventional cytogenetics, only dividing cells can be examined as metaphase spreads. Conventional cytogenetics cannot analyze cells in interphase. Furthermore, conventional cytogenetics requires fresh tissue and is most easily performed on relatively pure populations of rapidly growing tumors, such as those of hematolymphoid origin. Slowly growing solid tumors are more difficult to karyotype, as the cells are more difficult to induce into mitosis. Furthermore, in tissue biopsy specimens that also contain admixed reactive cells, the more rapidly growing reactive cells may overgrow the culture and represent the majority of cells in mitosis. When examining the metaphases, one cannot distinguish the malignant from the benign cells.

The great advantage of FISH is that it allows direct visualization of the signal within the cell nuclei of both dividing and *interphase* cells.[74] FISH can be performed on blood and bone marrow aspirate smears, cytospin cell preparations, and fixed, paraffin-embedded sections. In tissue sections FISH allows correlation of cytogenetic abnormalities with tissue architecture. As in ISH, a labeled probe with other ingredients necessary for hybridization is overlaid on the slides, followed by appropriate washing steps. Probes labeled with fluorochromes are popular, as they can easily be seen with an ultraviolet microscope. Other detection systems also may be used.

Fluorescence Immunophenotyping Combined with Interphase Cytogenetics

This technique more commonly has been referred to as *f*luorescence *i*mmunophenotyping and interphase *c*ytogenetics as a *t*ool for *i*nvestigation *o*f *n*eoplasms, leading to the convenient acronym FICTION. As is stated in the name, the advantage of this method is that immunophenotyping is used simultaneously with FISH to identify more accurately the cells with cytogenetic abnormalities. The FICTION method is discussed extensively by others elsewhere.[75,76]

Comparative Genomic Hybridization

Comparative genomic hybridization is a powerful method to assess globally for chromosomal gains or losses that has been recently applied to the study of lymphoid neoplasms. As has been reviewed by others,[77] test and reference genomic DNAs are labeled with different fluorochromes, co-hybridized with normal human metaphase chromosomes, and then computer analyzed by fluorescence microscopy. Differential fluorescent hybridization signals represent changes (i.e., gain or loss of chromosomes) of test DNA relative to the reference DNA.

Comparative genomic hybridization is an excellent method for screening chromosomes to detect segments likely to carry important but unknown genes, which can be subsequently characterized by molecular methods. It also has been applied to the study of formalin-fixed, paraffin-embedded tumors.[78]

In Situ PCR

In this method, PCR is done on tissue sections to amplify target DNA.[79,80] Thus, similar to standard PCR, specific oligonucleotide primers are designed, and all necessary reagents including DNA polymerase are combined in appropriate buffer and overlaid on tissue sections. Following amplification, a labeled internal probe is hybridized with the tissue section using an ISH protocol.

The sensitivity of in situ PCR is much greater than the sensitivity of standard ISH and is particularly helpful for the detection of target sequences present in low copy number.[79,80] Amplified product also can be related to tissue architecture and cytologic features. Thus, in situ PCR combines the best features of ISH and PCR. The method allows direct observation of target sequences in cells and tissues with the sensitivity of PCR.

Single Stranded Conformational Polymorphism

As the numbers of known oncogenes and tumor suppressor genes have increased, methods became needed to screen specific target DNA sequences for potential gene mutations. A number of methods that accomplish this goal exist, with single-stranded conformational polymorphism (SSCP) perhaps being the most popular because it is relatively simple and rapid and can be applied to the study of routinely processed, paraffin-embedded tissue blocks. Most SSCP assays also include the use of PCR to initially amplify the DNA target sequence. This method has been extensively reviewed by others.[81] PCR SSCP is briefly reviewed here.

The PCR SSCP technique is based on the principle that single stranded DNA migrates in a nondenaturing gel as a function of its size and its secondary structure. This secondary structure results from intrastrand nucleotide interactions and, therefore, is a result of the base sequence. A single base mutation will change the sequence, which often alters the secondary structure and the electrophoretic mobility of single stranded DNA. The detection of a mobility shift suggests that a mutation is present. However, single base mutations may result in a gel shift and yet the base substitution may not change the predicted amino acid (since the genetic code is degenerate). Conversely, since the secondary structure of single stranded DNA is difficult to predict, it seems reasonable to assume that not all base substitutions will result in a change in mobility, although this is probably not a common occurrence. Thus, the detection of mobility shifts using PCR SSCP is an excellent screening tool but is not a definitive test for gene mutations. The "gold standard" for this purpose remains DNA sequencing.

Method

Using the example of analyzing a tumor for *p53* gene mutation, genomic DNA is extracted from tumor tissue, preferably from as pure a population of tumor cells as possible. For biopsy specimens with abundant reactive tissue, microdissection can be done to isolate the tumor for analysis. Then routine PCR methods are used to amplify the target DNA, in this case the *p53* gene. Since this gene has known mutational hot spots that occur in exons 5 through 9, different primer sets are used that amplify each of these exons. In most studies the primers are radioactively labeled, and the signal is incorporated into the PCR products. Next, the PCR amplified products are electrophoresed in a denaturing (formamide added), high resolution polyacrylamide gel. Denaturation is needed to ensure that the DNA will run through the gel as single strands. The PCR products of each amplified exon of the *p53* gene are then run in separate lanes. After the gel is dried (water quenches radioactivity) and fixed to a support such as firm blotting paper, x-ray film is laid over the gel and autoradiography is performed. The expected result for a homozygous gene sequence, theoretically, is that two complementary single strands of DNA will result in two bands in a lane. For a patient sample that is heterozygous for the gene analyzed, theoretically four different single strands of DNA result in four bands per lane. Any change in the mobility of one of these expected bands implies the presence of a mutation that altered the secondary structure of single stranded DNA. Of course, it is not this simple, since more than one single stranded DNA can migrate a similar distance in the gel and be superimposed as one band. Furthermore, there are technical issues and artifacts of the assay that can complicate analysis.

For a sample with a mobility shift that is to be sequenced, the abnormally migrating band can be cut out of the gel, eluted, and reamplified, either by PCR or by cloning the fragment into a cloning vector. The products are then sequenced using the dideoxynucleotide method described below.

Sensitivity

The sensitivity of PCR SSCP is not an issue if a pure cell population such as a cell line is analyzed. Sensitivity is an issue when patient biopsy samples are analyzed in which normal reactive cells are always present to some degree. Sensitivity also depends on the goals of the assay. For the example of screening the *p53* gene, the sensitivity is at least 10 percent.[75] In other words, one cell with a mobility shift can be detected in a population of 10 normal cells. Others have reported even greater sensitivity, down to 1 percent.[81]

DNA Sequencing

A complete discussion of DNA sequencing is beyond the scope of this chapter. However, as mentioned above, DNA sequencing is the next step after PCR SSCP (or another screening method) to confirm the presence or absence of gene mutations. Thus, DNA sequencing is discussed briefly.

Most current DNA sequencing protocols rely on the Sanger dideoxynucleotide method.[82] This method exploits the fact that dideoxynucleotides (ddNTP) can be incorporated into DNA being actively synthesized, but their incorporation then halts DNA synthesis because phosphodiester bonds cannot be formed with ddNTPs.

To employ the Sanger method, the DNA fragment to be sequenced is divided into four aliquots, each combined with two labeled oligonucleotides (to prime synthesis of each DNA strand), a low ratio of one ddNTP to its normal deoxynucleotide (dNTP) counterpart, the other three dNTPs, and DNA polymerase. Each aliquot will contain ddATP, ddCTP, ddGTP, or ddTTP. As normal DNA synthesis begins, nucleotides will be incorporated. When a ddNTP is incorporated, synthesis will stop. If the appropriate ratio of ddNTP to dNTP is used, a series of DNA strands of different lengths will result, each ending with a ddNTP. The four aliquots are then analyzed in a high resolution polyacrylamide gel, in four different and adjacent lanes, with each lane containing a different ddNTP (ddATP, ddCTP, ddGTP, or ddTTP). Following drying of the gel and autoradiography, the end result will be a ladder of bands in each lane, each band corresponding to the site where a ddNTP was incorporated, for example, an A in the ddATP lane, a C in the ddCTP lane, and so forth. When the procedure is technically well done, one can read across the four lanes on the film identifying the position of the various nucleotides.

EPSTEIN-BARR VIRUS

Epstein-Barr virus (EBV) is a human herpes type virus. The EBV genome has been entirely cloned and sequenced and is a linear, double-stranded, 172 kb length of DNA.[83] The exact size of the virion differs from molecule to molecule because of a variable number of tandemly repeated segments, each 500 bp long, present at either end of the virus.[84,85] The virus also has a number of repeated sequences, one of the largest being a 3,072 bp internal repeat sequence.[83] Two major viral strains of EBV are known, types A and B (also known as 1 and 2).[86]

Epstein-Barr virus infects cells in linear form (Fig. 1-8). After infection, the virus may follow

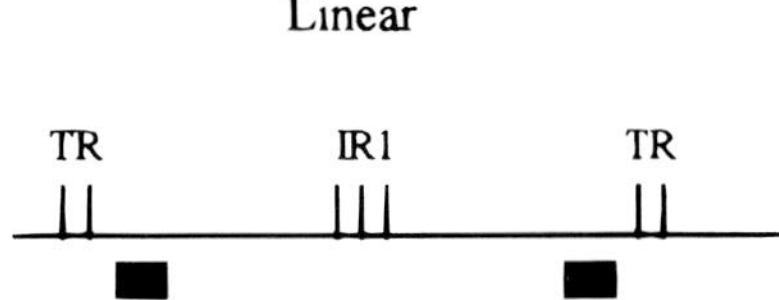

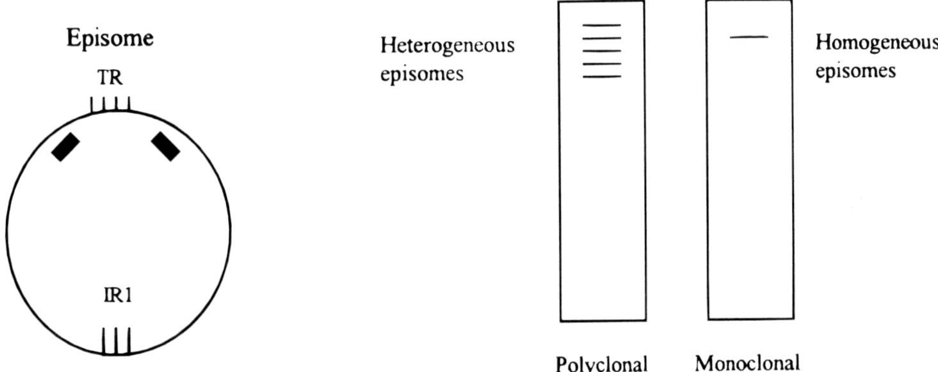

Fig. 1-8. Schematic illustration of the EBV genome. EBV infects cells as a linear molecule, which, in latent infection, circularizes into an episome. Usually only one virion infects a cell. Using genomic terminal repeat (TR) region probes (*boxes*), Southern blot hybridization analysis, and *Bam*HI-digested genomic DNA, a polyclonal population of cells contains many differently sized EBV episomes resulting in a heterogeneous ladder of bands. In contrast, a monoclonal population of cells contains identically sized EBV episomes that result in a single band. IR1, internal repeat region 1. (Modified from Raab-Traub and Flynn,[84] with permission.)

two possible courses.[85] The virus may actively replicate, ultimately resulting in cell death and the release of many virions, causing lytic infection. In lytic infection, the virus expresses a number of viral proteins representing the majority of the viral genome.[87] Alternatively, the virus may circularize by fusion of the termini to form an episome resulting in latent infection. The EBV episome is analogous to a plasmid in a bacterial cell and is exactly replicated in all progeny. In latent infection, only a limited number of viral proteins are expressed, including the nuclear antigen (EBNA) types 1, 2, 3A, 3B, and 3C and latent membrane protein types 1, 2A, and 2B.[87]

Southern Blot Hybridization

Southern blotting has been used to assess for the presence of virus. Usually a genomic probe derived from a highly repeated region, such as the *Bam*HI-W fragment from the internal repeat sequence, is used.[88] Probes derived from highly repeated sequences are preferred because the sensitivity is greater than with a probe specific for a single copy viral sequence. Southern blot methods to determine the presence of EBV are of historical more than practical interest, since other methods such as PCR are much more sensitive and easier to perform.[85]

Southern blot hybridization is currently more useful as a means to assess the clonality of EBV-infected cells.[84,85] At the time of EBV circularization in latent infection, random deletion of one or more tandemly repeated terminal DNA segments occurs as the termini of EBV fuse (Fig. 1-8). As a result, EBV virions may circularize into approximately 20 differently sized episomes, each varying in size by 500 bp intervals.[85]

Remembering that an EBV episome is exactly reproduced in all cell progeny and assuming that only one virion infects a neoplastic cell, as is usually the case in vitro,[89] EBV probes may be used to assess clonality. Genomic probes that have been cloned from unique DNA segments adjacent to the termini of the EBV molecule (known as terminal repeat region probes) are available.[84,85] Using these probes, a biopsy specimen that contains only one size of episomal EBV DNA is a monoclonal population (Fig. 1-8). This finding suggests that all cells arose from a single parent cell containing one EBV DNA episome that was exactly replicated. In contrast, a biopsy specimen containing different sized EBV DNA episomes, each fragment varying in length by 500 bp (a so-called ladder of fragments), is a polyclonal population of cells. In this case, the various cells probably arose from different precursor cells, each infected by a different EBV virion containing a different sized EBV DNA episome.[84,85]

Terminal repeat region probes from both ends of EBV may also allow determination of the integration status of EBV in some cases. For example, if left- and right-sided terminal repeat probes hybridize with identically sized restriction fragments, the EBV is episomal and is not integrated. If these probes detect different sized fragments, the virus is likely to be integrated.[89] The different size of the fragments is a function of the distance from the ends of the virus to the next restriction enzyme site in the host genome.[89] In lymphoid cells grown in tissue culture, EBV may be maintained as an episome or may be integrated into the host DNA. However, in most EBV-positive malignant lymphomas in vivo the virus is not integrated into the host cell genome.[85,89]

The use of EBV terminal repeat probes to assess clonality offers several advantages. These probes can assess clonality in nonhematopoietic EBV-positive neoplasms in which the antigen receptor genes do not rearrange. For example, this method has shown that nasopharyngeal carcinomas are monoclonal.[84] EBV terminal probes also may assess clonality in EBV-positive hematopoietic neoplasms independent of the antigen receptor genes (Fig. 1-9). For hematopoietic neoplasms in which multiple copies of episomal DNA are present in each malignant cell (e.g., Burkitt's lymphoma), analysis of the EBV termini for monoclonality may be more sensitive than analysis of the antigen receptor genes, with only one or two rearranged alleles per malignant cell. Finally, these methods have added to our understanding of the pathogenesis of EBV-positive tumors. The finding of identically sized EBV episomal DNA implies that the virus is present prior to monoclonal expansion and raises the possibility that EBV is involved in malignant transformation.

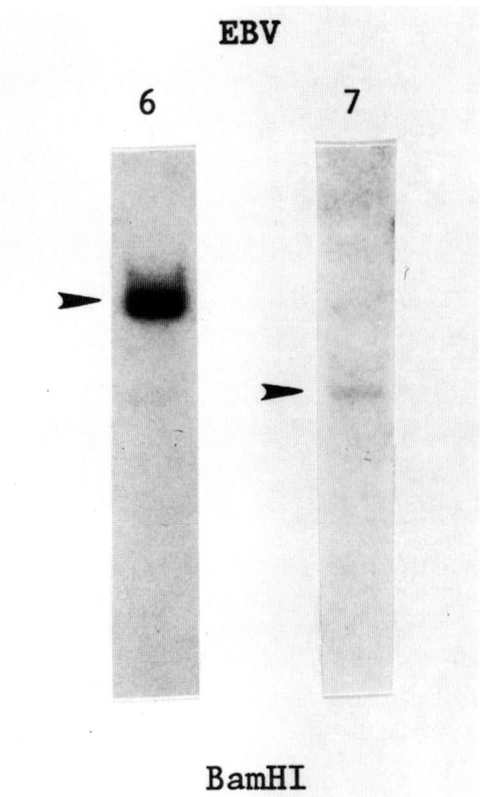

Fig. 1-9. Two malignant lymphomas studied using Southern blot hybridization, *Bam*HI-digested tumor genomic DNA, and an EBV terminal repeat region probe. Both tumors contain a homogeneous population of EBV episomes, consistent with the virus being monoclonal. Antigen receptor gene rearrangements were not identified by Southern blotting in these tumors. Lane 6, angiocentric T-cell lymphoma of nasopharynx; lane 7, lymphomatoid granulomatosis/lymphoma of lung.

Southern blotting to detect EBV in tissues has two main disadvantages. As alluded to previously, this method is much less sensitive than other methods. In addition, Southern blot results do not identify the cell population in which the virus resides.

Polymerase Chain Reaction

PCR is a very sensitive method for assessing the presence of EBV in tissues (Fig. 1-10). Primers have been designed to amplify a number of regions of EBV, and PCR methods can be used to analyze fixed, paraffin-embedded tissues.[85] However, like Southern blotting, PCR methods do not identify the cell population in which the virus resides. For this application, in situ hybridization is much more useful.[85]

PCR-based methods to detect EBV are more useful for two purposes: strain typing and analysis of the EBV latent membrane protein (LMP) gene. The A and B strains of EBV differ in the organization of their EBNA-2 and EBNA-3A–C genes and can be readily distinguished by using PCR with primers designed to amplify the EBNA-2 gene.[86,90] Both strains can be identified in oropharyngeal epithelium. However, peripheral blood lymphocytes usually contain type A unless the patients are immunosuppressed. Type A much more readily immortalizes lymphocytes in vitro and is most often identified in immunocompetent individuals.[86,90]

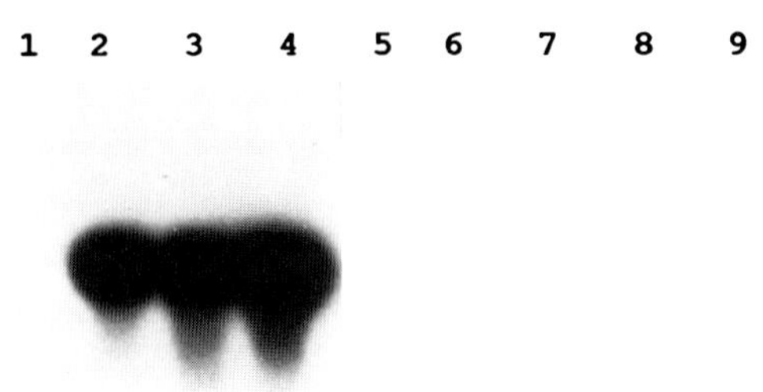

Fig. 1-10. Malignant lymphomas analyzed for EBV using the PCR technique. In this study, DNA was extracted from paraffin blocks, amplified for the presence of EBV using primers designed to amplify an 80 bp portion of the EBNA-1 gene, electrophoresed in agarose gels, transferred by the Southern method to nylon membranes, and hybridized with an internal ^{32}P-labeled oligonucleotide probe. Lane 1, negative control; lanes 2–4, three EBV-positive tumors; lanes 5–9, five EBV-negative tumors.

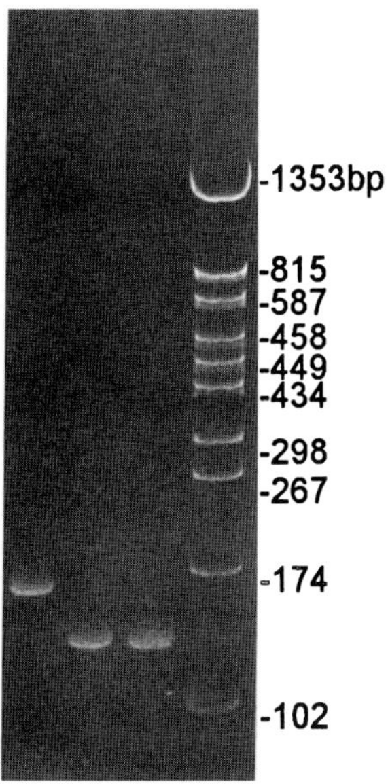

Fig. 1-11. Two malignant neoplasms analyzed for deletions in the 3′ end of the EBV latent membrane protein (*LMP*) gene. In this study, DNA was extracted from paraffin blocks, amplified for the presence of 3′ EBV *LMP* gene sequences with specific flanking primers, electrophoresed in agarose gels, and stained with ethidium bromide. Lane 1, EBV-positive control with nondeleted *LMP* gene, seen as a 161 bp product; lane 2, EBV-positive large cell lymphoma with deleted *LMP* gene, seen as a 131 bp product; lane 3, gastric carcinoma with deleted *LMP* gene; M, $\varnothing\chi$174 puc 19/*Hae*III size markers.

The EBV LMP gene is known to undergo deletion or mutations involving the 3′ end of the gene and affecting the carboxy terminus of the LMP1 protein in a variety of EBV-positive neoplasms, such as Burkitt's lymphoma, peripheral T-cell lymphomas, and Hodgkin's disease.[91,92] Using primers designed to amplify the relevant portion of the LMP gene, PCR is a convenient way to test for LMP gene deletions (Fig. 1-11). These deletions are usually 30 bp long and result in the loss of 10 amino acids from the cytoplasmic domain of the LMP.[91,92] Deletions in the LMP1 gene may render the protein more tumorigenic, as has been shown to be the case in a nasopharyngeal carcinoma cell line.[93]

Deletions of the EBV LMP1 gene also have been identified in lymphoid tissues from patients with infectious mononucleosis.[91] Thus, LMP1 gene deletions are not restricted to malignant neoplasms.

In Situ Hybridization

ISH for EBV may be done with DNA, RNA, or oligonucleotide probes. Initially, ISH studies for EBV used genomic DNA probes.[85] Although useful, a major disadvantage of DNA probes is that sensitivity is limited. Generally there is only one or a few copies of the virus per cell unless the virus is amplified multiple times, as may occur in Burkitt's lymphomas and Burkitt's lymphoma cell lines. Similarly, RNA or oligonucleotide probes designed to hybridize with EBV DNA are limited by low DNA copy number.

A major breakthrough in EBV ISH studies was the recognition that small EBV-encoded RNA molecules are abundantly transcribed in latent EBV infection and are present in greater than 10^7 copies per cell.[94] Thus, although cellular RNA is less well preserved than DNA, the extraordinary number of EBV-encoded RNA transcripts allows for very sensitive detection of EBV by ISH, with a sensitivity approximating PCR. However, theoretically the EBV-encoded RNA method will not detect cells in which only lytic infection by EBV has occurred.[95]

ISH for EBV provides significant advantages over Southern blotting and PCR.[85] First, and most important, ISH allows recognition of the cell population within which EBV resides (Fig. 1-12). Although not particularly important in Burkitt's lymphoma, where almost every cell is positive, in Hodgkin's disease ISH methods allowed the recognition of EBV preferentially located within the Reed-Sternberg cells and mononuclear variants.[96] Second, ISH can be done on routinely fixed and processed paraffin tissue blocks, which cannot be used for Southern blotting.

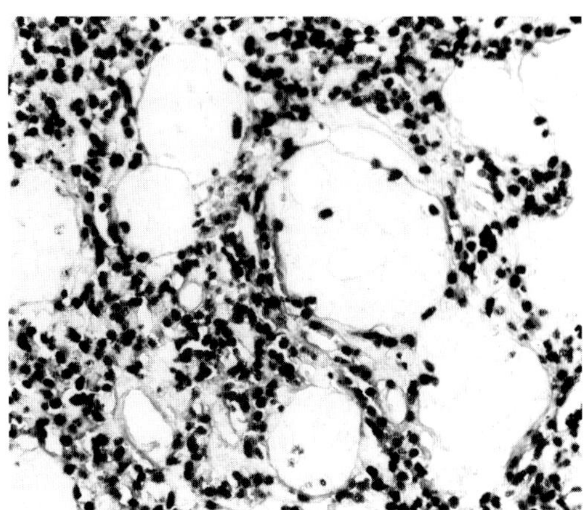

Fig. 1-12. Angiocentric T-cell lymphoma of nasopharynx assessed by ISH for EBV RNA. The neoplastic lymphoid cells contain abundant EBV RNA (black). Benign epithelial glands are negative for EBV RNA. This tumor is also illustrated in lane 6 of Fig. 1-9. (ISH for EBER, detected with an avidin-alkaline phosphatase conjugate followed by development of signal in McGadey's substrate, without counterstain, × 400.)

MOLECULAR GENETIC FINDINGS IN LYMPHOID NEOPLASMS

Acute Lymphoblastic Leukemia/Lymphoma

Acute lymphoblastic leukemia (ALL) and lymphoblastic lymphoma (LBL) are neoplasms of immature B cells or T cells, arrested at an early stage in lymphocyte maturation. Approximately 80 to 90 percent of ALLs are of immature B-cell lineage, and these cases include neoplasms once designated as "non-B, non-T," "null," and "common" ALL. The remainder of ALLs, 10 to 20 percent, are of immature T-cell lineage.[13] The converse is true for LBLs; approximately 70 to 80 percent arise from immature T cells and 20 to 30 percent arise from immature B cells.[13,97] The molecular findings in the majority of immature B-cell ALLs and LBLs are virtually identical, as are the molecular findings in ALLs and LBLs of immature T-cell lineage. The recently proposed Revised European-American Classification of Lymphoid Neoplasms recognizes this similarity with the designation of these tumors as precursor B-cell or T-cell lymphoblastic leukemia/lymphoma.[98]

Precursor B-Cell ALL/LBL

Virtually all precursor B-cell ALL/LBLs contain IgH gene rearrangements (Table 1-3). Approximately 40 to 50 percent of ALL/LBLs also carry Igκ gene rearrangements, and 20 to 25 percent carry Igκ gene rearrangements or deletions and Igλ gene rearrangements.[11,13]

The TCR genes are commonly rearranged in precursor B-cell neoplasms.[13,99] TCRδ is rearranged or deleted (following rearrangement) in up to 80 percent of cases. The TCRγ, TCRα, and TCRβ genes are rearranged in 50 to 60 percent, 40 to 50 percent, and 20 to 30 percent, respectively. As a result of lineage infidelity, TCR as well as Ig probes can be used to assess clonality in precursor B-cell ALL/LBL, although it also follows that assessment of individual antigen receptor genes is less useful for determination of lineage.

Conventional cytogenetic methods have demonstrated nonrandom chromosomal translocations in precursor B-cell ALL/LBLs.[28,100,101] In general, these translocations involve candidate or known oncogenes. Tumor suppressor genes are also involved in a subset of precursor B-cell ALL/LBLs. Some of the more common molecular abnormalities are as follows.

t(9;22)(q34;q11). The t(9;22)(q34;q11), also known as the Philadelphia chromosome, is one of the most common recurrent chromosomal translocations in ALL, detected in 5 percent of children and approximately 20 percent of adults with ALL.[101,102] This translocation, restricted to precursor B-cell neoplasms, joins the c-*abl* gene at chromosome 9q34 with the *bcr* locus at 22q11 (Fig. 1-13). The result is a chimeric mRNA transcript that encodes a fusion gene with increased tyrosine kinase activity. Two types of the t(9;22) occur. In approximately 25 to 50 percent of adults with ALL, the translocation is identical to that seen in chronic myeloid leukemia and the fusion protein is 210 kd, known as p210. In the remaining 50 to 75 percent of adults and the majority of children with ALL, the breakpoint on chromosome 22 is not in the *bcr* region but 100 kb 5′ or upstream, resulting in a different fusion protein of 190 kd. The p190 protein has greater tyrosine kinase activity and transforming capacity than p210. For translocations that produce p210, the breakpoints in the *bcr* gene are tightly clustered, amenable to Southern blot analysis. Translocations that result in the production of p190 have more widely scattered breakpoints that are less amenable to analysis by Southern blotting. Reverse transcriptase PCR assays are very useful for detecting either translocation.

t(1;19)(q23;q13). The t(1;19)(q23;q13) translocation occurs in approximately 6 percent of all ALLs and in up to 30 percent of precursor B-cell neoplasms.[101,103,104] The t(1;19) is most commonly identified in those tumors with a "pre-B cell" (cytoplasmic IgM positive) immunophenotype. In this translocation, the homeobox gene *Pbx1* on chromosome 1q23 is joined to the *E2A* gene on chromosome 19p13.[103,104] *E2A* is a gene that encodes an enhancer-binding transcription factor. The translocation creates a unique fusion gene that encodes for a chimeric transcription factor. The sequences involved in the t(1;19) have been cloned and sequenced, permitting detection using Southern blot analysis. For example, Kawamura and colleagues[105] used an *E2A* probe and Southern blot analysis and demonstrated *E2A* rearrangements in 15 of 16 (93.8 percent) cases shown to have the t(1;19) by conventional cytogenetics methods.[105] The breakpoints are also clustered and are suitable for detection using PCR.[106]

t(8;14). The t(8;14) and the variant translocations involving the Ig light chain genes t(2;8) and t(8;22) occur in approximately 6 percent of ALLs.[100,101] These tumors express monotypic surface Ig and are equivalent to Burkitt's lymphoma (discussed subsequently).

Table 1-3. Antigen Receptor Gene Rearrangements in Lymphoid Neoplasms

	Cases with Antigen Receptor Gene Rearrangement (%)					
	Immunoglobulin Genes			T-Cell Receptor Genes		
	IgH	Igκ[a]	Igλ	TCRβ	TCRγ	TCRδ[b]
B-cell neoplasms						
Precursor B-cell acute lymphoblastic leukemia/lymphoma	100	40–50	20–25	20–30	50–60	70–80
Chronic lymphocytic leukemia/CD5+ small lymphocytic lymphoma	100	100	30	<10	<10	<10
Prolymphocytic leukemia	100	100	30	Rare	Rare	NA
Hairy cell leukemia	100	100	50	Rare	NA	NA
Hairy cell leukemia variant	100	100	30	Rare	NA	NA
Lymphoplasmacytoid lymphoma/immunocytoma	100	100	30	Rare	NA	NA
Extranodal small lymphocytic lymphoma	100	100	30	<10	<10	NA
Marginal zone B-cell lymphoma						
Monocytoid B-cell lymphoma	100	>90	30	<10	Rare	NA
Low-grade B-cell lymphoma of mucosa-associated lymphoid tissue	100	100	30	<10	Rare	NA
Splenic marginal zone cell lymphoma	100	100	30	0	NA	NA
Splenic lymphoma with villous lymphocytes	100	100	30	Rare	NA	NA
Mantle cell lymphoma	100	100	50	Rare	NA	NA
Follicular lymphoma, all subtypes	100	100	30	<10	<10	<10
Diffuse aggressive B-cell lymphomas						
Mixed small and large cell	100	100	30	<10	<10	NA
Large cell	100	100	30	<10	<10	NA
Large cell immunoblastic	100	100	30	<10	<10	NA
T-cell-rich B-cell lymphoma	90	90	30	<10	Rare	NA
Primary mediastinal B-cell lymphoma	100	100	30	Rare	NA	NA
Small noncleaved cell lymphoma						
Burkitt's	100	100	30–40	Rare	Rare	NA
Non-Burkitt's	100	100	30	Rare	Rare	NA
Plasma cell myeloma	90	90	30	10	10	NA
T-cell neoplasms						
Precursor T-cell acute lymphoblastic leukemia/lymphoma	20	Rare	Rare	90–95	90–95	>95
Chronic lymphocytic leukemia/prolymphocytic leukemia	<10	0	0	100	100	>90
Large granular lymphocytic leukemia						
T-cell	Rare	0	0	>90	>90	>90
Natural killer cell	0	0	0	0	0	0
Peripheral T-cell lymphoma, unspecified	<10	Rare	0	>90	>90	>90

Continued

Table 1-3. Antigen Receptor Gene Rearrangements in Lymphoid Neoplasms *(continued)*

	Cases with Antigen Receptor Gene Rearrangement (%)					
	Immunoglobulin Genes			T-Cell Receptor Genes		
	IgH	Igκ[a]	Igλ	TCRβ	TCRγ	TCRδ[b]
Peripheral T-cell lymphoma, specific variants						
Adult T-cell leukemia/lymphoma	<10	0	0	100	>90	>90
Sinonasal angiocentric lymphoma	0	0	0	<10	0	Rare
Angioimmunoblastic T-cell lymphoma	20	10–20	10–20	90	90	90
Intestinal T-cell lymphoma	0	0	0	100	NA	NA
Anaplastic large cell lymphoma	10	Rare	0	60–70	60–70	90
Hepatosplenic γ/δ T-cell lymphoma	0	0	0	70–80	70–80	80–90
T-cell lymphoma involving subcutaneous tissue	0	0	0	>90	>90	50
Lennert's lymphoma	0	0	0	>90	60–70	>90
Mycosis fungoides/Sezary syndrome	0	0	0	70–80	70–80	>90
Uncertain lineage neoplasms						
Intravascular lymphomatosis	75	NA	NA	25	NA	NA

[a] Igκ includes deletion and rearrangement.
[b] TCRδ includes deletion and rearrangement.

11q23. To date, 25 different chromosomal bands have been reported to be involved in rearrangements of the 11q23 locus, with these abnormalities occurring in a variety of lymphoid and myeloid hematopoietic neoplasms.[107] In most of these tumors, however, the breakpoints within the 11q23 locus are localized to a 9.0 kb region and involve the *MLL* gene (also known as *ALL1*, *HTRX1*, and *HRX*).[101,107]

The *MLL* gene spans 100 kb and contains at least 21 exons.[107] It encodes a protein that is thought to be involved in transcriptional regulation. Translocations involving the 11q23 region usually result in the formation of fusion transcripts that code for chimeric proteins.[107]

In ALLs, 11q23 abnormalities are usually detected as translocations involving the following partner chromosome loci: 9p11, 9p21–22, 4q21, 19p13, 1q21, 1p32, 6q27, 12p13, 17q21, 17q25, 20q13, and Xq13.[107] The t(4;11), t(9;11), and t(11;19) are probably the most common. The majority of cases of ALL with 11q23 abnormalities are of immature B-cell type, but a small subset of tumors has been of immature T-cell lineage.

In the t(4;11)(q21;q23), the gene located at 4q21 is known as *AF4* or *FEL*. In the t(9;11)(p22;q23), the gene located at 9p22 is named *AF9*. In the t(11;19), the gene located on chromosome band 19p13 is named *ENL*.[107] In all three translocations, chimeric proteins are formed that have nuclear targeting sequences that are thought to facilitate transcriptional regulation.

The t(4;11) occurs in approximately 2 percent of childhood ALLs and in 5 to 6 percent of adult ALLs and is associated with a poor prognosis.[101] In infants with precursor B-cell ALL, 11q23 abnormalities have been correlated with an age of less than 6 months, a high leukocyte count, absence of the CD10 antigen, and frequent co-expression of myeloid antigens, with the CD15 antigen being most frequently co-expressed.[108]

The *MLL* gene has been cloned, and probes are available that can be used to detect rearrangements or deletions with Southern blot hybridization or FISH methods.[107,108]

Deletions and novel inversions of the 11q23 locus also occur in a subset of ALLs. These tumors, unlike the cases with 11q23 transloca-

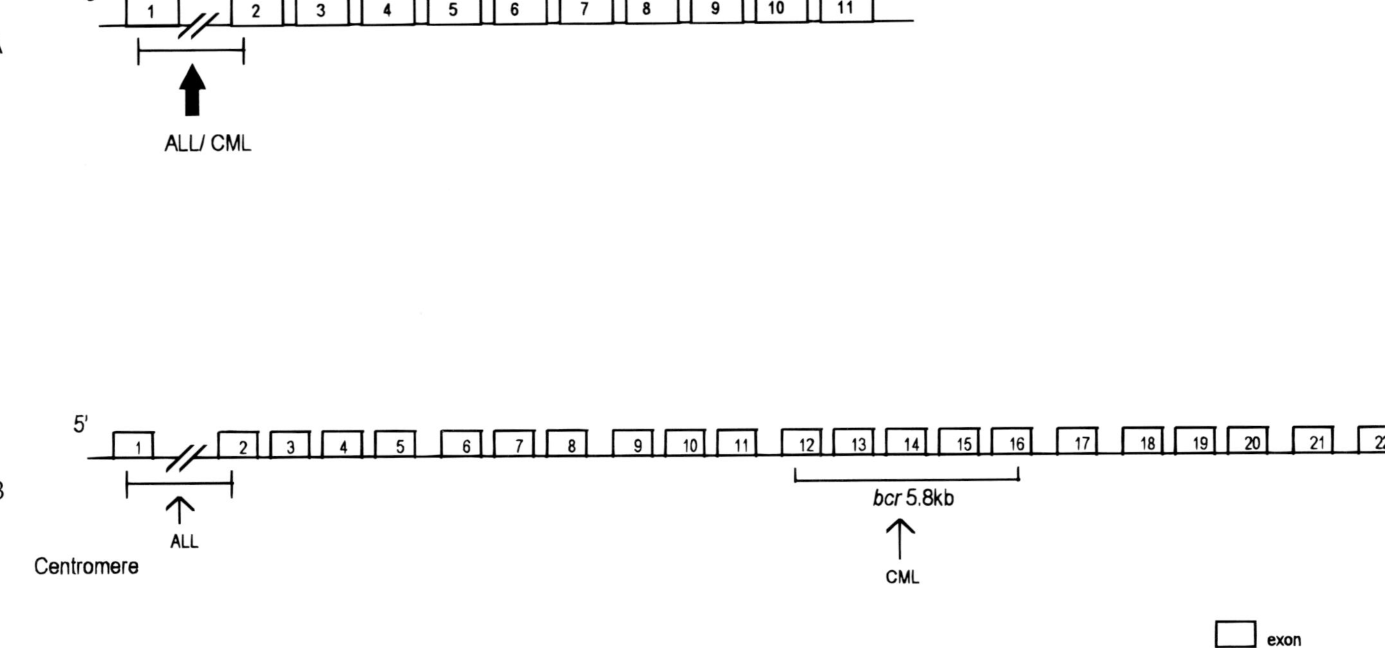

Fig. 1-13. Germline configuration of (**A**) c-*abl* and (**B**) *bcr* genes and breakpoints involved in the t(9;22)(q34;q11). In both acute lymphoblastic leukemia (ALL) and chronic myeloid leukemia (CML) the breakpoints in c-*abl* span the same region. In contrast, the *bcr* gene breakpoints may occur either in the 5.8 kb *bcr* region (most CML and 25 to 50 percent adult ALL) or 100 kb 5′ (50 to 75 percent adult and most pediatric ALL), resulting in p210 and p190 kd proteins, respectively.

tions, do not have *MLL* gene rearrangements and have a relatively better prognosis.[109]

12p13. A variety of unbalanced translocations and interstitial deletions occur in the 12p13 region in a variety of hematopoietic neoplasms, including a subset of childhood ALLs.[110] In this locus two genes have been identified, *TEL* and *KIP1*. *TEL* is a transcription factor. *KIP1* enodes for a p27 product that inhibits the cyclin E–cdk2 complex. Both *TEL* and *KIP1* are candidate tumor suppressor genes. Translocations and deletions involving the 12p13 locus are typically heterozygous and may be detected using Southern blotting and FISH methods.[110,111]

t(5;14)(q31;q32). Precursor B-cell ALL/LBLs may be associated with eosinophilia and carry the t(5;14)(q31;q32) chromosomal translocation.[112,113] In two such cases, Meeker and colleagues[113] demonstrated that the breakpoints on chromosome 5 are tightly clustered within the promoter region of the interleukin-3 (IL-3) receptor gene and the chromosome 14 breakpoints occur within the J region of the IgH gene.[113] The translocation results in the head-to-head juxtaposition of the IL-3 gene with the Ig heavy chain gene J region. Presumably the t(5;14) results in overexpression of IL-3 mRNA, with IL-3 inducing eosinophilia.

p53. Some *p53* gene mutations have been identified in a small subset of t(1;19) ALLs. In one study, 2 of 22 (9.1 percent) cases at diagnosis and three additional cases at time of relapse had mutations. The *p53* gene mutations appeared to correlate with a worse prognosis.[105]

ras. N-*ras* gene mutations have been reported in 6 of 33 (18 percent) null cell (precursor B-cell) ALLs.[114] Neri and colleagues[114] reported that N-*ras* gene mutations preferentially involve codons 12 or 13. Kawamura and colleagues[105] also identified an N-*ras* gene mutation in 1 of 22 (4.5 percent) cases of t(1;19)-positive ALL.[105] K-*ras* and H-*ras* gene mutations are rare in precursor B-cell ALLs.

Precursor T-Cell ALL/LBL

Gene rearrangement studies of precursor T-cell ALL/LBLs have shown various patterns of TCR gene rearrangement corresponding to the stage of differentiation of the neoplasm. These stages may be divided into three groups, early, middle, and late thymic, in accord with the maturation of normal T cells in the thymus.[12,97] In general, ALLs are arrested at an earlier stage of differentiation than LBLs.

In a subset of early thymic T-cell ALL/LBLs, only rearrangements of the TCRδ gene or both the TCRδ and TCRγ genes are identified with the TCRβ gene in the germline configuration[12] (Table 1-3). In the remaining early thymic cases and in all of the middle and late thymic ALL/LBLs, all of the TCR genes are rearranged. The TCRδ gene is often deleted following rearrangement.[12] Although the TCRα gene is difficult to analyze using Southern blotting, TCRα gene transcripts have been detected in late thymic T-cell ALL/LBLs with Northern blot hybridization. These findings suggest a hierarchy of TCR gene rearrangements in normal developing T lymphocytes: the TCRδ gene rearranges first, followed by rearrangement of the TCRγ and the TCRβ genes, lastly followed by rearrangement of the TCRα locus.[12]

Lineage infidelity is common in precursor T-cell precursor ALL/LBLs. IgH gene rearrangements occur in approximately 20 percent of precursor T-cell neoplasms.[115] However, Ig light chain gene rearrangements are exceptionally rare.

A number of nonrandom chromosomal translocations involving candidate oncogenes have been identified in precursor T-cell ALL/LBLs. Tumor suppressor genes also may be involved. Some of the more common abnormalities are specifically addressed as follows.

***tal*-1.** The *tal*-1 gene, also known as *SCL* and *tcl*-5, is located at chromosome 1p32 and encodes a transcription factor with a basic helix-loop-helix domain. This gene is a member of a family of transcription factor genes involved in growth regulation and differentiation. The *tal*-1 gene is rearranged in 25 to 30 percent of precursor T-cell ALL/LBLs.[116,117] In most cases with *tal*-1 gene rearrangements, representing approximately 25 percent of all T-cell ALLs, small interstitial deletions in the *tal*-1 locus result in the *tal*-1 gene being joined with the *SIL* gene. This joining is thought to be an example of illegitimate recombination mediated by the V-(D)-J recombinase mechanism using heptamer-nonamer-like sequences flanking each gene.[29,116] In these cases no abnormalities are detectable by conventional cytogenetics. In a smaller subset of cases, representing 3 to 5 percent of all T-cell ALLs, the t(1;14)(p32;q11) is present, which brings the *tal*-1 gene into continuity with the TCRα/δ locus. The *tal*-1 gene rearrangements, both deletions and translocations, are readily identified by Southern blot and PCR analyses.

A monoclonal antibody that reacts with the tal-1/SCL protein has been produced.[118] Initial immunohistochemical studies have shown that tal-1/SCL protein expression can occur independently of *tal*-1 gene rearrangement.[118] Thus, mechanisms in addition to *tal*-1 gene rearrangement, such as point mutations, may be involved in protein expression.

del 9p21–22. Approximately 10 percent of cases of precursor ALL/LBLs, most often of T-cell lineage, have deletions of chromosome 9p21–22 as shown by conventional cytogenetics.[119,120] Recent studies have identified two closely related candidate tumor suppressor genes at this locus, *p16* (also known as *MTS1, CDK4I,* and *CDKN2*) and *p15* (*MTS2*).[121] Both genes encode 16 and 15 kd proteins, respectively, that inhibit cyclin D-dependent kinases 4 and 6. These cyclins are involved in regulating cell cycle progression from the G1 to the S phase, and their inhibition would be expected to provide a cell with a growth advantage.[121]

Using a variety of methods, homozygous (and, less frequently, heterozygous) deletions of the *p16* locus have been identified almost exclusively in precursor ALLs among hematopoietic tumors, with the vast majority of cases being of immature T-cell lineage.[121–124] The *p16* deletions have been identified in most cases with 9p21–22 deletion as shown by conventional cytogenetics as well as in cases in which conventional cytogenetics are normal.[121] The *p15* locus has a similar frequency of homozygous deletions in immature T-cell ALLs, although this locus has been analyzed less commonly.[121] Occasional immature B-cell ALLs with *p16* and *p15* homozygous deletions also have been described.[121–124]

The *p16* and *p15* gene deletions, in addition to correlating strongly with immature T-cell lineage, correlate with a poorer survival and are uncommon in hyperdiploid (more than 50 chromosomes) ALLs.[121,122]

t(10;14)(q24;q11). Approximately 5 to 10 percent of T-cell ALLs carry the t(10;14), involving the *HOX11* gene situated on chromosome 10q24. The *HOX11* gene (also known as *tcl*-3) has been characterized as a homeobox gene involved in transcriptional regulation.[125] In the majority of cases, the breakpoint on chromosome 10 is 5′ to the *HOX11* gene, resulting in deregulation and increased expression of qualitatively normal HOX11 protein.[125] DNA probes to detect *HOX11* gene rearrangements can be obtained.

An antibody reactive with HOX11 protein has been developed.[126] Immunohistochemical studies have shown that HOX11 protein is maximally expressed at the transition from G1 to S phases of the cell cycle.[126]

t(8;13)(p11;q11). Rare cases of precursor T-cell LBL are associated with peripheral blood or tissue eosinophilia and carry the t(8;13)(p11; q11) translocation.[127–129] Clinical follow-up of these patients has shown that they have a high risk for developing myeloid hyperplasia, myelodysplastic syndromes, or acute myeloid leukemia. The genes involved in this translocation are not yet cloned. However, 13q12 is the site of the *FLT3* and *FLT1* genes that encode receptor tyrosine kinases.[129]

Miscellaneous. Other translocations have been identified in precursor T-cell ALL/LBLs by conventional cytogenetics, often involving the T-cell antigen receptor loci TCRδ/α at 14q11, TCRβ at 7q34, and TCRγ at 7p15.[101] These translocations, present in small subsets of precursor T-cell ALL/LBL, involve known or candidate oncogenes brought into continuity with the antigen receptor locus, with dysregulation and inappropriate overexpression of the oncogene product. For example, the c-*myc* gene may be rearranged in T-cell ALLs as a result of translocation to the TCRδ locus.[130] Also, *Ttg*-1 is a candidate oncogene located at chromosome 11p15 that is juxtaposed with the TCRδ locus via the t(11;14)(p15;q11).[131] The *Ttg*-1 gene (also known as rhombotin 1) is a zinc finger protein.[132] There are many other candidate oncogenes cloned from T-cell ALLs, including *Ttg*-2 (rhombotin 2). *lyl*-1, and *TAN*-1.[133–135] The *Ttg*-1, *Ttg*-2, and *lyl*-1 genes are transcription factor genes. *TAN*-1 encodes for an integral membrane protein.

Mature B-cell Lymphomas and Leukemias

Chronic Lymphocytic Leukemia/ Nodal Small Lymphocytic Lymphoma

Chronic lymphocytic leukemia (CLL) and nodal small lymphocytic lymphoma (SLL) are mature B-cell neoplasms that are immunophenotypically and genetically similar. Thus, these diseases are discussed together as one entity that may have different clinical manifestations.

Virtually all cases of CLL/SLL have Ig heavy and light chain gene rearrangements.[136] Either one or both IgH genes may be rearranged. In tumors with two rearranged bands, presumably one rearranged allele is nonfunctional and the other allele is functionally rearranged. More CLL/SLLs express Igκ than Igλ. Thus, in the majority of CLL/SLLs, the Igκ light chain gene is rearranged and the Igλ light chain is germline. In Igλ positive tumors, both the Igκ and Igλ genes are rearranged, although the Igκ light chain gene also may be subsequently deleted.[1,3,136] The TCR genes are usually in the germline configuration; less than 10 percent of CLL/SLLs have TCR gene rearrangements (i.e., lineage infidelity).[136]

Biased use of IgH gene variable segments (V_H) has been reported in CLL/SLL. For example, Mayer and colleagues[137] reported that the V_{H6} family is preferentially used in CLL, whereas the V_{H5} family is used more frequently in SLL. The Igκ gene V_{HIIIb} family also has been reported to be used more often in CLL than can be explained by chance alone.[138]

DNA sequence analysis of the D and J segments involved in IgH gene rearrangement has shown a low frequency of somatic mutations.[139] Analysis of the Igκ gene V segments has similarly shown that somatic mutations are infrequent.[138] These findings suggest that CLL/SLLs arise from B cells that have not been exposed to antigen selection.[138]

Chromosomal abnormalities have been shown in CLL/SLL. Trisomy 12 is most common, found in approximately one third of cases, and the 12q13–22 region is likely to be most important.[140–142] Complex karyotypes are associated with a poor prognosis.[143] A major problem encountered in conventional cytogenetic analysis is that the neoplastic cells are poorly proliferative, even with exposure to mitogens, and thus many cases are negative using this method. Chromosome abnormalities are more commonly detected using FISH and comparative genomic hybridization. For example, Bentz and colleagues[144] compared conventional cytogenetics with genomic hybridization in 28 cases of CLL/SLL: in 13 of 28 (46 percent) tumors, comparative genomic hybridization detected chromosomal abnormalities involving a variety of chromosomes not detected by routine karyotyping. Loss of chromosome 17p was most common, occurring in 9 of 28 (32 percent) cases.[144]

Conventional cytogenetics studies have rarely identified the t(14;18)(q32;q21) in CLL/SLL.[145] More commonly, Southern blot hybridization studies have shown *bcl*-2 involvement, in approximately 5 to 10 percent of cases of CLL/SLL. In these cases the *bcl*-2 oncogene at 18q21 is involved in either the t(2;18)(p11;q21) or the t(18;22)(q21;q11) translocations, involving the Igκ (chromosome 2p13) or Igλ (chromosome 22q11) gene loci.[145–147] The breakpoint on chromosome 18 usually occurs within the variant cluster region, 5′ to the *bcl*-2 gene, but may also occur 3′ to the *bcl*-2 gene at a location intermediate between the major and minor breakpoint cluster regions.[145–147] These translocations result in deregulation of the *bcl*-2 gene with a quantitative increase of qualitatively normal bcl-

2 protein. Errors in the V-(D)-J recombination process may be involved in the generation of the t(2;18) and t(18;22), as Tashiro and colleagues[147] have identified a hepatamer-like sequence 5′ to the *bcl*-2 gene. Conventional cytogenetics studies also have shown the presence of either the t(2;18)(p11;q21) or the t(18;22)(q21; q11) in occasional cases of CLL/SLL.[147] The higher incidence of *bcl*-2 gene rearrangement detected by Southern blot analysis than with conventional cytogenetics may be related to technical difficulties associated with karyotyping poorly proliferative tumors.

In a small subset of CLL/SLLs, other chromosomal translocations have been found, including the t(14;19)(q32;q13) and t(11;14)(q13;q32). In both translocations oncogenes are juxtaposed with the Ig heavy chain gene at chromosome 14q32.[140,148] The t(14;19), rare in CLL/SLL, involves the *bcl*-3 oncogene at chromosome 19q13.[148] The t(11;14), involving the *bcl*-1 oncogene at chromosome 11q13, also has been reported. However, this translocation is rare in CLL/SLL and common in mantle cell lymphomas.[149] It seems likely that at least some cases of CLL/SLL with the t(11;14) previously reported were incorrectly classified histologically.

The *bcl*-6 gene was not rearranged in four cases of CLL/SLL analyzed.[150] The c-*myc* oncogene is not rearranged in typical cases of CLL/SLL and when found usually correlates with histologic transformation.[149]

Various tumor suppressor genes have been analyzed for mutations in CLL/SLL. Of these, the *Rb* locus or another tumor suppressor cell gene telomeric to the *Rb* locus is deleted commonly in B-cell CLL. Liu and colleagues[151] have reported 13q14 deletions using Southern blotting in 33 of 75 (44 percent) cases of CLL. Studies using FISH and comparative genomic hybridization also have frequently shown *Rb*-1 and 13q deletions.[144,152] Other tumor suppressor cell gene abnormalities reported include *p53* gene mutations, identified in approximately 10 percent of cases,[153] and deletions of the *p16* and *p15* genes at the 9p21 locus, which have been found in 5 to 10 percent of cases of CLL/SLL.[154] Comparative genomic hybridization studies have shown additional chromosome abnormalities, such as loss of 17p, that may be the site of currently unknown tumor suppressor genes.[144]

Richter Syndrome

CLL/SLL also may transform into high grade diffuse lymphoma; this phenomenon has been given the eponym Richter syndrome.[156] The high grade lymphoma most often resembles diffuse large cell or large cell immunoblastic lymphoma; small noncleaved cell lymphomas also have been reported.

In the majority of cases of Richter syndrome, conventional cytogenetics or Southern blot analysis has demonstrated that both the CLL/SLL and the high grade lymphoma components have common chromosomal abnormalities and/or identically sized Ig gene rearrangements, indicating that both tumors arose from the same neoplastic B-cell clone.[156] However, in other patients, Southern blot studies have shown different patterns of Ig gene rearrangement in the low and high grade lymphomas. Since the Ig genes frequently undergo somatic mutation and may also undergo reiterative Ig gene rearrangements (so-called Ig receptor editing), these changes may alter restriction enzyme sites and the size of the rearranged fragments.[157,158] In support of this hypothesis, Aoki and colleagues[139] have shown a higher frequency of somatic mutation in IgH D and J segments in Richter syndrome than in CLL/SLL. Thus, these cases may still represent origin from the same B-cell clone. The presence of common cytogenetic abnormalities or common DNA sequences within the rearranged Ig genes in both the CLL/SLL and the high grade lymphoma have proven a common clonal origin for at least some Richter syndrome cases with dissimilar Southern blot results.[158] However, it is possible that in a subset of patients with Richter syndrome the high grade lymphomas arise as a second B-cell clone, independent from the initial CLL/SLL clone.[156]

In many cases of Richter syndrome, cytogenetic abnormalities not present in the CLL/SLL have been found in the high grade lymphoma, a reflection of the genomic instability of the neoplastic cells at the time of histologic transformation.[140,159] There is no consistent pattern of cytogenetic abnormalities. In one recent study, Brynes and colleagues showed that trisomy 12 not initially present in the low grade component was acquired at the time of transformation. Occasionally, specific translocations have been identified only in the high grade component, such as the t(8;14)(q24;q32).[140] The *p53* gene mutations are also commonly found in the high grade lymphomas of Richter syndrome but not in the CLL/SLL,[153,160] and in a small subset of cases EBV has been found only in the high grade lymphoma.[161]

In rare cases of Richter syndrome, patients have developed high grade T-cell lymphomas.[162,163] The high grade T-cell lymphomas analyzed using molecular methods have had TCR gene rearrangements with germline Ig genes.[162] EBV has been absent.[163] The relationship of these T-cell lymphomas to the CLL/SLL is uncertain, although most likely coincidental.

B-Cell Prolymphocytic Leukemia

As in CLL/SLL, the Ig heavy and light chain genes are rearranged in B-cell prolymphocytic leukemia. The TCR genes are rarely rearranged. Unlike CLL/SLL, the Ig genes demonstrate a higher frequency of somatic mutation, and trisomy 12 is rare.[164] Both the t(11;14)(q13;q32) translocation and *bcl*-1 gene rearrangements have been reported in rare cases of B-cell prolymphocytic leukemia.[164,165] The t(14;18)(q32; q21) and *bcl*-2 gene rearrangements have not been identified.[145] Other known oncogenes such as *bcl*-3, *bcl*-6, and c-*myc* have not been reported to be rearranged.

Hairy Cell Leukemia

Molecular genetic studies were essential in establishing the mature B-cell lineage of hairy cell leukemia (HCL).[166] These neoplasms have rearrangements of the Ig heavy and light chain genes.[166,167] In contrast with most other B-cell lymphoid neoplasms, which express Igκ more often than Igλ, the Igλ light chain is expressed as often as or more than Igκ in HCL.[166] Accordingly, the Igλ gene is productively rearranged and the Igκ gene is rearranged and subsequently deleted in some cases. The TCRβ gene is usually in the germline configuration, although lineage infidelity has been reported.[167] The Ig genes commonly undergo somatic mutations, consistent with these tumors arising from cells influenced by antigen selection.[168]

No specific chromosomal translocations are known, and known B-cell oncogenes such as *bcl*-1, *bcl*-2, *bcl*-3, *bcl*-6, and c-*myc* are not known to be involved in HCL.[145]

With the advent of 2-chlorodeoxyadenosine as a very effective therapy for patients with HCL, complete remissions as determined using clinical and histologic criteria are common. Nevertheless, in these patients immunohistochemical and molecular studies have shown persistent low level, stable disease in the bone marrow, often representing less than 1 percent of all cells within the bone marrow biopsy.[169,170] The molecular study used the PCR technique to amplify IgH gene rearrangements successfully in HCL patients who were in complete clinical remission following therapy.[170]

Hairy Cell Leukemia-Variant

The variant form of hairy cell leukemia (HCL-V) is a low grade lymphoproliferative disorder with clinical features intermediate between typical HCL and B-cell prolymphocytic leukemia. Unlike HCL, patients with HCL-V often present with an elevated white blood cell count, the peripheral monocyte count is normal, and the tumor cells often lack tartrate-resistant acid phosphatase. These tumors have a mature B-cell immunophenotype.[171]

Relatively few cases of HCL-V have been analyzed using molecular methods. As expected in mature B-cell tumors, in HCL-V Ig heavy and light chain gene rearrangements are found. The

TCR genes are usually in the germline configuration. Relatively few oncogenes have been assessed in HCL-V. Dyer and colleagues[145] did not identify *bcl*-2 gene rearrangements in 12 cases of HCL-V.

Lymphoplasmacytoid Lymphoma/ Immunocytoma

The Ig heavy and light chain genes are rearranged and the TCR genes are usually in the germline configuration in lymphoplasmacytoid lymphoma/immunocytoma (LPL/I).[136] The IgH and Igκ genes have been shown to frequently undergo somatic mutation.[139,168]

A del(7)(32) has been identified in neoplasms designated as small lymphocytic lymphoma with plasmacytoid features, some of which are probably LPL/I.[172] There are no other characteristic chromosomal abnormalities known to occur in LPL/I, although rarely numerical abnormalities have been reported. The *bcl*-1, *bcl*-2, *bcl*-3, *bcl*-6, and c-*myc* oncogenes do not appear to be involved. In one case, a t(8;14)(q24;q32) was reported in LPI/I, which probably represented evidence of clonal evolution of LPL/I to a high grade lymphoma.[173]

Extranodal Small Lymphocytic Lymphoma

The application of immunophenotypic methods to the diagnosis of extranodal small lymphocytic and lymphoplasmacytic infiltrates, lesions once referred to as *pseudolymphomas,* has shown that approximately two thirds of these cases express monotypic Ig light chain.[174,175] Monotypic Ig light chain expression by these lesions correlates with an increased risk of subsequent systemic lymphoma, although not survival, justifying the reclassification of these lesions as low grade B-cell lymphomas.[174] Using the Working Formulation, many of these tumors have been classified as small lymphocytic lymphoma and many also have histologic features typical of low grade B-cell lymphomas of MALT.[98]

Southern blot analysis has shown Ig heavy and light chain gene rearrangements in monotypic extranodal small lymphocytic lymphoma.[174,175] The TCRβ gene is usually in the germline configuration. Other TCR genes have been analyzed rarely. Known oncogenes such as *bcl*-1, *bcl*-2, and c-*myc* have been in the germline configuration.[175,176] The t(11;18)(q21;q21) translocation has been identified in four cases of extranodal small lymphocytic lymphoma; the *bcl*-2 gene, located at 18q21, was in the germline configuration in these four tumors.[177]

Ig gene rearrangements also have been found in extranodal small lymphocytic or lymphoplasmacytic infiltrates that express polytypic Ig light chains.[175,176,178] Usually, the size of the monoclonal population in these lesions is much smaller than that found in monotypic extranodal small lymphocytic lymphoma. In addition, extranodal lesions that histologically demonstrate marked reactive lymphoid hyperplasia also may have small oligoclonal or monoclonal Ig gene rearrangements. Clinical follow-up studies of patients with these lesions have shown that the patients usually do not develop malignant lymphoma.[175,176,178] One explanation proposed for these findings is that monoclonal populations of B cells may arise in reactive lesions, under the influence of chronic antigen stimulation. Progression to overt malignant lymphoma is associated with the accumulation of a much larger monoclonal B-cell population or the occurrence of other genetic alterations.

Marginal Zone B-Cell Lymphomas

In the recently proposed Revised European-American Classification of Lymphoid Neoplasms, the term *marginal zone B-cell lymphoma* was suggested to encompass both monocytoid B-cell lymphoma and low grade B-cell lymphoma of MALT.[98] Both tumors are thought to arise from the nodal marginal zone or the extranodal equivalent of the marginal zone, respectively. Splenic marginal zone cell lymphomas are another closely related entity that are thought to arise from the marginal zone of the spleen.

Monocytoid B-Cell Lymphoma. A limited number of monocytoid B-cell lymphomas have been analyzed and reported. The Ig heavy and light chain genes are rearranged.[179,180] The TCRβ chain gene is usually in the germline configuration, although lineage infidelity has been rarely reported.[181] The *bcl*-2 gene rearrangements have not been identified by Southern blot hybridization studies, although Ngan and associates[180] detected the t(14;18)(q32;q21) in one neoplasm using PCR. The significance of this finding is uncertain. Sheibani and Ben-Ezra[182] used PCR to amplify HTLV-I, HTLV-II, and HIV genomes in monocytoid B-cell lymphomas. HTLV-I and HTLV-II genomes were negative. One monocytoid B-cell lymphoma was positive for HIV DNA; most are negative for EBV.

Conventional cytogenetic studies have been performed on very few monocytoid B-cell lymphomas. One of the larger studies analyzed them in association with other non-Hodgkin's lymphomas (composite lymphomas).[183] No abnormalities common to all monocytoid B-cell lymphomas were reported. Using FISH, Brynes and colleagues[184] reported trisomy 3 in a majority of monocytoid B-cell lymphomas, with detection of trisomy 12 in approximately one third of cases.

Low Grade B-Cell Lymphoma of Mucosa-Associated Lymphoid Tissue. Low grade B-cell lymphomas of MALT are mature B-cell neoplasms that have rearrangements of the Ig heavy and light chain genes.[185–187] The TCRβ chain is usually in the germline configuration; lineage infidelity is rare.[187] Analysis of other TCR genes in low grade B-cell MALT lymphomas has been reported rarely. The Ig genes can undergo somatic mutations.[188]

Using PCR, EBV may be identified in a subset of cases (less than 10 percent), but it is unclear from these studies whether the EBV is localized within the neoplastic cells.[189] Using ISH, EBV has been identified within the neoplastic cells of MALT lymphomas in a smaller subset of tumors[190] and may be associated with histologic transformation to large cell lymphoma in rare cases (unpublished observations).

Conventional cytogenetic studies have identified numerical abnormalities involving chromosomes 3, 6, 7, 8, 12, 16, and 18 in MALT lymphomas, with trisomy 3 being the most common finding.[191,192] Recently, Wotherspoon and colleagues[193] followed up these findings by performing FISH on 70 B-cell MALT lymphomas. Trisomy 3 was found in 42 (60 percent) cases. They also identified trisomy 18, trisomy 12, and trisomy 7 in 12, 13, and 3 percent of cases, respectively.[193]

Chromosomal translocations have been found in only a few low grade B-cell lymphomas of MALT. The t(11;18)(q21;q21) translocation has been reported in two MALT lymphomas[194] and in four other extranodal small lymphocytic lymphomas that were probably low grade B-cell lymphomas of MALT.[177] A t(1;14)(p22;q32) was reported in one low grade B-cell lymphoma of the pulmonary MALT.[195] One study of lymphomas involving the parotid gland reported the t(14;18)(q32;q21) in three of seven cases.[196] However, in most studies the t(14;18) has not been identified in MALT lymphomas, including low grade MALT lymphomas of the parotid gland.[189] It seems likely that most parotid gland lymphomas with the t(14;18) are follicular lymphomas involving intraparotid gland lymph nodes.

Using Southern blot hybridization, the *bcl*-1, *bcl*-3, and c-*myc* loci have been in the germline configuration. Most studies assessing the *bcl*-2 gene using either Southern blotting or PCR have reported that the *bcl*-2 gene is not rearranged.[197,198] Rare cases reported with *bcl*-2 gene rearrangement may be attributable to lymphomas in extranodal sites that are not truly of MALT origin. Studies of the *bcl*-6 gene in MALT lymphomas have not yet been reported. A recent study reported in abstract form did not identify *p53* gene mutations.[199]

Patients with low grade B-cell lymphomas of MALT may have multiple sites of disease at presentation, involving one or more organ system. Elenitoba-Johnson and colleagues[24] recently reported a lung B-cell MALT lymphoma in which there were three distinct tumor nodules associated with multiple tiny nodules composed of histologically benign lymphoid tissue. PCR detected an identical Ig heavy chain gene rearrangement in all three tumor nodules as well as the histologically benign sites sampled.[24]

Patients with MALT lymphomas commonly relapse in other extranodal sites. Are the relapse sites involved by the same clone, or are patients susceptible to multiple extranodal MALT lymphomas arising from different B-cell clones? Diss and colleagues[200] recently reported an elderly woman with Sjögren syndrome who underwent a lip biopsy and developed gastric B-cell MALT lymphoma 2 years later. PCR with direct sequencing of the amplified products detected an identical Ig heavy chain gene rearrangement in both sites.[200] Similar cases have since been reported by others.[201]

Patients with *Helicobacter pylori*-induced gastritis analyzed by PCR have been shown in a small subset of cases to have IgH rearrangements in the absence of histologic or clinical follow-up evidence of malignant lymphoma.[25,202] Southern blot analysis of reactive processes in the gastrointestinal tract also has revealed an oligoclonal pattern of Ig heavy chain gene and/or TCRβ chain gene rearrangements in a subset of cases.[187] When found, the rearranged bands are typically small and multiple, with each band representing less than 10 percent of the entire cell population in the biopsy specimen. These results suggest that small B-cell clones arise in histologically benign lymphoid hyperplasias, perhaps under the influence of chronic antigenic stimulation. The finding of a small B-cell clone by Southern blotting or PCR must be correlated with clinical and histologic data before the diagnosis of lymphoma can be established.

Splenic Marginal Zone Cell Lymphoma. These are B-cell neoplasms that are thought to arise from splenic marginal zone cells and are closely related to other marginal zone B-cell lymphomas.[203,204] Splenic marginal zone cell lymphomas are probably more common than has been appreciated in the literature and most likely were classifed as other types of non-Hodgkin's lymphoma in the past.

Relatively few cases have been studied using molecular techniques. Splenic marginal zone cell lymphomas are mature B-cell neoplasms that contain Ig heavy and light chain gene rearrangements.[203,205] The TCRβ chain gene and the *bcl*-1 and *bcl*-2 oncogenes have not been rearranged using either Southern blotting or PCR methods.[205] One study suggested that mutations of the *p53* gene are common in splenic marginal zone cell lymphomas.[206] However, a subsequent study did not confirm this finding.[205]

Splenic Lymphoma With Villous Lymphocytes. This disorder was initially described by Melo and colleagues[207] prior to the recognition of splenic marginal zone cell lymphomas. Patients usually have an absolute peripheral blood lymphocytosis and the lymphocytes are slightly larger than normal, with unevenly distributed cytoplasmic villi morphologically (but not immunophenotypically) resembling hairy cells. These patients also have prominent splenomegaly, and Isaacson and colleagues[204] have recently concluded that splenic lymphoma with villous lymphocytes and splenic marginal zone cell lymphoma represent the same disease, the former with more prominent peripheral blood involvement.[204]

Cytogenetic studies of splenic lymphoma with villous lymphocytes have commonly shown chromosomal abnormalities, that may be single or complex. Oscier and colleagues[208] identified abnormalities in 27 of 31 cases (87 percent), the most common findings being an abnormal 7q locus in 7 tumors (22 percent), the t(11;14)(q13;q32) in 5 neoplasms (16 percent), and translocations involving 2p11 or an isochromosome 17q in 4 cases each (13 percent). Trisomy 12 is rare, and the t(14;18)(q32;q21) has not been found. Southern blot hybridization analysis of splenic lymphoma with villous lymphocytes has shown Ig gene rearrangements.[209] The *bcl*-1 gene has been rearranged as shown by both Southern blotting and pulsed field gel electrophoresis, almost exclusively in cases shown to have the t(11;14) by conventional cytogenetic methods.[209] The *bcl*-2 gene is in the germline configuration.[145]

Mantle Cell Lymphoma

Mantle cell lymphoma (MCL), also known as centrocytic lymphoma and intermediate lymphocytic lymphoma, is a neoplasm of mature B-cell lineage. Thus, the Ig heavy and light chain genes are rearranged, and the TCR genes are usually in the germline configuration.[210–212] Unlike most other non-Hodgkin's lymphomas, and similar to hairy cell leukemia, MCLs more often express Igλ light chain, with a Igκ to Igλ ratio of approximately 1:1. (The normal Igκ to Igλ ratio is 2 to 1.) In MCLs, the V genes used in IgH gene rearrangement rarely show evidence of somatic mutations, consistent with origin from "virgin" pre-germinal center B cells not exposed to antigen selection.[213]

Conventional cytogenetic studies have demonstrated that the t(11;14)(q13;q32) is commonly found in MCLs and is rare in other types of non-Hodgkin's lymphoma.[214–217] For example, in two survey studies of non-Hodgkin's lymphoma, the t(11;14) was identified in 17 of 214 (8 percent) non-Hodgkin's lymphoma; 15 of the 17 (88 percent) were MCLs.[215,216] This translocation juxtaposes the *bcl*-1 locus at chromosome 11q13 with an enhancer region of the Ig heavy chain gene locus at chromosome 14q32, with deregulation of the *bcl*-1 gene.[155,218]

There are multiple chromosome 11 breakpoints involved in the t(11;14). Initial attempts to identify the *bcl*-1 gene (also known as *PRAD-1, D11S287E,* and *CCND1*) were frustrated by the distance between the gene and the initially cloned major translocation cluster region, which is present approximately 110 kb upstream (5′) to the *bcl*-1 gene (Fig. 1-14).[218] Other breakpoint sites are known as minor translocation cluster regions, which are also upstream but relatively closer to the *bcl*-1 gene (Fig. 1-14).[219–221]

The *bcl*-1 gene spans 15 kb and contains five exons.[222] The gene encodes for a cyclin D1 protein that, by binding to a cyclin-dependent kinase, regulates the transition of the cell from G1 to S phase. In the t(11;14), despite the various chromosome 11 breakpoint sites, the coding region of the *bcl*-1 gene is not interrupted, and thus the translocation results in a quantitative increase of qualitatively normal cyclin D1 mRNA and protein.

Using Southern blot hybridization analysis, approximately 70 percent of MCLs have been shown to have *bcl*-1 gene rearrangements.[220] The majority of these, over half, occur in the major translocation cluster region of chromosome 11q13.[210,211,220] Probes specific for other breakpoint sites are needed to detect additional cases with *bcl*-1 gene rearrangement.[220] Of these, the p94PS probe specific for the minor translocation cluster 22 kb 5′ to the major translocation cluster detects the greatest number of cases.[220] Also, cases of MCL are reported with cytogenetic evidence of the t(11;14) but no evidence of *bcl*-1 gene rearrangement detected by Southern blotting. Thus, other breakpoints exist outside the regions detected by currently available probes.[223]

PCR may be used to detect *bcl*-1 gene rearrangements in MCL. These protocols have focused on the major translocation cluster region since the breakpoints on chromosome 11 in this region are tightly clustered and amenable to PCR analysis.[220] These assays detect most cases with

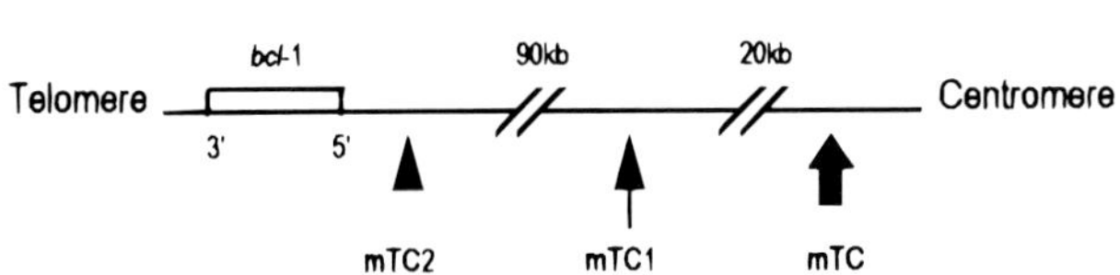

Fig. 1-14. Germline configuration of the chromosome 11q13 region involved in the t(11;14)(q13;q32). The *bcl*-1 gene is indicated as an open box. The major translocation cluster region (mTC) and two minor translocation cluster regions (mTC1, mTC2) are shown.

bcl-1 gene rearrangements occurring in the major translocation cluster region, approximately 40 to 50 percent of all MCLs.[224–227]

The cyclin D1 protein is a 35 kd protein that is a member of the cyclin G1 family. Overexpression of cyclin D1 is thought to disturb the transition between the G1 and S phases of the cell cycle, resulting in an expanded B-cell compartment.[228,229] Other molecular events are probably also necessary for neoplastic transformation.

Both polyclonal and monoclonal antibodies reactive with cyclin D1 protein have been developed and applied to tissue sections of MCLs and other low grade B-cell lymphomas. Nuclear cyclin D1 expression is almost specific for MCLs and occurs in tumors with and without molecular evidence of the t(11;14).[229,230]

The *bcl*-2 gene has been in the germline configuration in almost all MCLs studied.[210,211] In rare cases *bcl*-2 gene rearrangements and the t(14;18)(q32;q21) have been identified in MCLs that also carry *bcl*-1 gene rearrangements. The *bcl*-3 gene is not rearranged in MCLs.[148] Bastard and colleagues[150] reported a *bcl*-6 gene rearrangement in one of five diffuse small cleaved cell lymphomas, the category in the Working Formulation where MCL is most commonly placed. However, no *bcl*-6 gene rearrangements have been identified in MCLs by others.[231]

Some *p53* gene mutations have been identified in a subset of cases of MCL, more often in the blastic (high grade) variant.[232–234] For example, in abstract form, Greiner and colleagues identified *p53* gene mutations in 9 of 24 (38 percent) blastic and 2 of 31 (6.5 percent) typical cases of MCL.[232] The *p53* gene mutations also may correlate with a poorer prognosis, although it is not yet clear if *p53* gene mutations correlate with prognosis independent of blastic histologic findings.

Follicular Lymphoma

All follicular lymphomas, regardless of histologic subdivision, are mature B-cell tumors with similar molecular findings and therefore are discussed as a group.

In most cases, both IgH genes are rearranged.[136] One IgH allele is involved in the t(14;18)(q32;q21) chromosomal translocation, which is present in 70 to 90 percent of cases.[235,236] Since the majority of follicular lymphomas express surface Ig, the other IgH allele is involved in functional gene arrangement. The Ig light chain genes are also rearranged. The TCR genes are most often in the germline configuration, although occasional follicular lymphomas have been reported with TCRβ gene rearrangements.[136] Numerous polyclonal T cells, often outnumbering the malignant B cells, are commonly present in lymph nodes involved by follicular lymphoma. Thus, a polyclonal pattern of TCRγ gene rearrangements may be found in these lymphomas, which should not be confused with monoclonal TCRγ gene rearrangements.[43]

Application of PCR to detect Ig heavy chain gene rearrangements in follicular lymphomas is problematic. Unlike analysis of B-cell CLL/SLL or MCL in which somatic hypermutations within the Ig heavy chain gene variable regions (V_H) is relatively infrequent, somatic hypermutations within the V_H genes are common in follicular lymphomas.[49,62,213] These mutations result in a large subset of Ig heavy chain gene rearrangements not being amplified, probably because the Ig heavy chain gene variable region consensus primer selected will not anneal with the V_H region involved in rearrangement.[49,50] Using multiple primers the sensitivity of the method is increased, but even in optimum conditions PCR cannot detect Ig heavy chain gene rearrangements in approximately 30 percent of follicular lymphomas.[49,50] The sensitivity of detection of monoclonality can be increased to over 80 percent if primers designed to amplify the t(14;18) are combined with Ig heavy chain gene analysis.[49]

The t(14;18)(q32;q21) chromosomal translocation has been identified in approximately 80 percent of follicular lymphomas using routine karyotyping methods.[237] The t(14;18) is a reciprocal translocation that juxtaposes the *bcl*-2 oncogene on chromosome 18q21 with the IgH gene on chromosome 14q32. As a result, transcription of the *bcl*-2 gene is brought under the control

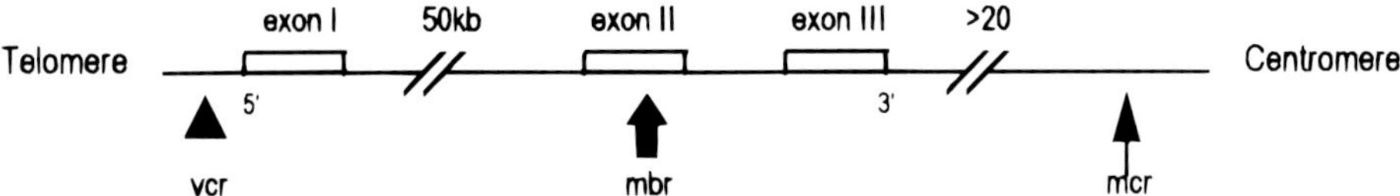

Fig. 1-15. Germline configuration of the chromosome 18q21 region involved in the t(14;18)(q32;q21), t(2;18)(p13;q21), and t(18;22)(q21;q11) translocations. The three exons of the *bcl*-2 gene are indicated as open boxes. In the t(14;18), the majority of breakpoints occur in the major breakpoint cluster (MBR) and minor breakpoint cluster (MCR) regions. In the t(2;18) and t(18;22), the breakpoints occur in the variant translocation cluster region (VCR).

of the IgH gene regulatory elements, most likely an enhancer region, resulting in constitutive overexpression of the *bcl*-2 gene.[235,236,238] The *bcl*-2 gene is composed of three exons and two introns.[238] The first exon is not translated as the open reading frame begins in the second exon.[238]

There are a number of molecularly distinct t(14;18) translocations. The chromosome 14 breakpoint is relatively constant and involves the Ig heavy chain gene J region. The chromosome 18 breakpoint is variable; at least four breakpoint regions have been identified (Fig. 1-15).[235,236] However, the majority of tumors involve two tightly clustered breakpoint regions, known as the major and minor breakpoint cluster regions. The major breakpoint cluster region is a 150 bp sequence within the 3′ untranslated region of the third exon of the gene, where 50 to 60 percent of follicular lymphoma breakpoints are clustered.[235,236] An additional 20 to 25 percent of follicular lymphomas have breakpoints clustered in the minor cluster region, which is 20 to 30 kb further 3′ to the *bcl*-2 gene.[235] Other minor chromosome 18 breakpoints occur in areas both 3′ and 5′ to the *bcl*-2 gene in less than 20 percent of follicular lymphomas.[235,236] The 5′ breakpoint region is known as the *variant cluster region*.[239]

The clustering of the chromosome 18 breakpoints allows the detection of the t(14;18) using Southern blotting and PCR. Most efforts have focused on the detection of translocations involving the major or minor cluster regions, since these represent the majority of t(14;18) translocations. For example, Horsman and colleagues[240] used Southern blot hybridization and PCR to detect the t(14;18) in follicular lymphomas with genomic probes or primer sets specific for the major and minor breakpoint clusters, respectively. Of 91 cytogenetically t(14;18)-positive cases, 78 (86 percent) cases were positive by Southern blotting and 68 (75 percent) cases were positive by PCR. These results indicate that both Southern blotting and PCR may be used as an alternative to conventional cytogenetics for detecting the t(14;18), particularly for cases with known breakpoints within the major or minor cluster regions. However, there remains a subset of t(14;18)-positive cases, approximately 15 percent by Southern blotting and 25 percent by PCR, in which the t(14;18) is not detected. Presumably, in the tumors negative by Southern blotting the chromosome 18 breakpoints do not occur in either cluster region.[240]

Regardless of the sites involved in the t(14;18), the open reading frame of the *bcl*-2 gene in the second exon is not disrupted. Thus, the t(14;18) results in a quantitative increase of qualitatively normal bcl-2 protein.[238]

The bcl-2 protein is 25 kD and has been localized to subcellular membranes such as the inner mitochondrial membrane.[241,242] The bcl-2 protein is now known to play a prominent role in protecting the cell from apoptosis (i.e., programmed cell death).[241] Cells that overexpress bcl-2 protein have a prolonged half-life, making these cells more susceptible to secondary genetic events that may result in transformation to a more aggressive phenotype.

A variety of immunohistochemical studies have analyzed bcl-2 protein expression in normal and neoplastic lymphoid tissues using either polyclonal or monoclonal antibodies.[243–245] In normal tissues, B cells in the mantle and marginal zones are bcl-2 positive. Normal germinal center B cells are negative. T cells also strongly express bcl-2. In neoplastic tissues, approximately 80 percent of follicular lymphomas express bcl-2, in contrast with reactive germinal centers. Furthermore, a variety of other B-cell lymphomas, particularly low grade B-cell tumors, express bcl-2 protein, although these tumors do not carry *bcl*-2 gene rearrangements.[243–245] Thus, bcl-2 protein expression occurs independently of the t(14;18).

Cases of follicular lymphoma without the t(14;18) or *bcl*-2 gene rearrangements represent 10 to 20 percent of all follicular lymphomas.[235–237,240] A subset of these cases may carry the t(14;18), that occurs in breakpoints not detectable by conventional cytogenetics, Southern blotting, or PCR. For example, Zelenetz and colleagues[246] used pulsed-field gel electrophoresis to detect the t(14;18) in follicular lymphomas negative for the translocation by other methods. Nevertheless, approximately 10 percent of all follicular lymphomas are negative for the t(14; 18) by all methods. Thus, there appear to be other molecular pathways that can result in follicular lymphoma, apparently independent of the t(14;18). Distinctive molecular abnormalities that have been described in t(14;18)-negative follicular lymphomas include translocations involving 3q27 and the *bcl*-6 gene, a distinctive t(8;14), and tumors with a t(2;18).

***bcl*-6.** Some *bcl*-6 gene rearrangements have been found in a subset of follicular lymphomas (approximately 5 to 15 percent).[150,231,247,248] Follicular lymphomas with *bcl*-6 gene rearrangements are clinically and histologically similar to *bcl*-2 rearranged follicular lymphomas. The *bcl*-6 and *bcl*-2 gene rearrangements are not mutually exclusive, as rearrangements of both genes have been identified in a subset of cases.[231] In two studies, *bcl*-6 gene rearrangements were not associated with histologic transformation to high grade lymphoma.[231,248]

t(8;14). In occasional cases of follicular lymphoma, a t(8;14)(q24;q32) or t(8;22)(q24; q11) has been identified in addition to the t(14; 18).[249] The presence of the t(8;14) or t(8;22) correlated with an aggressive clinical course.[250] More commonly, there is a subset (less than 10 percent) of follicular lymphomas with the t(8; 14)(q24;q32) and without evidence of the t(14; 18). Rearrangements of *bcl*-2 and c-*myc* genes were also not identified.[251] The patients with these tumors had an indolent clinical course, and molecular analysis of these cases suggested that the t(8;14) is structurally distinct and does not deregulate c-*myc,* in contrast with the t(8;14) in Burkitt's lymphomas. Other chromosomal abnormalities were also found in these cases, including trisomy 3, trisomy 8, and structural alterations in chromosomes 1 and 6.[251]

t(2;18). In a small subset of cases of follicular lymphoma, the t(2;18)(p11;q21) has been identified.[239,252] In one such neoplasm, the molecular breakpoints of this translocation were cloned and sequenced.[239] The breakpoint on chromosome 2 occurred in the J_{H4} region of Igκ. The breakpoint on chromosome 18 occurred 13 kb 5′ to the *bcl*-2 gene and involved another gene, named *FVT*-1 (follicular lymphoma variant translocation). The *FVT*-1 gene is composed of at least four exons and encodes for a protein predicted to be 36 kD. The function of this protein is not clear.[239] The t(2;18) juxtaposes *FVT*-1 with an Igκ gene enhancer, resulting in a quantitative increase in normal *FVT*-1 mRNA and protein, thought to be involved in lymphomagenesis.

t(14;18) in Benign Lymphoid Tissues

The t(14;18)(q32;q21) has been unequivocally demonstrated in benign tonsils and lymph nodes. Both Limpens et al.[26] and Aster and colleagues[27] have amplified the t(14;18) in over half of the hyperplastic lymphoid tissues studied and proven that the amplified products are unique translocations (and not contaminants) by DNA sequencing. Similarly, Limpens and colleagues[253] also identified the t(14;18) in the peripheral blood of normal blood donors. The patients had no histologic or clinical evidence of malignant lymphoma. These findings indicate that the t(14;18) by itself is insufficient to cause follicular lymphoma.

However, these findings are probably not a practical problem in routine molecular diagnosis. Others were only able to demonstrate the t(14;18) by employing a number of modifications of the PCR technique that greatly enhanced its sensitivity.[26,27,253] Routine PCR analysis of lymphoid tissues for the t(14;18) rarely detects the translocation in biopsy specimens and amplifies a strong signal in many follicular lymphomas.[254] The interpretation of t(14;18) results in the setting of minimal residual disease detection may be confounded.

Diffuse Aggressive Lymphomas

The designation *diffuse aggressive lymphoma* has been used for a group of malignant lymphomas that present with common clinical features and similarly respond to combination chemotherapy but otherwise are immunologically and molecularly heterogeneous. Included in this group are lymphomas classified in the Working Formulation categories of diffuse mixed small and large cell, diffuse large cell, and large cell immunoblastic. This discussion is focused on B-cell tumors. Diffuse aggressive lymphomas of T-cell lineage are discussed subsequently in this chapter.

B-cell diffuse aggressive lymphomas are mature B-cell neoplasms that have rearrangements of the Ig heavy and light chain genes. The TCR genes are usually in the germline configuration.[136] Prior to gene rearrangement analysis, diffuse aggressive lymphomas that lacked monotypic Ig expression were referred to as *null cell* lymphomas. The vast majority of these tumors have been shown to have Ig gene rearrangements and are of B-cell lineage.[255]

Diffuse aggressive lymphomas are for the purpose of discussion further divided into two groups: de novo neoplasms and tumors occurring in patients with a history of low grade lymphoma (i.e., secondary).

de Novo B-Cell Diffuse Aggressive Lymphomas. Conventional cytogenetic studies of de novo diffuse aggressive lymphomas have revealed a number of abnormalities. The two most common abnormalities are translocations involving the 3q27 locus and the t(14;18)(q32;q21), the latter identical to that found in follicular lymphoma.[237,256,257] Translocations involving the 3 q27 locus most commonly include the t(3;14)(q27;q32), t(2;3)(p12;q27), and t(3;22)(q27;q11).[257] In these translocations the gene located at 3q27 has been cloned and named *bcl-6/LAZ3*.[258–260] This gene was also designated *bcl*-5 by one group of investigators.[261] Via translocation, the *bcl*-6 gene is juxtaposed with either the Ig heavy chain gene at 14q32 or the Igκ and Igλ genes located at 2p12 and 22q11, respectively.[258–261] This allows the *bcl*-6 gene to come under the influence of the immunoglobulin enhancer region or other regulatory elements, resulting in constitutive expression of *bcl*-6, which is then involved in lymphomagenesis. In a small subset of cases, translocations involving *bcl*-6 at 3q27 involve loci other than the Ig genes, such as 1p32, 1p34, 3p14, 5q3, 6q23, 8q24, 11q13, 12p13, 14q11, and 16p13.[248]

The *bcl*-6 gene is composed of 10 exons. In tumors with the t(3;14), t(2;3), or t(3;22), the breakpoints on chromosome 3 are 5′ to the *bcl*-6 coding region (exons 2 to 10), clustered within a 10 kb segment, leaving the coding region intact. Thus, the translocation results in a quantitative increase of normal *bcl*-6 protein, which is then involved in lymphomagenesis. The breakpoints on chromosome 14 in some neoplasms have been mapped to the Ig switch region.[258,262]

The *bcl*-6 gene has a zinc finger motif and is thought to encode a DNA-binding transcription factor.[259] The *bcl*-6 protein is predicted to be 79 kd, but is phosphorylated and migrates in gels as 92 to 98 kd.[263–265] The activity of bcl-6 protein is likely to be regulated by phosphorylation. Antibodies reactive with bcl-6 protein have been produced; the protein is expressed in normal tissues in germinal center B cells and CD4-positive T cells. In non-Hodgkin's lymphomas, bcl-6 protein expression occurs in tumors with and without *bcl*-6 gene rearrangement.[263–265]

Southern blotting studies have shown that the *bcl*-6 gene is commonly rearranged in de novo diffuse aggressive lymphomas, ranging from 28.6 to 37 percent in three studies.[150,231,247] In one large study, the presence of *bcl*-6 gene rearrangements in diffuse large cell lymphoma correlated with extranodal sites of presentation and infrequent bone marrow involvement.[266] Furthermore, following appropriate therapy, patients with diffuse large cell lymphomas with *bcl*-6 gene rearrangement had improved freedom from progression of disease and survival compared with patients who had diffuse large cell lymphomas with germline *bcl*-6 and *bcl*-2 genes or neoplasms with only *bcl*-2 gene rearrangements.[266]

The *bcl*-2 gene is also rearranged in approximately 20 percent of de novo B-cell diffuse large cell and large cell immunoblastic lymphomas.[236,267] Presumably, these lymphomas have the t(14;18)(q32;q21) when studied using conventional cytogenetics and may represent diffuse progression of an occult follicular lymphoma. Patients with de novo diffuse large cell or large cell immunoblastic lymphomas with *bcl*-2 gene rearrangements appear to have an increased likelihood of relapse (responsive to additional chemotherapy) compared with patients with histologically similar lymphomas without *bcl*-2 gene rearrangements, more in keeping with the behavior of follicular lymphomas.[266–268]

The *bcl*-2 and *bcl*-6 gene rearrangements are not mutually exclusive, and diffuse aggressive lymphomas have been reported with rearrangements of both oncogenes.[266]

The c-*myc* gene at 8q24 is not rearranged in the majority of nodal diffuse aggressive lymphomas. However, c-*myc* gene rearrangements have been identified in approximately 10 to 20 percent of cases, particularly diffuse large cell and large cell immunoblastic lymphomas occurring in patients with AIDS and in primary gastric large cell lymphomas.[269,270]

The *lyt*-10 oncogene was cloned from a diffuse intermediate grade B-cell lymphoma with a t(10;14)(q24;q32) translocation.[271] In this tumor, the *lyt*-10 gene is brought into proximity with the Cα1 region of the Ig heavy chain gene, resulting in the production of a *lyt*-10–Cα1 fusion gene. The *lyt*-10 protein is a transcription regulation factor and is a member of the NF-κB family. In one study, the *lyt*-10 gene was shown to be rearranged in two additional diffuse B-cell lymphomas and one case of B-cell chronic lymphocytic leukemia.[271]

The *lyt*-10 oncogene is closely related to the c-*rel* oncogene, located at chromosome 2p11.2–14. Yunis and colleagues[272] have reported abnormalities in the 2p11.2–14 locus in 8 of 74 (12 percent) diffuse large cell lymphomas. The c-*rel* oncogene was cloned from a cell line derived from a diffuse large cell lymphoma and is a member of the NF-κB family of transcription regulation factors.[273] Chromosome 2p11.2–14 abnormalities also have been detected in secondary diffuse aggressive lymphomas, arising in patients with a history of follicular lymphoma.[272]

The *bcl*-1 and *bcl*-3 oncogenes are rarely rearranged in diffuse aggressive lymphomas. The *p16* and *p15* genes have been homozygously deleted in a small subset of tumors.[274] EBV may be identified within the neoplastic cells of a small subset of diffuse aggressive lymphomas, 7 of 67 (10.4 percent) cases in one study.[275] EBV is found with higher frequency in diffuse aggressive lymphomas arising in immunocompromised patients, particularly central nervous system lymphomas.[276]

The 9p21–22 and 9q31–34 chromosome regions also have been reported to be deleted in a subset of diffuse aggressive lymphomas.[277] The *p16* tumor suppressor gene, located at chromosome 9p21, has been reported to be deleted in approximately 10 percent of these tumors.[278] The 9q31–34 locus may be the site of a tumor suppressor gene that is currently not characterized.

Secondary B-Cell Diffuse Aggressive Lymphomas. These tumors occur in patients with a history of low grade lymphoma and have molecular characteristics similar to those found in the low grade lymphoma. In addition, in many cases molecular abnormalities unique to the diffuse aggressive lymphoma have been identified that may have been involved in histologic transformation. For example, *p53* gene mutations have been identified in diffuse large cell lymphomas occurring in patients who previously had *p53*-negative CLL/SLL or follicular lymphoma.[160,279,280]

Anaplastic large cell lymphomas of B-cell lineage also commonly occur as another form of secondary diffuse aggressive lymphoma. Although the majority of anaplastic large cell lymphomas are of T-cell or null cell lineage (discussed subsequently), a small subset of cases are of B-cell lineage.[281] For example, Penny and colleagues[282] reported cases of B-cell anaplastic large cell lymphomas that arose in patients with a history of low grade B-cell lymphoma and suggested that anaplastic histologic features may represent one common manifestation of histologic transformation of low grade lymphomas.

B-cell anaplastic large cell lymphomas have Ig heavy chain gene rearrangements, with Ig light chain gene rearrangements in some cases. The TCR genes are usually in the germline configuration.[281]

Oncogenes have been infrequently studied in B-cell anaplastic large cell lymphomas. Inghirami and colleagues[283] reported that the c-*myc* gene may be rearranged, amplified, or mutated in a subset of cases. These authors did not identify *bcl*-2 gene rearrangements or N-, K- or H-*ras* gene mutations.[283]

T-Cell-Rich B-Cell Lymphoma

T-cell-rich B-cell lymphomas are malignant lymphomas of B-cell origin in which the majority of cells in the biopsy are reactive cells, predominantly T lymphocytes.[284,285] The predominant T-cell population may lead to the erroneous diagnosis of T-cell lymphoma, and in the past some of these tumors were classified as T-cell lymphomas.[284,285]

With the advent of gene rearrangement analysis, T-cell-rich B-cell lymphomas were recognized. Both Southern blotting and PCR have been used to demonstrate that the Ig heavy and light chain genes are rearranged (Fig. 1-16).[284–287] The TCRβ is usually in the germline configuration, although lineage infidelity has been reported.[286,287] Using Southern blot hybridization, the Ig rearrangements are of much less intensity than the germline bands, consistent with the clonal population being the minority cell population in the biopsy.[286] However, in some cases the malignant cell population is so sparse that Ig gene rearrangements may not be detected by Southern blotting.[285–287]

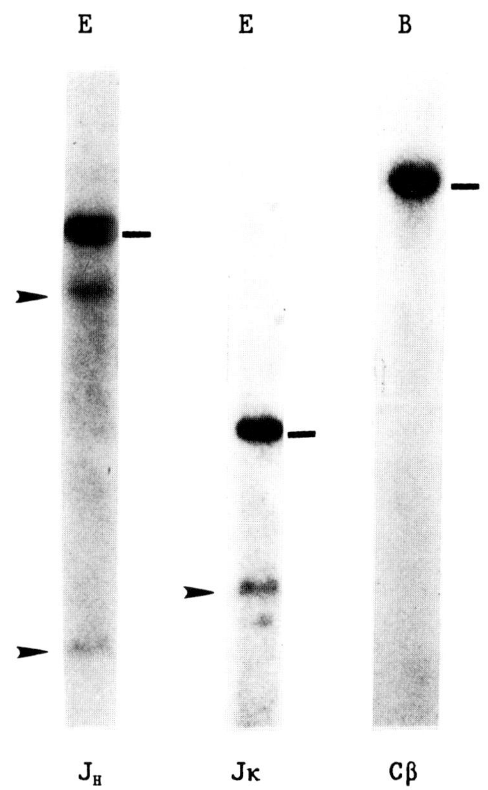

Fig. 1-16. T-cell-rich B-cell lymphoma. In this case the intensity of the signals of the rearranged fragments (*arrows*) is substantially less than the signal intensity of the germline fragments (*dashes*), indicating that the monoclonal B-cell population represents a minority of the total cell population in the biopsy specimen. Southern blot hybridization analysis was performed with *Eco*RI (E) and *Bam*HI (B) digested genomic DNA and ^{32}P-labeled probes specific for the joining regions of the IgH (JH) and Igκ (Jκ) genes and the constant region of the TCRβ gene (Cβ).

Analysis of the TCRβ and TCRγ genes can

also be used to assess the many T cells present in these tumors. As mentioned earlier, using a Cβ probe and *Eco*R1-digested DNA the 11 kb germline band is decreased, consistent with the presence of numerous polyclonal T cells.[286] Similarly, a Jγ probe typically demonstrates a ladder of bands, consistent with the presence of numerous polyclonal T cells.[286]

A subset of T-cell-rich B-cell lymphomas have had *bcl*-2 gene rearrangements or the t(14; 18) as amplified by PCR.[285] EBV has been identified in occasional cases[287,288] and may be present as a monoclonal episome.[288]

The variable presence of *bcl*-2 gene rearrangements and EBV, combined with clinical and histologic evidence, suggest that T-cell-rich B-cell lymphomas do not represent a distinct clinicopathologic entity. Instead, T-cell-rich B-cell lymphomas represent a heterogeneous group of B-cell neoplasms, all of which are histologically characterized by the presence of many reactive T cells.[284,285]

Primary Mediastinal Large B-Cell Lymphoma

Mediastinal lymphomas may be either primary, localized to the mediastinum, or secondary, as a part of widespread nodal disease. Primary mediastinal large B-cell lymphomas have unique clinicopathologic and histologic features and therefore may represent a distinct entity. Although over 200 cases have been reported in the literature, relatively few have been analyzed molecularly.[289–291]

Primary mediastinal large B-cell lymphomas are neoplasms of mature B-cell lineage. Thus, these tumors have Ig heavy and light chain gene rearrangements. These neoplasms commonly do not express Ig protein; in these tumors usually both alleles of the Ig genes are rearranged nonfunctionally.[289] The TCR genes are usually in the germline configuration.

Rearrangements or mutations of the c-*myc* gene have been reported in 6 of 25 (24 percent) cases in two recent studies.[290,291] A subset of cases, approximately 20 percent, have *p53* gene mutations and rarely K-*ras* gene mutations.[291] The *bcl*-2 gene is in the germline configuration.[290] Cesarman and colleagues[291] reported *bcl*-6 gene rearrangements in 1 of 16 (6 percent) cases, in contrast with nodal large cell lymphomas, in which the *bcl*-6 gene is rearranged in approximately 30 to 40 percent of cases.[291] EBV is usually absent.[290]

Small Noncleaved Cell Lymphoma

Burkitt's Type. Small noncleaved cell Burkitt's lymphomas are neoplasms of mature B-cell lineage. As expected, in virtually all cases the Ig heavy and light chain genes are rearranged, and the TCR genes are usually in the germline configuration.[136] Lineage infidelity is rare in Burkitt's lymphomas.[136]

Burkitt's lymphomas have been further subdivided into at least three groups based on geographic and clinicopathologic features: endemic (equatorial Africa), sporadic (industrialized countries such as the United States, Europe), and AIDS associated.[292,293] Using serologic and molecular techniques, EBV has been found in over 90 percent of cases of endemic Burkitt's lymphoma. In contrast, approximately 20 to 40 percent of sporadic Burkitt's lymphomas and Burkitt's lymphomas associated with AIDS have contained EBV.[269,293–295] In South America, in countries such as Brazil, EBV is present with a frequency intermediate between equatorial Africa and industrialized countries, 71 percent in one recent study.[296] In endemic, sporadic, and AIDS-associated Burkitt's lymphomas, the EBV is monoclonal, indicating that viral infection preceded and may contribute to clonal expansion.[293,294]

There are differences in the strain of EBV found in patients with Burkitt's lymphoma from different geographic regions. In patients from equatorial Africa, both types A and B EBV are found.[297] Normal patients in these regions also have a relatively high frequency of type B EBV.[297] In contrast, in South America and industrialized countries most patients have type A EBV.[86,298] Deletions of the EBV *LMP1* gene have been found commonly in Burkitt's lymphomas in Brazilian patients, even though these tumors do not express LMP protein and the significance of these deletions is uncertain.[298]

Conventional cytogenetic studies have shown that virtually all Burkitt's lymphomas are characterized by reciprocal chromosomal translocations involving the c-*myc* oncogene locus at chromosome 8q24 juxtaposed with one of the Ig gene loci.[299,300] In approximately 70 to 80 percent of cases, the t(8;14)(q24;q32) is present. In the remaining cases, the c-*myc* gene is juxtaposed with either the Igκ or Igλ light chain genes, forming the t(2;8)(p11;q24) or t(8;22)(q24;q11), respectively.[299]

The c-*myc* gene is composed of three exons (Fig. 1-17), the second and third exons encoding a protein of 49 kd.[299,300] The c-myc protein, via binding to DNA, is thought to control transcription and cell proliferation, although its function is not completely known. Translocations involving c-*myc* do not interupt either the second or third exons of the gene and thus result in a quantitative increase in transcription and translation of normal c-myc protein.[299,300]

The t(8;14) has been extensively analyzed with molecular techniques that have shown differences in the site of chromosome 8 breakpoints in Burkitt's lymphomas (Fig. 1-17).[292,293,300,301] Approximately 75 percent of endemic Burkitt's lymphomas have chromosome 8 breakpoints significantly upstream (5′) to the c-*myc* gene. In contrast, in sporadic Burkitt's lymphomas the chromosome 8 breakpoint is within or in close proximity to the c-*myc* gene. The chromosome 14 breakpoint occurs within the Ig heavy chain gene, commonly in the joining region (JH), but also may occur in the IgM switch (Sμ) or constant (Cμ) regions or in switch or constant regions of other Ig subclasses.[300]

These differences in the chromosome 8 and 14 breakpoints have important implications regarding the pathogenesis of Burkitt's lymphoma.[300,301] For example, chromosome 8 breakpoints far 5′ to the c-*myc* gene leave the regulatory regions of c-*myc* intact. In contrast, breakpoints within or close to the c-*myc* gene separate the regulatory region (located on chromosome 14 after the translocation) from the remainder of the gene. These structural differences probably affect the mechanism by which c-*myc* is deregulated. Similarly, although chromosome 14 breakpoints do not correlate with geography, these breakpoints may correlate with chromosome 8 breakpoints.[301] For example, cases with chromosome 14 breakpoints in the Sμ region are more common in tumors in which the chromosome 8 breakpoint occurs within or near the c-*myc* gene.[301] One rationale to explain this association is that the Ig enhancer elements between the JH and Sμ regions are translocated to chromosome 8 and juxtaposed with c-*myc*, thereby being involved in c-*myc* deregulation. In contrast, chromosome 14 breakpoints in the JH region result in these enhancer regions remaining on chromosome 14. In these cases the regulatory elements of c-*myc* need to remain on chromosome 8, and thus the chromosome 8 breakpoint is more commonly (but not exclusively) far 5′ to c-*myc*, leaving the gene intact.[300,301] The presence of EBV in most endemic but in only 20 to 40 percent of sporadic Burkitt's lymphomas also may be explained by the anatomy of the t(8;14) by being involved in

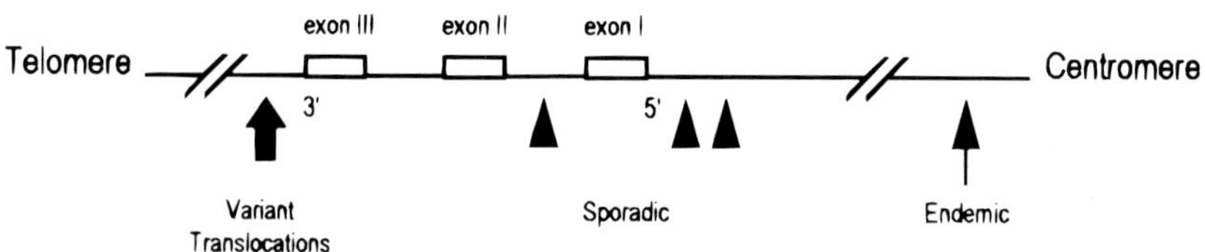

Fig. 1-17. Germline configuration of the chromosome 8q24 region involved in the t(8;14)(q24;q32), t(2;8)(p13;q24), and t(8;22)(q24;q11) translocations in Burkitt's lymphoma. The three exons of the c-*myc* gene are indicated as open boxes. The location of the chromosome 8 breakpoints in the t(8;14) differs in endemic and sporadic cases as well as in tumors with the t(2;8) and t(8;22) variant translocations.

the mechanism of c-*myc* deregulation, although its role is currently uncertain.

These differences at the molecular level in Burkitt's lymphoma suggest that these tumors may arise from B cells at different stages of maturation. Furthermore, these molecular findings demonstrate that endemic, sporadic, or AIDS-associated Burkitt's lymphomas are not homogeneous at the molecular level. For this reason, Magrath[300] has suggested that Burkitt's lymphomas be subdivided into groups on the basis of the chromosome 8 and 14 breakpoints.

The heterogeneity of the t(8;14) breakpoints in Burkitt's lymphomas has practical implications for the detection of the translocation by Southern blot analysis. For example, c-*myc* probes do not detect c-*myc* rearrangements in approximately 75 percent of endemic Burkitt's lymphomas, whereas they usually do in sporadic Burkitt's lymphomas. The breakpoint site, beyond the analyzable restriction fragment sizes in endemic but not sporadic Burkitt's lymphoma, explains these results. Similarly, the standard JH probes will not detect IgH gene rearrangements in cases in which the chromosome 14 breakpoint is in Sμ or further 3′ sites.

In addition to the t(8;14), other molecular abnormalities have been reported in Burkitt's lymphomas that may be involved in deregulating c-*myc*. For example, mutations commonly occur within the first exon of the c-*myc* gene.[300] These mutations occur in close proximity to a *Pvu*II restriction enzyme site and are found in most tumors in which the chromosome 8 breakpoint is far 5′ to the c-*myc* gene. Mutations also have been reported in the second exon of the c-*myc* gene in sporadic Burkitt's lymphomas.[302] Although the role of these mutations is unknown, they are clustered in regions of the exon associated with transcriptional activation and thus may alter c-myc protein activity.[302]

The t(2;8) and t(8;22) in Burkitt's lymphoma are also referred to as the *variant translocations*. The variant translocations have been reported in endemic, sporadic, and AIDS-associated Burkitt's lymphomas with approximately equal frequency. Usually, Burkitt's lymphomas with the t(2;8) express Igκ light chain, whereas those tumors with the t(8;22) express Igλ light chain.[303] However, exceptions to this general rule have been described.[300] Analysis of the variant translocations has revealed further heterogeneity in the site of chromosome 8 breakpoints. In Burkitt's lymphomas with either the t(2;8) or the t(8;22), the breakpoint on chromosome 8 usually occurs relatively far downstream (3′) to the c-*myc* locus, in some cases at the site of a transcription unit known as *PVT*.[300,304] As a result, Southern blot studies with a c-*myc* probe will not detect rearrangement in tumors with the variant translocations.

In one study of six endemic Burkitt's lymphomas, the reverse transcriptase PCR method and DNA sequencing were used to analyze the V_H regions involved in IgH gene rearrangement.[305] In all six cases, somatic point mutations were identified within the V_H genes. These results suggest that Burkitt's lymphomas arise in B cells that traversed the germinal center and were exposed to antigen selection.[305]

Other B-cell oncogenes, such as *bcl*-1, *bcl*-2, *bcl*-3, and *bcl*-6, are rarely rearranged in Burkitt's lymphomas.[247,293] The *p53* gene mutations have been reported in approximately 20 to 30 percent of Burkitt's lymphomas, in both the endemic and sporadic types.[153,306] In one study of 16 AIDS-associated small noncleaved cell lymphomas with c-*myc* gene rearrangements (the histologic distinction between Burkitt's and non-Burkitt's was not specified), *p53* gene mutations were found in 10 (62.5 percent) cases.[295] In the same study *ras* gene mutations were identified in 3 (18.8 percent) cases, and the *Rb* gene was not mutated.

Non-Burkitt's Type (Burkitt-Like). Small, noncleaved cell lymphomas of the non-Burkitt's type (SNCNB) are also mature B-cell neoplasms. Thus, these tumors carry Ig heavy and light chain gene rearrangements.[136,293] The TCR genes are usually in the germline configuration.

Unlike Burkitt's lymphomas, a study of 11 SNCNB lymphomas did not identify c-*myc* gene rearrangements nor were mutations in the first exon of c-*myc* found. Interestingly, three cases had *bcl*-2 gene rearrangements and each tumor presented as peripheral lymphadenopathy.[293] In contrast, most other patients presented with extensive extranodal disease. These findings suggest that tumors designated as SNCNB lymphoma are a heterogeneous group, and molecular findings may correlate with different clinical features.[293] Furthermore, cases with *bcl*-2 gene rearrangements could be closely related to diffuse large cell lymphomas with *bcl*-2 gene rearrangements.

The *bcl*-1 and *bcl*-3 genes have been rarely studied and have not been rearranged in SNCNB lymphomas. The *bcl*-6 gene has not been studied. In one study, EBV was detected in 1 of 11 cases (9 percent).[293]

Plasma Cell Myeloma

Plasma cell neoplasms may involve the bone marrow as plasma cell myeloma, become leukemic usually in the late stages of disease, or involve lymph nodes or extranodal sites as an extramedullary plasamacytoma. Furthermore, monoclonal gammopathy of undetermined significance is clinically benign, but a part of the spectrum of plasma cell tumors. Most molecular data available regarding plasma cell neoplasms have been derived from the analysis of plasma cell myeloma.

As expected in neoplasms derived from terminally differentiated B cells, the Ig heavy and light chain genes are usually rearranged, and TCR gene rearrangements are uncommon.[136,307–309] Since plasma cell IgH genes commonly undergo IgH class switching, *Bam*HI and *Eco*RI enzyme digests may miss Ig gene rearrangements, since the normal location of the 3′ restriction enzyme sites for these enzymes may be altered by IgH switching.[308] In patients with newly diagnosed and low stage tumors, Ig gene rearrangements also may not be detected.[307] One possible explanation for the absence of Ig gene rearrangements may be that only a subpopulation of the plasma cells observed in bone marrow aspirates of these cases are actually monoclonal, this number being below the sensitivity of Southern blot analysis.[307] In some cases of monoclonal gammopathy of undetermined significance, Ig gene rearrangements also may not be detected by Southern blot analysis because of insufficient sensitivity. Use of PCR with its increased sensitivity would address this possibility in these cases.

In large studies of plasma cell myelomas, cytogenetic studies have identified abnormalities in 40 to 50 percent of all cases.[310–312] In one recent study, numerical chromosome abnormalities were most frequent.[310] The chromosomes most often gained were 3, 5, 7, 9, 11, 15, and 19. Chromosome 13 was most frequently lost (15 percent), followed by 8, 14, and X. Structural abnormalities of chromosomes 1 and 14 (15 and 10 percent, respectively), were also common. The t(11;14)(q13;q32) translocation has been found in a subset of plasma cell myelomas, less than 5 percent in most studies, but reported to be as high as 20 percent in one abstract.[311–313] The t(14;18) and other translocations associated with other B-cell lymphomas are rare or absent.[310,312]

The c-*myc* gene has been rearranged in a small subset of plasma cell tumors (less than 5 percent).[315,316] Also, increased c-*myc* expression has been observed in plasma cell myelomas without gene rearrangements, which has been correlated with an aggressive clinical course.[317] One abstract reported that c-*myc* transcripts in plasma cell myeloma were longer than those found in normal bone marrow and peripheral blood samples.[318] Palumbo and colleagues[319] have reported that the human homolog of the Moloney leukemia virus integration-4 locus is rearranged in 20 percent of plasma cell myelomas. Since this locus is 20 kb 3′ to the c-*myc* locus, perhaps these rearrangements result in increased c-*myc* expression.

Various oncogenes have been reported to be rearranged or mutated in plasma cell tumors. For example, *bcl*-1 gene rearrangements have been identified in 5 to 16 percent of cases by some groups.[311,314] However, Fiedler and colleagues[313] did not find *bcl*-1 gene rearrangements using a major translocation cluster probe in 17 tumors, including two tumors with the t(11;

14). In one study, Corradini and colleagues[320] identified N-*ras* and K-*ras* oncogene mutations in 9 percent of plasma cell myelomas and 30.7 percent of plasma cell leukemias, but not in solitary plasmacytomas or monoclonal gammopathy of undetermined significance N-*ras* mutations were most common, involved codons 61, 12, and 13 with decreasing frequency, and appeared to correlate with advanced stage disease. The authors suggested that *ras* gene mutations were a late event in the plasma cell tumorigenesis.[320] The *bcl*-2, *bcl*-3, and *bcl*-6 oncogenes are not reported to be involved in plasma cell tumors.

The *p53* tumor suppressor gene is mutated in a subset of plasma cell tumors. For example, Neri and colleagues[321] identified *p53* gene mutations in 7 of 52 (13 percent) tumors, including 7 of 16 (43 percent) clinically aggressive neoplasms. They suggested that *p53* gene mutations may also be a late event involved in tumor progression.[321] The *Rb* gene has been reported to be deleted in 12 of 23 (52 percent) cases of plasma cell myeloma, shown using FISH methods.[322]

EBV genomes have been detected in occasional cases of plasmacytoma that occurred in the setting of immunodeficiency.[323] However, most plasma cell myelomas are EBV negative (unpublished observations).

Mature T-Cell Lymphomas and Leukemias

T-Cell Chronic Lymphocytic Leukemia/T-Cell Prolymphocytic Leukemia

Some investigators consider T-cell chronic lymphocytic leukemia (CLL) and T-cell prolymphocytic leukemia (PLL) to be separate diseases. However, these tumors share common immunophenotypic and molecular findings, leading others to group these neoplasms together. These neoplasms characteristically involve the peripheral blood, but the spleen is usually involved and lymph nodes, liver, and skin may also be involved. PLLs occur with increased frequency in patients with ataxia-telangiectasia.[324] CLL/PLLs are neoplasms of mature T-cell lineage.[325] Molecular studies have shown rearrangements of the TCRβ and TCRγ genes. The TCRδ gene is usually deleted. The Ig heavy and light chain genes are usually in the germline configuration.[326]

A characteristic chromosomal abnormality, inv(14)(q11;q32), occurs in approximately two thirds of T-cell CLL/PLLs.[327] A subset of cases also has been described with chromosomal translocations, such as the t(14;14)(q11;q32) and the t(7;14)(q35;q32).[328] These translocations juxtapose the *tcl*-1 gene at 14q32 with either the TCRγ/δ or TCRβ genes. The *tcl*-1 gene is then thought to come under the influence of the TCRα regulatory elements, deregulating the *tcl*-1 gene. A qualitatively normal increase of tcl-1 protein provides the cell with a growth advantage.[329]

A t(X;14)(q28;q11) has been identified in cases of T-cell PLL.[330,331] Trisomy 8 also has been reported.[325]

Large Granular Lymphocytic Leukemia

These tumors have been designated previously as T-cell CLL (Kiel and French-American-British classification), Tγ lymphoproliferative disease, and T8 lymphocytosis with neutropenia.[332] Immunophenotypic studies have shown T-cell and natural killer cell subtypes.[332,333] Although most cases involve the peripheral blood, bone marrow and lymph nodes may be involved.

Molecular studies have shown that T-cell large granular lymphocyte leukemias have rearrangements of the TCRγ, TCRα, and TCRβ chain genes.[334,335] The TCRδ genes are usually deleted. Natural killer cell large granular lymphocyte leukemias do not have TCR gene rearrangements. In both subtypes, the Ig genes are usually in the germline configuration.[334,335] No characteristic chromosomal abnormalities have been described, and known oncogenes do not appear to be involved.

Peripheral T-Cell Lymphomas, Unspecified

The term *peripheral T-cell lymphoma* was coined by Waldron and colleagues[336] to describe lymphoid neoplasms of mature T-cell lineage as opposed to tumors of thymic or "central" origin. The terms *post-thymic* and *mature* T-cell lymphoma have also been used to describe these tumors. In the Working Formulation, most tumors fit within the diffuse mixed small and large cell, diffuse large cell, and large cell immunoblastic categories.

Molecular studies have shown TCRβ and TCRγ gene rearrangements in most cases. The TCRα gene has been rearranged in the few cases analyzed.[2,136] The TCRδ gene is usually deleted, and the Ig genes are usually in the germline configuration.[337] Approximately 5 to 10 percent of peripheral T-cell lymphomas lack TCR gene rearrangements.[338] Two specific types of peripheral T-cell lymphoma, angiocentric lymphoma and anaplastic large cell lymphoma, most commonly lack TCR gene rearrangements (discussed subsequently). Two likely explanations for the absence of TCR gene rearrangements in these tumors are neoplastic transformation of an early precursor T-cell prior to the stage of TCR gene rearrangement or clonal expansion of a cell that shares antigens with T cells but does not normally rearrange its TCR genes, such as a natural killer cell.

EBV has been identified in a subset of peripheral T-cell lymphomas, more commonly in Asian than in Western patients.[339] In Asian patients, the presence of EBV may correlate with a more aggressive clinical course.[339] Sandvej and colleagues[92] have reported that EBV-positive peripheral T-cell lymphomas have a high frequency of 30 bp deletions in the 3′ end of the *LMP1* gene, with a higher frequency in Malaysian than in Danish cases.[92] Perhaps the mutant form of the EBV LMP1 protein plays a role in the more aggressive course of EBV-positive T-cell lymphomas in Asia. Single base mutations in the 3′ end of the *LMP1* gene, occurring in specific codons or "hot spots," are also common.

One group has reported that the *p53* gene is mutated in approximately 10 percent of peripheral T-cell lymphomas.[340] However, the authors found that p53 protein expression is more common in these tumors and occurs independently of the presence of gene mutations. Since only exons 5 to 9 of the *p53* gene were analyzed, it is possible that the mutations occurred in different exons, resulting in *p53* staining. However, since exons 5 to 8 are evolutionarily conserved and are the sites where most mutations occur (the so-called hot spots), other explanations need to be considered. The *p16* and *p15* genes have been shown to be homozygously deleted in a small subset of peripheral T-cell lymphomas.[274]

Peripheral T-Cell Lymphomas, Specific Types

Adult T-Cell Leukemia/Lymphoma. Adult T-cell leukemia/lymphoma (ATLL) is a distinct clinicopathologic entity associated with infection by the human T-cell leukemia/lymphoma retrovirus type 1 (HTLV-I).[342] Immunophenotypic studies have shown that ATLLs are mature T-cell neoplasms, almost always with a T-helper cell immunophenotype.[342]

The hallmark of ATLL is the demonstration of HTLV-I, either serologically by detection of serum antibodies or using molecular methods to detect the virus in the neoplastic cells.[342] Using Southern blot hybridization, HTLV-I has been shown to be clonally integrated into the host cell genome.[343,344] Most studies have reported that the site of HTLV-I integration is random.[343] However, in a recent report of Japanese cases, Shimamoto and colleagues[344] showed that the site of viral integration was similar in the majority of cases. In 83 of 89 (93.3 percent) patients with ATLL, studied by Southern blot analysis using *Eco*RI-digested DNA, an identical 9 kb band was found, suggesting that the site of HTLV-I integration into the host cell genome is the same in these cases. Differently sized restriction fragments in six cases, suggestive of unusual sites of viral integration, correlated with a poorer prognosis.[344]

Antigen receptor gene rearrangement analyses have shown rearrangements of the TCRβ and TCRγ chain genes in most cases of ATLL.[345] The TCRα chain gene has been rearranged in a small number of cases studied.[346] The TCRδ chain genes are usually deleted and the Ig genes are most often in the germline configuration.[337,347]

Cytogenetic studies commonly show abnormalities in ATLL, including trisomy 12, 6q−, and translocations involving the chromosome 14q11 (TCR α/β locus) or 7p14–15 loci (TCRγ locus).[348]

Tumor suppressor genes are reported to be mutated or deleted in ATLL. For example, *p53* gene mutations have been detected in 30 to 40 percent of cases of ATLL.[349,350] The *p15* and *p16* tumor suppressor genes located also may be deleted in ATLL. These genes are reported to be deleted, either homozygously or heterozygously, in approximately 20 percent of ATLLs.[351] The *p15* and *p16* gene deletions are much more common in the acute and lymphomatous forms as opposed to the chronic variant of ATLL, suggesting that these deletions may be involved in transformation.[351] Point mutations of the *p15* and *p16* genes in ATLL are uncommon. The $p27^{KIP1}$ gene is rarely deleted in ATLL.[352] The N-*ras,* K-*ras,* and H-*ras* genes were examined in a series of 10 ATLLs and did not exhibit mutations.[349] Also in that study c-*myc* gene rearrangements and mutations were not detected.[349]

EBV has been identified in a subset of ATLL cases in Japan. Tokunaga and colleagues[353] studied 96 cases of ATLL: ISH for EBV EBER1 was positive within the neoplastic cells of 16 (16.7 percent) cases, 15 of which also expressed EBV latent membrane protein as detected immunohistochemically.

Angiocentric Lymphoma. Previously, the term *angiocentric immunoproliferative lesion* was proposed as a generic, unifying name to emphasize both the angiocentric and immunoproliferative aspects of these lesions regardless of anatomic site.[354] Included under the umbrella of angiocentric immunoproliferative lesion were lesions of the upper respiratory tract, also known in the literature as lethal midline granuloma, polymorphic reticulosis, midline malignant reticulosis, and sinonasal lymphomas, as well as lesions of the lung known as lymphomatoid granulomatosis.[354] However, recent evidence suggests that a subset of cases of pulmonary lymphomatoid granulomatosis may be of B-cell lineage.[355,356] Thus, despite their histologic similarity, a subset of lymphomatoid granulomatosis lesions of the lung are probably not equivalent to angiocentric lymphomas of the upper respiratory tract.

Sinonasal Angiocentric Lymphoma. Immunohistochemical studies have shown that the neoplastic cells commonly express T-cell markers, including CD2, CD7, and CD3, in a subset of cases.[357–359] The tumors are also commonly positive for CD56, a natural killer cell-associated antigen.[359] Although cell surface CD3 expression is specific for T-cell lineage, cytoplasmic CD3 may be found in natural killer cells, particularly the CD3ϵ subunit in activated natural killer cells and the CD3ϵ, CD3γ, and CD3δ subunits in fetal natural killer cells.[359]

Molecular studies of sinonasal angiocentric lymphomas have demonstrated an absence of TCR and Ig gene rearrangements in the majority of cases studied.[357–360] Rare cases reported have had rearrangements of the TCRγ, TCRβ, or TCRδ genes.[357–359] The TCRδ gene is rarely deleted.[337] An occasional sinonasal angiocentric lymphoma reported has been of B-cell lineage with Ig gene rearrangements.[360]

The presence of germline TCR genes and CD56 antigen positivity in sinonasal angiocentric lymphomas, combined with the recent knowledge that cytoplasmic CD3 may be present in natural killer cells, has led to the attractive hypothesis that the majority of sinonasal lymphomas arise from natural killer cells. Since occasional tumors rearrange the TCR genes and are probably of true T-cell lineage, Lanier and colleagues[361,362] have suggested that sinonasal angiocentric lymphomas arise from a T-cell/natural killer cell progenitor cells population.

EBV genomes have been identified in sinonasal angiocentric lymphomas using Southern blot, PCR, and ISH techniques (Figs. 1-9, 1-10, 1-12).[357,359–367] Southern blot studies have shown that the virus is monoclonal (Fig. 1-9), most commonly in high grade lesions, suggesting that the virus is present in the neoplastic cells prior to clonal expansion and may be involved in pathogenesis.[357,360] ISH studies have demonstrated EBV within the neoplastic cells, also most commonly in high grade lesions (Fig. 1-12).[364–367]

Lymphomatoid Granulomatosis. Lymphomatoid granulomatosis shares histologic features with sinonasal lymphoma. These lesions are angiocentric with angioinvasion and necrosis and encompass a spectrum of histologic findings in which early lesions have relatively few cytologically malignant cells, which then accrue over time until the malignant cells represent the majority of the cells in the specimen.

Southern blot hybridization studies analyzing the antigen receptor genes have shown that the TCR and Ig genes are usually in the germline configuration.[357,368,39] Rare cases are reported with TCRβ gene rearrangements.[370] However, using PCR, Guinee and colleagues[355] reported IgH gene rearrangements in six of nine cases; the TCRγ gene was not rearranged in three cases analyzed. Myers and colleagues[356] have reported similar results. In one case conventional cytogenetics identified an abnormal clone, characterized by a t(1;6)(p35;q23), t(1;19)(q23;p24; q13) abnormality.[369]

EBV is commonly present in lymphomatoid granulomatosis. Peiper and Katzenstein[371] were the first investigators to demonstrate EBV, in 21 of 29 (72.4 percent) cases, using PCR. ISH methods have localized EBV to the neoplastic cells, most easily appreciated in high grade lesions, and Southern blot studies in high grade lesions have shown that the virus is monoclonal, suggesting that EBV is present in the neoplastic cells prior to monoclonal expansion (Fig. 1-9).[357]

Recently, two groups used ISH for EBV EBER combined with immunohistochemical techniques to show that the EBV-positive cells in some cases of lymphomatoid granulomatosis are B cells.[355,356] This finding, combined with the PCR results of their studies that showed Ig heavy chain rearrangements, suggests that at least some cases of lymphomatoid granulomatosis may be EBV-positive B-cell neoplasms associated with numerous reactive T cells.[355,356]

Angioimmunoblastic T-Cell Lymphoma. Angioimmunoblastic T-Cell lymphoma, originally described as angioimmunoblastic lymphadenopathy with dysproteinemia (AILD) in 1974, was initially viewed as a preneoplastic disorder associated with immunologic dysfunction.[372] However, shortly after the recognition of this disease, patients with AILD were shown to be at increased risk of developing malignant lymphoma.

Molecular methods have been extensively applied to the analysis of both AILD and lymphomas arising in AILD. These studies have demonstrated that the majority of cases of AILD as well as lymphomas arising in AILD are monoclonal. Thus, AILD is now referred to as *angioimmunoblastic T-cell lymphoma* in the Revised European-American Classification of Lymphoid Neoplasms.[98]

The majority of cases of angioimmunoblastic T-cell lymphoma have rearrangements of the TCRγ and TCRβ chain genes.[16,373–375] The TCRδ gene is commonly deleted.[337] The Ig heavy chain gene is rearranged in 10 to 20 percent of cases. Ig light chain gene rearrangements are less common. Nonrandom chromosomal abnormalities, most often involving chromosomes 3, 5, or X, have been identified commonly.[376–378] For example, Schlegelberger and colleagues[378] used conventional cytogenetics and FISH methods to demonstrate aberrant clones in 32 of 36 (89 percent) patients with angioimmunoblastic T-cell lymphoma and, in many cases, more than one clone indicating the presence of an oligoclonal population of cells. At the time of progression to high grade lymphoma, additional clonal populations of T cells or B cells are often recognized, and the high grade lymphomas may be of T-cell or B-cell lineage.[16]

EBV is commonly associated with angioimmunoblastic T-cell lymphomas, as shown by a variety of molecular methods.[379–381] ISH studies have shown that EBV is particularly abundant in B-cell lymphomas arising in the patients with angioimmunoblastic T-cell lymphoma.[381] The EBV is also monoclonal, indicating that the virus is present before clonal expansion and suggesting that EBV may play a role in the pathogenesis of the B-cell lymphoma.[381,382] One hypothesis to explain this finding is that immunosuppression associated with angioimmunoblastic T-cell lymphoma predisposes to EBV infection of B cells. These cells, as a result of viral infection, have a prolonged lifespan, increasing the likelihood of secondary molecular aberrations that result in high grade B-cell lymphoma.[381]

Nevertheless, a subset of cases of angioimmunoblastic T-cell lymphoma do not have molecular evidence of monoclonality or evidence of an oligoclonal population, leading others to maintain that lesions without molecular abnormalities are preneoplastic and are better designated as AILD. For example, Frizzera and colleagues[383] suggested that these lesions be classified into three groups: AILD, AILD-like T-cell lymphoma, and AILD-like dyscrasias. In AILD, the lesions lack histologic, immunophenotypic, or molecular evidence of clonality and may represent a primary hyperreactive immunologic disorder. In AILD-like T-cell lymphoma, the lesions exhibit histologic evidence of malignant lymphoma and both immunophenotypic and molecular evidence of monoclonality. In AILD-like dysplasias, histologic evidence of malignant lymphoma is absent or equivocal, but clonal populations of either T or B cells are present that may undergo spontaneous remission.

Intestinal T-Cell Lymphoma. These tumors, of mature T-cell lineage, may be associated with gluten-sensitive enteropathy and thus also have been reported in the literature as enteropathy-associated T-cell lymphoma.[384–386] However, many cases occur without clinical or histologic evidence of enteropathy.[386] These tumors may arise in the stomach as well as the small and large intestines. However, the majority of neoplasms arise in the small intestine/jejunum, and tumors at this site are most often associated with gluten-sensitive enteropathy.[386]

The TCRβ and TCRγ genes are usually rearranged. Studies of the TCRδ gene have not been reported. The Ig heavy and light chain genes are most often in the germline configuration.[384,385,387] One case of adult-onset celiac disease without histologic evidence of malignant lymphoma was found to have TCRβ and TCRγ gene rearrangements.[388] This finding raises the possibility that some cases of celiac disease may, in fact, be low grade, enteropathy-associated T-cell lymphoma. In addition, in a subset of patients with intestinal T-cell lymphoma, both normal mucosa and mucosa histologically involved by lymphoma were found to have identical TCR gene rearrangements.[387] These findings suggest that in some cases monoclonal populations of mucosal T cells arise secondary to chronic antigenic stimulation. Most likely, other molecular abnormalities are involved in the development of malignant lymphoma.

EBV is present within the neoplastic cells of a small subset of cases of intestinal T-cell lymphoma (less than 10 percent in three studies).[386,389,390] The presence of EBV did not correlate with the coexistence of gluten-sensitive enteropathy. PCR studies for EBV in intestinal T-cell lymphomas may demonstrate a much higher rate of positivity for EBV (over 50 percent of cases in one study).[386] Reactive small lymphocytes associated with these tumors are commonly EBV positive, probably explaining the discrepancy between the ISH and PCR results.

Anaplastic Large Cell Lymphoma. These tumors, also referred to as *Ki-1 lymphomas* because they usually express the CD30 (Ki-1) antigen, represent the majority of cases that were once considered to be malignant histiocytosis.[391,392] The majority of cases are of T-cell immunophenotype, but a minority of cases lack lineage-specific antigens (null cell). A small subset of histologically similar CD30+ tumors are of B-cell lineage (discussed previously).[282,393]

A significant number of anaplastic large cell lymphomas (ALCLs) lack antigen receptor gene rearrangements (20 to 33 percent).[281] This finding has led others to suggest that these tumors arise from lymphoid cells at an early stage of differentiation, prior to the time at which gene rearrangements occur.[281] In the remaining cases gene rearrangements are detected that generally correlate with immunophenotype. However, lineage infidelity is more common in ALCLs than in most other lymphomas of mature T-cell or B-cell lineage.[281]

T-cell ALCLs typically have rearrangements of the TCRβ and TCRγ genes.[281,337,393,394] The TCRδ gene may be rearranged or deleted.[337,395] The Ig heavy chain gene is commonly in the germline configuration, but also may be rearranged.[281,337,394] The Ig light chain genes are rarely rearranged. Null cell ALCLs have neither immunophenotypic nor gene rearrangement evidence of lineage.[281]

The chromosomal translocation t(2;5)(p23; q35) has been identified in a subset of of ALCLs (ranging from 13 to 50 percent of cases).[394,396–402] In this translocation, the nucleophosmin gene *NPM* at 5q35 is juxtaposed with an anaplastic lymphoma kinase gene, *ALK* at 2p23.[402] The *NPM* gene encodes a nucleolar phosphoprotein that shuttles ribosomal components between the nucleolus and cytoplasm in the later stages of ribosomal assembly. The *ALK* gene is homologous to other tyrosine kinase receptor genes and either is not transcribed or is transcribed at low levels in normal lymphoid cells. Morris and colleagues[402] have hypothesized that the *NPM* gene contributes an active promoter to drive the expression of the *ALK* gene in lymphoma cells containing the t(2;5).[402] As a result of the translocation a fusion gene is created, encoding a chimeric mRNA transcript and a correspondingly novel protein. ISH and immunohistochemical analysis for *ALK* gene products have shown these products in a subset of ALCLs, most commonly T-cell or null cell tumors occurring in younger patients.[403–405]

Importantly, the t(2;5)(p23;q35) is not specific for ALCL. Using reverse transcriptase PCR methods, this translocation has been found in B-cell and T-cell lymphomas that are CD30 antigen negative and do not have histologic features of ALCL.[406]

In one study, the H-, K-, and N-*ras* oncogenes were not mutated in T-cell and null cell ALCLs.[283] The *Rb* and *p53* tumor suppressor genes also have been analyzed. The *Rb* gene is not rearranged. The *p53* gene is uncommonly mutated, although immunohistochemical studies have shown that ALCLs are commonly positive for p53 protein.[283,407] For example, Cesarman and colleagues[407] studied a group of 17 ALCLs, over 80 percent immunohistochemically positive for p53 protein. Only one neoplasm (5.9 percent) had a missense point mutation within the *p53* gene, shown by PCR-SSCP and confirmed by sequencing. Cesarman and colleagues[407] correlated *p53* staining with Ki-67 staining and suggested that the *p53* immunohistochemical positivity may be related to high cell proliferation.

EBV has been identified within biopsy specimens of ALCL. With PCR, EBV has been commonly identified in ALCLs, although the cell population containing the virus in these studies is uncertain.[408] ISH studies have localized EBV within the neoplastic cells in a much smaller percentage of cases, approximately 10 to 15 percent of ALCLs, in two studies.[283,409]

In an area endemic for HTLV-I in Japan, HTLV-I proviral DNA was shown to be clonally integrated into the host cell genome in 17 of 43 T-cell ALCLs (39.5 percent).[410] Patients with HTLV-I-positive ALCL had a shorter median survival than did patients with HTLV-I-negative ALCLs.[410] HTLV-I viral sequences were not identified in one series of ALCLs in patients from the United States.[283]

Cutaneous Anaplastic Large Cell Lymphoma. These neoplasms are closely related to lymphomatoid papulosis and, most likely, lymphomatoid papulosis and cutaneous (C) ALCL represent two opposite extremes of a continuous spectrum.[98] This hypothesis is supported by the clinical indolence of C-ALCL, the histologic similarity between lymphomatoid papulosis and C-ALCL, and patients who present with lymphomatoid papulosis and subsequently develop C-ALCL, or vice versa.[98,411]

Molecular analysis of the antigen receptor genes has shown TCRβ and TCRγ gene rearrangements in C-ALCL.[98] The Ig genes are usually in the germline configuration. Unlike systemic ALCL, the t(2;5)(p23;q35) has been rarely identified in C-ALCLs.[397]

Conventional cytogenetic studies of C-ALCL have been reported infrequently. Kadin and colleagues[411] reported 9q34 and 1p36 breakpoints and an isochromosome 17q in C-ALCLs that arose in patients who also had lymphomatoid papulosis preceding C-ALCL. A 9p abnormality has been reported in a single case.

Anagnostopoulos and colleagues,[412] using Southern blotting and PCR methods, found HTLV-I proviral sequences in six C-ALCLs. EBV is rarely found within the tumor cells of C-ALCLs.[409]

Hepatosplenic γ/δ T-Cell Lymphoma. These neoplasms represent a relatively recently recognized type of mature T-cell lymphoma that preferentially involves the hepatic sinusoids, splenic red pulp, and bone marrow. Characteristically, the neoplastic cells express the TCR γ/δ receptor.[413,414]

Molecular studies to date are limited, performed on approximately 15 cases.[414–419] The TCRδ gene is usually functionally rearranged. The TCRγ gene has been rearranged in a smaller number of cases studied, and the TCRβ gene also may be rearranged nonproductively. The IgH gene has been in the germline configuration. Isochromosome 7q and trisomy 8 were identified in three cases in one report.[418] One case occurred in the clinical setting of a renal transplant.[419] In this case, both TCRβ and TCRγ gene rearrangements were found, and a t(7;9)(p15; q13) translocation was identified.[419]

T-Cell Lymphoma Involving Subcutaneous Tissue. This is another relatively recently recognized type of mature T-cell lymphoma that preferentially involves the subcutaneous tissue and commonly is associated with a hemophagocytic syndrome.[420]

Southern blot analysis demonstrated TCRβ or TCRγ gene rearrangements in a small number of cases analyzed.[420–422] The Ig genes have been in the germline configuration. The TCRδ gene was rearranged in one case that also expressed the TCRγ/δ receptor.[423] Using paraffin tissue blocks and PCR, TCRγ gene rearrangements have been identified in a subset of cases.[421] ISH for EBV EBER1 is negative in the majority of cases.[421] Occasional cases are reported in which serologic or PCR evidence of EBV has been found.[424,425]

Lennert's Lymphoma. The majority of neoplasms reported as Lennert's lymphoma are T-cell neoplasms, but rarely B-cell lymphomas may be histologically similar. The characteristic histologic finding is the presence of numerous epithelioid histiocytes, often obscuring the neoplastic cell population.

Molecular studies of Lennert's lymphomas of T-cell lineage have shown rearrangements of the TCRβ gene.[286,337,426] The TCRγ gene is also commonly rearranged. Since many reactive T cells are also intermixed within these tumors, a polyclonal pattern of TCRγ rearrangements may be detected using either Southern blotting or PCR. If enough polyclonal T cells are present in large numbers, as is commonly the case, a monoclonal TCRγ rearrangement may be obscured.[43] The TCRδ genes are usually deleted in the tumor cells, although this may be difficult to appreciate because of the large number of non-T cells present without deleted TCRδ genes.[337] The Ig genes are usually in the germline configuration.

Mycosis Fungoides/Sezary Syndrome. Mycosis fungoides/Sezary syndrome (MF/SS) is a distinctive type of mature T-cell lymphoma/ leukemia, almost always of T-helper cell immunophenotype.[98]

With Southern blot hybridization, the ability to detect monoclonal TCR gene rearrangements is dependent on the stage of the disease. Almost all cases of the tumor form and high clinical stage MF, as well as SS, have TCRβ and TCRγ

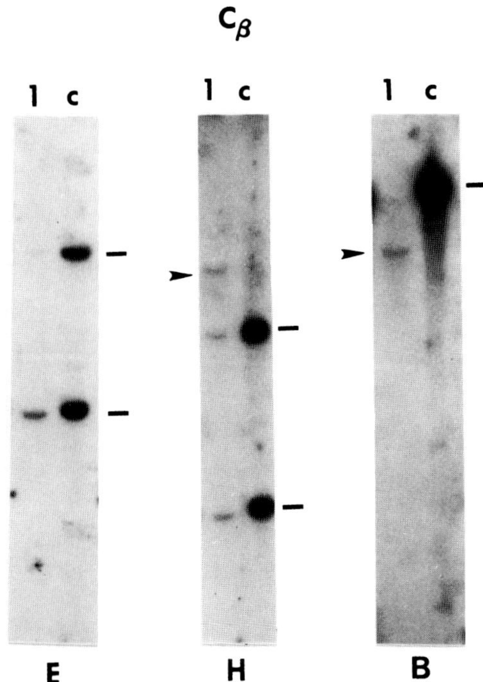

Fig. 1-18. Mycosis fungoides (lane 1) and control (c) placental DNA. TCRβ gene rearrangements are detected with all restriction enzymes used. Southern blot hybridization analysis was performed with *Eco*RI (E), *Hin*dIII (H), and *Bam*HI (B) digested genomic DNA and a ^{32}P-labeled probe specific for the constant region of the TCRβ gene. (*Dashes,* germline fragments; *arrows,* rearranged fragments.)

gene rearrangements (Fig. 1-18).[427–429] The TCRδ chain genes are usually deleted.[427,429] The Ig genes are usually in the germline configuration. By contrast, TCR gene rearrangements may not be detected in biopsies of early (patch or plaque) stage MF/SS.[427,428] Thus, cases of early stage MF/SS may represent polyclonal infiltrates within which a clonal T-cell population subsequently arises. Alternatively and more likely, MF/SS may be monoclonal at onset, but the monoclonal population is present in insufficient numbers to be detected by Southern blot analysis.

Multiple sites of MF/SS obtained from the same patient have identical TCR gene rearrangements.[429] Thus, these separate skin lesions arise from the same monoclonal process. Identical TCR gene rearrangements also have been found in skin lesions and regional lymph nodes.[429] Furthermore, TCR gene rearrangements have been found in lymph nodes unequivocally involved by MF/SS as well as in lymph nodes that histologically resemble dermatopathic lymphadenopathy, without histologically obvious tumor.[429] These results may explain why the presence of palpable lymphadenopathy, even when histologic examination of the lymph node biopsy reveals only dermatopathic lymphadenopathy, is a poor prognostic finding.[430]

Gene rearrangement analysis appears to be a better method than morphologic evaluation for assessing peripheral blood involvement, particularly when the number of circulating malignant cells is low. For example, in one study of 26 patients with MF/SS, TCR gene rearrangements were found in the peripheral blood specimens that were negative morphologically.[431]

Although patients with MF/SS are seronegative for HTLV-I antibodies by ELISA and Western blotting methods, PCR-based assays have demonstrated the virus in both peripheral blood mononuclear cells and skin biopsies in 10 to 30 percent of patients.[432–435] Reverse transcript PCR studies have shown the *tax, rex,* and *pol* but not the *gag* genes of HTLV-I.[410–412] The absence of seropositivity also suggests that the virus is defective: either viral DNA is deleted or viral replication is inadequate.[432] The HTLV-I is integrated into the host cell genome in MF/SS, and viral DNA may also be present in episomal form.[434]

Intravascular Lymphomatosis

Intravascular lymphomatosis, also known as *malignant angioendotheliomatosis* or *angiotropic large cell lymphoma,* is a rare lymphoproliferative disorder in which large neoplastic cells are found predominantly within small blood vessels in a variety of organs.[436] Immunophenotypic studies have shown that the neoplasms are most often of B-cell lineage, although a small subset of cases have been of T-cell lineage.[436]

Molecular studies have been performed on very few cases. In accord with the immunophenotypic findings, the Ig heavy chain gene is rearranged and the TCRβ and TCRγ genes are in the germline configuration in most cases.[437–439] However, in one T-cell case the TCRβ gene was rearranged.[440] The PCR technique was used in one B-cell tumor that demonstrated an IgH gene rearrangement; the *bcl*-2 gene was not involved.[439]

One case studied by conventional cytogenetics revealed a complex, hyperdiploid karyotype with a t(1;3)(p22;p21) translocation.[441]

REFERENCES

1. Cossman J, Uppenkamp M, Sundeen J et al: Molecular genetics and the diagnosis of lymphoma. Arch Pathol Lab Med 112:117, 1988
2. Knowles DM: Immunophenotypic and antigen receptor gene rearrangement analysis in T cell neoplasia. Am J Pathol 134:761, 1989
3. Kirsch IR, Kuehl WM: Gene rearrangements in lymphoid cells. P. 381. In Stamatoyannopoulos G, Nienhuis AW, Majerus PW, Varmus H (eds): The Molecular Basis of Blood Diseases. 2nd Ed. WB Saunders, Philadelphia, 1994
4. Pascual V, Capra JD: Human immunoglobulin heavy-chain variable region genes: organization, polymorphism, and expression. Adv Immunol 49:1, 1990
5. Forster A, Huck S, Ghanem N et al: New subgroups in the human T cell rearranging Vγ gene locus. EMBO J 6:1945, 1987
6. Cossman J, Zehnbauer BM, Garrett CT et al: Gene rearrangements in the diagnosis of lymphoma/leukemia: guidelines for use based on a multi-institutional study. Am J Clin Pathol 95: 347, 1991
7. Pauza ME, Rehmann JA, LeBien TW: Unusual patterns of immunoglobulin gene rearrangement and expression during human B-cell ontogeny: human B-cells can simultaneously express surface κ and λ light chains. J Exp Med 178:139, 1993
8. Tonegawa S: Somatic generation of antibody diversity. Nature 302:575, 1983
9. Oettinger MA, Schatz DG, Gorka C, Baltimore D. RAG-1 and RAG-2, adjacent genes that synergistically activate V(D)J recombination. Science 248:1517, 1990
10. deVillartay J-P, Hockett R, Coran D et al: Deletion of the human T-cell receptor δ-gene by a site-specific recombination. Nature 335:170, 1988
11. Korsmeyer SJ, Hieter PA, Ravetch JV et al: Developmental hierarchy of immunoglobulin gene rearrangements in human leukemic pre-B-cells. Proc Natl Acad Sci USA 78:7096, 1981
12. deVillartay J-P, Pullman AB, Andrade RE et al: γ/δ lineage relationship within a consecutive series of human precursor T-cell neoplasms. Blood 74:2508, 1989
13. Felix CA, Poplack DG, Reaman GH et al: Characterization of immunoglobulin and T-cell receptor gene patterns in B-cell precursor acute lymphoblastic leukemia of childhood. J Clin Oncol 8:431, 1990
14. Pelicci P, Knowles DM, Dalla Favera R: Lymphoid tumors displaying rearrangements of both immunoglobulin and T-cell receptor genes. J Exp Med 162:1015, 1985
15. Raffeld M, Wright JJ, Lipford E et al: Clonal evolution of t(14;18) follicular lymphomas demonstrated by immunoglobulin genes and the 18q21 major breakpoint region. Cancer Res 47: 2537, 1987
16. Lipford EH, Smith HR, Pittaluga S et al: Clonality of angioimmunoblastic lymphadenopathy and implications for its evolution to malignant lymphoma. J Clin Invest 79:637, 1987
17. Arnold A, Cossman J, Bakhshi A et al: Immunoglobulin gene rearrangements as unique clonal markers in human lymphoid neoplasms. N Engl J Med 309:1593, 1983
18. Hall PA, Donaghy M, Cotter FE et al: An immunohistological and genotypic study of the plasma cell form of Castleman's disease. Histopathology 14:333, 1989
19. Soulier J, Grollet L, Oksenhendler E et al: Molecular analysis of clonality in Castleman's disease. Blood 86:1131, 1995
20. Fishleder A, Tubbs R, Hesse B, Levine H: Uniform detection of immunoglobulin gene rearrangement in benign lymphoepithelial lesions. N Engl J Med 316:1118, 1987
21. Locker J, Nalesnik M: Molecular genetic analysis of lymphoid tumors arising after organ transplantation. Am J Pathol 135:977, 1989
22. Pelicci P-G, Knowles DM, Arlin ZA et al: Multiple monoclonal B cell expansions and c-*myc* oncogene rearrangements in acquired immune deficiency syndrome-related lymphoprolifera-

tive disorders: implications for lymphomagenesis. J Exp Med 164:2049, 1986
23. Kamel OW, Van de Rijn M, Weiss LM et al: Brief report: reversible lymphomas associated with Epstein-Barr virus occurring during methotrexate therapy for rheumatoid arthritis and dermatomyositis. N Engl J Med 328:1317, 1993
24. Elenitoba-Johnson K, Medeiros LJ, Khorsand J, King TC: Lymphoma of the mucosa-associated lymphoid tissue of the lung: a multifocal case of common clonal origin. Am J Clin Pathol 103: 341, 1995
25. Hsi ED, Greenson JK, Singleton TP et al: Detection of immunoglobulin heavy chain (IgH) gene rearrangement by polymerase chain reaction (PCR) in chronic active gastritis (CAG-Hp), abstracted. Lab Invest 72:113A, 1995
26. Limpens J, deJong D, Van Krieken JHJM et al: *Bcl*-2/J_H rearrangements in benign lymphoid tissues with follicular hyperplasia. Oncogene 6: 2271, 1991
27. Aster JC, Kobayashi Y, Shiota M et al: Detection of the t(14;18) at similar frequencies in hyperplastic lymphoid tissues from American and Japanese patients. Am J Pathol 141:291, 1992
28. Rabbitts TH: Chromosomal translocations in human cancer. Nature 372:143, 1994
29. Aplan PD, Lombardi DP, Ginsberg AM et al: Disruption of the human SCL locus by ''illegitimate'' V(D)J recombinase activity. Science 250:1426, 1990
30. Wyatt RT, Rudders RA, Zelenetz A et al: BCL2 oncogene translocation is mediated by a χ-like consensus. J Exp Med 175:1575, 1992
31. Boehm T, Mengle-Gaw L, Kees UR et al: Alternating purine-pyrimidine tracts may promote chromosomal translocations seen in a variety of human lymphoid tumors. EMBO J 8:2621, 1989
32. Lipkowitz S, Stern M-H, Kirsch IR: Hybrid T cell receptor genes formed by interlocus recombination in normal and ataxia-telangiectasia lymphocytes. J Exp Med 172:409, 1990
33. Gaidano G, Dalla-Favera R: Protooncogenes and tumor suppressor genes. p. 245. In Knowles DM (ed): Neoplastic Hematopathology. Williams & Wilkins, Baltimore, 1992
34. Weinberg RA: Oncogenes, anti-oncogenes, and the molecular basis of multistep carcinogenesis. Cancer Res 49:3713, 1989
35. Friend SH, Dryja TP, Weinberg RA: Oncogenes and tumor-suppressing genes. N Engl J Med 318:618, 1988
36. Marshall CJ: Tumor suppressor genes. Cell 64: 313, 1991
37. Haber DA, Housman DE: Rate limiting steps: the genetics of pediatric cancers. Cell 64:5, 1991
38. Levine AJ, Momand J, Finlay CA: The p53 tumour suppressor gene. Nature 351:453, 1991
39. Malkin D, Li FP, Strong LC et al: Germline p53 mutations in a familial syndrome of breast cancer, sarcomas and other neoplasms. Science 250:1233, 1990
40. Macgeoch C, Turner G, Bobrow LG et al: Heterogeneity in Li-Fraumeni families: *p53* mutation analysis and immunohistochemical staining. J Med Genet 32:186, 1995
41. Cleary ML, Chao J, Warnke R, Sklar J: Immunoglobulin gene rearrangement as a diagnostic criterion of B-cell lymphoma. Proc Natl Acad Sci USA 81:593, 1984
42. Pittaluga SM, Raffeld M, Lipford E, Cossman J: 3A1 (CD7) expression precedes Tβ gene rearrangements in precursor T (lymphoblastic) neoplasms. Blood 68:134, 1986
43. Uppenkamp M, Andrade R, Sundeen J et al: Diagnostic interpretation of T_γ gene rearrangement: effect of polyclonal T cells. Hematol Pathol 2:15, 1988
44. Eisenstein BI: The polymerase chain reaction: a new method of using molecular genetics for medical diagnosis. N Engl J Med 322:178, 1990
45. Templeton NS: The polymerase chain reaction: history, methods, and applications. Diagn Mol Pathol 1:58, 1992
46. Stetler-Stevenson M, Raffeld M, Cohen P, Cossman J: Detection of occult follicular lymphoma by specific DNA amplification. Blood 72:1822, 1988
47. Segal GH, Jorgensen T, Scott M, Braylan RC: Optimal primer selection for clonality assessment by polymerase chain reaction analysis: II. Follicular lymphomas. Hum Pathol 25:1276, 1994
48. Burgart LJ, Robinson RA, Heller MJ et al: Multiplex polymerase chain reaction. Mod Pathol 5: 320, 1992
49. Diss TC, Peng H, Wotherspoon AC et al: Detection of monoclonality in low-grade B-cell lymphomas using the polymerase chain reaction is dependent on primer selection and lymphoma type. J Pathol 169:291, 1993
50. Ling FC, Clarke CE, Corbett WEN, Lillicrap DP: Sensitivity of PCR in detecting monoclonal B cell proliferations. J Clin Pathol 46:624, 1993

51. Albrecht S, Bruner JM, SeGall GK: Immunoglobulin heavy chain rearrangements in primary brain lymphomas: a study using PCR to amplify CDR-III. J Pathol 169:297, 1993
52. Inghirami G, Szabolcs MJ, Yee HT et al: Detection of immunoglobulin gene rearrangement of B cell nonHodgkin's lymphomas and leukemias in fresh, unfixed and formalin-fixed, paraffin-embedded tissue by polymerase chain reaction. Lab Invest 68:746, 1993
53. Ilyas M, Jalal H, Linton C, Rooney N: The use of the polymerase chain reaction in the diagnosis of B-cell lymphomas from formalin-fixed paraffin-embedded tissue. Histopathology 26:333, 1995
54. Lehman CM, Sarago C, Nasim S et al: Comparison of PCR with Southern blot hybridization for the routine detection of immunoglobulin heavy chain gene rearrangements. Am J Clin Pathol 103:171, 1995
55. Sioutos N, Bagg A, Michaud GY et al: Polymerase chain reaction versus Southern blot hybridization: detection of immunoglobulin heavy-chain gene rearrangements. Diagn Mol Pathol 4:8, 1995
56. Achille A, Scarpa A, Montresor M et al: Routine application of polymerase chain reaction in the diagnosis of monoclonality of B-cell lymphoid proliferations. Diagn Mol Pathol 4:14, 1995
57. Slack DN, McCarthy KP, Wiedemann LM, Sloane JP: Evaluation of sensitivity, specificity and reproducibility of an optimized method for detecting clonal rearrangements of immunoglobulin and T cell receptor genes in formalin-fixed, paraffin-embedded sections. Diagn Mol Pathol 2:223, 1993
58. Kuppers R, Zhao M, Rajewsky K, Hansmann M-L: Detection of clonal B cell populations in paraffin-embedded tissues by polymerase chain reaction. Am J Pathol 143:230, 1993
59. Kuppers R, Willenbrock K, Rajewsky K, Hansmann M-L: Detection of clonal λ light chain gene rearrangements in frozen and paraffin-embedded tissues by polymerase chain reaction. Am J Pathol 147:806, 1995
60. Lorenzen J, Jux G, Zhao-Hohn M et al: Detection of T-cell clonality in paraffin-embedded tissues. Diagn Mol Pathol 3:93, 1994
61. Greiner TC, Raffeld M, Lutz C et al: Analysis of T cell receptor-γ gene rearrangements by denaturing gradient gel electrophoresis of GC-clamped polymerase chain reaction products: correlation with tumor-specific sequences. Am J Pathol 146:46, 1995
62. Segal GH, Jorgensen T, Masih AS, Braylan RC: Optimal primer selection for clonality assessment by polymerase chain reaction analysis: I. Low grade B-cell lymphoproliferative disorders of nonfollicular center cell type. Hum Pathol 25: 1269, 1994
63. Yamada M, Hudson S, Tournay O et al: Detection of minimal disease in hematopoietic malignancies of the B-cell lineage by using third-complementarity-determining region (CDR-III) probes. Proc Natl Acad Sci USA 86:5123, 1989
64. Tycko B, Palmer JD, Link MP et al: Polymerase chain reaction amplification of rearranged antigen receptor genes using junction-specific oligonucleotides: possible application for detection of minimal residual disease in acute lymphoblastic leukemia. Cancer Cells 7:49, 1989
65. Gribben JG, Freedman AS, Woo SD et al: All advanced stage non-Hodgkin's lymphomas with a polymerase chain reaction amplifiable breakpoint of *bcl*-2 have residual cells containing the *bcl*-2 rearrangement at evaluation and after treatment. J Clin Oncol 78:3275, 1991
66. Price CGA, Meerabux J, Murtagh S et al: The significance of circulating cells carrying t(14; 18) in long remission from follicular lymphoma. J Clin Oncol 9:1527, 1991
67. Campana D, Pui C-H: Detection of minimal residual disease in acute leukemia: methodologic advances and clinical significance. Blood 85: 1416, 1995
68. Ito Y, Wasserman R, Galili N et al: Molecular residual disease status at the end of chemotherapy fails to predict subsequent relapse in children with B-lineage acute lymphoblastic leukemia. J Clin Oncol 11:546, 1993
69. Kawasaki E, Clark S, Coyne M et al: Diagnosis of chronic myeloid and lymphocytic leukemias by detection of leukemia-specific mRNA sequences amplified in vivo. Proc Natl Acad Sci USA 85:5698, 1988
70. Ehlich A, Kuppers R: Analysis of immunoglobulin gene rearrangements in single B cells. Curr Opin Immunol 7:281, 1995
71. Sukpanichnant S, Vnencak-Jones CL, McCurley TL: Detection of clonal immunoglobulin heavy chain gene rearrangements by polymerase chain reaction in scrapings from archival hematoxylin and eosin-stained histologic sec-

tions: implications for molecular genetic studies of focal pathologic lesions. Diagn Mol Pathol 2:168, 1993
72. Greer CE, Peterson SL, Kiviat NB, Manos MM: PCR amplification from paraffin-embedded tissues: effects of fixative and fixation time. Am J Clin Pathol 95:117, 1991
73. Grody WW, Cheng L, Lewin KJ: Application of in situ DNA hybridization technology to diagnostic surgical pathology. Pathol Annu 22(Pt. 2):151, 1987
74. Anastasi J: Interphase cytogenetic analysis in the diagnosis and study of neoplastic disorders. Am J Clin Pathol (Suppl 1):S22, 1991
75. Weber-Matthiesen K, Winkemann M, Muller-Hermelink A et al: Rapid immunophenotypic characterization of chromosomally aberrant cells by the new FICTION method. Cytogenet Cell Genet 63:123, 1993
76. Weber-Matthiesen K, Pressl S, Schlegelberger B, Grote W: Combined immunophenotyping and interphase cytogenetics on cryostat sections by the new FICTION method. Leukemia 7:646, 1993
77. Houldsworth J, Chaganti RSK: Comparative genomic hybridization: an overview. Am J Pathol 145:1253, 1994
78. Isola J, DeVries S, Chu L et al: Analysis of changes in DNA sequence copy number by comparative genomic hybridization in archival paraffin-embedded tumor samples. Am J Pathol 145:1301, 1994
79. Nuovo G, MacConnell P, Forde A, Delvenne P: Detection of human papillomavirus DNA in formalin-fixed tissues by in situ hybridization after amplification by polymerase chain reaction. Am J Pathol 139:847, 1991
80. Komminoth P, Long AA, Ray R, Wolfe HJ: In situ polymerase chain reaction detection of viral DNA, single-copy genes, gene rearrangements in cell suspensions and cytospins. Diagn Mol Pathol 1:85, 1992
81. Spagnolo DV, Turbett GR, Dix B, Iacopetta B: Polymerase chain reaction and single-strand conformation polymorphism analysis (PCR-SSCP): a novel means of detecting DNA mutations. Adv Anat Pathol 1:61, 1994
82. Sanger F, Nicklen S, Coulson AR: DNA sequencing with chain-terminating inhibitors. Proc Natl Acad Sci USA 74:5463, 1977
83. Baer R, Bankier AT, Biggin MD et al: DNA sequence and expression of the B95-8 Epstein-Barr virus genome. Nature 310:207, 1984
84. Raab-Traub N, Flynn K: The structure of the termini of the Epstein-Barr virus as a marker of clonal cellular proliferation. Cell 47:883, 1986
85. Gulley ML, Raab-Traub N: Detection of Epstein-Barr virus in human tissues by molecular genetic techniques. Arch Pathol Lab Med 117: 1115, 1993
86. Sixbey JW, Shurley P, Chesney PJ et al: Detection of a second widespread strain of Epstein-Barr virus. Lancet 2:761, 1989
87. Raab-Traub N, Pagano JS: Epstein-Barr virus and its antigens. p. 477. In Litwin SD (ed): Human Immunogenetics: Basic Principles and Clinical Relevance. Marcel Dekker, New York, 1989
88. Weiss LM, Strickler JG, Warnke RA et al: Epstein-Barr viral DNA in tissues of Hodgkin's disease. Am J Pathol 129:86, 1987
89. Gulley ML, Raphael M, Lutz CT et al: Epstein-Barr virus integration in human lymphomas and lymphoid cell lines. Cancer 70:185, 1992
90. Jilg W, Sieger E, Alliger P, Wolf H: Identification of type A and B isolates of Epstein-Barr virus by polymerase chain reaction. J Virol Methods 30:319, 1990
91. Knecht H, Bachmann E, Joske DJL et al: Molecular analysis of the LMP (latent membrane protein) in Hodgkin's disease. Leukemia 7:580, 1993
92. Sandjev K, Peh S-C, Andresen BS, Pallesen G: Identification of potential hot spots in the carboxy-terminal part of the Epstein-Barr virus (EBV) BNLF-1 gene in both malignant and benign EBV-associated diseases: high frequency of a 30-bp deletion in Malaysian and Danish peripheral T-cell lymphomas. Blood 84:4053, 1994
93. Hu LF, Chen F, Zheng Z et al: Clonability and tumorigenicity of human epithelial cells expressing the EBV encoded membrane protein LMP1. Oncogene 8:1575, 1993
94. Glickman JN, Howe JG, Steitz JA: Structural analysis of EBER-1 and EBER-2 ribonucleoprotein particles present in Epstein-Barr virus-infected cells. J Virol 62:902, 1988
95. Gilligan K, Rajadurai P, Resnick L, Raab-Traub N: Epstein-Barr virus small nuclear RNAs are not expressed in permissively infected cells in AIDS-associated leukoplakia. Proc Natl Acad Sci USA 87:8790, 1990

96. Weiss LM, Movahed LA, Warnke RA, Sklar J: Detection of Epstein-Barr viral genomes in Reed-Sternberg cells of Hodgkin's disease. N Engl J Med 320:502, 1989
97. Weiss LM, Bindl JM, Picozzi VJ et al: Lymphoblastic lymphoma: an immunophenotype study of 26 cases with comparison to T cell acute lymphoblastic leukemia. Blood 67:474, 1986
98. Harris NL, Jaffe ES, Stein H et al: A revised European-American classification of lymphoid neoplasms: a proposal from the International Lymphoma Study Group. Blood 84:1361, 1994
99. Yano T, Pullman A, Andrade R et al: A common Vδ2-Dδ2-Dδ3 T-cell receptor gene rearrangement in precursor B acute lymphoblastic leukemia. Br J Haematol 79:44, 1991
100. Heim S, Mitelmann F: Cytogenetic analysis in the differential diagnosis of acute leukemia. Cancer 70:1701, 1992
101. Cline MJ: The molecular basis of leukemia. N Engl J Med 330:328, 1994
102. Preti H, O'Brien S, Giralt S et al: Philadelphia-chromosome-positive adult acute lymphocytic leukemia: characteristics, treatment results, and prognosis in 41 patients. Am J Med 97:60, 1994
103. Mellentin JD, Murre C, Donlon TA et al: The gene for enhancer binding proteins E12/E47 lies at the t(1;19) breakpoint in acute leukemias. Science 246:379, 1989
104. Nourse J, Mellentin JD, Galili N et al: Chromosomal translocation t(1;19) results in synthesis of a homeobox fusion mRNA that codes for a potential chimeric transcription factor. Cell 60: 535, 1990
105. Kawamura M, Kikuchi A, Kobayashi S et al: Mutations of the *p53* and *ras* genes in childhood t(1;19)-acute lymphoblastic leukemia. Blood 85:2546, 1995
106. Hunger SP, Galili N, Carroll AJ et al: The t(1; 19)(q23;p13) results in consistent fusion of E2a and PBX1 coding sequences in acute lymphoblastic leukemias. Blood 77:687, 1991
107. Bernard OA, Berger R: Molecular basis of 11q23 rearrangements in hematopoietic malignant proliferations. Genes Chromosom Cancer 13:75, 1995
108. Pui C-H, Behm FG, Downing JR et al: 11q23/ MLL rearrangement confers a poor prognosis in infants with acute lymphoblastic leukemia. J Clin Oncol 12:909, 1994
109. Raimondi SC, Frestedt JL, Pui C-H et al: Acute lymphoblastic leukemias with deletion of 11q23 or a novel inversion (11)(p13q23) lack *MLL* gene rearrangements and have favorable clinical features. Blood 86:1881, 1995
110. Raimondi SC, Williams DL, Callihan T et al: Nonrandom involvement of the 12p12 breakpoint in chromosome abnormalities of childhood acute lymphoblastic leukemia. Blood 68: 69, 1986
111. Sato Y, Suto Y, Pietenpol J et al: *TEL* and *KIP1* define the smallest region of deletions of 12p13 in hematopoietic malignancies. Blood 86:1525, 1995
112. Hogan T, Koss W, Murgo A et al: Acute lymphoblastic leukemia with chromosomal 5;14 translocation and hypereosinophilia: case report and literature review. J Clin Oncol 5:382, 1987
113. Meeker TC, Hardy D, Willman C et al: Activation of the interleukin-3 gene by chromosome translocation in acute lymphocytic leukemia with eosinophilia. Blood 76:285, 1990
114. Neri A, Knowles DM, Greco A et al: Analysis of RAS oncogene mutations in human lymphoid malignancies. Proc Natl Acad Sci USA 85:9268, 1988
115. Kitchingman GR, Rovigatti U, Mauer AM et al: Rearrangement of immunoglobulin heavy chain genes in T-cell acute lymphoblastic leukemia. Blood 65:725, 1985
116. Brown L, Cheng J-T, Chen Q et al: Site-specific recombination of the *tal*-1 gene is a common occurrence in human T cell leukemia. EMBO J 9:3343, 1990
117. Kikuchi A, Hayashi Y, Kobayashi S et al: Clinical significance of TAL1 gene alteration in childhood T-cell acute lymphoblastic leukemia and lymphoma. Leukemia 7:933, 1993
118. Chetty R, Pulford K, Jones M et al: SCL/Tal-1 expression in T-acute lymphoblastic leukemia: an immunohistochemical and genotypic study. Hum Pathol 26:994, 1995
119. Chilcote RR, Brown E, Rowley JD: Lymphoblastic leukemia with lymphomatous features associated with abnormalities of the short arm of chromosome 9. N Engl J Med 313:286, 1985
120. Murphy SB, Raimondi SC, Rivera GK et al: Nonrandom abnormalities of chromosome 9p in childhood acute lymphoblastic leukemia: association with high-risk clinical features. Blood 74:409, 1989
121. Okuda T, Shurtleff SA, Valentine MB et al: Frequent deletion of $p16^{INK4a}$/*MTS1* and $p15^{INK4b}$/

MTS2 in pediatric acute lymphoblastic leukemia. Blood 85:2321, 1995

122. Hebert J, Cayuela JM, Berkeley J, Sigaux F: Candidate tumor suppressor genes *MTS1* (*p16*^{INK4A}) and *MTS2* (*p15*^{INK4B}) display frequent homozygous deletions in primary cells from T- but not B-cell lineage acute lymphoblastic leukemias. Blood 84:4038, 1994
123. Fizzotti M, Cimino G, Pisegna S et al: Detection of homozygous deletions of the cyclin-dependent kinase 4 inhibitor (p16) in acute lymphoblastic leukemia and association with adverse prognostic features. Blood 85:2685, 1995
124. Ogawa S, Hirano N, Sato N et al: Homozygous loss of the cyclin-dependent kinase 4-inhibitor (p16) gene in human leukemias. Blood 84:2431, 1994
125. Hatano M, Roberts CWM, Minden M et al: Deregulation of a homeobox gene, *HOX11*, by the t(10;14) in T-cell leukemia. Science 253:79, 1991
126. Zhang N, Gong Z-Z, Minden M, Lu M: The HOX-11 (TCL-3) homeobox proto-oncogene encodes a nuclear protein that undergoes cell cycle-dependent regulation. Oncogene 8:3265, 1993
127. Abruzzo LV, Jaffe ES, Cotelingam JD et al: T-cell lymphoblastic lymphoma with eosinophilia associated with subsequent myeloid malignancy. Am J Surg Pathol 16:236, 1992
128. Inhorn RC, Aster JC, Roach SA et al: A syndrome of lymphoblastic lymphoma, eosinophilia, and myeloid hyperplasia/malignancy associated with t(8;13(p11;q11): description of a distinctive clinicopathologic entity. Blood 85: 1881, 1995
129. Naeem R, Singer S, Fletcher JA: Translocation t(8;13)(p11;q11–12) in stem cell leukemia/lymphoma of T-cell and myeloid lineages. Genes Chromosom Cancer 12:148, 1995
130. Erikson J, Finger L, Sun L et al: Deregulation of c-*myc* by translocation of the α-locus of T-cell receptor in T-cell leukemias. Science 232: 884, 1986
131. Boehm T, Baer R, Lavenir I et al: The mechanism of chromosomal translocation t(11;14) involving the T-cell receptor Cα locus on chromosome 14q11 and a transcribed region of chromosome 11p15. EMBO J 7:385, 1988
132. McGuire EA, Hockett RD, Pollock KM et al: The t(11;14)(p15;q11) in a T-cell acute lymphoblastic leukemia cell line activates multiple transcripts, including *Ttg*-1, a gene encoding a potential zinc finger protein. Mol Cell Biol 9: 2124, 1989
133. Boehm T, Foroni L, Kaneko Y et al: The rhombotin family of cystein-rich LIM-domain oncogenes: distinct members are involved in T-cell translocations to human chromosomes 11p15 and 11p13. Proc Natl Acad Sci USA 88: 4367, 1991
134. Mellentin JD, Smith SD, Cleary ML: *Lyl*-1, a novel gene altered by chromosomal translocation in T cell leukemia, codes for a protein with a helix-loop-helix DNA binding motif. Cell 58: 77, 1989
135. Ellisen LW, Bird J, West DC et al: *TAN*-1, the human homolog of the *Drosophila* notch gene, is broken by chromosomal translocations in T lymphoblastic neoplasms. Cell 66:649, 1991
136. Medeiros LJ, Bagg A, Cossman J: Molecular genetics in the diagnosis and classification of lymphoid neoplasms. p. 58. In Jaffe ES (ed): Surgical Pathology of the Lymph Nodes and Related Organs. Major Problems in Pathology Series. Vol. 16, 2nd Ed. WB Saunders, Philadelphia, 1994
137. Mayer R, Logtenberg T, Strauchen J et al: CD5 and immunoglobulin V gene expression in B-cell lymphomas and chronic lymphocytic leukemia. Blood 75:1518, 1990
138. Kipps TJ, Tomhave E, Chen PP, Carson D: Autoantibody-associated κ light chain variable region gene expressed in chronic lymphocytic leukemia with little or no somatic mutation: implications for etiology and immunotherapy. J Exp Med 167:840, 1988
139. Aoki H, Takishita M, Kosaka M, Saito S: Frequent somatic mutations in D and/or J_H segments of Ig gene in Waldenstrom's macroglobulinemia and chronic lymphocytic leukemia (CLL) with Richter's syndrome but not in common CLL. Blood 85:1913, 1995
140. Bird ML, Ueshima Y, Rowley JD et al: Chromosome abnormalities in B cell chronic lymphocytic leukemia and their clinical correlations. Leukemia 3:182, 1989
141. Escudier SM, Pereira-Leahy JM, Drach JW et al: Fluorescent in situ hybridization and cytogenetic studies of trisomy 12 in chronic lymphocytic leukemia. Blood 81:2702, 1993
142. Dohner H, Pohl S, Bulgay-Morschel M et al: Trisomy 12 in chronic lymphoid leukemias—a

metaphase and interphase cytogenetic analysis. Leukemia 7:716, 1993

143. Juliusson G, Oscier DG, Fitchett M et al: Prognostic subgroups in B-cell chronic lymphocytic leukemia defined by specific chromosomal abnormalities. N Engl J Med 323:720, 1990
144. Bentz M, Huck K, duManoir S et al: Comparative genomic hybridization in chronic B-cell leukemias shows a high incidence of chromosomal gains and losses. Blood 85:3610, 1995
145. Dyer MJS, Zani VJ, Lu WZ et al: *BCL2* translocations in leukemias of mature B cells. Blood 83:3682, 1994
146. Adachi M, Teffrei A, Greipp PR et al: Preferential linkage of *bcl*-2 to immunoglobulin light chain in chronic lymphocytic leukemia. J Exp Med 171:559, 1990
147. Tashiro S, Takechi M, Asou H et al: Cytogenetic 2;18 and 18;22 translocation in chronic lymphocytic leukemia with juxtaposition of *bcl*-2 and immunoglobulin light chain genes. Oncogene 7: 573, 1992
148. Raghoebier S, Van Krieken JHJM, Kluin-Nelemans JC et al: Oncogene rearrangements in chronic B-cell leukemia. Blood 77:1560, 1991
149. Rechavi G, Katzir N, Brok-Simoni F et al: A search for *bcl1, bcl2,* and c-*myc* oncogene rearrangements in chronic lymphocytic leukemia. Leukemia 3:57, 1989
150. Bastard C, Deweindt C, Kerkaert JP et al: LAZ3 rearrangements in non-Hodgkin's lymphoma: correlation with histology, immunophenotype, karyotype, and clinical outcome in 217 patients. Blood 83:2423, 1994
151. Liu Y, Hermanson M, Grander D et al: 13q deletions in lymphoid malignancies. Blood 86:1911, 1995
152. Dohner H, Pilz T, Fischer K et al: Molecular cytogenetic analysis of RB-1 deletions in chronic B-cell leukemias. Leuk Lymphoma 16: 97, 1994
153. Gaidano G, Ballerini P, Gong JZ et al: *p53* mutations in human lymphoid malignancies: association with Burkitt lymphoma and chronic lymphocytic leukemia. Proc Natl Acad Sci USA 88:5413, 1991
154. Haidar MA, Cao X-B, Manshouri T et al: $p16^{INK4A}$ and $p15^{INK4B}$ gene deletions in primary leukemias. Blood 86:311, 1995
155. Tsujimoto Y, Jaffe E, Cossman J et al: Clustering of breakpoints on chromosome 11 in human B-cell neoplasms with the t(11;14) chromosome translocation. Nature 315:340, 1985
156. Foon KA, Thiruvengadam R, Saven A et al: Genetic relatedness of lymphoid malignancies: transformation of chronic lymphocytic leukemia as a model. Ann Intern Med 119:63, 1993
157. Gay D, Saunders T, Camper S, Weigert M: Receptor editing: an approach by autoreactive B cells to escape tolerance. J Exp Med 177:999, 1993
158. Cherepakhin V, Baird SM, Meisenholder GW, Kipps TJ: Common clonal origin of chronic lymphocytic leukemia and high-grade lymphoma of Richter's syndrome. Blood 82:3141, 1993
159. Brynes RK, McCourty A, Sun NCJ, Koo CE: Trisomy 12 in Richter's transformation of chronic lymphocytic leukemia. Am J Clin Pathol 104:199, 1995
160. Matolcsy A, Inghirami G, Knowles DM. Molecular genetic demonstration of the diverse evolution of Richter's syndrome (chronic lymphocytic leukemia and subsequent large cell lymphoma). Blood 83:1363, 1994
161. Khan G, Norton AJ, Slavin G. Epstein-Barr virus in Reed-Sternberg-like cells in non-Hodgkin's lymphomas. J Pathol 169:9, 1993
162. Strickler JG, Amsden TW, Kurtin PJ. Small B-cell lymphoid neoplasms coexisting with T-cell lymphoma. Am J Clin Pathol 98:242, 1992
163. Lee A, Skelly ME, Kingma DW, Medeiros LJ. B-cell chronic lymphocytic leukemia followed by high grade T-cell lymphoma: an unusual variant of Richter's syndrome. Am J Clin Pathol 103:348, 1995
164. Brito-Babapulle V, Pittman S, Melo JV et al: Cytogenetic studies on prolymphocytic leukemia. I. B-cell prolymphocytic leukemia. Hematol Pathol 1:27, 1987
165. Louie E, Tsujimoto Y, Heubner K, Croce C: Molecular cloning of the chromosomal breakpoint isolated from a B-prolymphocytic leukemia patient carrying t(11;14)(q13;q32). Am J Hum Genet, Suppl 41:31, 1987
166. Korsmeyer SJ, Greene W, Cossman J et al: Rearrangement and expression of immunoglobulin genes and expression of Tac antigen in hairy cell leukemia. Proc Natl Acad Sci USA 80:4522, 1983
167. Narni F, Mariano MT, Moretti L et al: Atypical pattern of light chain gene rearrangement in hairy cell leukemia. Hematol Pathol 5:11, 1991

168. Wagner SD, Martinelli V, Luzzatto L. Similar patterns of V_κ gene usage but different degrees of somatic mutation in hairy cell leukemia, Waldenstrom's macroglobulinemia, and myeloma. Blood 83:3647, 1994
169. Ellison DJ, Sharpe RW, Robbins BA et al: Immunomorphologic analysis of bone marrow biopsies after treatment with 2-chlorodeoxyadenosine for hairy cell leukemia. Blood 84:4310, 1994
170. Filleul B, Delannoy A, Ferrant A et al: A single course of 2-chlorodeoxyadenosine (2-CDA) does not eradicate leukemic cells in hairy cell leukemia (HCL) patients achieving complete remission, abstracted. Blood, suppl 82:142A, 1993
171. Sainati L, Matutes E, Mulligan S et al: A variant form of hairy cell leukemia resistant to α-interferon: clinical and phenotypic characteristics of 17 patients. Blood 76:157, 1990
172. Offit K, Louie DC, Parsa NC et al: del(7)(32) is associated with a subset of small lymphocytic lymphoma with plasmacytoid features. Blood 86:2365, 1995
173. San Roman C, Ferro T, Guzman M, Odriozola J: Clonal abnormalities in patients with Waldenstrom's macroglobulinemia with special reference to a Burkitt-type t(8;14). Cancer Genet Cytogenet 18:155, 1985
174. Medeiros LJ, Harmon DC, Linggood RM, Harris NL: Immunohistologic features predict clinical behavior of orbital and conjunctival lymphoid infiltrates. Blood 74:2121, 1989
175. Knowles DM, Athan E, Ubriaco A et al: Extranodal noncutaneous lymphoid hyperplasias represent a continuous spectrum of B-cell neoplasia: demonstration by molecular genetic analysis. Blood 73:1635, 1989
176. Medeiros LJ, Andrade RE, Harris NL, Cossman J: Lymphoid infiltrates of the orbit and conjunctiva: comparison of immunologic and gene rearrangement data. Lab Invest 60:61A, 1989
177. Griffin CA, Zehnbauer BA, Beschorner WE et al: t(11;18)(q21;q21) is a recurrent chromosome abnormality in small lymphocytic lymphoma. Genes Chromosom Cancer 4:153, 1992
178. Wood GS, Ngan B-Y, Tung R et al: Clonal rearrangements of immunoglobulin genes and progression to B cell lymphoma in cutaneous lymphoid hyperplasia. Am J Pathol 135:13, 1989
179. Sheibani K, Sohn CC, Burke JS et al: Monocytoid B-cell lymphoma: a novel B-cell neoplasm. Am J Pathol 124:310, 1986
180. Ngan B-Y, Warnke RA, Wilson M et al: Monocytoid B-cell lymphoma: a study of 36 cases. Hum Pathol 22:409, 1991
181. Xerri L, Horchowski N, Lejeune C et al: Rearrangement of the β T-cell receptor gene in a monocytoid B-cell lymphoma. Arch Pathol Lab Med 114:109, 1990
182. Sheibani K, Ben-Ezra J: Molecular biology of monocytoid B-cell lymphoma: absence of HTLV-I, HTLV-II, and HIV genome and rearranged *bcl*-2 genes in neoplastic monocytoid B cells. Lab Invest 62:92A, 1990
183. Slovak ML, Weiss LM, Nathwani BN et al: Cytogenetic studies of composite lymphomas: monocytoid B-cell lymphoma and other B-cell non-Hodgkin's lymphomas. Hum Pathol 24: 1086, 1990
184. Brynes RK, Almaguer PD, McCourty A, Nathwani BN: Numerical cytogenetic abnormalities of chromosomes 3, 7, and 12 in monocytoid B-cell lymphoma (MBCL). Lab Invest 72:107A, 1995
185. Spencer J, Diss TC, Isaacson PG: Primary B cell gastric lymphoma: a genotypic analysis. Am J Pathol 135:557, 1989
186. Wotherspoon AC, Pan L, Diss TC, Isaacson PG: A genotypic study of low grade B-cell lymphomas, including lymphomas of mucosa associated lymphoid tissue (MALT). J Pathol 162: 135, 1990
187. Kossakowska AE, Eyton-Jones S, Urbanski SJ: Immunoglobulin and T-cell receptor gene rearrangements in lesions of mucosa-associated lymphoid tissue. Diagn Mol Pathol 2:233, 1993
188. Qin Y, Greiner A, Trunk MJF et al: Somatic hypermutation in low-grade mucosa-associated lymphoid tissue-type B-cell lymphoma. Blood 86:3528, 1995
189. Diss TC, Wotherspoon AC, Speight P et al: B-cell monoclonality, Epstein-Barr virus, and t(14; 18) in myoepithelial sialadenitis and low-grade B-cell MALT lymphoma of the parotid gland. Am J Surg Pathol 19:531, 1995
190. Liu Q, Ohshima K, Masuda Y, Kikuchi M: Detection of the Epstein-Barr virus in primary gastric lymphoma by in situ hybridization. Pathol Int 45:131, 1995
191. Clark HM, Jones DB, Wright DH: Cytogenetic and molecular studies of t(14;18) and t(14;19) in

nodal and extranodal B-cell lymphoma. J Pathol 166:129, 1992

192. Wotherspoon AC, Pan L, Diss TC, Isaacson PG: Cytogenetic study of B-cell lymphoma of mucosa-associated lymphoid tissue. Cancer Genet Cytogenet 58:35, 1992
193. Wotherspoon AC, Finn TM, Isaacson PG: Trisomy 3 in low-grade B-cell lymphomas of mucosa-associated lymphoid tissue. Blood 85: 2000, 1995
194. Horsman D, Gascoyne R, Klasa R, Coupland R: t(11;18)(q21;q21.1): a recurring translocation in lymphomas of mucosa-associated lymphoid tissue (MALT). Genes Chromosom Cancer 4:183, 1992
195. Wotherspoon AC, Soosay GN, Diss TC, Isaacson PG: Low-grade primary B-cell lymphoma of the lung: an immunohistochemical, molecular, and cytogenetic study of a single case. Am J Clin Pathol 94:655, 1990
196. Kerrigan DP, Irons J, Chen IM. *bcl*-2 gene rearrangement in salivary gland lymphoma. Am J Surg Pathol 14:1133, 1990
197. Hey MM, Feller AC, Kirchner T et al: Genomic analysis of T-cell receptor and immunoglobulin antigen receptor genes and breakpoint cluster regions in gastrointestinal tract lymphomas. Hum Pathol 21:1283, 1990
198. Shepherd NA, McCarthy KP, Hall PA: 14;18 translocation in primary intestinal lymphoma: detection by polymerase chain reaction in routinely processed tissue. Histopathology 18:415, 1991
199. Levy V, Miller C, Koeffler HP, Said JW: *p53* in lymphomas of mucosal associated lymphoid tissues (MALT), abstracted. Lab Invest 72: 114A, 1995
200. Diss TC, Peng H, Wotherspoon AC et al: Brief report: a single neoplastic clone in sequential biopsy specimens from a patient with primary gastric-mucosa-associated lymphoid-tissue lymphoma and Sjogren's syndrome. N Engl J Med 329:172, 1993
201. Montalban C, Manzanal A, Castrillo JM et al: Low grade gastric B-cell MALT lymphoma progressing into high grade lymphoma. Clonal identity of the two stages of the tumor, unusual bone involvement, and leukaemic dissemination. Histopathology 27:89, 1995
202. Wotherspoon AC, Savio A, Diss TC et al: Diagnosis and treatment of *H. pylori* positive gastric MALT lymphoma, abstracted. Lab Invest 72: 124A, 1995
203. Schmid C, Kirkham N, Diss T, Isaacson PG: Splenic marginal zone cell lymphoma. Am J Surg Pathol 16:455, 1992
204. Isaacson PG, Matutes E, Burke M, Catovsky D: The histopathology of splenic lymphoma with villous lymphocytes. Blood 84:3832, 1994
205. Wu CD, Jackson CL, Medeiros LJ: Splenic marginal zone cell lymphoma: an immunophenotypic and molecular study of five cases. Am J Clin Pathol 105:277, 1996
206. Ballerini L, Fracchiola NS, Cro L et al: Frequent *p53* gene involvement in splenic B-cell leukemia/lymphomas of possible marginal zone origin. Blood 84:270, 1994
207. Melo JV, Robinson DSF, Gregory C, Catovsky D: Splenic B cell lymphoma with "villous" lymphocytes in the peripheral blood: a disorder distinct from hairy cell leukemia. Leukemia 1: 294, 1987
208. Oscier DG, Matutes E, Gardiner A et al: Cytogenetic studies in splenic lymphoma with villous lymphocytes. Br J Haematol 85:487, 1993
209. Jadayel D, Matutes E, Dyer MJS et al: Splenic lymphoma with villous lymphocytes: analysis of *BCL*-1 rearrangements and expression of the cyclin D1 gene. Blood 83:3664, 1994
210. Medeiros LJ, Van Krieken JH, Jaffe ES, Raffeld M: Association of *bcl*-1 rearrangements with lymphocytic lymphoma of intermediate differentiation. Blood 76:2086, 1990
211. Williams ME, Meeker TC, Swerdlow SH: Rearrangement of the chromosome 11 *bcl*-1 locus in centrocytic lymphoma: analysis with multiple breakpoint probes. Blood 78:493, 1991
212. Banks PM, Chan JM, Cleary ML et al: Mantle cell lymphoma. A proposal for unification of morphologic, immunologic, and molecular data. Am J Surg Pathol 16:637, 1992
213. Hummel M, Tamaru J-I, Kalvelage B, Stein H: Mantle cell (previously centrocytic) lymphomas express V_H genes with no or very little somatic mutations like the physiologic cells of the follicle mantle. Blood 84:403, 1994
214. Vandenburghe E, de Wolf-Peeters C, Van den Oord J et al: Translocation (11;14): a cytogenetic anomaly associated with B-cell lymphomas of non-follicle centre cell lineage. J Pathol 163:13, 1991
215. Leroux D, Le Marc'hadour F, Gressin R et al: Non-Hodgkin's lymphomas with t(11;14)(q13;

q32): a subset of mantle zone/intermediate lymphocytic lymphoma? Br J Haematol 77:346, 1991

216. Frizzera G, Sakurai M, Notohara K, Konishi H: t(11;14)(q13;q32) in B-cell lymphomas (intermediately differentiated lymphocytic and follicular): a report of four cases. Am J Clin Pathol 95:684, 1991
217. Weisenburger DD, Sanger WG, Armitage JO, Purtilo DT: Intermediate lymphocytic lymphoma: immunophenotypic and cytogenetic findings. Blood 69:1617, 1987
218. Tsujimoto Y, Yunis J, Onorato-Showe L et al: Molecular cloning of the chromosomal breakpoint of B-cell lymphomas and leukemias with the t(11;14) chromosome translocation. Science 224:1403, 1984
219. Motokura T, Bloom T, Kim HG et al: A novel cyclin encoded by a *bcl*-1-linked candidate oncogene. Nature 350:512, 1991
220. Williams ME, Zukerberg LR, Harris NL et al: Mantle cell/centrocytic lymphoma: molecular and phenotypic analysis including analysis of the *bcl*-1 major translocation cluster by PCR. Mechanisms in B-cell neoplasia. Curr Top Microbiol Immunol 194:341, 1994
221. Rimokh R, Berger F, Delsol G et al: Rearrangement and overexpression of the *BCL*-1/*PRAD*-1 gene in intermediate lymphocytic lymphomas and in t(11q13)-bearing leukemias. Blood 81: 3063, 1993
222. Motokura T, Arnold A: *PRAD*1/cyclin D1 proto-oncogene: genomic organization, 5′ DNA sequence, and sequence of a tumor-specific rearrangement breakpoint. Genes Chromosom Cancer 7:89, 1993
223. Raynaud S, Bekri S, Leroux D et al: Expanded range of 11q13 breakpoints with differing patterns of cyclin D1 expression in B-cell malignancies. Genes Chromosom Cancer 8:80, 1993
224. Molot RJ, Meeker TC, Wittwer CT et al: Antigen expression and polymerase chain reaction amplification of mantle cell lymphomas. Blood 83:1626, 1994
225. Rimokh R, Berger F, Delsol G et al: Detection of the chromosomal translocation t(11;14) by polymerase chain reaction in mantle cell lymphomas. Blood 83:1871, 1994
226. Luthra R, Hai S, Pugh WC: Polymerase chain reaction detection of the t(11;14) translocation involving the *bcl*-1 major translocation cluster in mantle cell lymphoma. Diagn Mol Pathol 4: 4, 1995
227. Campo E, Pinyol M, Nadal A et al: Detection of the *bd*-1 rearrangement (MTC) in frozen and paraffin-embedded tissues of mantle cell lymphomas by polymerase chain reaction, abstracted. Mod Pathol 9:108A, 1996
228. Rosenberg CL, Wong E, Petty EM et al: *PRAD*-1, a candidate *bcl*-1 oncogene: mapping and expression in centrocytic lymphoma. Proc Natl Acad Sci USA 88:9638, 1991
229. Yang W-I, Zukerberg LR, Motokura T et al: Cyclin D1 (BCL-1, PRAD1) protein expression in low-grade B-cell lymphomas and reactive hyperplasia. Am J Pathol 145:86, 1994
230. deBoer CJ, Schuuring E, Dreef E et al: Cyclin D1 protein analysis in the diagnosis of mantle cell lymphoma. Blood 86:2715, 1995
231. Otsuki T, Yano T, Clark HM et al: Analysis of LAZ3 (BCL-6) status in B-cell non-Hodgkin's lymphomas: results of rearrangement and gene expression studies and a mutational analysis of coding region sequences. Blood 85:2877, 1995
232. Greiner TC, Moynihan MJ, Chan WC et al: *p53* mutations in mantle cell lymphoma, abstracted. Lab Invest 72:111A, 1995
233. Louie D, Jaslow R, Offit K et al: Prognostic significance of *p53* overexpression in non-Hodgkin's lymphomas with t(11;14)(q13;q32), abstracted. Lab Invest 72:115A, 1995
234. Zoldan MC, Inghirami G, Masuda Y et al: Large cell variants of mantle cell lymphoma (MCL): cytologic characteristics predict poor outcome, abstracted. Lab Invest 72:124A, 1995
235. Tsujimoto Y, Cossman J, Jaffe E, Croce C: Involvement of the *bcl*-2 gene in human follicular lymphoma. Science 228:1440, 1985
236. Weiss LM, Warnke RA, Sklar J, Cleary ML: Molecular analysis of the t(14;18) chromosomal translocation in malignant lymphomas. N Engl J Med 317:1185, 1987
237. Yunis JJ, Oken MM, Theologides A et al: Recurrent chromosomal defects are found in most patients with non-Hodgkin's lymphoma. Cancer Genet Cytogenet 13:17, 1984
238. Seto M, Jaeger U, Hockett RD et al: Alternative promoters and exons, somatic mutation and deregulation of the *bcl*-2–Ig fusion gene in lymphoma. EMBO J 7:123, 1988
239. Rimokh R, Gadoux M, Bertheas M-F et al: *FVT*-1, a novel human transcription unit affected by

variant translocation t(2;18)(p11;q21) of follicular lymphoma. Blood 81:136, 1993

240. Horsman DE, Gascoyne RD, Coupland RW et al: Comparison of cytogenetic analysis, Southern analysis, and polymerase chain reaction for the detection of t(14;18) in follicular lymphoma. Am J Clin Pathol 103:472, 1995
241. Hockenberry D, Nunez G, Milliman C et al: *bcl*-2 is an inner mitochondrial membrane protein that blocks programmed cell death. Nature 348: 334, 1990
242. deJong D, Pring FA, Mason DY et al: Subcellular localization of the bcl-2 protein in malignant and normal lymphoid cells. Cancer Res 54:256, 1994
243. Ngan B-Y, Chen-Levy Z, Weiss LM et al: Expression in non-Hodgkin's lymphoma of the bcl-2 protein associated with the t(14;18) chromosomal translocation. N Engl J Med 318:1638, 1988
244. Pezzella F, Tse AGD, Cordell JL et al: Expression of the *bcl*-2 oncogene protein is not specific for the 14;18 chromosomal translocation. Am J Pathol 137:225, 1990
245. Zutter M, Hockenbery D, Silverman GA, Korsmeyer SJ: Immunolocalization of the *bcl*-2 protein within hematopoietic neoplasms. Blood 78: 1062, 1991
246. Zelenetz AD, Chu G, Galili N et al: Enhanced detection of the t(14;18) translocation in malignant lymphoma using pulsed-field gel electrophoresis. Blood 78:1552, 1991
247. Le Coco F, Ye BH, Lista F et al: Rearrangements of the BCL6 gene in diffuse large cell non-Hodgkin's lymphoma. Blood 83:1757, 1994
248. Wlodarska I, Mecucci C, Stul M et al: Fluorescence in situ hybridization identifies new chromosomal changes involving 3q27 in non-Hodgkin's lymphomas with BCL6/LAZ3 rearrangement. Genes Chromosom Cancer 14:1, 1995
249. Thangavelu M, Olopade O, Beckman E et al: Clinical, morphologic, and cytogenetic characteristics of patients with lymphoid malignancies characterized by both t(14;18)(q32;q21) and t(8; 14)(q24;q32) or t(8;22)(q32;q21). Genes Chromosom Cancer 2:147, 1990
250. Lee JT, Innes DJ, Williams ME: Sequential *bcl*-2 and c-*myc* oncogene rearrangements associated with the clinical transformation of non-Hodgkin's lymphoma. J Clin Invest 84:1454, 1989
251. Ladanyi M, Offit K, Parsa NZ et al: Follicular lymphoma with t(8;14)(q24;q32): a distinct clinical and molecular subset of t(8;14)-bearing lymphomas. Blood 79:2124, 1992
252. Hillion J, Mecucci C, Aventin A et al: A variant translocation t(2;18) in follicular lymphoma involves the 5′ end of *bcl*-2 and Igκ light chain gene. Oncogene 6:169, 1991
253. Limpens J, Stad R, Vos C et al: Lymphoma-associated translocation t(14;18) in blood B cells of normal individuals. Blood 85:2528, 1995
254. Segal GH, Scott M, Jorgensen T, Braylan RC: Standard polymerase chain reaction analysis does not detect t(14;18) in reactive lymphoid hyperplasia. Arch Pathol Lab Med 118:791, 1994
255. Cleary ML, Trela MJ, Weiss LM et al: Most null large cell lymphomas are B lineage neoplasms. Lab Invest 53:521, 1985
256. Offit K, Jhanwar S, Ebrahim SAD et al: t(3; 22)(q27;q11): a novel translocation associated with diffuse non-Hodgkin's lymphoma. Blood 74:1876, 1989
257. Bastard C, Tilly H, Lenormand B et al: Translocations involving band 3q27 and Ig gene regions in non-Hodgkin's lymphoma. Blood 79:2527, 1992
258. Baron BW, Nucifora G, McCabe N et al: Identification of the gene associated with the recurring chromosomal translocations t(3;14)(q27;q32) and t(3;22)(q27;q11). Proc Natl Acad Sci USA 90:5262, 1993
259. Kerckaert J-P, Deweindt C, Tilly H et al: *LAZ3*, a novel zinc-finger encoding gene, is disrupted by recurring chromosome 3q27 translocations in human lymphomas. Nature Genetics 5:66, 1993
260. Ye BH, Lista F, Lo Coco F et al: Alterations of a zinc finger-encoding gene, BCL-6, in diffuse large-cell lymphoma. Science 262:747, 1993
261. Miki T, Kawamata N, Hirosawa S, Aoki N: Gene involved in the 3q27 translocation with B-cell lymphoma, BCL5, encodes a Kruppel-like zinc-finger protein. Blood 83:26, 1994
262. Ye BH, Rao PH, Chaganti RSK, Dalla Favera R: Cloning of *bcl*-6, the locus involved in chromosome translocations affecting 3q27 of B-cell lymphoma. Cancer Res 53:2732, 1993
263. Onizuka T, Moriyama M, Yamochi T et al: *bcl*-6 gene product, a 92- to 98-kD nuclear phospho-

protein, is highly expressed in germinal center B cells and their neoplastic counterparts. Blood 86:28–37, 1995
264. Cattoretti G, Chang C-C, Cechova K et al: BCL-6 protein is expressed in germinal-center B cells. Blood 86:45–53, 1995
265. Flenghi L, Ye BH, Fizzotti M et al: A specific monoclonal antibody (PG-B6) detects expression of the BCL-6 protein in germinal center B cells. Am J Pathol 147:405, 1995
266. Offit K, Lo Coco F, Louie DC et al: Rearrangement of the *bcl*-6 gene as a prognostic marker in diffuse large-cell lymphoma. N Engl J Med 331:74, 1994
267. Offit K, Koduru PRK, Hollis R et al: 18q21 rearrangement in diffuse large cell lymphoma: incidence and clinical significance. Br J Haematol 72:178, 1989
268. Jacobson JO, Wilkes BM, Kwiatkowski DJ et al: *bcl*-2 rearrangements in de novo diffuse large cell lymphoma: association with distinctive clinical features. Cancer 72:231, 1993
269. Subar M, Neri A, Inghirami G et al: Frequent c-*myc* oncogene activation and infrequent presence of Epstein-Barr virus genome in AIDS-associated lymphoma. Blood 72:667, 1988
270. Van Krieken JHJM, Medeiros LJ, Pals ST et al: Diffuse aggressive B-cell lymphomas of the gastrointestinal tract: an immunophenotypic and gene rearrangement analysis of 22 cases. Am J Clin Pathol 97:170, 1992
271. Neri A, Chang C-C, Lombardi L et al: B cell lymphoma-associated chromosomal translocation involves candidate oncogene *lyt*-10, homologous to NF-κB p50. Cell 67:1075, 1991
272. Yunis JJ, Mayer MG, Arnesen MA et al: *bcl*-2 and other genomic alterations in the prognosis of large-cell lymphoma. N Engl J Med 320: 1047, 1989
273. Lu D, Thompson JD, Gorski GK et al: Alterations at the *rel* locus in human lymphoma. Oncogene 6:1235, 1991
274. Gombert AF, Morosetti R, Miller CW et al: Deletions of the cyclin-dependent kinase inhibitor genes $p16^{INK4A}$ and $p15^{INK4B}$ in non-Hodgkin's lymphomas. Blood 86:1534, 1995
275. Hummel M, Anagnostopoulos I, Korbjuhn P, Stein H: Epstein-Barr virus in B-cell non-Hodgkin's lymphomas: unexpected infection patterns and different infection incidence in low- and high-grade types. J Pathol 175:263, 1995
276. Chang KL, Flaris N, Hickey WF et al: Brain lymphomas of immunocompetent and immunocompromised patients: study of the association with Epstein-Barr virus. Mod Pathol 6:427, 1993
277. Chaganti SR, Gaidano G, Louie DC et al: Diffuse large cell lymphomas exhibit frequent deletions in 9p21–22 and 9q31–34. Genes Chromosom Cancer 12:32, 1995
278. Uchida T, Watanabe T, Kinoshita T et al: Mutational analysis of the CDKN2 (*MTS1/p16*^{ink4A}) gene in primary B-cell lymphomas. Blood 86: 2724, 1995
279. Lo Coco F, Gaidano G, Louie DC et al: *p53* mutations are associated with histologic transformation of follicular lymphoma. Blood 82: 2289, 1993
280. Ichikawa A, Hotta T, Takagi N et al: Mutations of *p53* gene and their relation to disease progression in B-cell lymphoma. Blood 79:2701, 1992
281. Herbst H, Tippelmann G, Anagnostopoulos I et al: Immunoglobulin and T-cell receptor gene rearrangements in Hodgkin's disease and Ki-1-positive anaplastic large cell lymphoma: dissociation between phenotype and genotype. Leuk Res 13:103, 1989
282. Penny R, Blaustein J, Longtine J et al: Ki-1 positive large cell lymphomas, a heterogeneous group of neoplasms. Cancer 68:362, 1991
283. Inghirami G, Macri L, Cesarman E et al: Molecular characterization of CD30+ anaplastic large-cell lymphoma: high frequency of c-*myc* proto-oncogene activation. Blood 83:3581, 1994
284. Greer JP, Macon WR, Lamar RE et al: T-cell-rich B-cell lymphomas: diagnosis and response to therapy in 44 patients. J Clin Oncol 13:1742, 1995
285. Krishnan J, Wallberg K, Frizzera G: T-cell-rich large B-cell lymphoma: a study of 30 cases supporting its histologic heterogeneity and lack of clinical distinctiveness. Am J Surg Pathol 18: 455, 1994
286. Medeiros LJ, Lardelli P, Stetler-Stevenson M et al: Genotypic analysis of diffuse, mixed cell lymphomas: comparison with morphologic and immunophenotypic findings. Am J Clin Pathol 95:547, 1991
287. Baddoura FK, Chan WC, Masih AS et al: T-cell-rich B-cell lymphoma: a clinicopathologic study of eight cases. Am J Clin Pathol 103:65, 1995
288. Loke SL, Ho F, Srivastava G et al: Clonal Ep-

stein-Barr virus genome in T-cell-rich lymphomas of B or probable B lineage. Am J Pathol 16:981, 1992

289. Scarpa A, Bonetti F, Menestrina F: Mediastinal large cell lymphoma with sclerosis: genotypic analysis establishes its B nature. Virchows Arch [A] 412:17, 1987
290. Scarpa A, Borgato L, Chilosi M et al: Evidence of c-*myc* gene abnormalities in mediastinal large B-cell lymphoma of young adult age. Blood 78: 780, 1991
291. Cesarman E, Chadburn A, Liu YF et al: Molecular characterization of primary mediastinal B cell lymphoma, abstracted. Lab Invest 72:122A, 1995
292. Pelicci P-G, Knowles DM, Magrath I, Dalla-Favera R: Chromosomal breakpoints and structural alterations of the c-*myc* locus differ in endemic and sporadic forms of Burkitt lymphoma. Proc Natl Acad Sci USA 83:2984, 1986
293. Yano T, Van Krieken JHJM, Magrath IT et al: Histogenetic correlations between subcategories of small non-cleaved cell lymphomas. Blood 79: 1282, 1992
294. Neri A, Barriga F, Inghirami G et al: Epstein-Barr virus infection precedes clonal expansion in Burkitt's and acquired immunodeficiency syndrome-associated lymphoma. Blood 77: 1092, 1991
295. Ballerini P, Gaidano G, Gong JZ et al: Multiple genetic lesions in acquired immunodeficiency syndrome-related non-Hodgkin's lymphoma. Blood 81:166, 1993
296. Bacchi MM, Bacchi CE, Alvarenga M et al: Burkitt's lymphoma in Brazil: strong association with Epstein-Barr virus. Mod Pathol 9:63, 1996
297. Young LS, Yao QY, Roponey CM et al: New type B isolate of Epstein-Barr virus from Burkitt's lymphoma and normal individuals in endemic areas. J Gen Virol 68:2853, 1987
298. Chen W-G, Chen Y-Y, Bacchi MM et al: Genotyping of Epstein-Barr virus in Brazilian Burkitt lymphoma and reactive lymphoid tissue: type A with a high prevalence of deletions within the latent membrane protein gene. Am J Pathol 148: 17, 1996
299. Leder P, Battey J, Lenoir G et al: Translocations among antibody genes in human cancer. Science 222:765, 1983
300. Magrath I: The pathogenesis of Burkitt's lymphoma. Adv Cancer Res 53:133, 1990
301. Shiramizu B, Barriga F, Neequaye J et al: Patterns of chromosomal breakpoint locations in Burkitt's lymphoma: relevance to geography and Epstein-Barr virus association. Blood 77: 1516, 1991
302. Yano T, Sander CA, Clark HM et al: Clustered mutations in the second exon of the *MYC* gene in sporadic Burkitt's lymphoma. Oncogene 8: 2741, 1993
303. Lenoir G, Preud'homme JL, Bernheim A, Berger T: Correlation between immunoglobulin light chain expression and variant translocation in Burkitt's lymphoma. Nature 298:474, 1982
304. Shtivelman E, Henglein B, Groitl P et al: Identification of a human transcription unit affected by the variant chromosomal translocations 2;8 and 8;22 of Burkitt lymphoma. Proc Natl Acad Sci USA 86:3257, 1989
305. Chapman CJ, Mockridge CI, Rowe M et al: Analysis of V_H genes by neoplastic B cells in endemic Burkitt's lymphoma shows somatic hypermutation and intraclonal heterogeneity. Blood 85:2176, 1995
306. Preudhomme C, Dervite I, Wattel E et al: Clinical significance of *p53* mutations in newly diagnosed Burkitt's lymphoma and acute lymphoblastic leukemia: a report of 48 cases. J Clin Oncol 13:812, 1995
307. Humphries JE, Dressman HK, Williams ME: Immunoglobulin gene rearrangement in multiple myeloma: limitations of Southern blot analysis. Hum Pathol 22:966, 1991
308. Palumbo A, Battaglio S, Astolfi M et al: Multiple independent immunoglobulin class-switch recombinations occurring within the same clone in myeloma. Br J Haematol 82:676, 1992
309. Berenson J, Lichtenstein A: Clonal rearrangement of the beta-T cell receptor gene in multiple myeloma. Leukemia 3:133, 1989
310. Lai JL, Zandecki M, Mary JY et al: Improved cytogenetics in multiple myeloma: a study of 151 patients including 117 patients at diagnosis. Blood 85:2490, 1995
311. Travis P, Sawyer J, Lary C et al: Translocation 11;14 and *bcl*-1 gene abnormalities in multiple myeloma (MM), abstracted. Blood 82 (suppl 1): 261A, 1993
312. Dewald GW, Kyle RA, Hicks GA, Griepp PR: The clinical significance of cytogenetic studies in 100 patients with multiple myeloma, plasma cell leukemia, or amyloidosis. Blood 66:380, 1985

313. Fiedler W, Weh HJ, Hossfeld DK: Comparison of chromosome analysis and BCL-1 rearrangement in a series of patients with multiple myeloma. Br J Haematol 81:58, 1992
314. Selvanayagam P, Goodacre A, Strong L et al: Alterations of the *bcl*-1 oncogene in human multiple myeloma, abstracted. Proc Am Assoc Cancer Res 28:19A, 1987
315. Selvanayagam P, Blick M, Narni F et al: Alteration and abnormal expression of the c-*myc* oncogene in human multiple myeloma. Blood 71: 30, 1988
316. Neri A, Murphy JP, Cro L et al: *ras* oncogene mutation in multiple myeloma. J Exp Med 170: 1715, 1989
317. Nobuyoshi M, Kawano M, Tanaka H et al: Increased expression of the c-*myc* gene may be related to the aggressive transformation of human myeloma cells. Br J Haematol 77:523, 1991
318. Travis P, Kaushal V, Baltz B et al: Abnormal c-*myc* transcript size in 70 percent of patients with multiple myeloma (MM), abstracted. Blood, suppl 82:261A, 1993
319. Palumbo AP, Boccadoro M, Battaglio S et al: Human homologue of Moloney leukemia virus integration-4 locus (MLVI-4), located 20 kilobases 3′ of the *myc* gene, is rearranged in multiple myelomas. Cancer Res 50:6478, 1990
320. Corradini P, Ladetto M, Voena C et al: Mutational activation of N- and K-*ras* oncogenes in plasma cell dyscrasias. Blood 81:2708, 1993
321. Neri A, Baldini L, Trecca D et al: *p53* gene mutations in multiple myeloma are associated with advanced forms of malignancy. Blood 81: 128, 1993
322. Tricot G, Dao D, Gazitt Y et al: Deletion of the retinoblastoma gene (*Rb*-1) in multiple myeloma (MM), abstracted. Blood, suppl 82:261A, 1993
323. Joseph G, Barker RL, Yuan B et al: Posttransplant plasma cell dyscrasias. Cancer 74:1959, 1994
324. Gatti RA, McConville CM, Taylor AMR: Sixth international workshop on ataxia-telangiectasia. Cancer Res 54:6007, 1994
325. Matutes E, Brito-Babapulle V, Swansbury J et al: Clinical and laboratory features of 78 cases of T-prolymphocytic leukemia. Blood 78:3269, 1991
326. Knowles DM: The human T-cell leukemias: clinical, cytomorphologic, immunophenotypic and genotypic characteristics. Hum Pathol 17: 14, 1986
327. Brito-Babapulle V, Pomfret M, Matutes E et al: Cytogenetic studies on prolymphocytic leukemia. II. T cell prolymphocytic leukemia. Blood 70:926, 1987
328. Matutes E, Brito-Babapulle V, Swansbury J et al: Clinical and laboratory features of 78 cases of T-prolymphocytic leukemia. Blood 78:3269, 1991
329. Fu T, Virgilio L, Narducci MG et al: Characterization and localization of the TCL-1 oncogene product. Cancer Res 56:6297, 1994
330. Fish P, Forster A, Sherrington PD et al: The chromosomal translocation t(X;14)(q28;q11) in T-cell prolymphocytic leukemia breaks within one gene and activates another. Oncogene 8: 3271, 1993
331. Thick J, Mak YF, Metcalfe J et al: A gene on chromosome Xq28 associated with T-cell prolymphocytic leukemia in two patients with ataxia-telangiectasia. Leukemia 8:564, 1994
332. Agnarsson B, Loughran TP, Starkebaum G et al: The pathology of large granular lymphocyte leukemia. Hum Pathol 20:643, 1989
333. Sheridan W, Winton EF, Chan WC et al: Leukemia of non-T lineage natural killer cells. Blood 72:1701, 1988
334. Rambaldi A, Pelicci P, Allavena P et al: T-cell receptor β chain gene rearrangements in lymphoproliferative disorders of large granular lymphocytes/natural killer cells. J Exp Med 162: 2156, 1985
335. Pelicci P, Allavena P, Alessandro R et al: T-cell receptor (α,β,γ) gene rearrangements and expression distinguish large granular lymphocyte/natural killer cells and T-cells. Blood 70: 1500, 1987
336. Waldron JA, Leech JH, Glick AD et al: Malignant lymphoma of peripheral T-lymphocyte origin: immunologic, pathologic and clinical features in six patients. Cancer 40:1604, 1977
337. Van Krieken JHJM, Elwood L, Andrade RE et al: Rearrangement of the T-cell receptor delta chain gene in T-cell lymphomas with a mature phenotype. Am J Pathol 139:161, 1991
338. Weiss LM, Picker LJ, Grogan T et al: Absence of clonal beta and gamma T-cell receptor gene rearrangements in a subset of peripheral T-cell lymphomas. Am J Pathol 130:436, 1988
339. Zhou XG, Hamilton-Dutoit SJ, Yan QH, Pallesen G: High frequency of Epstein-Barr virus

in Chinese peripheral T-cell lymphoma. Histopathology 24:115, 1994

340. Matshushima AY, Cesarman E, Chadburn A, Knowles DM: Post-thymic T cell lymphomas frequently overexpress p53 protein but infrequently exhibit *p53* gene mutations. Am J Pathol 144:573, 1994
341. Su IJ, Hsieh HG: Clinicopathologic spectrum of Epstein-Barr virus-associated T-cell malignancies. Leuk Lymphoma 7:47, 1992
342. Shimoyama M and The Lymphoma Study Group: Diagnostic criteria and classification of clinical subtypes of adult T-cell leukemia/lymphoma. Br J Haematol 79:428, 1991
343. Seiki M, Eddy R, Shows TB, Yoshida M: Nonspecific integration of the HTLV provirus genome into adult T-cell leukemia cells. Nature 309:640, 1984
344. Shimamoto Y, Suga K, Shibata K et al: Clinical importance of extraordinary integration patterns of human T-cell lymphotrophic virus type I proviral DNA in adult T-cell leukemia/lymphoma. Blood 84:853, 1994
345. Matsuoka M, Hagiya T, Hattori T et al: Gene rearrangements of T cell receptor β and γ chains in HTLV-I infected primary neoplastic T cells. Leukemia 2:84, 1988
346. Isobe M, Sadamori N, Russo G et al: Rearrangements in the human T-cell-receptor α-chain locus in patients with adult T-cell leukemia carrying translocations involving chromosome 14q11. Cancer Res 50:6171, 1990
347. Kimura N, Takihara Y, Akiyoshi T et al: Rearrangement of T-cell receptor δ chain gene as a marker of lineage and clonality in T-cell lymphoproliferative disorders. Cancer Res 49:4488, 1989
348. Fifth International Workshop on Chromosomes in Leukemia-Lymphoma: Correlation of chromosome abnormalities with histologic and immunologic characteristics in non-Hodgkin's lymphoma and adult T-cell leukemia lymphoma. Blood 70:1554, 1988
349. Cesarman E, Chadburn A, Inghirami G et al: Structural and functional analysis of oncogenes and tumor suppressor genes in adult T-cell leukemia/lymphoma shows frequent *p53* mutations. Blood 80:3205, 1992
350. Sakashita A, Hattori T, Miller CW et al: Mutation of *p53* gene in adult T-cell leukemia. Blood 79:477, 1992
351. Hatta Y, Hirama T, Miller CW et al: Homozygous deletions of the *p15* (*MTS2*) and *p16* (*CDKN2/MTS1*) genes in adult T-cell leukemia. Blood 85:2699, 1995
352. Morosetti R, Kawamata N, Gombart AF et al: Alterations of the $p27^{KIP1}$ gene in non-Hodgkin's lymphomas and adult T-cell leukemia/lymphoma. Blood 86:1924, 1995
353. Tokunaga M, Imai S, Uemura Y et al: Epstein-Barr virus in adult T-cell leukemia/lymphoma. Am J Pathol 143:1263, 1993
354. Lipford EH, Margolick JB, Longo DL et al: Angiocentric immunoproliferative lesions: a clinicopathologic spectrum of post-thymic T-cell proliferations. Blood 72:1674, 1988
355. Guinee D, Jaffe E, Kingma D et al: Pulmonary lymphomatoid granulomatosis: evidence for a proliferation of Epstein-Barr virus infected B-lymphocytes with a prominent T-cell component and vasculitis. Am J Surg Pathol 18:753, 1994
356. Myers JL, Kurtin PJ, Katzenstein A-L et al: Lymphomatoid granulomatosis: evidence of immunophenotypic diversity and relationship to Epstein-Barr virus infection. Am J Surg Pathol 19:1300, 1995
357. Medeiros LJ, Peiper SC, Elwood L et al: Angiocentric immunoproliferative lesions: a molecular analysis of 8 cases. Hum Pathol 22:1150, 1991
358. Suzumiya J, Takeshita M, Kimura N et al: Expression of adult and fetal natural killer cell markers in sinonasal lymphomas. Blood 83: 2255, 1994
359. Kanavaros P, Lescs M-C, Briere J et al: Nasal T-cell lymphoma: a clinicopathologic entity associated with peculiar phenotype and with Epstein-Barr virus. Blood 81:2688, 1993
360. Ho FCS, Srivastava G, Loke SL et al: Presence of Epstein-Barr virus DNA in nasal lymphomas of B and "T" cell type. Hematol Oncol 8:271, 1990
361. Lanier LL, Chang C, Spits H, Phillips JH: Expression of cytoplasmic CD3ϵ proteins in activated human adult natural killer (NK) cells and CD3γ, δ, ϵ complexes in fetal NK cells. J Immunol 149:1876, 1992
362. Lanier LL, Spits H, Phillips JH: The developmental relationship between NK cells and T cells. Immunol Today 13:392, 1992
363. Harabuchi Y, Yamanaka N, Kataura A et al: Epstein-Barr virus in nasal T-cell lymphomas

in patients with lethal midline granuloma. Lancet 1:128, 1990

364. Medeiros LJ, Jaffe ES, Chen Y-Y, Weiss LM: Localization of Epstein-Barr viral genomes in angiocentric immunoproliferative lesions. Am J Surg Pathol 16:439, 1992
365. Chan JKC, Yip TTC, Tsang WYW et al: Detection of Epstein-Barr viral RNA in malignant lymphomas of the upper aerodigestive tract. Am J Surg Pathol 18:938, 1994
366. Arber DA, Weiss LM, Albujar PF et al: Nasal lymphomas in Peru: high incidence of T-cell immunophenotype and Epstein-Barr virus infection. Am J Surg Pathol 17:392, 1993
367. Tao Q, Ho FCS, Loke SL, Srivastava G: Epstein-Barr virus is localized in the tumour cells of nasal lymphomas of NK, T or B cell type. Int J Cancer 60:315, 1995
368. Bleiweiss IJ, Strauchen JA: Lymphomatoid granulomatosis of the lung: report of a case and gene rearrangement studies. Hum Pathol 19: 1109, 1988
369. Donner LR, Dobin S, Harrington D et al: Angiocentric immunoproliferative lesions (lymphomatoid granulomatosis): a cytogenetic, immunophenotypic, and genotypic study. Cancer 65: 249, 1990
370. Gaulard P, Henni T, Marolleau J-P et al: Lethal midline granuloma (polymorphic reticulosis) and lymphomatoid granulomatosis: evidence for a monoclonal T-cell lymphoproliferative disorder. Cancer 62:705, 1988
371. Katzenstein AA, Peiper SC: Detection of Epstein-Barr virus genomes in lymphomatoid granulomatosis: analysis of 29 cases by the polymerase chain reaction technique. Mod Pathol 3:435, 1990
372. Frizzera G, Moran EM, Rappaport H: Angioimmunoblastic lymphadenopathy with dysproteinemia. Lancet 1:1070, 1974
373. Feller AC, Griesser H, Schilling CV et al: Clonal gene rearrangement patterns correlate with immunophenotype and clinical parameters in patients with angioimmunoblastic lymphadenopathy. Am J Pathol 133:549, 1988
374. Weiss LM, Strickler JG, Dorfman RF et al: Clonal T-cell populations in angioimmunoblastic lymphadenopathy and angioimmunoblastic lymphadenopathy-like T-cell lymphoma. Am J Pathol 122:392, 1986
375. Suzuki H, Namikawa R, Ueda R et al: Clonal T cell population in angioimmunoblastic lymphadenonpathy and related lesions. Jpn J Cancer Res 78:712, 1987
376. Godde-Salz E, Feller AC, Lennert K: Chromosomal abnormalities in lymphogranulomatosis X (Lgr X/angioimmunoblastic lymphadenopathy (AILD). Leuk Res 11:181, 1987
377. Schlegelberger B, Feller A, Godde E et al: Stepwise development of chromosomal abnormalities in angioimmunoblastic lymphadenopathy. Cancer Genet Cytogenet 50:15, 1990
378. Schlegelberger B, Zhang Y, Weber-Matthiesen K, Grote W: Detection of aberrant clones in nearly all cases of angioimmunoblastic lymphadenopathy with dysproteinemia-type T-cell lymphoma by combined interphase and metaphase cytogenetics. Blood 84:2640, 1994
379. Knecht H, Sahli R, Shaw P et al: Detection of Epstein-Barr virus DNA by polymerase chain reaction in lymph node biopsies from patients with angioimmunoblastic lymphadenopathy. Br J Haematol 75:610, 1990
380. Anagnostopoulos I, Hummel M, Finn T et al: Heterogeneous Epstein-Barr virus infection patterns in peripheral T-cell lymphoma of angioimmunoblastic lymphadenopathy type. Blood 80: 1804, 1992
381. Weiss LM, Jaffe E, Liu X et al: Detection and localization of Epstein-Barr viral genomes in angioimmunoblastic lymphadenopathy and angioimmunoblastic lymphadenopathy-like lymphomas. Blood 79:1789, 1992
382. Abruzzo LV, Schmidt K, Weiss LM et al: B cell lymphoma following angioimmunoblastic lymphadenopathy: a case with oligoclonal gene rearrangements associated with Epstein-Barr virus. Blood 82:241, 1993
383. Frizzera G, Kaneko Y, Sakurai M: Angioimmunoblastic lymphadenopathy and related disorders: a retrospective look in search of definitions. Leukemia 3:1, 1989
384. Isaacson P, Spencer J, Connolly C et al: Malignant histiocytosis of the intestine: a T-cell lymphoma. Lancet 2:688, 1985
385. Chott A, Dragosics B, Radaszkiewicz T: Peripheral T-cell lymphomas of the intestine. Am J Pathol 141:1361, 1992
386. deBruin PC, Oudejans JJ, Radasziewicz T, Meijer CJLM: Epstein-Barr virus in primary gastrointestinal T cell lymphomas: association with gluten-sensitive enteropathy, pathological features, and immunophenotype. Am J Pathol 146:861, 1995

387. Murray A, Cuevas EC, Jones DB, Wright DH: Study of the immunohistochemistry and T cell clonality of enteropathy-associated T cell lymphoma. Am J Pathol 146:509, 1995
388. Wright DH, Jones DB, Clark H et al: Is adult-onset coeliac disease due to a low-grade lymphoma of intraepithelial T lymphocytes? Lancet 337:1373, 1991
389. Walsh SV, Egan LJ, Connolly CE et al: Enteropathy-associated T-cell lymphoma in the west of Ireland: low-frequency of Epstein-Barr virus in these tumors. Mod Pathol 8:753, 1995
390. Ilyas M, Niedobitek G, Agathanggelou et al: Non-Hodgkin's lymphoma, coeliac disease, and Epstein-Barr virus: a study of 13 cases of enteropathy-associated T- and B-cell lymphoma. J Pathol 177:115, 1995
391. Bucsky P, Favara B, Feller AC et al: Malignant histiocytosis and large cell anaplastic (Ki-1) lymphoma in childhood: guidelines for differential diagnosis—report of the Histiocyte Society. Med Pediatr Oncol 22:200, 1994
392. Benz-Lemoine E, Brizard A, Huret J-L et al: Malignant histiocytosis: a specific t(2;5)(p23;q35) translocation? Review of the literature. Blood 72:1045, 1988
393. Xerri L, Horschowski N, Payan MJ et al: Genotypic analysis in large cell lymphomas expressing a restricted set of differentiation antigens. Pathol Res Pract 186:317, 1990
394. Ebrahim SAD, Ladanyi M, Desai SB et al: Immunohistochemical, molecular, and cytogenetic analysis of a consecutive series of 20 peripheral T-cell lymphomas and lymphomas of uncertain lineage, including 12 Ki-1 positive lymphomas. Genes Chromosom Cancer 2:27, 1990
395. Tkachuk DC, Griesser H, Takihara Y et al: Rearrangement of T-cell δ locus in lymphoproliferative disorders. Blood 72:353, 1988
396. Bullrich F, Morris SW, Hummel M et al: Nucleophosmin (NPM) gene rearrangement in Ki-1-positive lymphomas. Cancer Res 54:2873, 1994
397. Lopategui JR, Sun L-H, Chan JKC et al: Low frequency association of the t(2;5)(p23;q35) chromosomal translocation with CD30+ lymphomas from American and Asian patients: a reverse transcriptase-polymerase chain reaction study. Am J Pathol 146:323, 1995
398. McBride JA, Luthra RL, Sarris AH et al: Rearrangements of the NPM gene are selectively but infrequently associated with anaplastic large cell lymphoma (ALCL), abstracted. Lab Invest 72:116A, 1995
399. Yee HT, Ponzoni M, Merson A et al: Chimeric NPM-ALK transcripts of t(2;5) in anaplastic large cell lymphoma (ALCL) and Hodgkin's disease (HD), abstracted. Lab Invest 72:124A, 1995
400. Ngan B: The presence of transcripts of the fusion of kinase gene ALK to nucleophosmin gene NPM in the t(2;5)(p23;q35) translocation defines subsets of non-Hodgkin's lymphoma with or without CD30 (Ki-1) expression and Hodgkin's disease, abstracted. Lab Invest 72:118A, 1995
401. Wellman A, Otsuki T, Vogelbruch M et al: Analysis of the t(2;5)(p23;q35) translocation by reverse transcriptase-polymerase chain reaction in CD30+ anaplastic large-cell lymphomas, in other non-Hodgkin's lymphomas of T-cell phenotype, and in Hodgkin's disease. Blood 86: 2321, 1995
402. Morris SW, Kirstein MN, Valentine MB et al: Fusion of a kinase gene, *ALK*, to a nucleolar protein gene, *NPM*, in non-Hodgkin's lymphoma. Science 263:1281, 1994
403. Herbst H, Anagnostopoulos J, Heinze B et al: *ALK* gene products in anaplastic large cell lymphomas and Hodgkin's disease. Blood 86:1694, 1995
404. Shiota M, Fujimoto J, Takenaga M et al: Diagnosis of t(2;5)(p23;q35)-associated Ki-1 lymphoma with immunohistochemistry. Blood 84: 3648, 1994
405. Elmberger PG, Lozano MD, Weisenburger DD et al: Transcripts of the *npm-alk* fusion gene in anaplastic large cell lymphoma, Hodgkin's disease, and reactive lymphoid lesions. Blood 86:3517, 1995
406. Downing JR, Shurtleff SA, Zielenska M et al: Molecular detection of the t(2;5) translocation of non-Hodgkin's lymphoma by reverse transcriptase-polymerase chain reaction. Blood 85: 3416, 1995
407. Cesarman E, Inghirami G, Chadburn A, Knowles DM: High levels of p53 protein expression do not correlate with *p53* gene mutations in anaplastic large cell lymphoma. Am J Pathol 143:845, 1993
408. Kanavaros P, Jiwa NM, De Bruin PC et al: High incidence of EBV genome in CD30-positive non-Hodgkin's lymphomas. J Pathol 168:307, 1992

409. Lopategui JR, Gaffey MJ, Chan JKC et al: Infrequent association of Epstein-Barr virus with CD30-positive anaplastic large cell lymphomas from American and Asian patients. Am J Surg Pathol 19:42, 1995
410. Takeshita M, Ohshima K, Akamatsu M et al: CD30-positive anaplastic large cell lymphoma in a human T-cell lymphotropic virus-I endemic area. Hum Pathol 26:614, 619, 1995
411. Kadin ME, Peters K, Knoll JHM: Chromosome abnormalities in lymphomatoid papulosis (LyP) and cutaneous CD30+ anaplastic large cell lymphoma (ALCL), abstracted. Lab Invest 72: 113A, 1995
412. Anagnostopoulos I, Hummel M, Kaudewitz P et al: Detection of HTLV-I proviral sequences in CD30-positive large cell cutaneous T-cell lymphomas. Am J Pathol 137:1317, 1990
413. Gaulard P, Bourquelot P, Kanavaros P et al: Expression of the alpha/beta and gamma/delta T-cell receptors in 57 cases of peripheral T-cell lymphoma: identification of a subset of γ/δ T-cell lymphomas. Am J Pathol 137:617, 1990
414. Farcet J-P, Gaulard P, Marolleau J-P et al: Hepatosplenic T-cell lymphoma: sinus/sinusoidal localization of malignant cells expressing the T-cell receptor $\gamma\delta$. Blood 75:2213, 1990
415. Mastovich S, Ratech H, Ware RE et al: Hepatosplenic T-cell lymphoma: an unusual case of a $\gamma\delta$ T-cell lymphoma with a blast-like terminal transformation. Hum Pathol 25:102, 1994
416. Wong KF, Chan JKC, Matutes E et al: Hepatosplenic $\gamma\delta$T-cell lymphoma: a distinctive aggressive lymphoma type. Am J Surg Pathol 19:718, 1995
417. Garcia-Sanchez F, Menarguez J, Cristobal E et al: Hepatosplenic gamma-delta T-cell malignant lymphoma: report of the first case in childhood, including molecular minimal residual disease follow-up. Br J Haematol 90:943, 1995
418. Wang C-C, Tien H-F, Lin M-T et al: Consistent presence of isochromosome 7q in hepatosplenic T γ/δ lymphoma: a new cytogenetic-clinicopathologic entity. Genes Chromosom Cancer 12:161, 1995
419. Ross CW, Schnitzer B, Sheldon S et al: Gamma/delta T-cell posttransplantation lymphoproliferative disorder primarily in the spleen. Am J Clin Pathol 102:310, 1994
420. Gonzalez CL, Medeiros LJ, Braziel RM, Jaffe ES: T-cell lymphoma involving subcutaneous tissue: a clinicopathologic entity commonly associated with hemophagocytic syndrome. Am J Surg Pathol 15:17, 1991
421. Medeiros LJ, Greiner TC, Gonzalez CL et al: T-cell lymphoma involving subcutaneous tissue. Mod Pathology 7:116A, 1994
422. Perniciaro C, Zalla MJ, White JW, Menke DM: Subcutaneous T-cell lymphoma. Arch Dermatol 129:1171, 1993
423. Burg G, Dummer R, Wilhelm M et al: A subcutaneous delta-positive T-cell lymphoma that produces interferon gamma. N Engl J Med 325: 1078, 1991
424. Smith KJ, Skelton HG, Giblin WL, James WD: Cutaneous leions of hemophagocytic syndrome in a patient with T-cell lymphoma and active Epstein-Barr infection. J Am Acad Dermatol 25: 919, 1991
425. Harada H, Iwatsuki K, Kaneko F: Detection of Epstein-Barr virus genes in malignant lymphoma with clinical and histologic features of cytophagic histiocytic panniculitis. J Am Acad Dermatol 31:379, 1994
426. Feller AC, Griesser H, Mak TW, Lennert K: Lympho-epithelioid lymphoma (Lennert's lymphoma) is a monoclonal proliferation of helper/ inducer T cells. Blood 68:663, 1986
427. Whittaker SJ, Smith NP, Jones RR et al: Analysis of β, γ, and δ T-cell receptor genes in mycosis fungoides and Sezary syndrome. Cancer 68: 1572, 1991
428. Ralfkiaer E, O'Connor NTJ, Crick J et al: Genotypic analysis of cutaneous T-cell lymphomas. J Invest Dermatol 88:762, 1987
429. Weiss LM, Hu E, Wood GS et al: Clonal rearrangements of T-cell receptor genes in mycosis fungoides and dermatopathic lymphadenopathy. N Engl J Med 313:539, 1985
430. Colby TV, Burke JS, Hoppe RT: Lymph node biopsy in mycosis fungoides. Cancer 47:351, 1981
431. Weiss LM, Wood GS, Hu E et al: Detection of clonal T-cell receptor gene rearrangements in the peripheral blood of patients with mycosis fungoides/Sezary syndrome. J Invest Dermatol 92:601, 1989
432. Hall WW, Liu CR, Schneewind O et al: Deleted HTLV-I provirus in blood and cutaneous lesions of patient with mycosis fungoides. Science 253: 317, 1991
433. Pancake BA, Zucker-Franklin D: HTLV tax and mycosis fungoides. N Engl J Med 329:580, 1993
434. Ghosh SK, Abrams JT, Terunuma H et al:

Human T-cell leukemia virus type I *tax/rex* DNA and RNA in cutaneous T-cell lymphoma. Blood 84:2663, 1994

435. Manca N, Piacentini E, Gelmi M et al: Persistence of human T cell lymphotropic virus type 1 (HTLV-1) sequences in peripheral blood mononuclear cells from patients with mycosis fungoides. J Exp Med 180:1973, 1994
436. Stroup RM, Sheibani K, Moncada A et al: Angiotropic (intravascular) large cell lymphoma: a clinicopathologic study of seven cases with unique presentations. Cancer 66:1781, 1990
437. Kamesaki H, Matsui Y, Ohno Y et al: Angiocentric lymphoma with histologic features of neoplastic angioendotheliomatosis presenting with predominant respiratory and hematologic manifestations. Am J Clin Pathol 94:768, 1990
438. Otrakji CL, Voight W, Amador A et al: Malignant angioendotheliomatosis—a true lymphoma: a case of intravascular malignant lymphomatosis studied by Southern blot hybridization analysis. Hum Pathol 19:475, 1988
439. Sleater JP, Segal GH, Scott MD, Masih AS: Intravascular (angiotropic) large cell lymphoma: determination of monoclonality by polymerase chain reaction on paraffin-embedded tissues. Mod Pathol 7:593, 1994
440. Sepp N, Schuler G, Romani N et al: ''Intravascular lymphomatosis'' (angioendotheliomatosis): evidence for a T-cell origin in two cases. Hum Pathol 21:1051, 1990
441. Molina A, Lombard C, Donlon T et al: Immunohistochemical and cytogenetic studies indicate that malignant angioendotheliomatosis is a primary intravascular (angiotropic) lymphoma. Cancer 66:474, 1990

2

Reactive Lymphadenopathies

John K. C. Chan and William Y. W. Tsang

Because of widespread use of fine-needle aspiration cytology (FNAC) as the initial investigation for patients presenting with lymphadenopathy, lymph node excision specimens showing reactive changes are now much less frequently seen by surgical pathologists. Such lymph nodes are often observed for spontaneous resolution after the FNAC diagnosis is made and are therefore not biopsied at all. Biopsies are performed only if the lymphadenopathy persists despite an FNAC impression of benign lesion or if FNAC yields inconclusive or suspicious findings.

It is not possible to cover all forms of benign lymphadenopathies in this chapter given the limitation of space. Thus a general approach is given, and only selected newly recognized entities are described in some depth. For other new entities or established entities with new findings, only the relevant new information is highlighted because the basic information is already available widely in review articles and textbooks.[1–13] This chapter can therefore serve as a quick update on reactive lymphadenopathies for the practising surgical pathologist. The subjects of vasoproliferative and nonhematopoietic lesions of lymph nodes have been reviewed in depth elsewhere, and therefore most of these entities are not covered.[14,15]

THE COMPARTMENTS OF THE NORMAL LYMPH NODE AND THEIR REACTION TO STIMULI

The major compartments of the lymph node include the cortex, paracortex, medullary cords, sinuses, and connective tissue framework.[16–18]

The Cortex

The cortex is the predominantly B-cell region of the lymph node. Scattered in the cortex are primary follicles (rounded aggregates of small lymphocytes with round or slightly irregular nuclei) and secondary follicles (with germinal centers) (Fig. 2-1). Both the primary and secondary follicles are rich in follicular dendritic cells, which can be recognized by their pale "naked" nuclei (due to difficulties in defining the ramifying cell borders) with delicate violaceous nuclear membrane, a solitary small nucleolus, and occasional binucleated forms. They can be highlighted by immunostaining, such as CD21, CD35, and R4/23. In the germinal centers, besides the predominant component of follicle center B cells (large noncleaved cells [centroblasts] and small cleaved cells [centrocytes], which express IgG, IgM, or IgA but not IgD), there are some small T lymphocytes with a peculiar CD4+ CD57+ immunophenotype and tingible-body macrophages (Fig. 2-2). The mantle zone cells, which appear as small lymphocytes, comprise a heterogeneous population of cells that are not morphologically distinguishable. They include virgin nonstimulated B lymphocytes (IgD+ IgM+), recirculating B lymphocytes (IgD+ IgM+) generated in immune responses that are non-T-cell dependent, and memory B cells (IgD− and IgM+/IgG+) generated from the germinal centers.[19] Marginal zone cells (with nuclei slightly larger than those of small lymphocytes and with pale to clear cytoplasm) are rarely observed around the secondary follicles, except in some intraabdominal

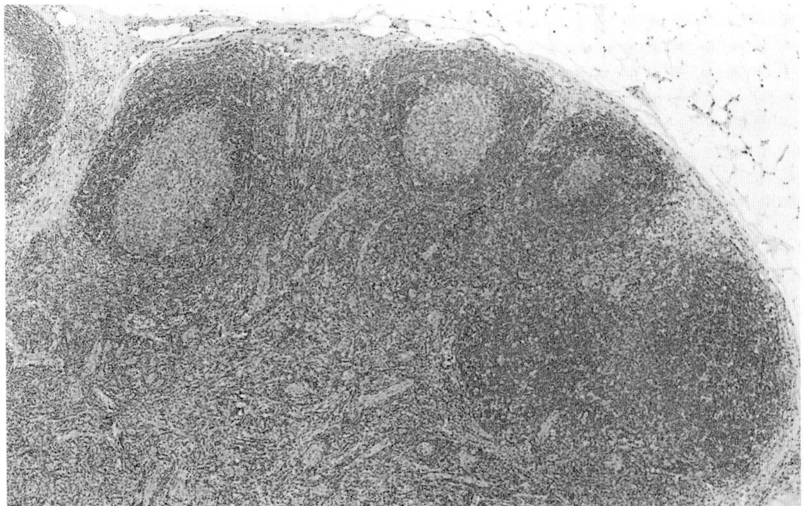

Fig. 2-1. Normal lymph node. Several secondary follicles are seen in the cortex. The paracortex, comprising small lymphocytes with interspersed light-staining high endothelial venules, is located between and deep to the cortex. The thin fibrous capsule that envelopes the node is barely visible under normal conditions.

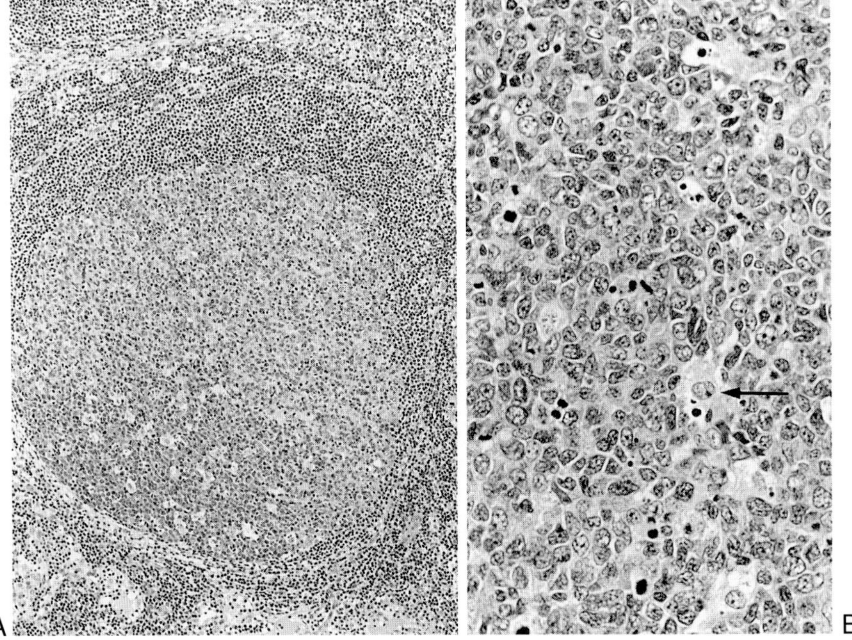

Fig. 2-2. Secondary lymphoid follicle. (**A**) This follicle shows polarity, that is, a dark zone at the bottom and a light zone on top. The starry-sky appearance is imparted by the interspersed tingible-body macrophages. The mantle is thicker on top, forming the so-called corona. (**B**) The germinal center comprises a mixture of small cleaved cells (centrocytes) and large noncleaved cells (centroblasts). Mitotic figures and apoptotic bodies are readily seen. A tingible-body macrophage is indicated by an arrow.

lymph nodes. They express an immunophenotype of IgM+ IgD−.

In a nonstimulated lymph node, most follicles are primary follicles. Secondary follicles are formed as a reaction to T-cell-dependent antigens. The germinal centers of the secondary follicles comprise a dark zone at the lower pole and a light zone toward the apical pole, where the mantle is thicker (corona) and faces the direction of antigen influx (marginal sinus) (Fig. 2-2A). In the dark zone, there is a higher proportion of large noncleaved cells (centroblasts) and more tingible-body macrophages. In the light zone, there are more small cleaved cells (centrocytes) (Fig. 2-2B). Occasionally, plasma cells can be found within germinal centers.

The Paracortex

The paracortex is the T zone of the lymph node. It is rich in high endothelial venules and populated predominantly by T cells (CD4+ more than CD8+), which are represented by small lymphocytes admixed with occasional immunoblasts (Fig. 2-1). Isolated B lymphocytes and plasma cells are also present. There are scattered S-100 protein-positive antigen-presenting cells (interdigitating reticulum cells and Langerhans cells); these cells possess deeply grooved or irregular contorted nuclei, delicate nuclear membrane, and abundant lightly eosinophilic cytoplasm. Scattered in the paracortex are rare isolated cytokeratin-positive dendritic cells, which cannot be definitively identified on morphologic grounds; they can potentially lead to a mistaken diagnosis of metastatic carcinoma on immunohistochemical evaluation.[20] These cells probably represent a subpopulation of fibroblastic reticulum cells.

Paracortical hyperplasia typically occurs in response to viral infection, hypersensitivity state, or regional tumor. Nodules (T nodules) are sometimes formed (Fig. 2-3), and they closely abut the B-cell follicles, together forming the so-called composite nodules.[17,21,22] High endothe-

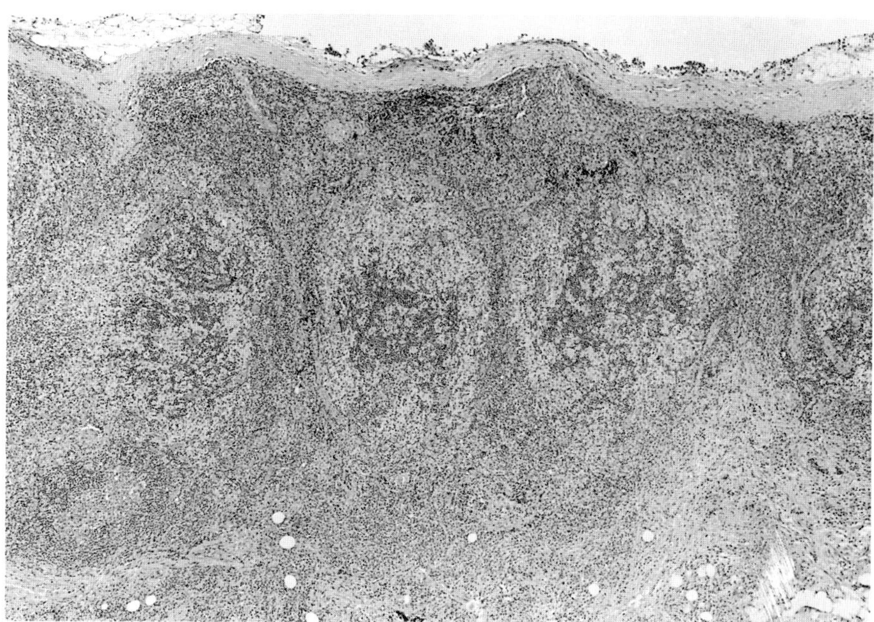

Fig. 2-3. Paracortical hyperplasia with formation of T nodules. The paracortex is expanded, forming pale-staining nodules. A lymphoid follicle is seen in the left lower corner. This node has a slightly thickened fibrous capsule.

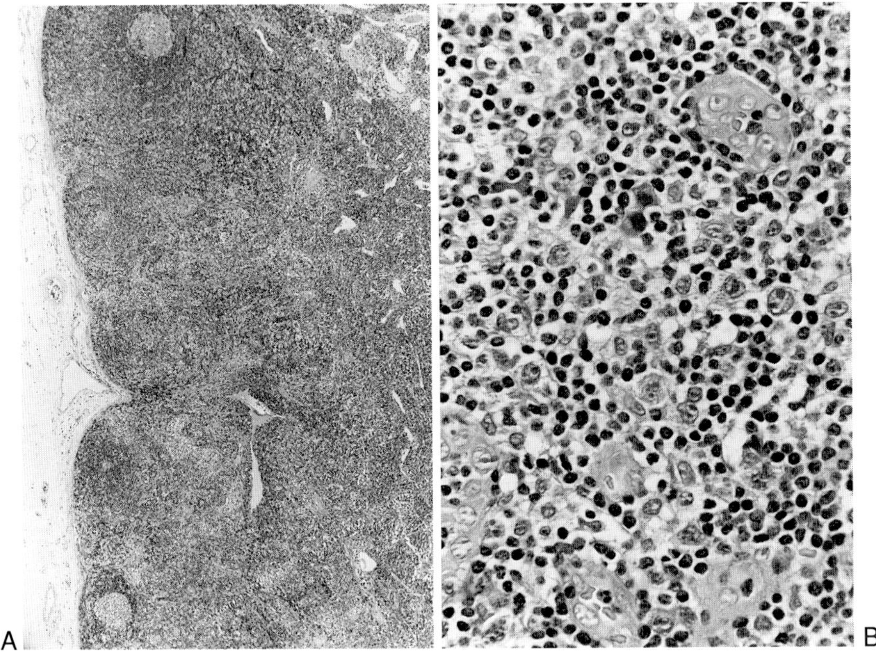

Fig. 2-4. Reactive paracortical hyperplasia, nonspecific. (**A**) The paracortex is markedly expanded, and only two lymphoid follicles are evident in this field. (**B**) The paracortex shows high endothelial venules, small lymphocytes, and interspersed immunoblasts with distinct nucleoli. Essentially there are two populations of lymphoid cells with few or no medium-sized cells.

lial venules are increased, and the lymphoid population consists of a variable mixture of small lymphocytes and immunoblasts (Fig. 2-4). Immunoblasts can occur in such large numbers that malignant lymphoma is mimicked. Most of the lymphoid cells in the paracortex are of T lineage, but there can be some intermixed small and large B cells. S-100 protein-positive interdigitating reticulum cells are also increased.

A distinctive form of paracortical reaction is seen in dermatopathic lymphadenopathy. Although this entity is widely believed to be associated with chronic itchy skin conditions, it is not uncommonly idiopathic or associated with conditions other than cutaneous lesions.[23] In the paracortex, there are irregular or nodular expansions of the paracortex (sometimes referred to as ''tertiary T nodules''), which has a characteristic pale and mottled (alopecia-like) appearance due to an abundance of interdigitating reticulum and Langerhans cells (Fig. 2-5). There are often some intermingled histiocytes with phagocytosed hemosiderin and melanin. The sinuses also show an increase in interdigitating reticulum cells and Langerhans cells. In dermatopathic lymphadenopathy, the increased histiocytes occur predominantly in the nodal parenchyma, contrasting with most other forms of histiocytosis, which usually show a predominant or exclusive sinusoidal distribution.

Medullary Cords

The medullary cords are packed with mature plasma cells. Depending on the plane of sectioning, the medullary cords may be inconspicuous (such as with tangential cutting through the cortex) or prominent (Figs. 2-5A, 2-6). The medullary cords can be expanded in conditions with B-cell reaction, such as reactive follicular hyper-

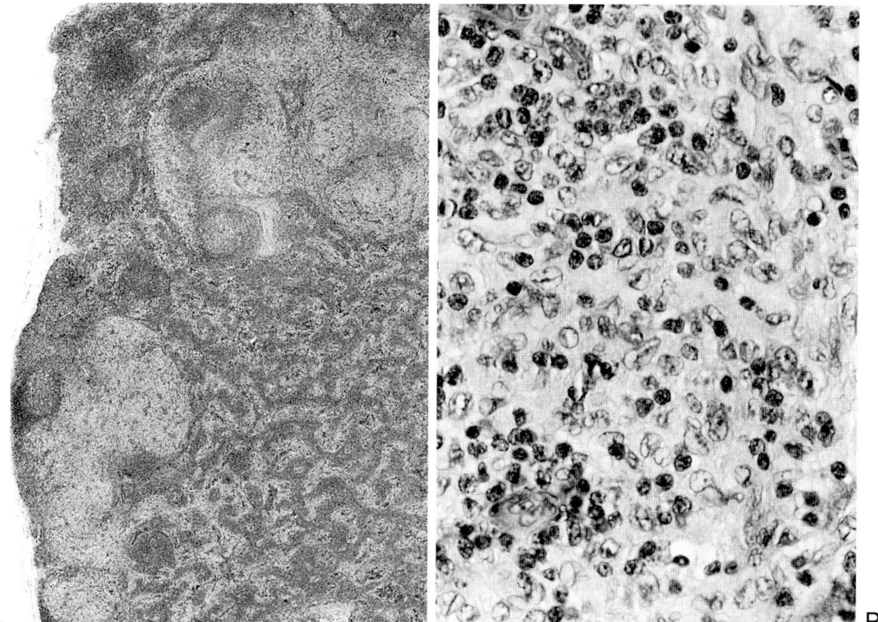

Fig. 2-5. Dermatopathic lymphadenopathy. (**A**) Multiple irregular, light-staining, alopecia-like patches characterize the low magnification appearance of dermatopathic lymphadenopathy. In this plane of section, the medullary cords and sinuses (right lower field) are evident. (**B**) Many interdigitating reticulum or Langerhans cells are seen within the pale foci. These cells have thin nuclear membranes that are grooved or contorted. The chromatin is very fine, and there is an appreciable amount of lightly eosinophilic cytoplasm.

plasia (particularly in association with rheumatoid arthritis) and plasma cell type Castleman's disease.

Sinuses

Multiple afferent lymphatics drain into the lymph node from the convex side. They drain into the subcapsular sinuses, which are connected with an elaborate network of intermediate sinuses and medullary sinuses and then drain out of the node via an efferent lymphatic at the nodal hilum. The sinuses are lined by flat sinus-lining cells probably of an endothelial nature. Some "reticulum cells" may cross the lumen to form a network. The sinuses often contain histiocytes and some lymphoid cells (Fig. 2-6).

Connective Tissue Framework

The lymph node is contained in a thin fibrous capsule, which is in continuity with fibrous trabeculae that penetrate the node. The blood vessels that supply and drain from the lymph node also follow the connective tissue framework. The fibrous trabeculae are normally inconspicuous, but can become prominent in various types of lymphadenopathy with a component of perilymphadenitis and in inflammatory pseudotumor.

SPECIAL CELL TYPES SEEN IN SOME REACTIVE CONDITIONS

Monocytoid B Cells

Monocytoid B cells, previously known as *immature sinus histiocytes,* are medium sized cells that form bands or arcs in the marginal zone around reactive follicles or occur in the sinuses.[24–30] They have indented or notched nuclei with moderately condensed chromatin and an appreciable amount of clear cytoplasm (Fig. 2-7). There may be intermingled isolated larger

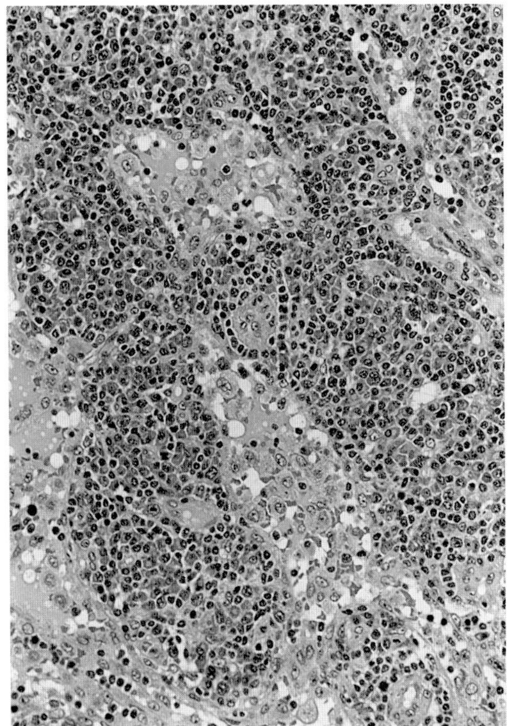

Fig. 2-6. Normal lymph node. The medullary cords, which are packed with plasma cells, are separated by sinuses. Some histiocytes are seen within the latter.

activated cells or neutrophils. Necrosis may occur in the center of the larger clusters. A large cell variant has recently been described, and the cells have rounder nuclei, vesicular chromatin, and more prominent nucleoli.[26]

Monocytoid B cells per se are not pathognomonic of any condition and can be seen in any lymph node showing B-zone reaction (reactive follicular hyperplasia). In a study of 566 consecutive reactive lymph nodes, monocytoid B cells were found in 78 cases (13.8 percent).[26] However, these cells are particularly prominent in the following[24,25,31]:

- Toxoplasmosis
- HIV-associated lymphadenopathy
- Cat scratch disease
- Lymphogranuloma venereum
- Cytomegalovirus lymphadenitis

Monocytoid B cells can be readily highlighted by immunostaining with B-cell markers. It has been suggested that they represent marginal zone cells[28,32] or postgerminal center cells that have not fully matured to marginal zone cells.[33]

When monocytoid B cells appear prominent, distinction between a reactive process and a neoplastic process (monocytoid B-cell lymphoma, which also typically shows patchy nodal involvement) can become difficult. The following features favor a diagnosis of monocytoid B-cell lymphoma over monocytoid B-cell hyperplasia[34]:

1. Monocytoid B cells forming the predominant population in the node
2. Marked confluence of monocytoid B-cell clusters
3. More transformed cells (with prominent nucleoli), higher mitotic rate, and more nuclear irregularities
4. Prominent plasma cell component

The distinction can be further aided by demonstration of light chain restriction by immunohistochemistry or in situ hybridization.[34,35]

Plasmacytoid Monocytes

Plasmacytoid monocytes, previously known as *plasmacytoid T cells* or *T-associated plasma cells,* can be identified on morphologic grounds in various types of reactive lymph nodes (10 to 17 percent of all nonspecific lymphadenopathies), but they are particularly common in the hyaline vascular type Castleman's disease and Kikuchi's lymphadenitis.[36–43] With the help of immunohistochemical techniques (such as MT1/CD43, LN2/CD74, and KP1/CD68), they can be detected in up to 87 percent of reactive lymph nodes.[36] It has been suggested that they represent precursors of epithelioid histiocytes.[44,45]

Plasmacytoid monocytes can be recognized as small, violaceous clusters in the paracortex, although they can also be individually dispersed (Fig. 2-8A). The cells are medium sized, with eccentrically placed round nuclei, moderately condensed chromatin, and a moderate amount of amphophilic cytoplasm. There are typically interspersed apoptotic cells, which may be ingested by macrophages (tingible-body macro-

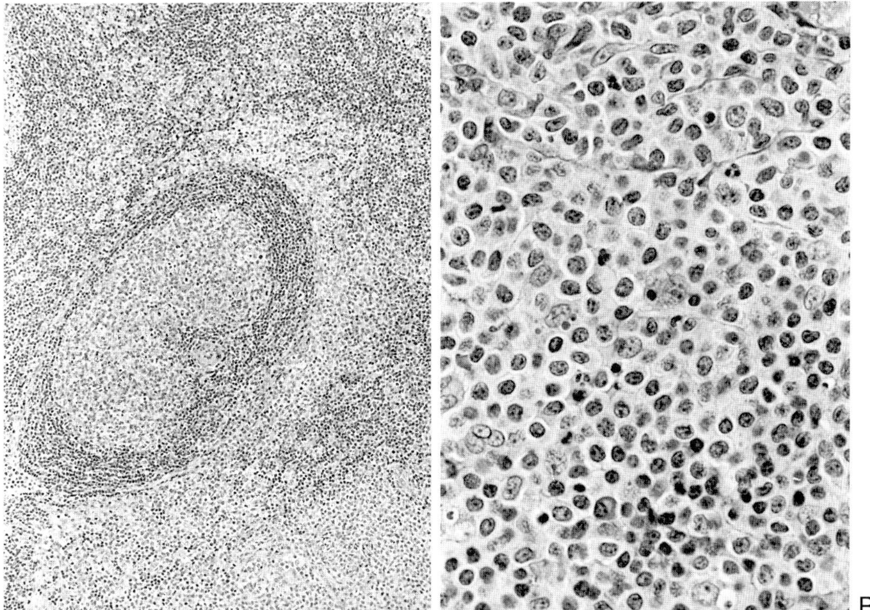

Fig. 2-7. Monocytoid B cell reaction. (**A**) Monocytoid B cells typically form pale-staining arcs around reactive follicles. (**B**) The monocytoid B cells are medium sized and possess slightly indented or notched nuclei. There can be occasional intermingled activated large cells.

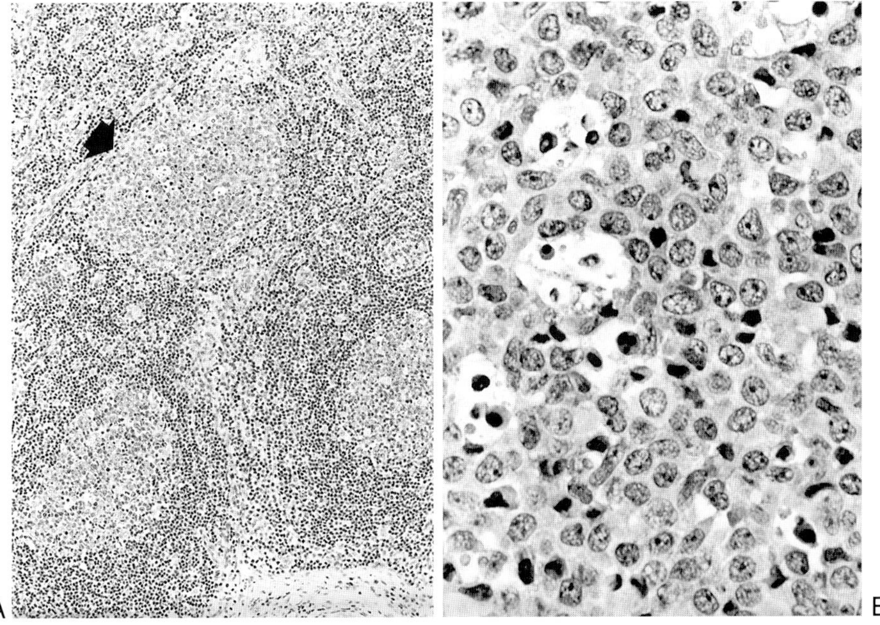

Fig. 2-8. Plasmacytoid monocytes in nonspecific lymphoid hyperplasia. (**A**) A discrete cluster of plasmacytoid monocytes is indicated by an arrow. In hematoxylin-eosin stained sections, these clusters have a violaceous quality. Contrast with the two lymphoid follicles in the lower field. (**B**) The plasmacytoid monocytes are medium-sized cells with round nuclei, somewhat granular but not very coarse chromatin, and a moderate amount of eccentrically placed cytoplasm. Apoptotic bodies are typically abundant.

phages) (Fig. 2-8B). The typical immunophenotype is CD2− CD3− CD4+ CD5− CD7− CD8− CD36+ CD43+ CD45RA+ CD68+ CD74+.[36,38–40,46–51] Although plasmacytoid monocytes are now widely believed to belong to the myelomonocytic series,[48] some authors consider them to be possible sessile terminally differentiated T cells.[52]

Plasmacytoid monocytes show a superficial resemblance to plasma cells, but can be distinguished by their higher nuclear-cytoplasmic ratio, lack of "clock face" condensed chromatin, and absence of a pale Golgi zone.

Polykaryocytes

Polykaryocytes, also known as *Warthin-Finkeldey giant cells,* are cells with multiple (4 to 60) nuclei clustered together in a grape-like pattern. The individual nuclei are round to ovoid, with clear chromatin and a small distinct nucleolus. Cytoplasm is scanty (Fig. 2-9). The nuclei may appear degenerated.[53,54] These cells commonly occur in the germinal centers,[54] although they can occur in the paracortex (found adjacent to venules) (Fig. 2-10).[53–55] They are particularly common in the following types of benign lymphadenopathies[53,54,56]:

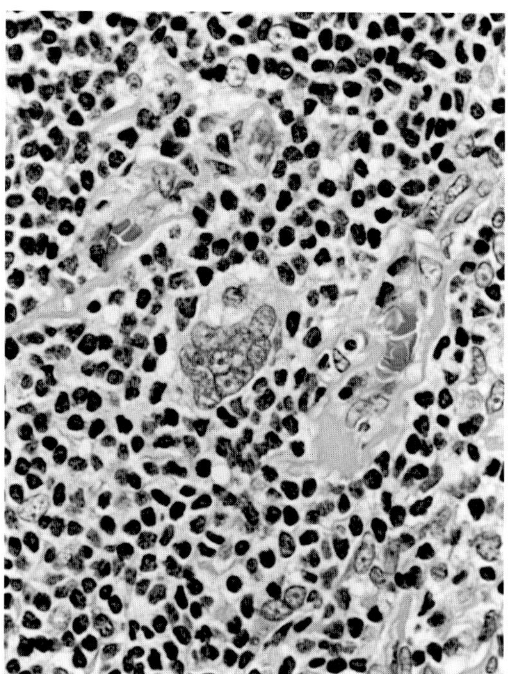

Fig. 2-10. Kimura's disease lymphadenopathy. A polykaryocyte is seen in the paracortex adjacent to the venules.

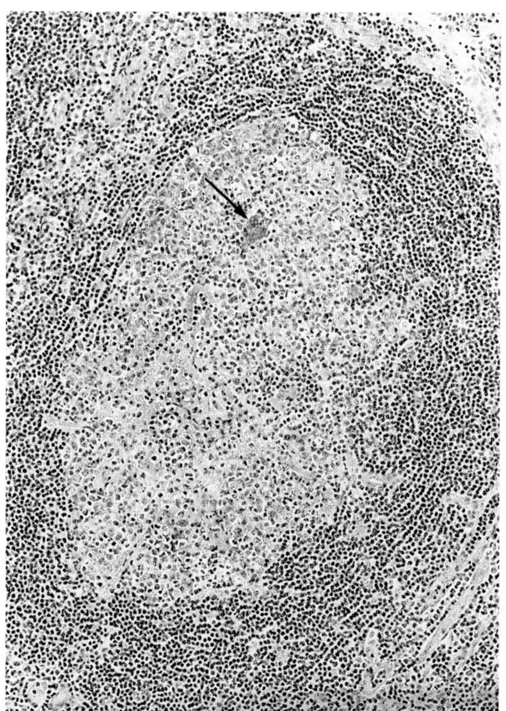

Fig. 2-9. Kimura's disease lymphadenopathy. This lymphoid follicle is penetrated by small venules and infiltrated by eosinophils. A polykaryocyte (*arrow*) is seen in the germinal center; this is a common phenomenon in this condition.

- HIV-associated lymphadenopathy
- Kimura's disease lymphadenopathy
- Measles infection

Their exact lineage is uncertain, although we suspect that some may represent fused follicular dendritic cells and others fused endothelial cells. One recent study on three cases demonstrated a T-cell immunophenotype (CD3+ CD43+ OPD4+) in the polykaryocytes, but the cells were located exclusively in the paracortex.[55]

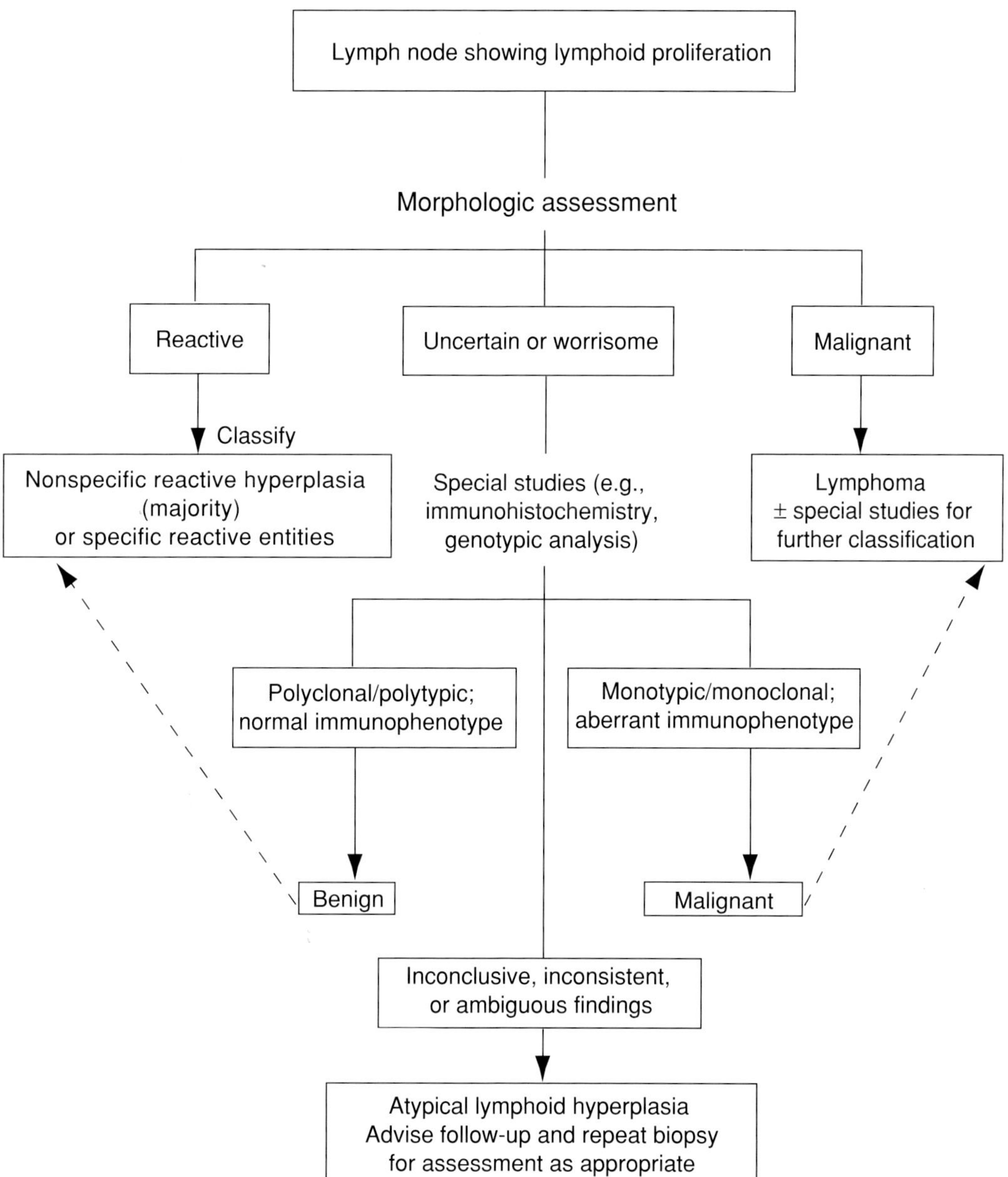

Fig. 2-11. Diagnostic approach to a lymphoid proliferation in a lymph node.

PRACTICAL APPROACH TO DIAGNOSIS OF REACTIVE LYMPHADENOPATHIES

The following questions should be asked when one evaluates a lymph node (Fig. 2-11): What is the major pattern? Are the changes indicative of a reactive or malignant process? If reactive, do the changes fall into a specific diagnostic category?

Patterns of Reaction in the Lymph Node and How Often a Specific Diagnosis Can Be Made

The major groups of reactive lymphadenopathies include (1) infective, (2) autoimmune, (3) hypersensitivity and iatrogenic, and (4) idiopathic. The various entities are listed in Table 2-1 according to the major pattern of reaction.[2,9,10,57–59]

Since there are only limited ways the lymphoid system can respond to stimuli or insults, it is sometimes frustrating that a more specific diagnosis cannot be made on lymph node biopsies. In a consecutive series of 186 patients with reactive lymphadenopathies studied by Pangalis et al.,[60] a specific diagnosis could be reached in 36.6 percent of cases (toxoplasmosis, 14 percent; infectious mononucleosis, 9.7 percent; tuberculosis, 8.6 percent; Kikuchi's lymphadenitis, 1.6 percent; others, 2.7 percent). In our experience, a specific diagnosis can be reached in 20 to 30 percent of all lymph node biopsies showing reactive changes. In places where infectious diseases (such as tuberculosis)

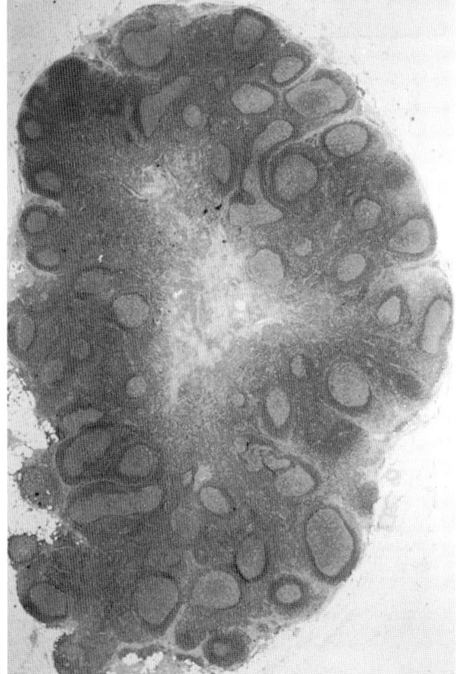

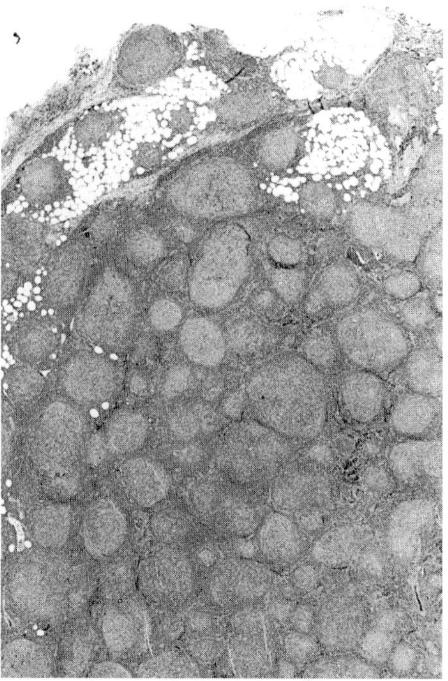

Fig. 2-12. Reactive follicular hyperplasia (rheumatoid arthritis) contrasted with follicular lymphoma. (**A**) In reactive follicular hyperplasia, the follicles are characteristically surrounded by discrete mantles and separated by an appreciable amount of interfollicular tissue. The follicles often vary in size and shape. (**B**) In a typical example of follicular lymphoma, the follicles are arranged in a back-to-back pattern. Mantles are indistinct, and there is scarcely any interfollicular tissue. The presence of many follicles in the perinodal fat also strongly favors a diagnosis of lymphoma over reactive hyperplasia.

Table 2-1. Major Forms of Reactive Lymphadenopathies Classified According to Pattern and Their Differential Diagnoses

Major Pattern	Reactive Lymphadenopathies	Neoplastic Hematolymphoid Proliferations to Consider in the Differential Diagnoses
Follicular (nodular)	Reactive follicular hyperplasia Nonspecific Specific entities (such as toxoplasmosis, syphilis, CMV infection, rheumatoid arthritis, plasma cell type of Castleman's disease, Kimura's disease, *Yersinia* infection, reaction to regional tumor, early phase of suppurative granulomatous lymphadenitis) HIV-associated lymphadenopathy Progressive transformation of germinal centers Castleman's disease, hyaline-vascular type Mantle zone hyperplasia	Follicular lymphoma Mantle cell lymphoma with nodular pattern Marginal zone cell lymphoma with follicular colonization Other types of non-Hodgkin's lymphoma (rare) Hodgkin's disease Nodular lymphocyte predominance Nodular sclerosis
Interfollicular or diffuse increase in large lymphoid cells	Reactive paracortical hyperplasia, nonspecific (including reaction to tumor in the drainage area) Interfollicular Hodgkinoid lymphadenitis Kikuchi's lymphadenitis Viral infection (e.g., EBV [infectious mononucleosis], herpes zoster, herpes simplex) Reactive immunoblastic proliferation (e.g., postvaccinial, drug hypersensitivity) Angioimmunoblastic lymphadenopathy	Post-thymic T-cell lymphoma Diffuse large B-cell lymphoma, including T-cell-rich large B-cell lymphoma Post-transplant lymphoproliferative disorder
Parenchymal histiocytic reaction, including granuloma formation	Granulomatous lymphadenitis[a] Tuberculosis and other infections (e.g., brucellosis, fungal infection, localized *Leishmania* lymphadenitis)[58,59] Sarcoidosis Berylliosis Crohn's disease, primary biliary cirrhosis Idiopathic (including reaction to tumors) Suppurative granulomatous lymphadenitis Cat scratch disease Lymphogranuloma venereum *Yersinia* infection Tularemia Fungal infection Atypical mycobacterial infection Chronic granulomatous disease of childhood Lepromatous leprosy lymphadenopathy *Mycobacterium avium-intracellulare* lymphadenitis Typhoid fever Dermatopathic lymphadenopathy Toxoplasmosis	Hodgkin's disease Lennert's T-cell lymphoma Other forms of lymphoma with prominent epithelioid histiocytic reaction Burkitt's lymphoma associated with necrotizing epithelioid granulomas Langerhans cell histiocytosis
Prominent necrosis	Infarction of lymph node Kikuchi's lymphadenitis Lupus erythematosus Kawasaki's disease Granulomatous lymphadenitis with necrosis (see above) Suppurative granulomatous lymphadenitis (see above) *Pneumocystis carinii* lymphadenitis	Lymphoma complicated by infarction Various types of lymphoma with focal necrosis Post-transplant lymphoproliferative disorders

Continued

Table 2-1. *(continued)*

Major Pattern	Reactive Lymphadenopathies	Neoplastic Hematolymphoid Proliferations to Consider in the Differential Diagnoses
Hypocellular appearance or lymphocyte depletion	HIV-associated lymphadenopathy (late phase) Reactive hemophagocytic syndrome Primary immunodeficiencies Angioimmunoblastic lymphadenopathy Vascular transformation of sinuses (some cases) Segmental infarction of lymph node Proteinaceous lymphadenopathy	Hodgkin's disease, lymphocyte depletion type and some cases of nodular sclerosis
Sinusoidal expansion	Sinus histiocytosis, nonspecific Sinus histiocytosis in reaction to tumor in the draining area Sinus histiocytosis with massive lymphadenopathy Reactive hemophagocytic syndrome Lymphangiogram effects Histiocytic reaction against foreign materials Whipple's disease lymphadenopathy Storage disease (e.g., Gaucher's disease, Niemann-Pick disease) Vascular transformation of sinuses Monocytoid B-cell hyperplasia (always invariably in combination with reactive follicular hyperplasia)	Malignant lymphoma (e.g., anaplastic large cell lymphoma, large cell lymphoma) Langerhans cell histiocytosis
Broadening of connective tissue framework	Perilymphadenitis (various causes) Inflammatory pseudotumor	Kaposi sarcoma

[a] Small granulomas are common in luetic lymphadenitis and HIV-associated lymphadenopathy, but they are not a major feature.

are prevalent, a specific diagnosis can probably be made in a higher proportion of reactive nodes.

Since there is no specific treatment for most forms of reactive lymphadenopathy, even a ''nonspecific'' diagnosis is helpful, because the main aim is to exclude a malignant process and treatable causes (in particular infection). The diagnostic label that can be applied in such circumstances depends on the most salient pattern of reaction observed:

- Reactive follicular hyperplasia (Fig. 2-12)
- Reactive paracortical hyperplasia (Fig. 2-4)
- Sinus histiocytosis (Fig. 2-13)
- Reactive lymphoid hyperplasia (for lymph nodes showing a mixed pattern of reaction, although the individual components present can be further mentioned) (Fig. 2-14)

Is This Lymphoid Proliferation Benign or Malignant?

Distinction between reactive lymphadenopathies and malignant lymphoma can range from very easy to very difficult. It is most important to have good quality histologic materials for assessment. Many mistakes in interpretation are committed because of the suboptimal quality of the histologic sections. If the tissue has not been well fixed or well processed, the following methods can improve the quality of the histologic sections, especially when coupled with cutting thin sections (less than 4 μm) to facilitate cytologic assessment:

1. Re-process the tissue after re-fixation in B5 solution[61]

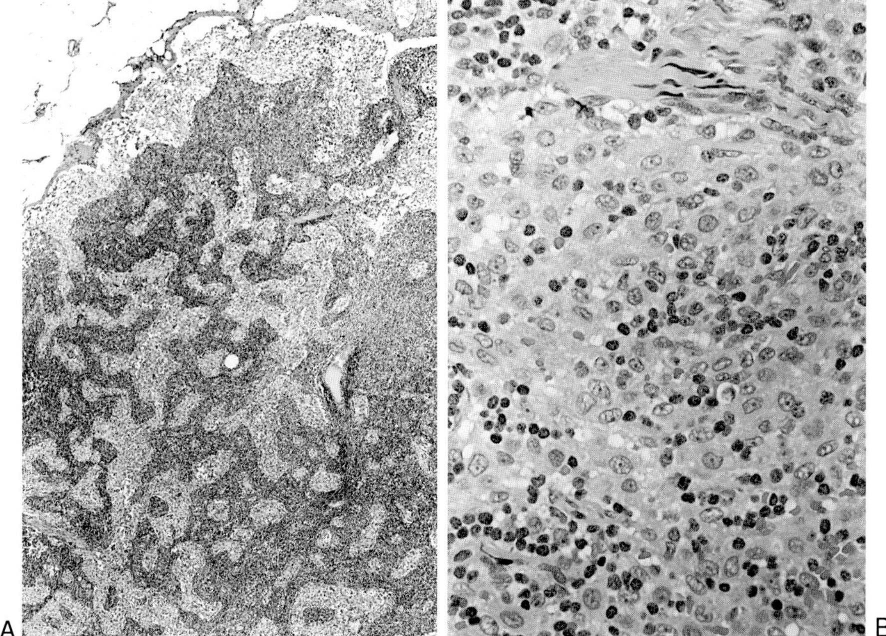

Fig. 2-13. Sinus histiocytosis, nonspecific. (**A**) The sinuses are distended with light-staining histiocytes. (**B**) The histiocytes differ from lymphoid cells in having delicate nuclear membrane, fine chromatin, and abundant cytoplasm.

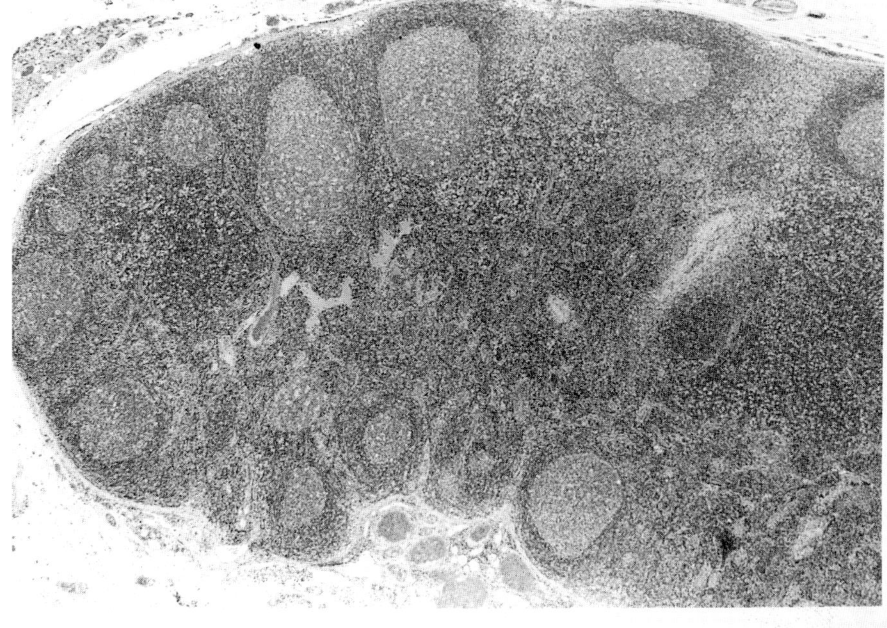

Fig. 2-14. Reactive lymphoid hyperplasia, nonspecific. This node shows a mixed pattern of reaction, with reactive follicles and an expanded paracortex. The follicles exhibit a starry-sky pattern and polarity, and the paracortex has a mottled appearance.

2. Cut paraffin sections from the incompletely fixed blocks, rehydrate, and then further fix in alcohol-acid-formalin fixative before staining[62]
3. Re-embed tissue in resin[63]

There are no simple criteria for distinction between reactive and malignant lymphoid proliferation. The criteria to be applied depend on the major pattern of reaction (see below). As a generalization, a reactive process usually

- Shows preserved (albeit sometimes distorted) architecture, with intact sinuses, reactive follicles, and a paracortical component (Figs. 2-13 through 2-15)
- Does not form any discrete expansile mass within the node
- Exhibits a mixture of lymphoid cell types (Fig. 2-4B)
- Lacks cellular atypia (i.e., not deviating from the appearances of the normal and reactive cells described above); presence of a significant population of cells with medium-sized nuclei, markedly folded nuclear membrane, abnormal granular chromatin, or clear cytoplasm usually suggests a diagnosis of lymphoma (Figs. 2-4, 2-16)

Exceptions to each of these ''rules,'' however, can occur. In difficult cases, ancillary studies can be very helpful (Table 2-2).[64–66]

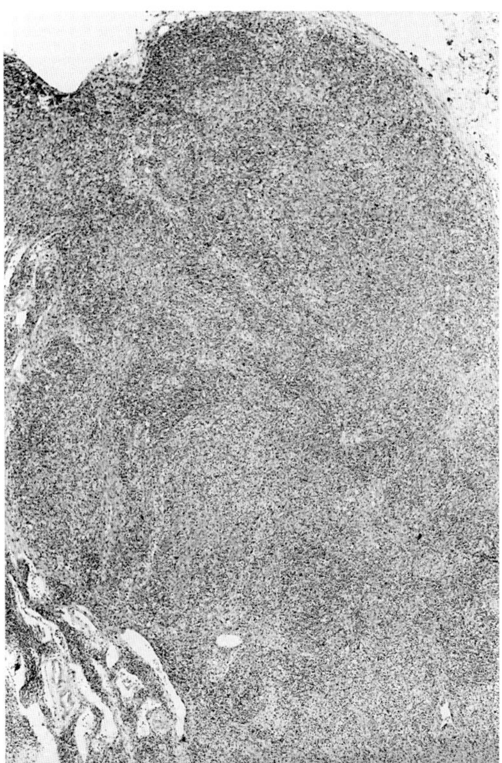

Fig. 2-15. Infectious mononucleosis. Despite marked expansion of the paracortex by large lymphoid cells (pale-staining areas), the presence of residual nodal architecture (sinuses in the left lower field) should at least lead one to consider the possibility of a benign process.

Distinction Between Reactive Follicular Hyperplasia and Follicular Lymphoma

It can be difficult to distinguish between florid reactive hyperplasia and follicular lymphoma. The most important criterion is the *architectural arrangement of the follicles at low magnification.* A pattern of back-to-back follicles disposed throughout the entire nodal parenchyma, with little interfollicular tissue, is diagnostic of follicular lymphoma (a pattern evident in 85 percent of all cases).[15,66,67] In contrast, the follicles in reactive follicular hyperplasia are characterized by the following features (Figs. 2-12 and 2-17 through 2-20).

- Discrete and well separated by at least some interfollicular lymphoid tissue
- Often variable in size and shape (not uncommonly dumbbell or serpentine)
- Well-defined mantles
- A heterogeneous population of follicular center cells (large cells often outnumbering small cells, especially for the large follicles) that are mitotically active and lack dysplastic features
- Interspersed tingible-body macrophages
- Cellular polarization seen in at least some follicles

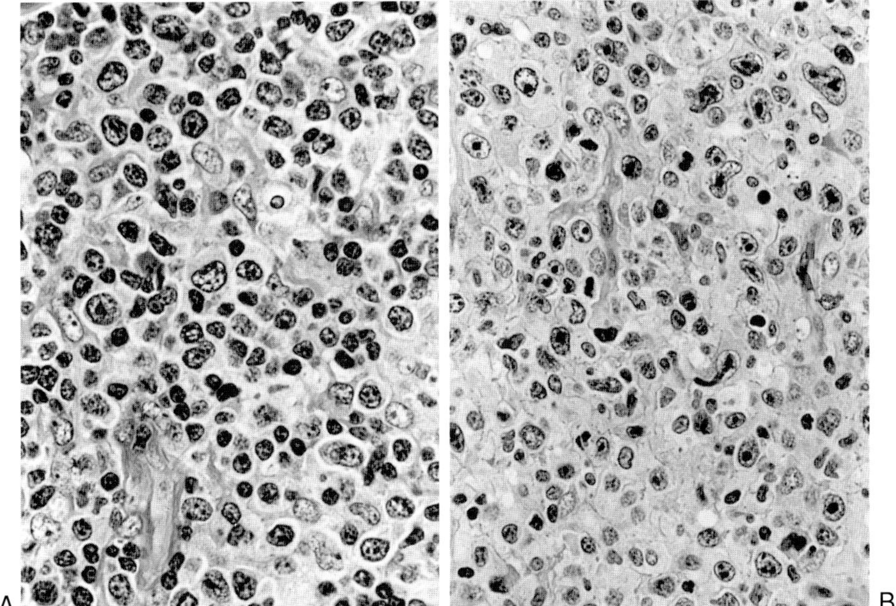

Fig. 2-16. Post-thymic T-cell lymphoma, illustrating atypia of the lymphoid cells. (**A**) There are many medium-sized and some large cells with coarse to granular chromatin. Some cells with clear cytoplasm are also evident. (**B**) In this example, the lymphoid cells show a continuous range of size rather than two distinct populations. Many have markedly folded nuclear membranes. Contrast with Fig. 2-4.

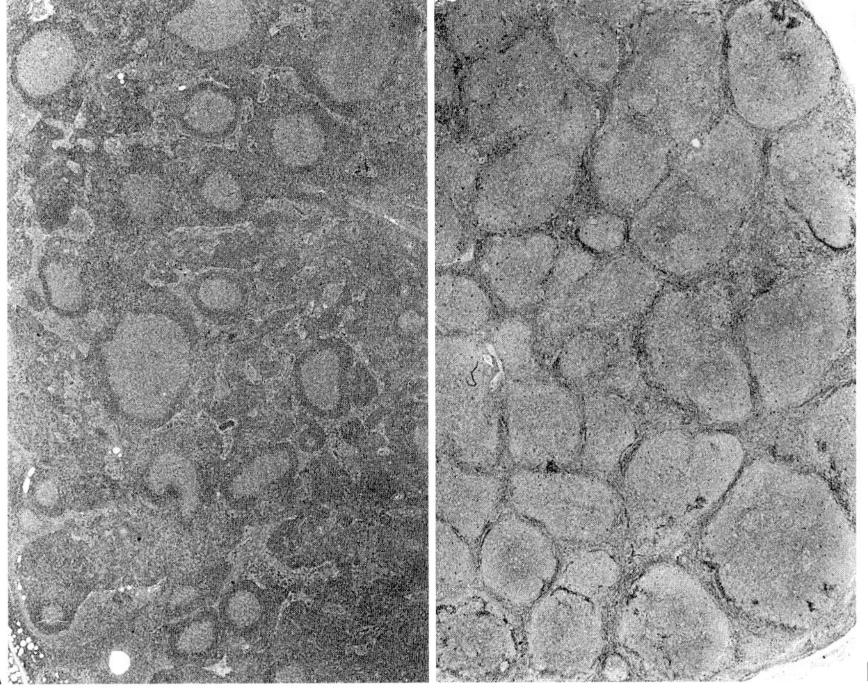

Fig. 2-17. Reactive follicular hyperplasia, nonspecific, contrasted with follicular lymphoma. (**A**) Note the discrete mantles in reactive follicular hyperplasia. The intervening sinuses are patent. (**B**) In this follicular lymphoma, the follicles are very closely packed.

Table 2-2. Special Studies for Distinguishing Between Neoplastic Versus Reactive Lymphoid Proliferations

Special Study	B-Cell Proliferation	T-Cell Proliferation
Demonstration of abnormal lymphocyte subsets	Immunohistochemical demonstration Ig light chain restriction favors a diagnosis of lymphoma. Normal $\kappa:\lambda$ ratio is 2:1 to 3:1. It has been suggested stringent criteria should be used to define light chain restriction (ratio >10:1 or >1:10) in order to avoid false positivity. Difficulties in interpretation of Ig immunostaining due to interstitial staining or passive absorption can sometimes be solved by using in situ hybridization to demonstrate light chain mRNA	Simple predominance of CD4+ or CD8+ cells in a T-cell proliferation cannot be taken as evidence of monoclonality. However, an aberrant immunophenotype of CD4+ CD8+ or CD4−CD8− in a mature T-cell proliferation supports a diagnosis of lymphoma
Aberrant immunophenotype	Aberrant B-cell immunophenotype, as evidenced by simultaneous staining for specific B-lineage markers (such as CD19, CD20, CD22, or CD79a) and markers not usually expressed in B cells (such as CD5 and CD43), supports a diagnosis of lymphoma	An anomalous T-cell immunophenotype, such as loss of pan-T markers (CD2, CD3, CD5, CD7 or α/β-TCR) or expression of CD56 in the majority of cells, supports a diagnosis of lymphoma. Loss of CD7 has to be interpreted with caution because subsets of normal T cells do not express CD7
Immature immunophenotype	Presence of large numbers of B cells with an immature phenotype (TdT+) favors a diagnosis of lymphoma (precursor B-cell lymphoblastic lymphoma/leukemia)	Outside the setting of the thymus or thymoma, a T-cell proliferation showing expression of precursor T-cell phenotype (TdT+ or CD1a+) represents a neoplastic rather than reactive process.
Abnormal immunoarchitecture	Diffuse sheets of B cells without any nodular architecture suggests a neoplastic rather than reactive process	Not applicable
Genotypic analysis by Southern blot technique or polymerase chain reaction	Demonstration of clonally rearranged Ig gene or rearranged oncogene supports a diagnosis of lymphoma	Demonstration of clonally rearranged TCR gene supports a diagnosis of lymphoma

- Follicle formation in perinodal tissue very rare

Some caveats have to be mentioned. Cellular polarization may not be evident even in reactive follicles; this may be attributable to the plane of sectioning. Mantles can be deficient in reactive follicles, in particular florid reactive hyperplasia in childhood and HIV-associated lymphadenopathy (Figs. 2-21, 2-22). On the other hand, some cases of follicular lymphoma can have thick mantles. Although reactive follicles are typically rich in large noncleaved cells (centroblasts) and are almost never predominated by small cleaved cells (centrocytes), the reactive follicle centers in rheumatoid arthritis lymphadenopathy can be paradoxically predominated by small cleaved cells (centrocytes), with few mitotic figures and few tingible-body macrophages.[68] Some cases of follicular lymphoma can exhibit an appreciable number of tingible-body macrophages. Thus, all features have to be integrated before reaching a conclusion.

Histologic assessment should be made in the well preserved portions of the specimen. In suboptimally fixed tissues (especially the central portion), even reactive follicles can appear worrisome because cellular polarization, lymphocytic mantles, and tingible-body macrophages often become inapparent, and the cellular shrinkage imparts an erroneous impression of small cleaved cell predominance (Fig. 2-23).

Besides histologic features, age of the patient is an important consideration. Since follicular

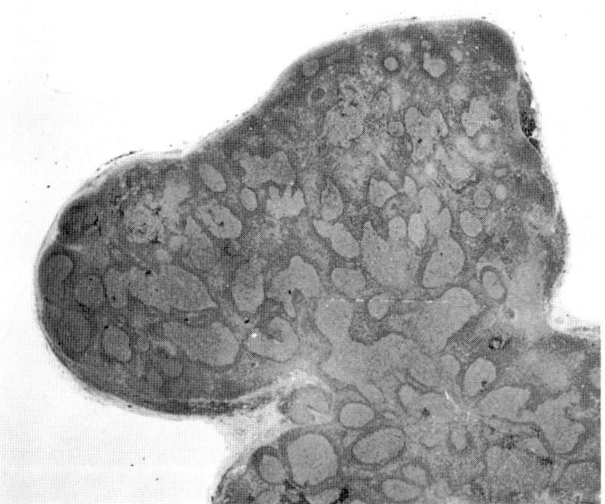

Fig. 2-18. Reactive follicular hyperplasia, nonspecific. The follicles not uncommonly assume irregular or bizarre contours. Note the discrete, albeit thin, mantles. A starry-sky pattern, imparted by the tingible-body macrophages, can be appreciated in some follicles.

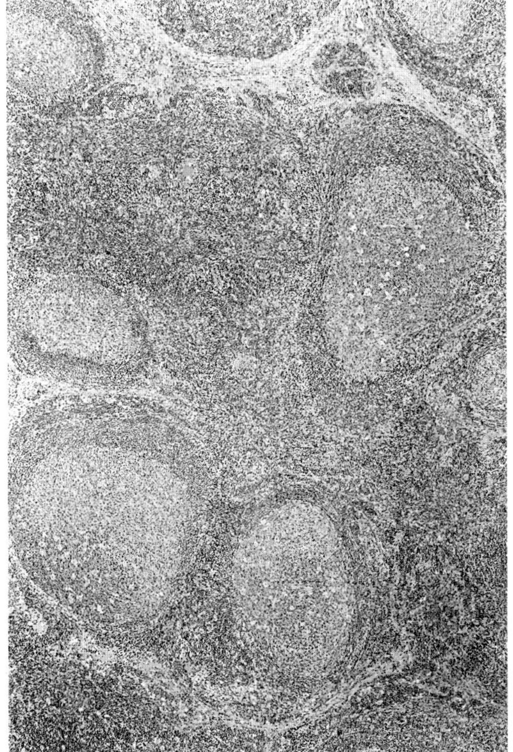

Fig. 2-19. Reactive follicular hyperplasia, nonspecific. The mantles are well developed. The tingible-body macrophages and polarity of the germinal centers are evident.

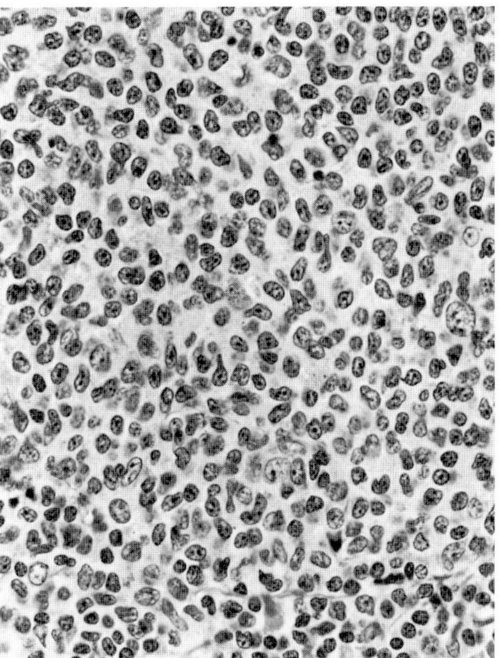

Fig. 2-20. Follicular lymphoma. The follicles comprise predominantly small cleaved cells (centrocytes) with no or few tingible-body macrophages. This cellular composition strongly favors a diagnosis of follicular lymphoma over reactive follicular hyperplasia. Compare with Fig. 2-2.

lymphoma is extremely rare below the age of 20 years, this diagnosis should be made with utmost caution and only with support by ancillary techniques.

Should there be any uncertainty, the following special studies are helpful in supporting a diagnosis of reactive follicular hyperplasia versus follicular lymphoma[15,66,69–78]:

- Immunohistochemical staining

  Lack of staining of the germinal center cells for bcl-2 protein (Fig. 2-24). In the germinal centers of reactive follicles, there can be small numbers of bcl-2-positive cells (mostly intrafollicular T cells). Follicular lymphoma is usually, but not invariably, bcl-2 positive. A potential pitfall in interpretation is that reactive lymphoid follicles can occasionally harbor an appreciable number of T lymphocytes, leading to a false

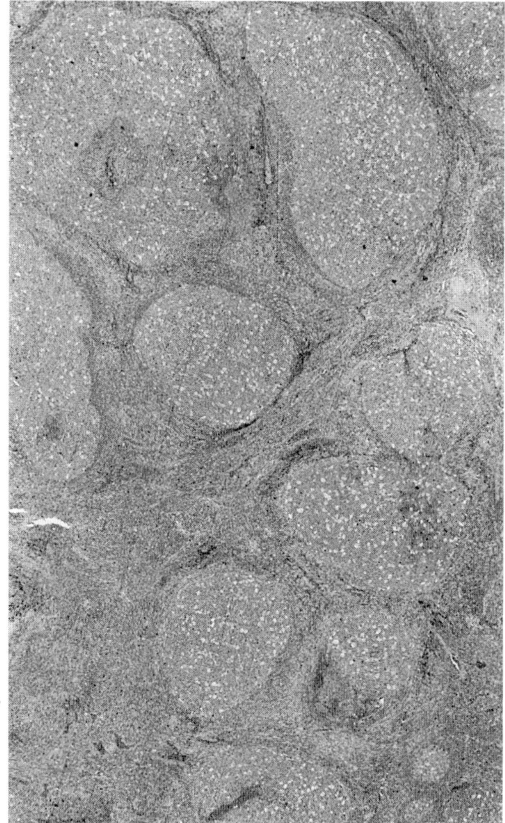

Fig. 2-21. Reactive follicular hyperplasia occurring in a child. In children, the reactive follicles are not uncommonly deficient in mantles. The benign nature of the process is suggested by the young age of the patient, prominent tingible-body macrophages, and presence of polarity (not evident in this field).

positive interpretation of staining: comparison with a corresponding section stained with a T-cell marker should obviate such a problem

Lack of staining of the germinal center cells with MT2

Polytypic staining for Ig light chain, often in a network pattern rather than discrete membrane staining of the follicular center cells. It is preferably performed on frozen tissues

Polarity as accentuated by immunostaining with MIB1 (Ki-67). In reactive follicles, a high proportion of the germinal center cells stain with proliferation markers, and there is a larger number of positive cells in the dark zone[78a]

- In situ hybridization for Ig mRNA to show polytypia
- Genotypic studies (Southern blot or polymerase chain reaction)

  Lack of immunoglobulin (Ig) gene rearrangement

  Lack of *bcl*-2 gene rearrangement

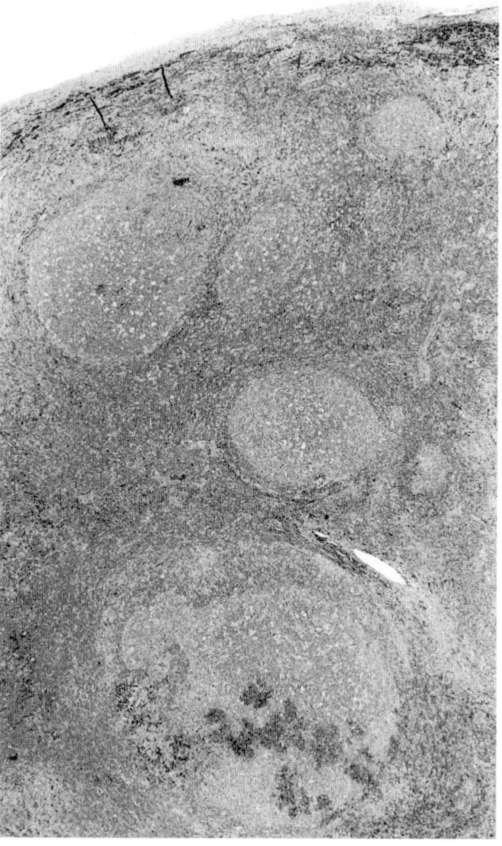

Fig. 2-22. HIV-associated lymphadenopathy. The follicles are typically deficient in mantles, but their reactive nature is betrayed by the presence of polarity and tingible-body macrophages (starry-sky appearance). The follicle in the lower field shows follicle lysis, with hemorrhage in the germinal center. Of further note is the thickened capsule on top, which on higher magnification reveals early Kaposi sarcoma. This combination of features is virtually pathognomonic of HIV-associated lymphadenopathy.

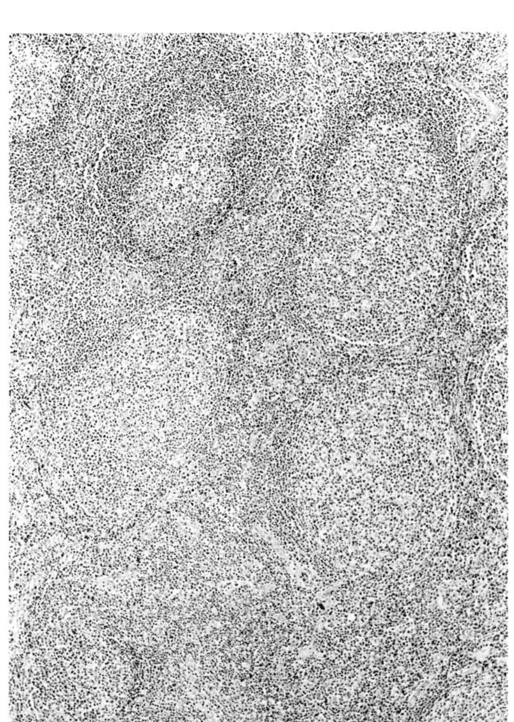

Fig. 2-23. Reactive follicular hyperplasia, nonspecific. Because of poor fixation, the follicles strongly mimic those seen in follicular lymphoma. Mantles appear to be deficient because the mantle cells fall apart and therefore do not appear well demarcated from the interfollicular small lymphocytes. Tingible-body macrophages appear less prominent, and polarity is often not seen. Examination of the follicles at the periphery of the specimen (where fixation is better and shown in the upper field) can be helpful to suggest that this is a benign process.

Distinction of Reactive Paracortical Hyperplasia from Malignant Lymphoma

In cases showing paracortical expansion with increase of large cells, the differential diagnosis would include reactive paracortical hyperplasia (including interfollicular Hodgkinoid lymphadenitis), post-thymic T-cell lymphoma, T-cell-rich large B-cell lymphoma, and Hodgkin's disease. The morphologic features favoring a benign process in this situation are

- No erosion of the mantles or germinal centers of the residual follicles (Fig. 2-25)
- The cellular proliferation comprises two distinct populations: small lymphocytes and large activated cells that lack atypical features such as marked irregular foldings or coarsely granular chromatin, rather than a continuous range of cell sizes (including medium sized cells)
- Absence of clear cells

In some instances of reactive paracortical hyperplasia, the proliferated cells are predominated by a fairly monotonous population of small lymphocytes with few admixed immunoblasts (Fig.

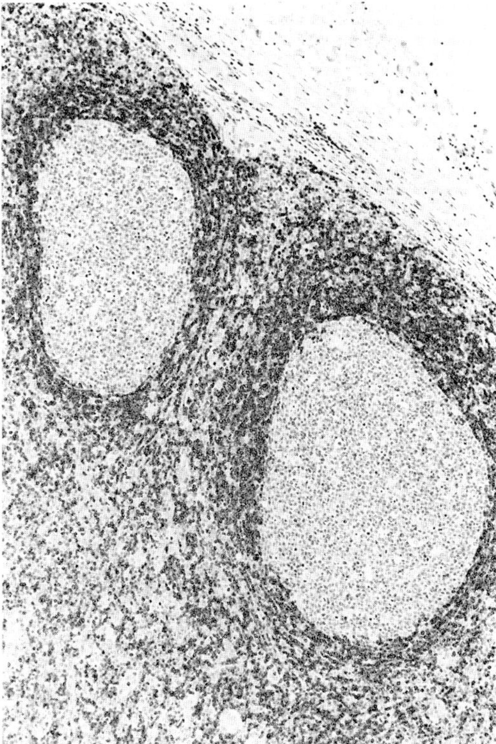

Fig. 2-24. Reactive follicular hyperplasia. Immunostaining with bcl-2 antibody shows that few or no cells within the germinal centers are positive. The mantle zone and interfollicular lymphocytes are typically positive.

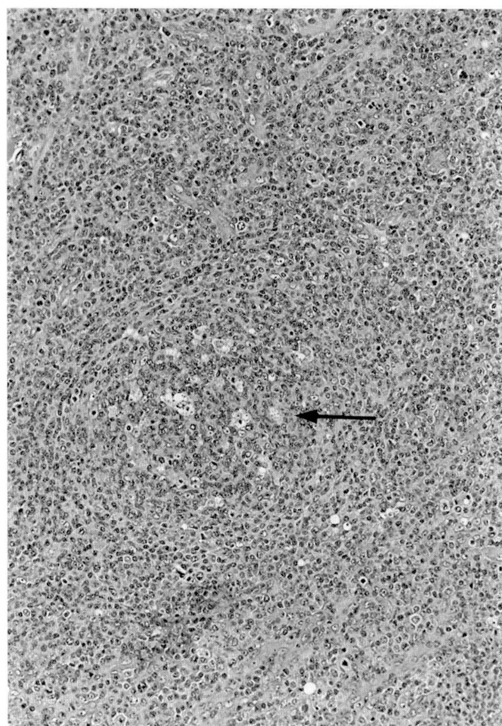

Fig. 2-25. Post-thymic T-cell lymphoma. The lymphoid infiltrate obliterates the preexisting lymphoid follicle, with erosion of its mantle (*arrow*). This feature is virtually never seen in reactive lymphoid hyperplasia.

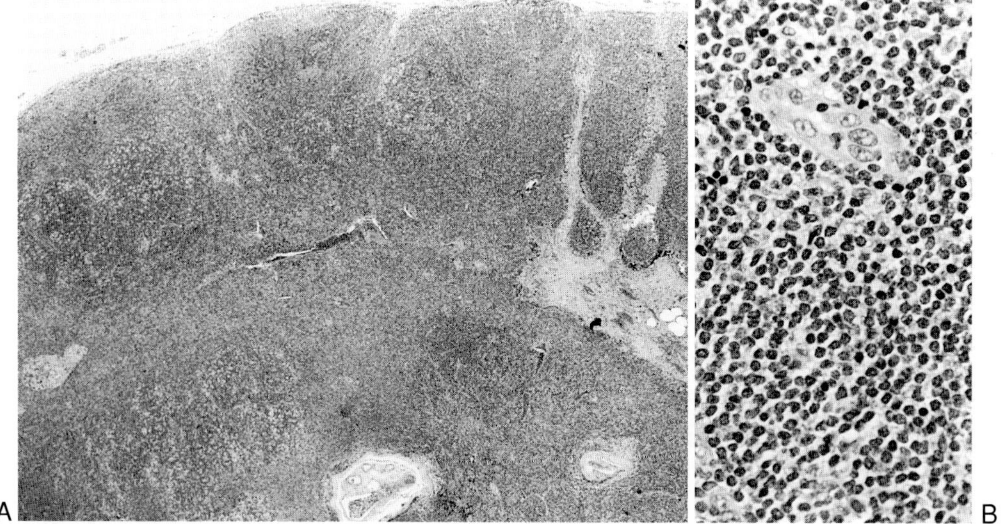

Fig. 2-26. Reactive paracortical hyperplasia, nonspecific. (**A**) There is marked expansion of the paracortex. (**B**) This unusual example is predominated by small lymphocytes with few activated cells.

2-26). This can potentially be mistaken for a small cell lymphoma. The clues to its benign nature are the normal appearances of the small lymphocytes (small round nuclei with at most mildly irregular foldings and dense chromatin) and lack of destructive growth pattern.

Distinction of Reactive Immunoblastic Proliferation from Diffuse Large Cell Lymphoma

For a lymphoid proliferation that is predominated by large activated lymphoid cells, the prototype of which is infectious mononucleosis, distinction between a reactive immunoblastic proliferation and diffuse large cell lymphoma can be exceedingly difficult (Fig. 2-27). There

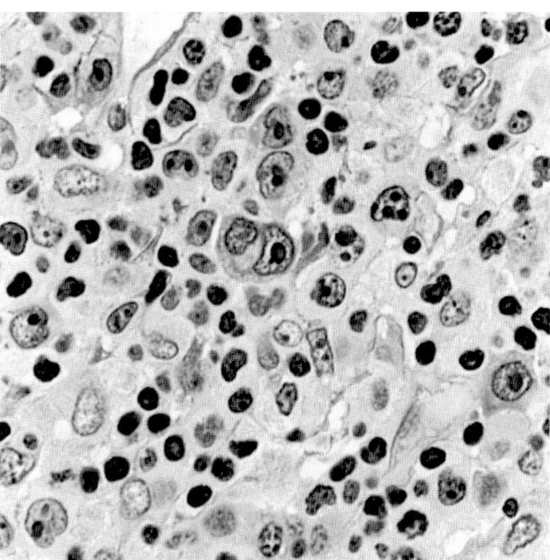

Fig. 2-28. Infectious mononucleosis. It is not uncommon to find binucleated cells (center of field) in this condition. These large cells may be mistaken for Reed-Sternberg cells by virtue of the prominent nucleoli.

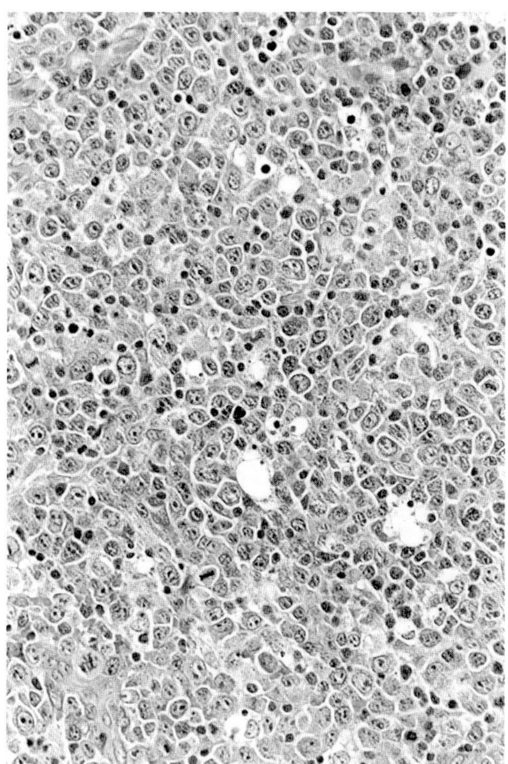

Fig. 2-27. Infectious mononucleosis. The presence of large lymphoid cells in sheets would certainly invite a misdiagnosis of malignant lymphoma. These cells, however, lack significant atypia.

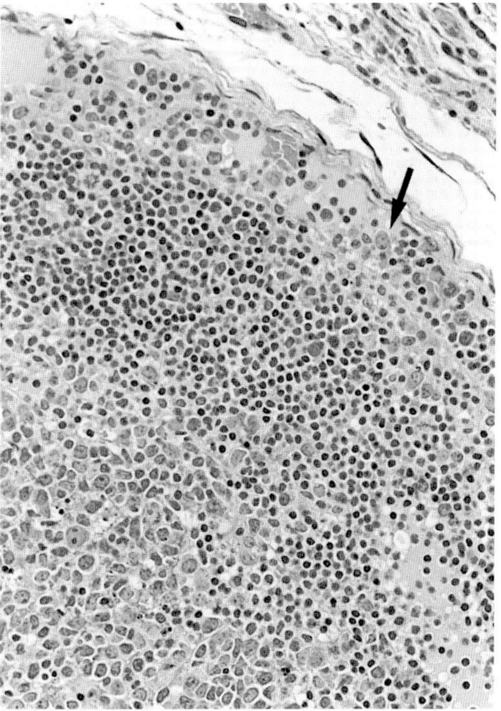

Fig. 2-29. Infectious mononucleosis. The parenchyma is extensively infiltrated by large lymphoid cells. The subcapsular sinus is patent (*arrow*) and contains some activated lymphoid cells.

can even be binucleated immunoblasts mimicking Reed-Sternberg cells (Fig. 2-28). The following features, present either in isolation or in combination, should at least raise a serious consideration for a reactive process despite the alarming histologic features[79–81]:

- Young age of patient
- Presence of some residual normal lymphoid architecture (e.g., preserved sinuses, residual lymphoid follicles, Figs. 2-15, 2-29)
- Necrosis of germinal centers (Fig. 2-30)
- Lack of atypia of the large transformed cells (such as marked irregular foldings of the nuclear membrane, coarse granular chromatin pattern; Fig. 2-31)
- Polymorphous appearance, with the immunoblasts showing a range of sizes and cytoplasmic basophilia, as well as transition to plasmablasts and plasma cells (Fig. 2-31)
- Immunoblastic proliferation merging imperceptibly with adjacent reactive follicles and paracortical zones
- Immunohistochemistry showing that the large lymphoid cells represent a mixture of B and T cells (note that presence of sheets of large B cells usually suggests a diagnosis of lymphoma) and polytypic B cells

In difficult cases, molecular analysis may help to determine the clonality.

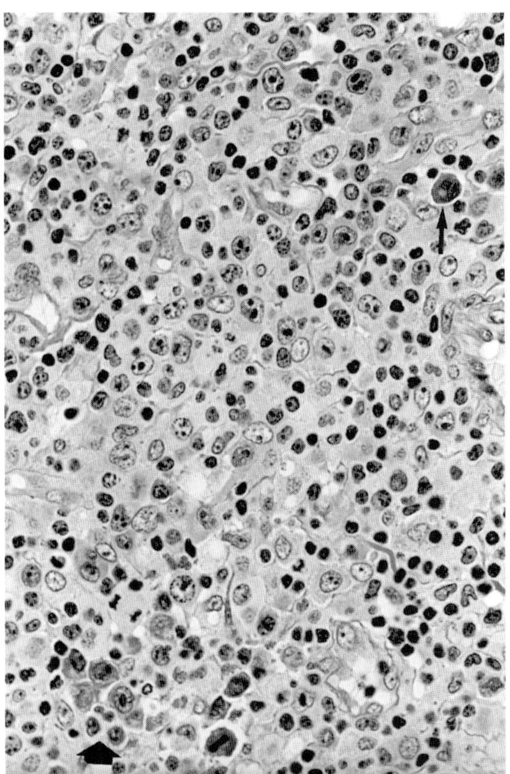

Fig. 2-31. Infectious mononucleosis. There is a polymorphous population of small and large lymphoid cells. The large cells look like reactive immunoblasts, and the nuclei are mostly round to ovoid. They typically exhibit a range of cytoplasmic staining, from pale to deeply basophilic (*broad arrow*). There are also intermingled plasma cells and plasmablasts (*thin arrow*).

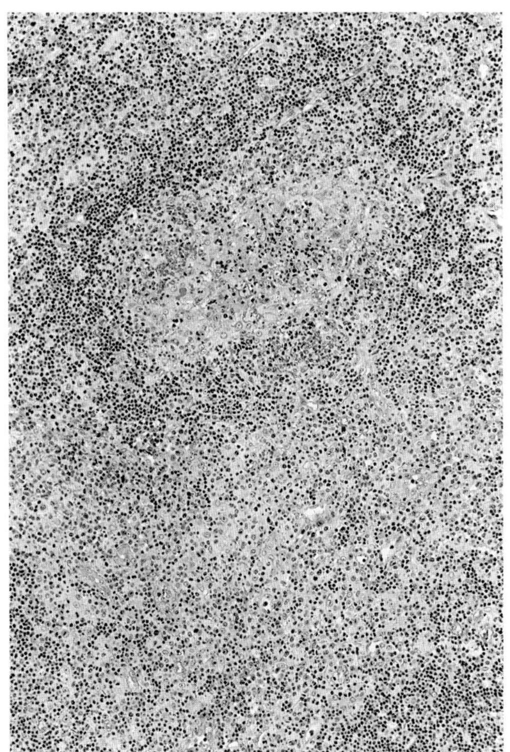

Fig. 2-30. Infectious mononucleosis. A partially necrotic germinal center (upper field) is seen in the lymphoid proliferation.

Clues for Recognizing Specific Types of Reactive Lymphadenopathies

After deciding that the lymph node changes are reactive, it is important look for features that may suggest specific forms of reactive lymphadenopathies (Table 2-1). Sometimes a specific diagnosis can only be made in conjunction with the clinical or serologic data, such as history of use of anticonvulsants, evidence of autoimmune disease.

For lymph nodes showing reactive follicular hyperplasia, the histologic features may suggest more specific diagnosis as shown in Table 2-3 (Figs. 2-22 and 2-32 through 2-35).[82–85] (see also a subsequent section on HIV-associated lymphadenopathy).

For lymph nodes showing reactive immuno-

Table 2-3. Clues To Recognizing Specific Entities in a Lymph Node Showing Reactive Follicular Hyperplasia

Histologic Features	Most Probable Diagnosis	Special Remarks
Mantle zones very thin or absent	HIV-associated lymphadenopathy; reactive follicular hyperplasia in children	Suggest serologic studies for HIV
Prominent follicle lysis	HIV-associated lymphadenopathy	Suggest serologic studies for HIV
"Granulomatous" change in many germinal centers ("epithelioid germinal centers")	Henoch-Schönlein purpura; *Yersinia* infection; children with overwhelming infection or shock[84,85]	
Selective accumulation of neutrophils in germinal centers	*Yersinia* infection	Need confirmation by culture or serology
Prominent interfollicular plasmacytosis	Plasma cell type of Castleman's disease or multicentric Castleman's disease; rheumatoid lymphadenopathy; luetic lymphadenitis	There can be some scattered hyaline-vascular follicles in plasma cell or multicentric type Castleman's disease; clinical correlation required for a firm diagnosis. Rheumatoid lymphadenopathy often shows in addition polymorphs in sinuses; diagnosis to be confirmed by clinical and serologic correlation. Also look for other features of luetic lymphadenitis
Prominent perilymphadenitis (capsule often thickened and nodal trabeculae often conspicuous), plasmacytosis, venulitis, small granulomas	Luetic lymphadenitis[82,83]	Confirm diagnosis by Warthin-Starry stain (spirochetes) and serologic studies
Prominent monocytoid B-cell reaction	Although not specific per se, it is worthwhile to exclude CMV infection	Examine multiple levels for CMV inclusions (which can be further confirmed by immunohistochemistry). An early phase of suppurative granulomatous lymphadenitis has also to be considered
Monocytoid B-cell reaction; small aggregates of epithelioid histiocytes with some encroaching on germinal centers	Toxoplasmosis; HIV-associated lymphadenopathy; Epstein-Barr virus infection (early phase)	Firm diagnosis of toxoplasmosis requires serologic studies
Prominent eosinophils (with some in the germinal centers), eosinophilic folliculolysis, vascularization of germinal centers	Kimura's disease lymphadenopathy	

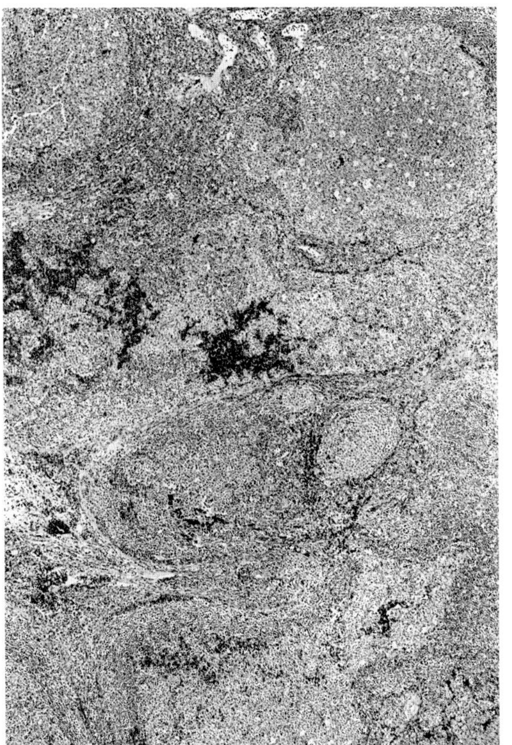

Fig. 2-32. HIV-associated lymphadenopathy. The follicles are large and irregularly shaped. The mantles are thin in many areas. In addition, there is prominent hemorrhage in the germinal centers (represented by the darkest areas).

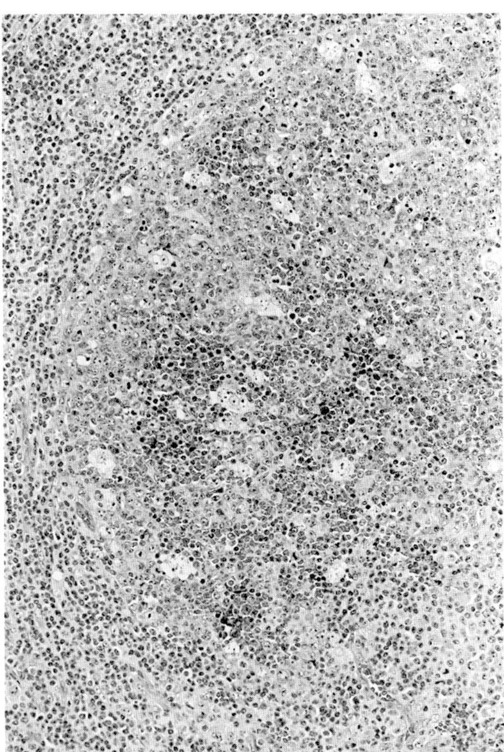

Fig. 2-33. HIV-associated lymphadenopathy. As characteristic of this condition, the mantle is absent. Clusters of degenerated cells and hemorrhage are evident in the germinal center, that is, follicle lysis. Some monocytoid B cells are seen in the right lower corner.

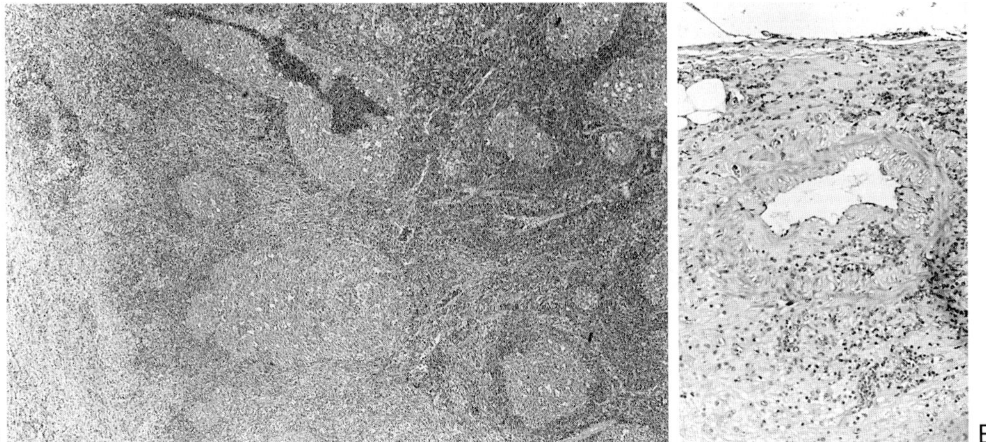

Fig. 2-34. Luetic lymphadenitis. (**A**) There is florid reactive follicular hyperplasia and thickening of the nodal capsule (left field). (**B**) Venulitis is evident in the perinodal tissue.

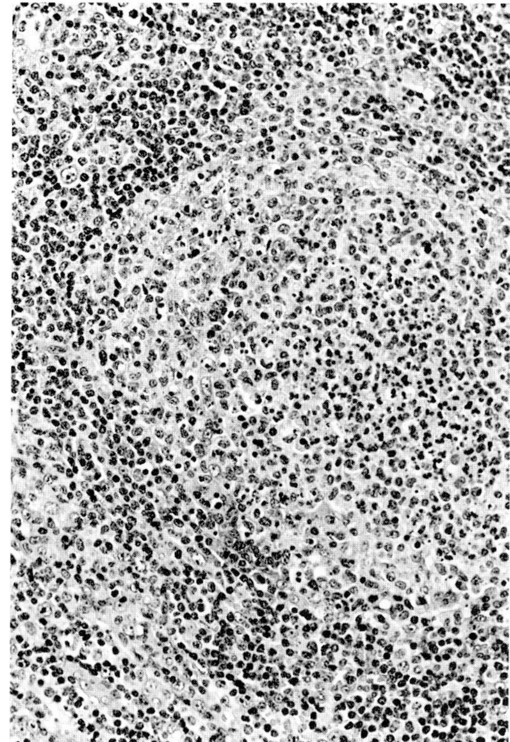

Fig. 2-35. *Yersinia* lymphadenitis. Neutrophils selectively infiltrate the germinal centers.

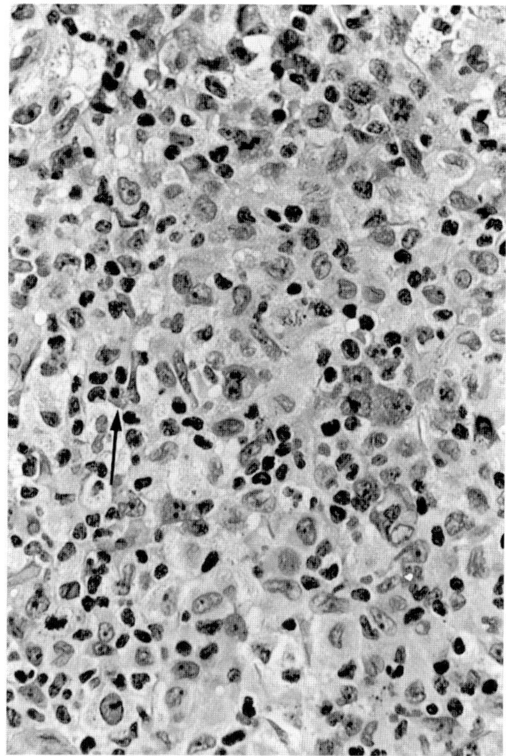

Fig. 2-36. Dilantin-associated lymphadenopathy. This lymphoid proliferation includes immunoblasts and interdigitating reticulum/Langerhans cells. Some eosinophils (*arrow*) are seen in the background.

blastic proliferation such as Epstein-Barr virus (EBV) infection (infectious mononucleosis), other viral infections, postvaccinial lymphadenitis, drug-associated lymphadenopathy, and hypersensitivity reaction, the etiology cannot be ascertained by morphologic assessment alone, except for the rare occasions in which viral inclusions can be identified (such as herpes simplex). Presence of an appreciable number of eosinophils may raise the possibility of postvaccinial lymphadenitis or drug hypersensitivity (Fig. 2-36).[86] A diagnosis of EBV infection can be aided by immunohistochemical staining for EBV latent membrane protein-1 (LMP-1) or in situ hybridization for EBV-encoded early nuclear RNA (EBER) or EBV DNA.[87–92] It is important to remember that while demonstration of EBV in a significant number of lymphoid cells supports a diagnosis of EBV infectious mononucleosis in a reactive immunoblastic proliferation, this technique cannot be used to distinguish between a reactive versus a neoplastic large lymphoid cell proliferation because some lymphomas are EBV positive. Kikuchi's lymphadenitis can show florid proliferation of immunoblasts, some of which may exhibit irregular nuclear foldings; it can be recognized by the characteristic discrete foci of involvement and prominence of admixed crescentic histiocytes and nuclear debris.

What Is Atypical Lymphoid Hyperplasia?

For lymphoid proliferations showing indeterminate features, the term *atypical lymphoid hyperplasia* can be applied (Fig. 2-11). Atypical lymphoid hyperplasia is neither a clinical nor a pathologic entity, but represents an interim designation for lymphoid proliferations for which the pathologist cannot decide with certainty whether it is benign or malignant.[93] It includes cases of reactive hyperplasia with some features worrisome of lymphoma, and cases of lymphoma with subtle cytologic atypia, partial nodal involvement, or other unusual features.

The terms *atypical paracortical hyperplasia, atypical lymphoplasmacytic and immunoblastic proliferation,* and *abnormal immune response* have also been applied by some authors to lymph node proliferations that resemble angioimmunoblastic lymphadenopathy (AILD), AILD-like T-cell lymphoma, or peripheral T-cell lymphomas but do not fulfill the criteria for any of these three diseases; these cases show a high incidence of an associated autoimmune disease, such as rheumatoid arthritis, autoimmune hemolytic anemia, mixed cryoglobulinemia, and positive serologic markers.[94,95] This lesion is considered by Nathwani and Brynes[81] to be potentially malignant.

The diagnostic term *atypical lymphoid hyperplasia* should certainly not be used if a more specific diagnosis can be made. Factors that may influence the need to apply this label are suboptimal histologic preparations, expertise of the pathologist, and availability of specialized studies to help in further analysis. Several studies published in the era before the availability of immunohistochemistry and molecular analysis indicate that 3 to 40 percent of all lymph nodes receive a diagnosis of "atypical hyperplasia" and lymphoma is eventually diagnosed in 30 to 60 percent of such cases based on follow-up biopsies.[93,96–99] Nowadays, the percentage of lymph nodes given this designation should be much lower because of better characterization of many reactive entities, refinement of diagnostic criteria in lymphoma, and availability of specialized techniques. In a recent study by Williams and colleagues[100] among 11 cases diagnosed as atypical lymphoid hyperplasia based on morphologic and immunohistochemical evaluation, 6 showed clonal Ig gene rearrangement, and a diagnosis of lymphoma was confirmed on subsequent biopsy in all such cases (at a median follow-up of 3.5 months). Among 5 patients without detectable clonal Ig or T-cell receptor (TCR) gene rearrangement, two subsequently developed lymphoma, and three had remained well on follow-up.[100] These findings illustrate that molecular studies can permit an earlier diagnosis of lymphoma to be made, although a negative result cannot totally rule out the possibility of a lymphoma or prelymphomatous state.

For patients given a label of *atypical lymphoid hyperplasia,* follow-up and repeat biopsy (immediate, or later if there are no more palpable nodes) should be advised. In repeat biopsies it is important to reserve materials for culture, immunohistochemistry, molecular analysis, and cytogenetic studies.

SELECTED REACTIVE LYMPHADENOPATHIES THAT ARE NEWLY CHARACTERIZED OR RECENTLY RE-EVALUATED

Kikuchi's Lymphadenitis

Clinical Features

Kikuchi's lymphadenitis, also known as Kikuchi's disease, Kikuchi-Fujimoto disease, histiocytic necrotizing lymphadenitis, and histiocytic necrotizing lymphadenitis without granulocytic infiltration, is an uncommon, self-limiting condition of unknown etiology that usually affects young female patients.[1,37,38,101–121] This disease appears to be more prevalent among Orientals. The female to male ratio ranges from 1 : 1 to 9 : 1, with the higher ratios being reported in Caucasian series. The age range is wide (mean 25.5 years), but most patients are less than 40 years. The patients usually present with solitary, or occasionally multiple, lymph node enlargement in the cervical region, but lymph nodes in other sites and rarely extranodal tissues (skin, bone marrow, salivary gland) can be involved.[122–124] Generalized lymphadenopathy is rare. Symptoms other than fever and tenderness in the affected lymph node are uncommon, and the general condition of the patient is almost invariably excellent. The onset may be preceded by flu-like symptoms. Sometimes more than one member of the family are affected.[110] Some cases present with fever of unknown origin or ''acute appendicitis'' (mesenteric lymph node involvement).[37,125–127] Occurrence in patients with AIDS and the regional lymph nodes of malignant tumor have also been reported.[117,128,129]

Laboratory tests may reveal neutropenia, raised erythrocyte sedimentation rate, and atypical lymphocytosis. The diagnosis is usually made by lymph node biopsy, but a reasonably firm diagnosis can also be made by FNAC.[101,130,131] However, it is prudent to perform serologic studies to exclude systemic lupus erythematosus because of the overlapping histologic features.[109,120]

Although an infective etiology (EBV, human herpesvirus 6, parainfluenza virus, parvovirus, yersina, or toxoplasma) has been suggested, the evidence is so far not convincing.[121,132–138] It has also been suggested that Kikuchi's lymphadenitis represents a self-limited form of lupus-like disease caused by autoimmune reaction to virus-transformed lymphoid cells.[109,113]

Natural History

Kikuchi's lymphadenitis usually resolves within 2 months (80 percent), but this process may take up to a few months or 1 year.[37,108,114,120] Although the fever can be controlled by antipyretics (but not antibiotics), such therapy is rarely required. Occasional patients with severe systemic symptoms have been reported to respond to steroid.[109,123] The disease can recur in a small proportion of patients (less than 4 percent).[37,108,110,111,120] Exceptional cases with systemic involvement and fatal outcome have also been reported.[139,140]

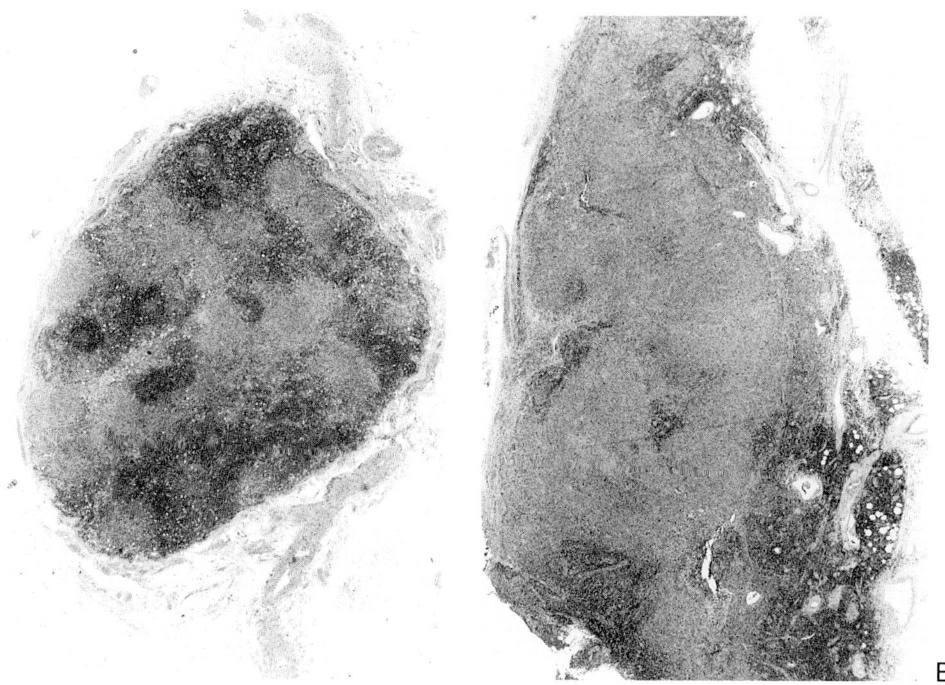

Fig. 2-37. Low-magnification appearance of Kikuchi's lymphadenitis. (**A**) In most cases, there are multiple, discrete, coalescing pale nodules without perinodal involvement. Some nodules are wedge-shaped and located immediately beneath the capsule. Note the starry-sky appearance of the uninvolved paracortex. (**B**) This case shows much more extensive involvement.

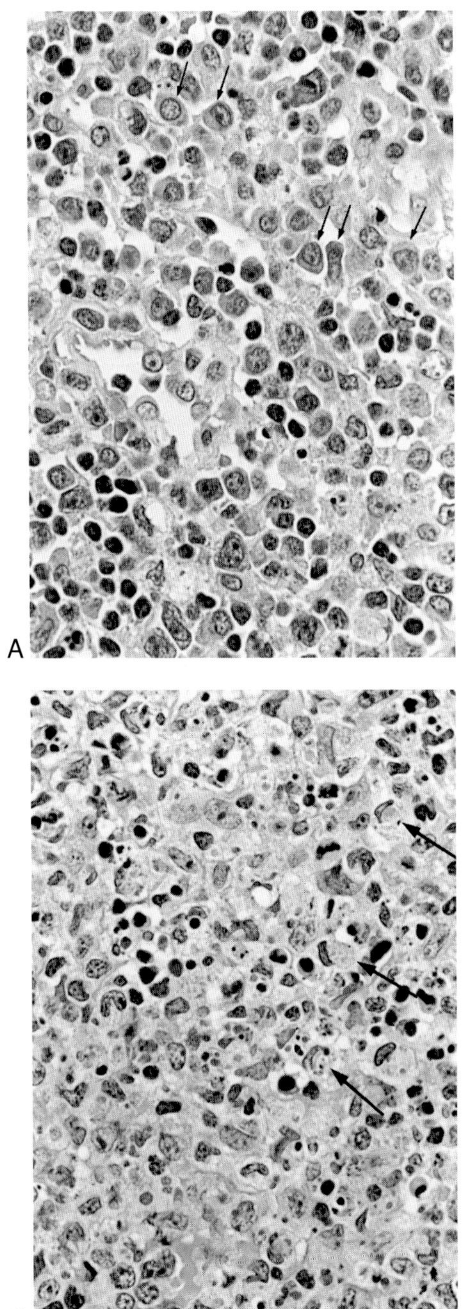

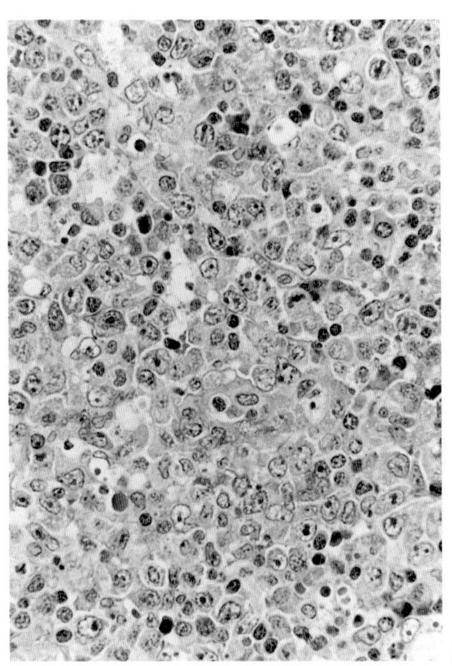

Fig. 2-38. Cytologic composition of the karyorrhectic foci in Kikuchi's lymphadenitis. (**A**) The earliest foci are characterized by abundant plasmacytoid monocytes (*arrows*), which are mixed with few karyorrhectic bodies, immunoblasts, and crescentic histiocytes. In most examples, the plasmacytoid monocytes are not as easy to appreciate and merely appear as medium-sized cells with round nuclei and poorly defined cellular borders. (**B**) This field is rich in immunoblasts with thick nuclear membrane and prominent nucleoli. There are admixed plasmacytoid monocytes (medium-sized cells with round nuclei), histiocytes, and karyorrhectic debris. Such cases can potentially be mistaken for malignant lymphoma. (**C**) This focus is predominated by karyorrhectic debris, histiocytes with twisted nuclei, and crescentic histiocytes (*arrows*).

Pathologic Features

The involved lymph node almost always measures less than 2 cm. On low power examination, it typically gives a mottled appearance due to multiple discrete, round to irregular, coalescing paracortical karyorrhectic foci, which are the hallmark of Kikuchi's lymphadenitis (Fig. 2-37). Coagulative necrosis is common, particularly in the larger foci, but is not a prerequisite for diagnosis. Perilymphadenitis is common, but extension of the karyorrhectic process beyond the nodal capsule occurs in only a minority of cases (Fig. 2-37B). Germinal centers are usually not prominent. The paracortex often shows a "starry-sky" appearance due to a lymphocyte-rich background decorated by scattered immunoblasts and histiocytes (Fig. 2-37A). Clusters of plasmacytoid monocytes are commonly found.

The cellular composition of the karyorrhectic foci varies with the size and presumably stage of development. The earliest recognizable foci are formed by plasmacytoid monocytes with interspersed karyorrhectic bodies and crescentic histiocytes (Fig. 2-38). The larger foci show a mixture of plasmacytoid monocytes, karyorrhectic debris, histiocytes, and immunoblasts. A zonation phenomenon can often be observed in these foci in that the center is predominated by histiocytes and karyorrhectic debris; the intermediate zone an admixture of various cell types but with less debris; and the outer zone lymphocytes and immunoblasts (Fig. 2-38). The histiocytes found in Kikuchi's lymphadenitis are distinctive.[37,130] Crescentic histiocytes possess peripherally placed, crescent-shaped, twisted nuclei and abundant cytoplasm that contains phagocytosed nuclear and cytoplasmic fragments; they therefore look different from tingible-body macrophages, which have centrally placed oval nuclei (Fig. 2-38C). Other histiocytes have centrally placed, elongated, and markedly twisted nuclei with or without phagocytic activity. Foamy histiocytes are also common, and lesions rich in these cells are sometimes referred to as *xanthomatous* or *foamy cell* type.[108,120] The histiocytes may even assume a signet-ring appearance, mimicking signet ring cell adenocarcinoma. The admixed immunoblasts are distinguishable from the histiocytes by their thick nuclear membrane, more clumped chromatin, prominent nucleoli, and amphophilic to basophilic cytoplasm (Fig. 2-38B). They are mitotically active and can show atypical features such as irregular nuclei and coarse chromatin. When present in abundance, they can mimic large cell lymphoma. Neutrophils are distinctly sparse or totally absent, and plasma cells are uncommon. Some cases (10 percent) may show wedge-shaped or irregular-shaped foci of fibrogranulation tissue formation, probably representing the repair phase of the lesion (Fig. 2-39).

Immunohistochemical studies show that the necrotizing foci are composed almost exclusively of T cells and histiocytes (including plasmacytoid monocytes) with remarkable paucity

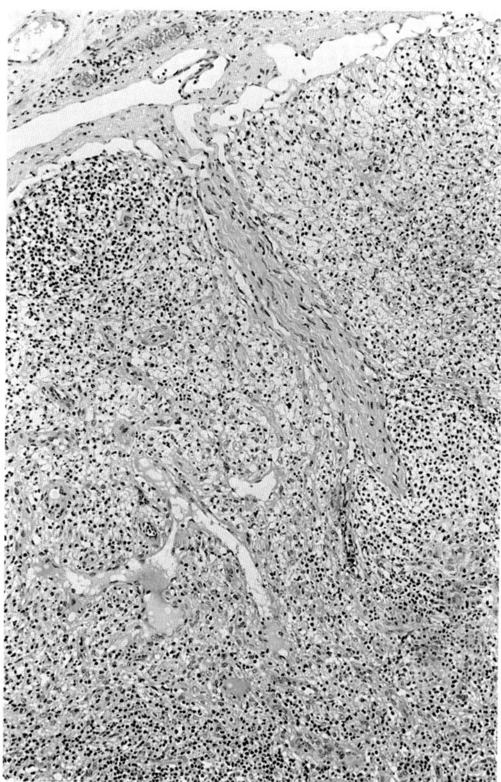

Fig. 2-39. Kikuchi's lymphadenitis with fibrovascular regeneration. This area is depleted of lymphoid cells and shows proliferation of fibrovascular stroma.

of B cells. The T cells present in karyorrhectic foci are mostly T-suppressor (CD8 +) cells, but they can be mixed with some CD4 + T lymphocytes.[115,141–145]

Differential Diagnosis

Since the histologic features of Kikuchi's lymphadenitis can be indistinguishable from lupus lymphadenitis, appropriate clinical tests and follow-up are indicated to exclude systemic lupus erythematosus. Furthermore, Kikuchi's disease may rarely coexist with systemic lupus and other connective tissue diseases.[37,140,146] Histologically, the presence of polymorphs, plasma cells, hematoxyphil bodies, and leukocytoclastic vasculitis should raise the possibility of lupus lymphadenitis, but only hematoxyphil bodies are pathognomonic.[147,148] Hematoxyphil bodies appear as blotches of extracellular violaceous materials, which are most commonly found in the sinuses (Fig. 2-40).

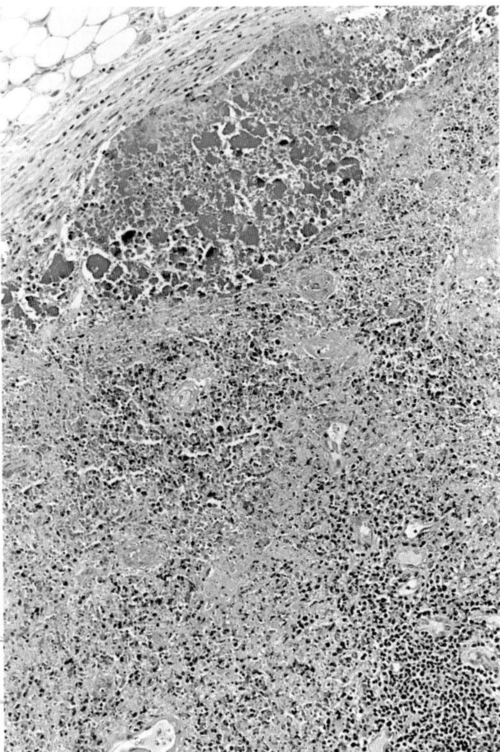

Fig. 2-40. Lupus lymphadenitis. The lymph node shows extensive coagulative necrosis and deposition of hematoxyphil bodies in the subcapsular sinuses (upper field).

Kawasaki's disease, a disease with necrotizing lymphadenitis, is characterized by more extensive, geographic rather than discrete focal necrosis and prominent fibrinoid thrombosis of blood vessels outside the necrotizing foci, both of which are not features of Kikuchi's lymphadenitis (Fig. 2-41). Furthermore, neutrophils, many of which are degenerated, are commonly found. The importance of distinction from Kikuchi's lymphadenitis lies in the need to initiate prompt therapy (such as aspirin and intravenous immunoglobulin) to reduce the incidence of coronary artery aneurysm.[149]

Kikuchi's lymphadenitis may be mistaken for malignant lymphoma due to the abundance of immunoblasts.[116,145] The distinguishing features are the discrete focal pattern of involvement, abundant karyorrhectic debris, prominence of plasmacytoid monocytes and histiocytes with twisted or crescentic nuclei, and zonation phenomena.

Histiocytic necrotizing lymphadenitis with granulocytic infiltration is morphologically identical to Kikuchi's lymphadenitis except for the plentiful neutrophils, which can be highlighted by chloroacetate esterase stain. Clinically, such nodes are often shown to drain foci of infection or to be associated with systemic lupus erythematosus.[104]

Kimura's Disease Lymphadenopathy

Clinical Features

Kimura's disease is an idiopathic, chronic allergic-inflammatory condition usually affecting young to middle-aged subjects and shows a striking male predominance. It is more prevalent but not exclusive among Orientals.[150–156] The patients usually present with slowly enlarging mass lesions in the head and neck region, with involvement of the subcutaneous and soft tis-

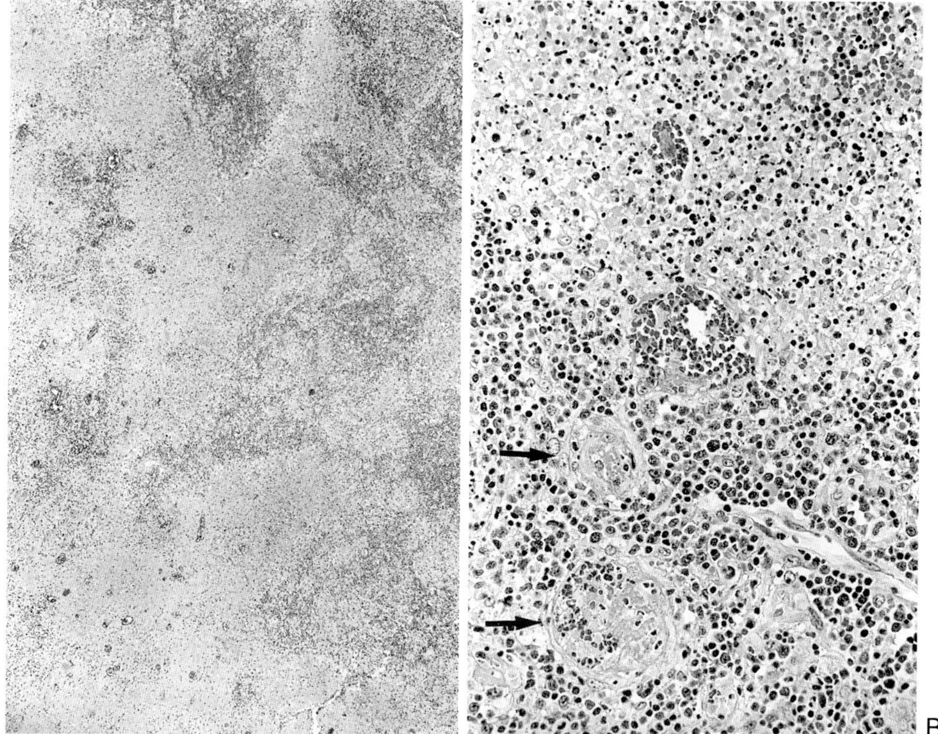

Fig. 2-41. Kawasaki's disease lymphadenitis. (**A**) There is prominent geographic necrosis. (**B**) The upper field shows necrosis and degenerated neutrophils. Fibrin thrombosis is evident in the blood vessels (*arrows*) situated outside the necrotic foci.

sues, major salivary glands, and lymph nodes. Lymph node involvement, sometimes multiple, may be the presenting symptom and can even be the only site of disease. Laboratory tests usually reveal eosinophilia and elevated serum IgE level. Renal complication in the form of proteinuria or nephrotic syndrome, attributable to circulating IgE immune complex deposition, has been reported in up to 12 percent, and apparently this complication is limited to the male sex.[157–159] Kimura's disease usually runs a self-limiting course. If left untreated, the lesion usually attains a static phase after years and may even show some degree of regression in size. Surgery is required only for diagnostic purposes and disfiguring lesions, but recurrences are common after excision. The etiology of Kimura's disease is unknown, but it is generally considered to be an aberrant allergic response, possibly through lymphocyte-mediated interleukin-5 production.[160,161]

Pathologic Features

The enlarged lymph nodes can measure up to a few centimeters in diameter. Multiple enlarged lymph nodes may become adherent to each other and the surrounding soft tissues, causing clinically alarming masses. Kimura's disease lymphadenopathy is characterized by a constellation of histologic features, none of which individually is pathognomonic. The nodal architecture is preserved. The florid reactive follicles have prominent germinal centers that are often rich in proteinaceous precipitate, and the well-defined mantles commonly show multiple tongues of intrusion into the germinal centers (Fig. 2-42). Immunohistochemical studies reveal IgE deposited in a network (dendritic) pattern in the follicles.[151] Some germinal centers are typically penetrated by multiple high endothelial venules (vascularization of germinal centers), a process

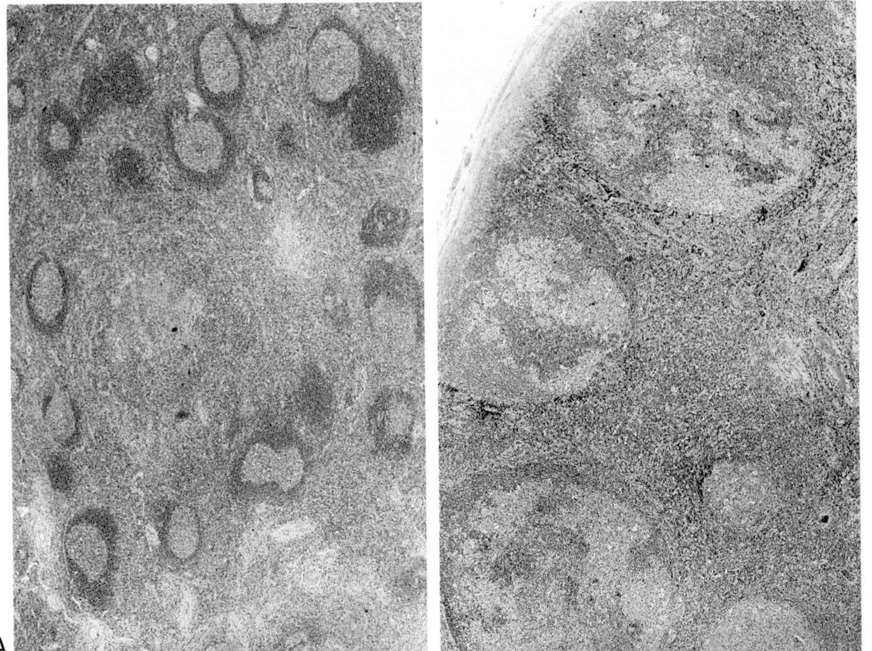

Fig. 2-42. Kimura's disease lymphadenopathy. (**A**) There is reactive follicular hyperplasia and patchy paracortical expansion (due to eosinophil infiltration and proliferation of high endothelial venules). (**B**) The germinal centers can be "intruded" by multiple tongues of mantle cells.

almost always accompanied by eosinophil infiltration of the germinal centers (Fig. 2-9). The eosinophils in the germinal centers can form abscesses and be associated with necrosis (eosinophil folliculolysis) (Fig. 2-43), although some germinal centers can show partial to total necrosis in the absence of eosinophil infiltration. The paracortex is patchily expanded, comprising high endothelial venules, numerous eosinophils, small lymphocytes, plasma cells, and mast cells (Fig. 2-42A, 2-44). The proliferated venules and eosinophils may form pale aggregates or nodules. Eosinophil abscesses are commonly found in the paracortex, although some of them have originated in the lymphoid follicles as evidenced by the presence of residual small clusters of germinal center cells (Fig. 2-45). Polykaryocytes are not uncommonly identified in the germinal centers and paracortex (Fig. 2-9). The sinuses are also typically infiltrated by eosinophils. Variable degrees of sclerosis are common, in particular around the venules.

Minimum Diagnostic Criteria and Differential Diagnosis

A histologic diagnosis of Kimura's disease requires the presence of florid reactive follicular hyperplasia, germinal center and paracortical vascularization, and marked eosinophil infiltration. The presence of all these features together distinguishes Kimura's disease from various lymphadenopathies with tissue eosinophilia, such as allergy, drug reaction, and parasitic infestation. Other specific lymphadenopathies with tissue eosinophilia, such as interfollicular Hodgkinoid lymphadenitis (see below) and dermatopathic lymphadenopathy, can be recognized by the features characteristic of these entities.

Eosinophils are often prominent in Langerhans' cell histiocytosis and Hodgkin's disease. The Langerhans cells with deeply grooved and contorted nuclei characteristic of the former, and Reed-Sternberg cells and their

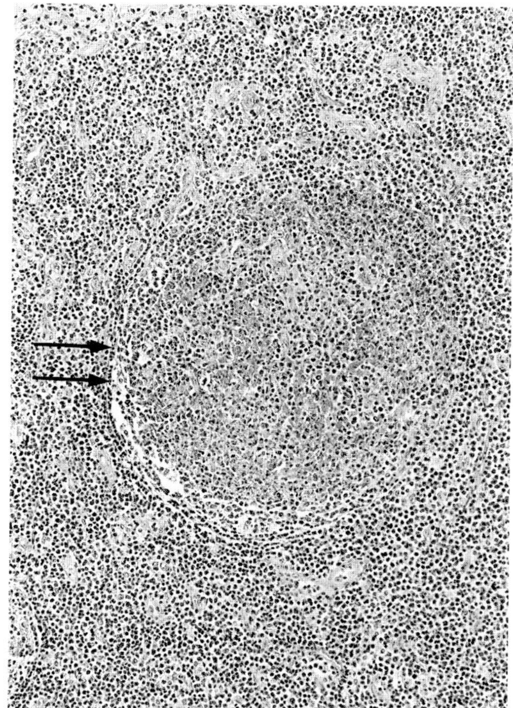

Fig. 2-43. Kimura's disease lymphadenopathy. A hyperplastic follicle shows eosinophilic folliculolysis.

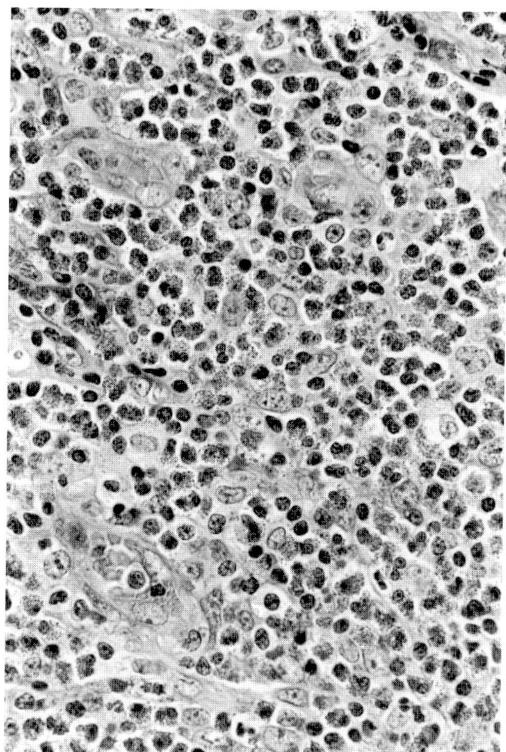

Fig. 2-44. Kimura's disease lymphadenopathy. The paracortex is heavily infiltrated by eosinophils. High endothelial venules are increased.

variants typical of the latter, are not seen in Kimura's disease. The polykaryocytes in Kimura's disease can be distinguished from Reed-Sternberg cells by their multiple, delicate, overlapping nuclei, absence of inclusion-like nucleoli, and paucity of cytoplasm (Fig. 2-9).

Kimura's disease has been most often confused with angiolymphoid hyperplasia with eosinophilia (ALHE, or epithelioid hemangioma).[150–153,162–167] ALHE is a tumor or tumor-like condition characterized by the proliferation of blood vessels lined by plump, oval to hobnail endothelial cells with abundant densely eosinophilic vacuolated cytoplasm and often accompanied by reactive lymphoid cells and eosinophils. In many cases, connection of the proliferated vessels with an adjacent damaged muscular artery or vein can be demonstrated.[150,162,168,169] The distinctive epithelioid (histiocytoid) appearance of the endothelial cells lining the proliferated vessels is the most important distinguishing feature of ALHE, differing from those of the venules of Kimura's disease, which have scanty cytoplasm.

Interfollicular Hodgkinoid Lymphadenitis

Clinical Features

Interfollicular Hodgkinoid lymphadenitis is a form of idiopathic lymphadenitis that can mimic Hodgkin's disease, especially the interfollicular variant, histologically.[170–172] Although patients of a wide age range can be affected, it typically occurs in young men, who present with otherwise asymptomatic lymph node enlargement. The lymph node may be enlarged up to 4 cm in diameter. The cervical region is most commonly

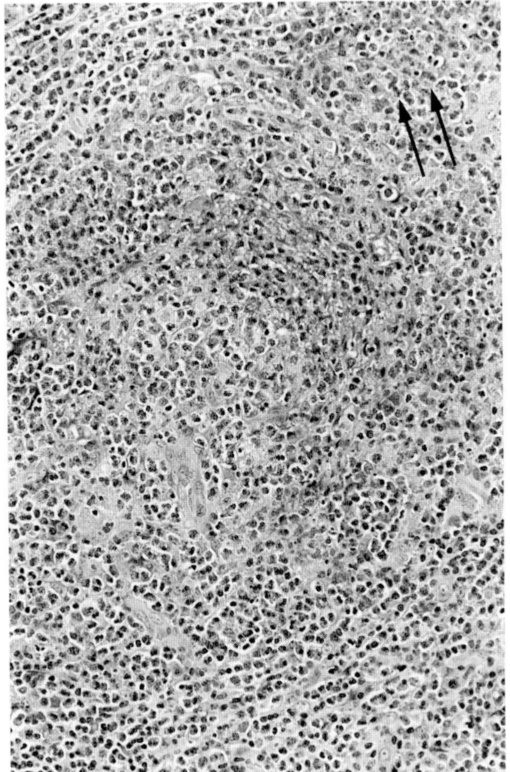

Fig. 2-45. Kimura's disease lymphadenopathy. This eosinophil abscess, which is apparently located in the paracortex, has actually originated in a lymphoid follicle, as evidenced by the whorled pattern of cellular arrangement and presence of residual germinal center cells (*arrows*).

affected. Multifocal disease can be seen in about one-third of cases.

On follow up, there is no progression to lymphoma. This condition probably represents a reaction pattern involving both the T- and B-cell compartments of lymph node rather than a distinctive clinicopathologic entity, and it merges morphologically with nonspecific reactive lymphoid hyperplasia.

Pathologic Findings

Histologically, the lymph node invariably shows preserved architecture, with reactive follicular hyperplasia and patent sinuses (Fig. 2-46). The most striking feature is the presence of pale, mottled patches in the interfollicular zone, composed of epithelioid histiocytes, lymphocytes, eosinophils, and immunoblasts intermingled with high endothelial venules. Some immunoblasts may possess inclusion-like nucleoli, mimicking Hodgkin cells. However, in contrast to the latter, they are smaller, the cytoplasm is basophilic or amphophilic, the chromatic pattern is more coarse, and nucleoli are smaller and basophilic. Furthermore, classic Reed-Sternberg cells are not found. Other inconsistent findings include progressive transformation of germinal centers and presence of plasmacytoid monocytes or monocytoid B-cell clusters. Immunohistochemistry clearly distinguishes this condition from conventional Hodgkin's disease, since the immunoblasts are either T- or B-cell marker positive but are uniformly negative for CD15 (Leu-M1).

B-Cell-Associated Granulomatous Reaction (Suppurative Granulomatous Lymphadenitis), Including Cat Scratch Disease

There is recent evidence that suppurative granulomatous lymphadenitis usually represents a B-cell-associated granulomatous reaction, contrasting with hypersensitivity-type (epithelioid) granulomas as seen in tuberculosis, leprosy, or sarcoidosis, which appear to be mediated by activated CD8+ T cells, dendritic cells, and monocyte-derived cells without the participation of B cells.[173–178]

There are many causes of suppurative granulomatous lymphadenitis (Table 2-1). The involved lymph nodes are usually the regional lymph nodes draining the portal of entry of the causative organism (e.g., cervical in cat scratch disease [CSD], mesenteric in *Yersinia* infection, inguinal in lymphogranuloma venereum).[4,173,179,180] Although these three diseases have been shown to be associated with B-cell reaction,[173] information is so far not available for other causes of suppurative granulomatous lymphadenitis, such as tularemia, atypical my-

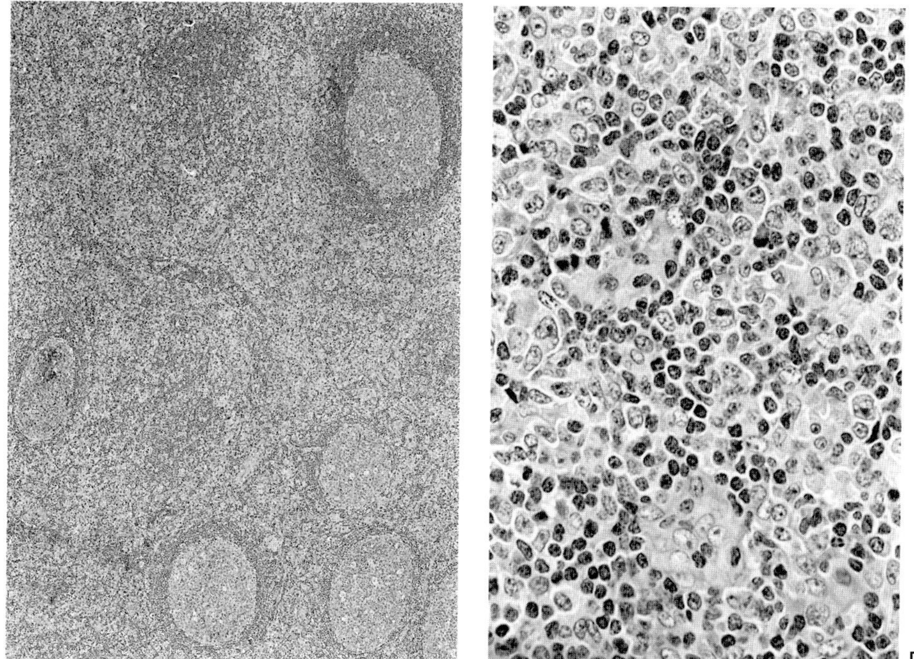

Fig. 2-46. Interfollicular Hodgkinoid lymphadenitis. (**A**) The paracortex is patchily expanded between hyperplastic follicles. It is mottled due to interspersed venules, immunoblasts, and solitary epithelioid histiocytes. (**B**) Some immunoblasts possess large inclusion-like nucleoli resembling mononuclear Hodgkin cells (center of field). The background comprises a mixture of small lymphocytes, plasma cells, histiocytes, and eosinophils.

cobacterial infection, and chronic granulomatous disease.

CSD typically affects children and young adults, who develop vesicular skin lesions (which may be inconspicuous) at the site of a cat scratch or bite, followed 2 weeks later by regional lymphadenopathy. The disease usually resolves in 2 to 4 months. However, up to 5 percent of patients may have atypical, prolonged, or recurrent disease, including, for example, Parinaud oculoglandular syndrome, erythema nodosa, osteolytic lesions, encephalitis, and systemic dissemination. Even such cases recover completely without specific therapy.[4,181,182]

Pathologic Features of B-Cell-Associated Granulomatous Lymphadenitis

The early phase is characterized by preserved nodal architecture, florid reactive follicular hyperplasia, and abundant monocytoid B cells in the sinuses and the parafollicular areas.[183] The intermediate phase is characterized by the appearance of small suppurative granulomas (histiocytic aggregates with central collections of neutrophils) that occur in close association with or appear to arise in the monocytoid B-cell clusters (Figs. 2-47, 2-48). There can also be scattered nonsuppurative granulomas (Fig. 2-49). The fully developed lesion is characterized by enlarging and coalescing suppurative granulomas that appear stellate or geographic, with the central hypocellular necrotic foci containing neutrophil debris and fibrinoid material, and the periphery showing palisades of histiocytes, with or without fibroblastic reaction (Figs. 2-50, 2-51). Multinucleated histiocytes are rare. Monocytoid B cells may be less prominent at this stage. In CSD, atypical plasma cells with large bizarre nuclei or multiple nuclei can be found in the interfollicular areas.[184] Vacuolated macrophages (shown on special studies to contain organisms) have recently been shown to be a highly characteristic

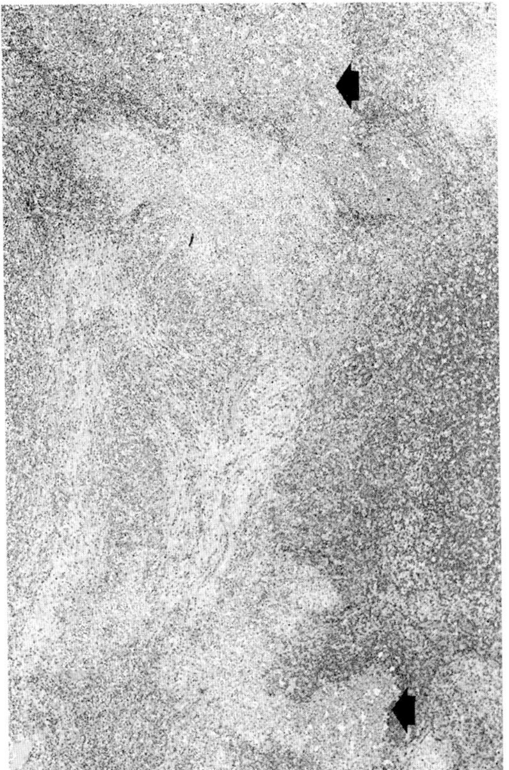

Fig. 2-47. B-cell-associated granuloma. There are irregular pale patches of monocytoid B cells with early granuloma formation. Note the close association with lymphoid follicles (*arrows*).

feature of lymphogranuloma venereum.[184a] These macrophages often occur around or within the supporative foci and monocytoid B-cell clusters. The perinodal connective tissue always shows marked edema with inflammatory infiltrates (perilymphadenitis) (Figs. 2-49, 2-51).

Immunohistochemistry shows that the suppurative granulomas are composed of an admixture of B cells, T cells, histiocytes, polymorphs and S-100 protein-positive dendritic cells.[173,174] B-cell markers remarkably highlight the clusters of monocytoid B cells, which, however, can be sparse in the smaller granulomas or large granulomas with extensive necrosis. The following sequence of changes has been suggested for the genesis of suppurative granulomas: granuloma formation, followed by recruitment of monocytoid B cells, which then lead to granulocytic infiltration (possibly via complement activation due to local immune complex formation) and necrosis.[173] Our own observation and that of Kojima et al.[174a] suggest that the lesion commences as foci of monocytoid B cells, where necrosis and suppuration develop in their centers, followed by formation of granuloma (Fig. 2-47).

Differential Diagnosis

The definitive diagnosis of suppurative granulomatous reaction requires demonstration of the infective agent (Table 2-1). Based on the results from three series of 140 lymph nodes showing suppurative granulomas, pleomorphic (CSD) bacilli can be demonstrated in 89 (63.6 percent).[175,185,186] Thus CSD appears to be the most significant cause of suppurative granulomatous lymphadenitis. The negative cases are due to other microorganisms or other causes (including idiopathic cases), although presumably some may still represent CSD in which the bacilli cannot be demonstrated because of prior antibiotic therapy, technical factors, focal distribution of the bacteria, and late phase of the disease. The CSD bacilli are gram negative. They appear as clumps of pleomorphic coccobacilli with occasional chains or L forms in Warthin-Starry stain or Dieterle stain (Fig. 2-52), and they can also be demonstrated by immunohistochemical technique.[179,186–190] The bacilli are patchy in distribution, but are found mostly in the necrotic foci, around the blood vessels, and in the macrophages lining the sinuses.[187,190,191] Ultrastructural studies reveal predominantly extracellular rod-shaped bacteria with thick trilaminar cell wall.[185,190,191] The Warthin-Starry stain can also confirm a diagnosis of lymphogranuloma venereum by demonstrating the fine, sand-like organisms (*Chlamydia trachomatis*) within the vacuolated macrophages.[184a] Serologic tests or culture can be performed in suspected CSD, lymphogranuloma venereum, tularemia, or atypical mycobacteria.[4,176,180]

Suppurative granuloma can be distinguished from hypersensitivity-type granuloma by the presence of polymorphs within the granuloma, frequent prominence of monocytoid B cells, and paucity of multinucleated giant cells. Furthermore, B lymphocytes are absent within hypersensitivity-type granulomas.

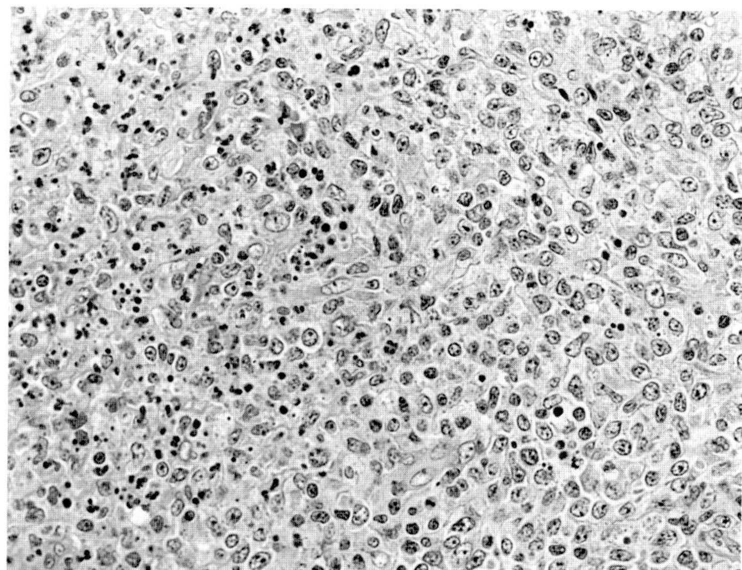

Fig. 2-48. B-cell-associated granuloma (cat scratch disease). In this granuloma, monocytoid B cells are evident in the right field and degenerated polymorphs in the left field.

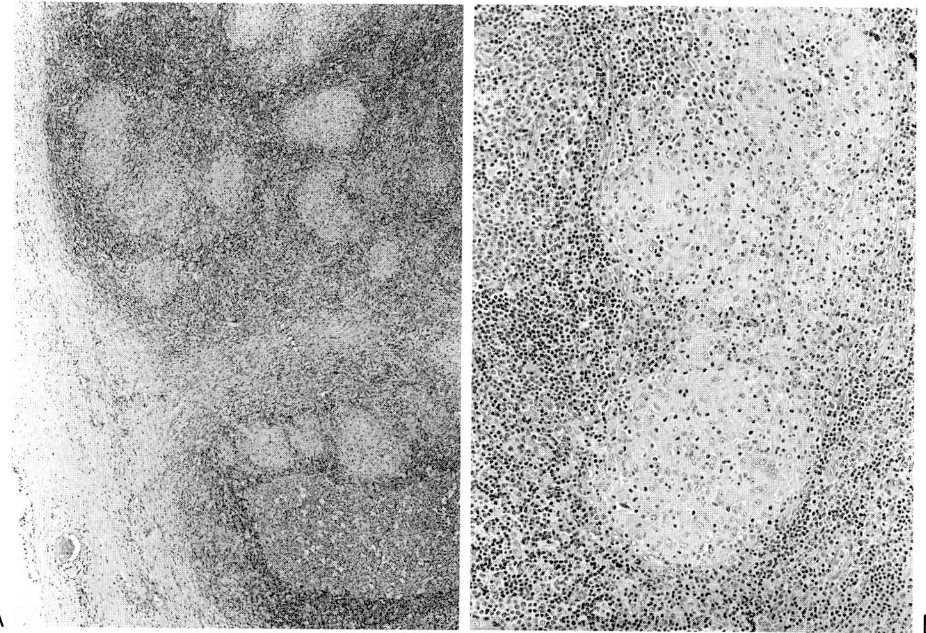

Fig. 2-49. B-cell-associated granuloma (lymphogranuloma venereum). (**A**) In this example, some epithelioid granulomas are found between reactive follicles. Suppurative granulomas are seen elsewhere in the node. The capsule (left field) is thickened as typical of this condition. (**B**) The granulomas are formed by epithelioid histiocytes without suppuration.

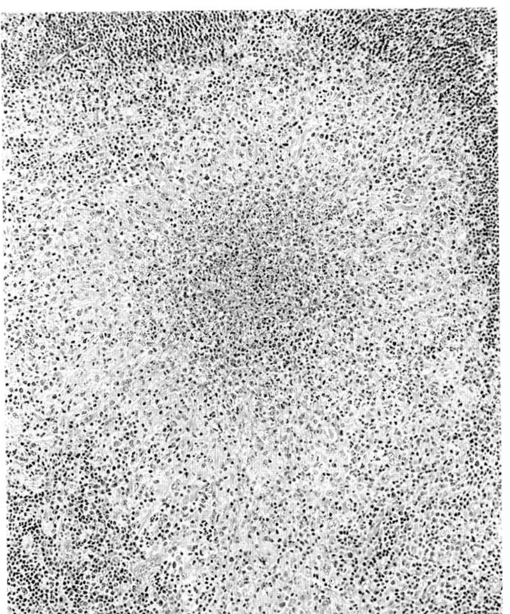

Fig. 2-50. B-cell-associated granuloma (cat scratch disease). A well-developed suppurative granuloma, with the center being formed by neutrophils with leukocytoclasis. The peripheral portion is formed by histiocytes and monocytoid B cells. The latter cells are best highlighted by immunostaining with a B-lineage marker.

Although both suppurative granulomatous lymphadenitis and Kikuchi's lymphadenitis are characterized by necrotizing lesion, they can be distinguished on morphologic grounds. The plasmacytoid monocytes seen in the latter differ from monocytoid B cells by their oval eccentrically placed nuclei and amphophilic to basophilic cytoplasm, presence of interspersed apoptotic bodies, and lack of admixed neutrophils. The cellular content of the necrotizing (karyorrhectic) foci of Kikuchi's lymphadenitis is different with admixture of debris, plasmacytoid monocytes, immunoblasts, and histiocytes (including crescentic histiocytes) but with no neutrophils; stellate-shaped granulomas with palisaded histiocytes are also absent.

Recent Advances on the Causative Agent of CSD

An infective cause for CSD was definitely proven in 1983 with demonstration of the organism in tissue sections.[187] The CSD organism was subsequently cultured.[189] Later, it was named *Afipia felis* and was thought to be unrelated to the causative agent of bacillary angiomatosis, *Bartonella henselae* (*Rochalimaea henselae* then).[192–194] Recent studies paradoxically show that *B. henselae* is a more important cause of CSD. Immunocytochemical staining with antibodies against *B. henselae* shows positive labeling of the pleomorphic bacilli in lymph nodes obtained from patients with CSD.[188] *B. henselae* has been cultured from lymph nodes showing classical features of CSD.[195] A high titer of antibodies against this organism is demonstrated in 88 percent of patients suffering from CSD as well as in their cats, while few patients have antibodies against *A. felis*.[196] Molecular analyses further support that both *B. henselae* and *A. felis* can cause CSD, with the former being much

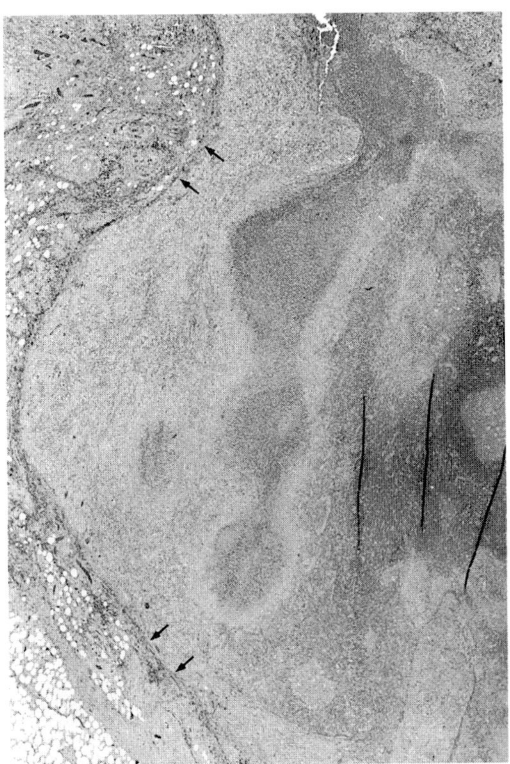

Fig. 2-51. B-cell-associated granuloma, established lesion (cat scratch disease). The node is replaced by granulomas with geographic or stellate outline and central fibrinoid necrosis with debris. There is also prominent perilymphadenitis (*arrows*).

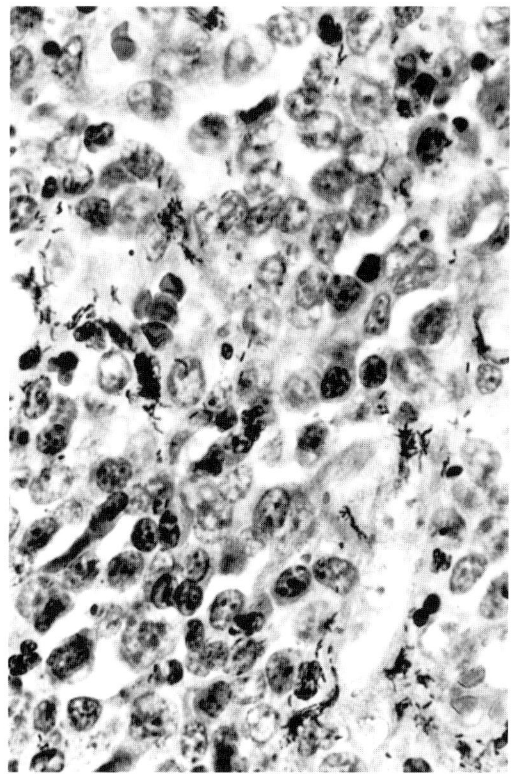

Fig. 2-52. Cat scratch disease. Numerous short bacilli are revealed by Warthin-Starry stain. Many bacilli are located around blood vessels.

more significant. In two studies on 59 cases fulfilling the clinical criteria of CSD, *B. henselae* was detected in 44 (74.6 percent).[197,198] In another study on 12 cases utilizing the polymerase chain reaction, *B. henselae* was detected in 5, *A. felis* in 3, both organisms in 2, and 2 were negative.[199]

Inflammatory Pseudotumor of Lymph Node

Clinical Features

Inflammatory pseudotumor of lymph node was first described by Perrone et al.[200] as a distinctive *pattern* of nodal reaction closely resembling its extranodal counterparts.[14,201–203] This condition usually affects young adults with no sex predilection. The patients present with lymphadenopathy of acute or insidious onset. The lymphadenopathy may be solitary or involve multiple regions (both superficial and deep), and rarely there is concomitant splenic involvement.[200,203] The enlarged lymph nodes can measure up to 9 cm and can be matted and adherent to the surrounding soft tissues, giving a clinical impression of malignancy. Systemic symptoms such as fever (including fever of unknown origin), night sweating, and anorexia are more likely to be found in cases with extensive disease. Laboratory investigations commonly show raised erythrocyte sedimentation rate, anemia, and hypergammaglobulinemia. The disease pursues a benign course. It may resolve spontaneously or after surgical excision of the enlarged lymph node(s). Surgery can occasionally result in a dramatic disappearance of the systemic symptoms. However, it can be persistent or relapsing, requiring steroid and anti-inflammatory drugs for control of symptoms. Partial response to antibiotics has also been documented.

Pathologic Findings

The most striking feature of nodal inflammatory pseudotumor is focal to subtotal *connective tissue framework involvement* with some spilling into the perinodal soft tissue (Figs. 2-53, 2-54). The nodal capsule, trabeculae, and hilum are expanded by edematous to sclerosed mesenchymal tissue containing bland-looking spindly or polygonal cells, small blood vessels, and inflammatory cells (mainly plasma cells and lymphocytes, mixed with some immunoblasts, eosinophils, and neutrophils) (Figs. 2-55, 2-56). Depending on the plane of section, the process may appear as anastomosing cords connected to the hilum or, on cross section, as multiple nodules (Fig. 2-54). The spindly and polygonal cells are arranged in a vague fascicular or storiform pattern and comprise a mixture of histiocytes possessing elongated vesicular nuclei and eosinophilic cytoplasm and fibroblasts/myofibroblasts with large oval vesicular nuclei, distinct central nucleoli, and abundant amphophilic cytoplasm (Figs. 2-55, 2-56). The proliferated blood vessels are well-formed and lined by flat or plump endothelium (Fig. 2-55); they may

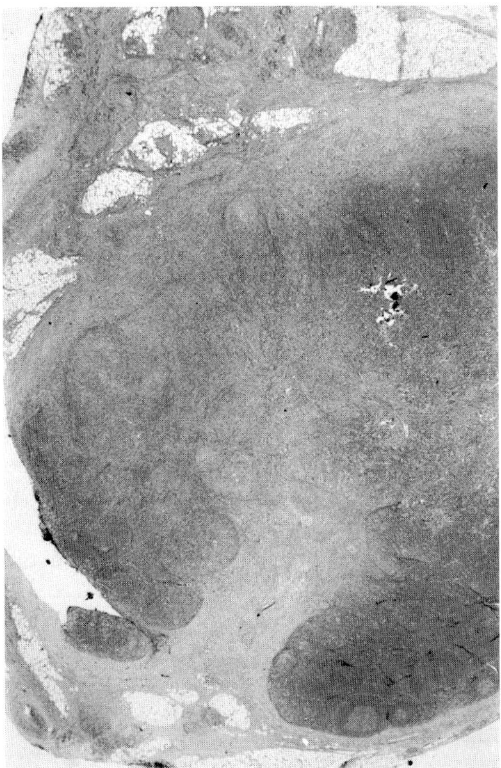

Fig. 2-53. Inflammatory pseudotumor of lymph node. In this example, there is marked broadening of the connective tissue framework of the node (pale areas). The hilum is also expanded (lower field). The process extends into the perinodal tissues (upper field).

merge with the high endothelial venules in the adjacent hyperplastic paracortex. The relative proportions of blood vessels, spindly cells, and inflammatory cells are highly variable. Exceptionally, histiocytes predominate and form aggregates that give an impression of a granulomatous reaction. Another characteristic feature is venulitis (which can be fibro-obliterative) involving the hilar and capsular blood vessels (Fig. 2-57). The sinuses are not uncommonly expanded or obliterated by the process. In almost all cases, lymphoid follicles are inconspicuous.

Differential Diagnosis

Early nodal involvement by Kaposi sarcoma also shows prominent capsular and trabecular involvement.[14] In contrast to nodal inflammatory pseudotumor, the vascular channels are slit-like, poorly formed, and irregularly anastomosing. Furthermore, periodic acid Schiff-positive eosinophilic hyaline globules are almost invariably present.

Mycobacterial spindle cell pseudotumor (see below) forms a space-occupying lesion in the lymph node rather than showing selective involvement of the connective tissue framework and is composed mainly of fascicles of spindly histiocytes and plasma cells.[204–207] A Ziehl-Neelsen stain is diagnostic.

The bland cytology of the proliferated spindly cells in nodal inflammatory pseudotumor allows its distinction from the mass-forming follicular dendritic or interdigitating reticulum cell sar-

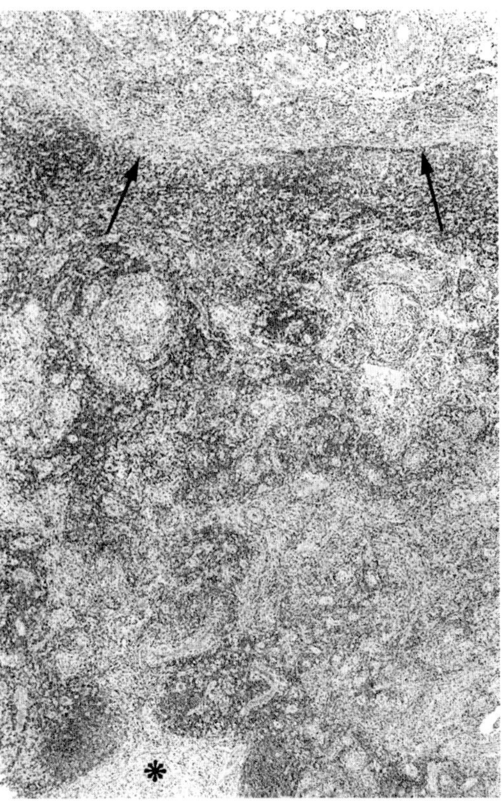

Fig. 2-54. Inflammatory pseudotumor of lymph node. This node shows thickening and inflammation of the capsule (*arrows*) and patchy pale areas within the node due to expansion and inflammation of the fibrous trabeculae. The hilum is indicated by an asterisk.

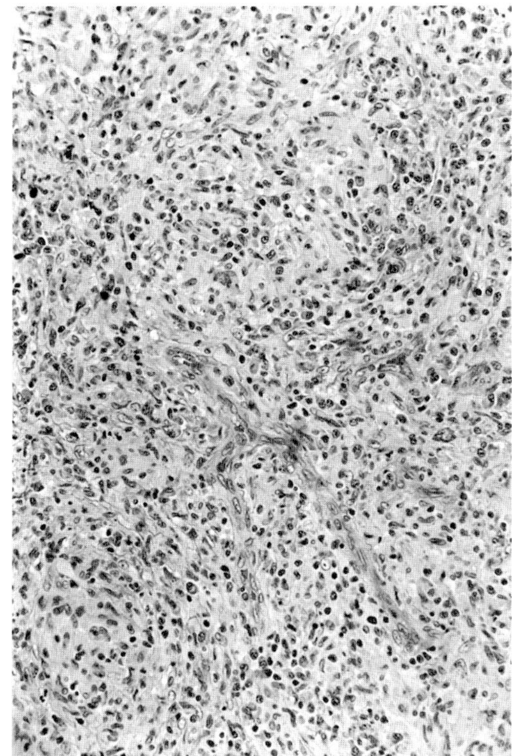

Fig. 2-55. Inflammatory pseudotumor of lymph node. The process is characterized by spindly cells with a vague storiform pattern, branching capillaries or venules, and chronic inflammatory cells.

comas to be made readily. The lack of atypia in the lymphoid cells and sparing of the nodal parenchyma proper (which shows reactive changes) allows the distinction from peripheral T-cell lymphoma.

Relationship of Nodal to Extranodal Inflammatory Pseudotumor: the Same or Different Entities?

Inflammatory pseudotumor has been described in various sites of the body such as the lung, liver, orbit, gastrointestinal tract, urogenital tract, spleen, and skin.[208–217] The unifying features of these lesions are their mass-forming properties and the mixed cellular composition, including variable proportions of plasma cells, lymphocytes, histiocytes, and myofibroblasts. However, extranodal inflammatory pseudotumor appears to be a heterogeneous entity, encompassing a number of lesions that cannot be reliably distinguished on morphologic grounds—some are clearly of inflammatory or infective origin,[214,218–220] while some are obviously reparative (akin to nodular fasciitis).[217] Some lesions are myofibroblastic neoplasms of low malignant potential (merging with fibrous histiocytoma and so-called inflammatory fibrosarcoma) as substantiated by demonstration of clonal cytogenetic aberrations or metastases in occasional cases,[216,221–224] and some hepatic and splenic inflammatory pseudotumors may represent EBV-positive follicular dendritic cell tumors or mesenchymal proliferations.[225,226]

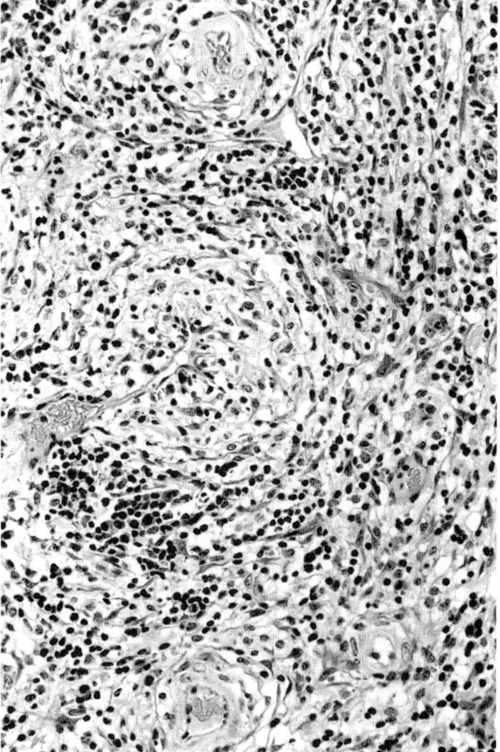

Fig. 2-56. Inflammatory pseudotumor of lymph node. In this case, there is more conspicuous chronic inflammatory infiltrate, with concentric proliferation of spindly cells around the blood vessels.

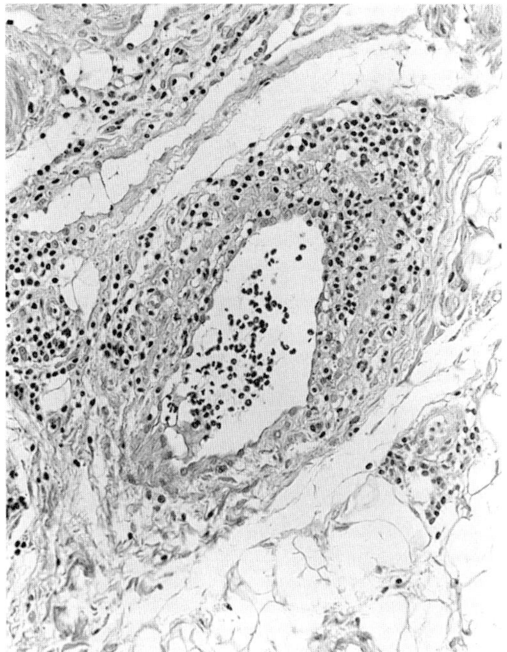

Fig. 2-57. Inflammatory pseudotumor of lymph node. Venulitis, as seen in this perinodal blood vessel, is a common occurrence.

Notwithstanding these uncertainties, nodal inflammatory pseudotumor should be conceptually distinguished from the extranodal counterparts, since the pattern of connective tissue framework involvement with sparing of nodal parenchyma is different from the solid spindle cell proliferation and dense plasma cell infiltration characteristic of extranodal lesions.[226a] The histologic features, occasional documentation of response to antibiotics, and occasional identification of an infective etiology in nodal inflammatory pseudotumor suggest that it is an exaggerated form of perilymphadenitis associated with lymphoid hyperplasia, caused by an inflammatory or infective process.[200,202] In approximately 20 percent of cases, EBV can be detected in some lymphoid cells within the lesion, suggesting a possible etiologic role of the virus in some cases.[225] The rare examples of extranodal inflammatory pseudotumor with regional lymph node involvement look completely different, with space-occupying lesions replacing the nodal parenchyma (Fig. 2-58).[208]

Vascular Transformation of Sinuses

Clinical Features

Vascular transformation of sinuses (VTS) is a reactive vasoformative condition characterized by conversion of lymph node sinuses into vascular channels of variable complexities.[227–232] Although VTS is by itself innocuous, it is important to recognize this entity because it is commonly associated with neoplasms in the vicinity or drainage area. Furthermore, the more complex and solid examples of VTS may be mistaken for Kaposi sarcoma. On the other hand, it is important not to mistake bacillary angiomatosis, an eminently treatable condition, for VTS. In the literature, lesions identical to or closely simulating VTS have been described under a plethora of designations such as nodal angiomatosis, hemangiomatoid, plexiform vascularization, and stasis lymphadenopathy.[233–235]

The age range of the patients is wide, and there is no sex predilection. Most commonly, the involved lymph nodes are deliberately sampled or found incidentally during investigation or surgical treatment of tumors. Some patients present with lymphadenopathy alone. Both superficial and deep nodes may be affected.

It has been suggested that venous obstruction is an important cause of VTS.[227] However, experimental models have shown that changes of VTS can be produced in lymph nodes by obstruction of the efferent lymphatics, irrespective of the patency of the venous channels, suggesting that lymphatic obstruction plays a pivotal role in the pathogenesis.[236] In a study of 76 cases, 71 percent are found to show definite or probable lymphovascular obstruction, such as tumor in the same node or in the vicinity, venous thrombosis, and a sluggish circulation (such as heart failure or constrictive pericarditis).[229] Angiogenic factors may be implicated in other cases, as suggested by the association with cancer or hemangioma in the drainage area.[229,237,238]

Pathologic Findings

The lymph node architecture is invariably preserved, although extensive involvement may result in architectural distortion. The capsule is

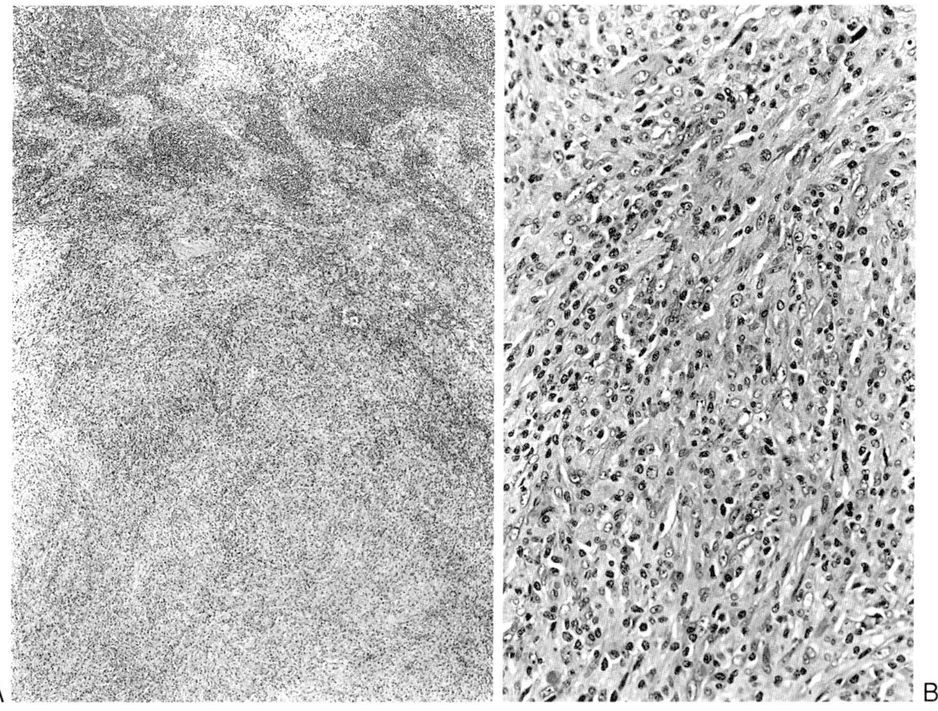

Fig. 2-58. Regional lymph node involvement by a colonic inflammatory pseudotumor. (**A**) The pattern is that of a space-occupying lesion replacing the nodal parenchyma. Residual lymphoid tissue is seen in the upper field. (**B**) The cellular constituent is identical to the primary lesion in the colon, being composed of spindly fibrohistiocytic cells admixed with lymphocytes and plasma cells.

not involved, and the prominent perinodal blood vessels may show thrombosis or thickening of the muscle coat. The hallmark of VTS is expansion of the subcapsular, intermediate, and medullary sinuses in a diffuse or segmental fashion by blood vessels and fibrous tissue (Fig. 2-59). The lymphoid parenchyma is often atrophic, which is more striking in examples showing florid VTS (Fig. 2-59B).

The proliferated vessels may show a range of appearances (Figs. 2-60, 2-61). Most often they are ectatic, rounded, thin-walled spaces lined by flat or plump endothelium or slit-like with a straight or sinuous configuration. Within the vascular spaces, there may be scanty to abundant red cells or amorphous lymph-like material. The blood vessels are typically embedded in a sclerotic stroma (Fig. 2-61A), and extravasation of red cells is common. Fibrin deposition can be seen in rare cases. In some cases, the VTS has an almost solid appearance, either focally or extensively (Figs. 2-60, 2-61B,C). This can be due to the presence of very plump endothelium with regular oval nuclei; the interspersed vascular spaces can be inconspicuous. Alternatively, this is produced by bland-looking spindly cells that form haphazard arrays or short fascicles, typically interspersed with irregular *branching* vascular spaces (Fig. 2-61B). The solid foci usually exhibit "maturation" into well-formed or ectatic channels in the subcapsular sinuses (Fig. 2-60).

The plexiform variant is a rare pattern of VTS that has so far been observed only in intra-abdominal lymph nodes (Fig. 2-61D). The involved node shows dilatation of the sinuses, which contain anastomosing, labyrinth-like, empty, or lymph-filled vascular channels lined by flat endothelium. This pattern is identical to what has been described in cats as "plexiform vascularization" of lymph nodes.

The nodular spindle cell variant is character-

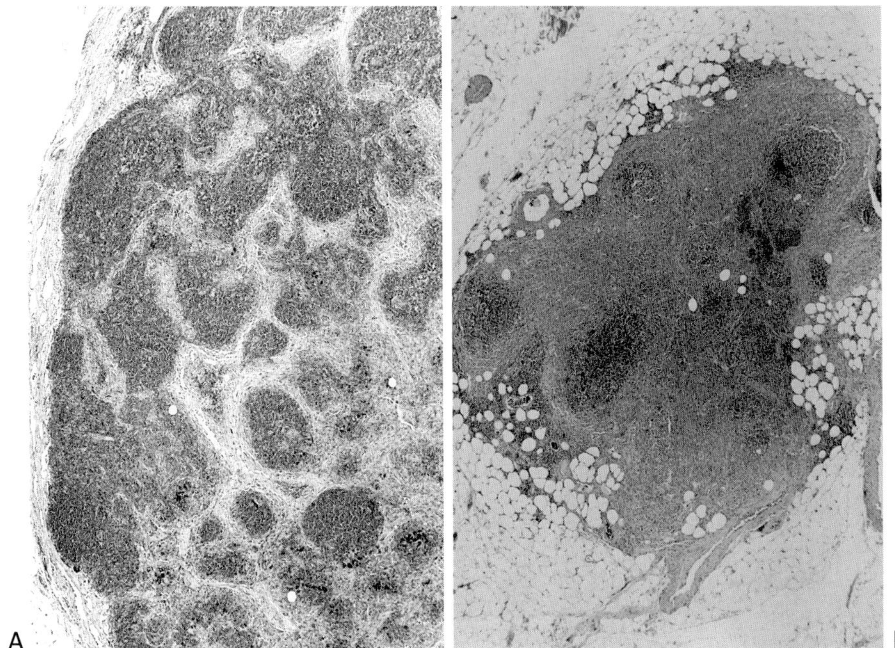

Fig. 2-59. Vascular transformation of sinuses. (**A**) The sinuses are expanded by the vasoproliferative process with sparing of the parenchyma and capsule. (**B**) A florid example, which is associated with lymphoid atrophy. The markedly expanded sinuses appear pale on low magnification.

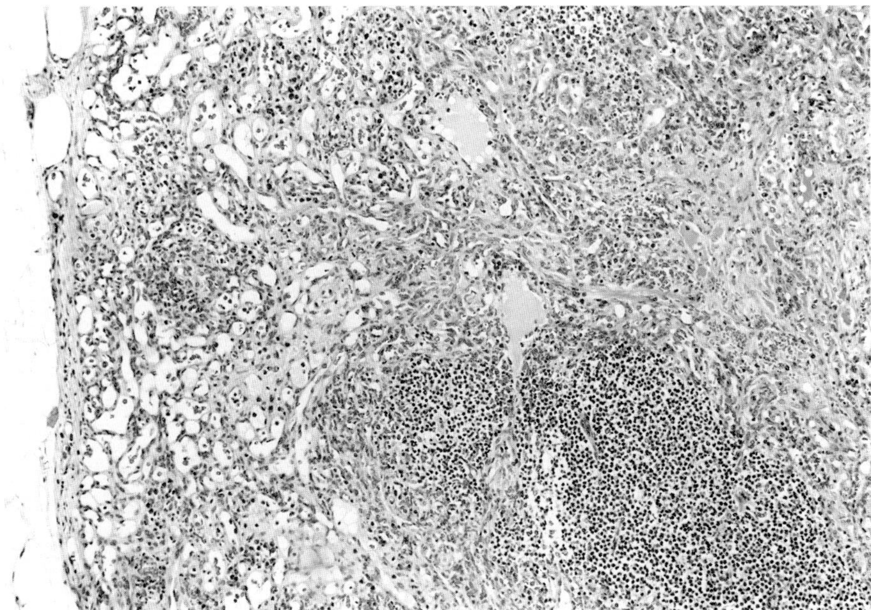

Fig. 2-60. Vascular transformation of sinuses. The fairly solid cellular proliferation in the intermediate sinuses (right field) gradually merges into well-formed rounded vascular spaces toward the subcapsular sinuses (left field). Irregular, arborizing, narrow vascular spaces are seen within the former.

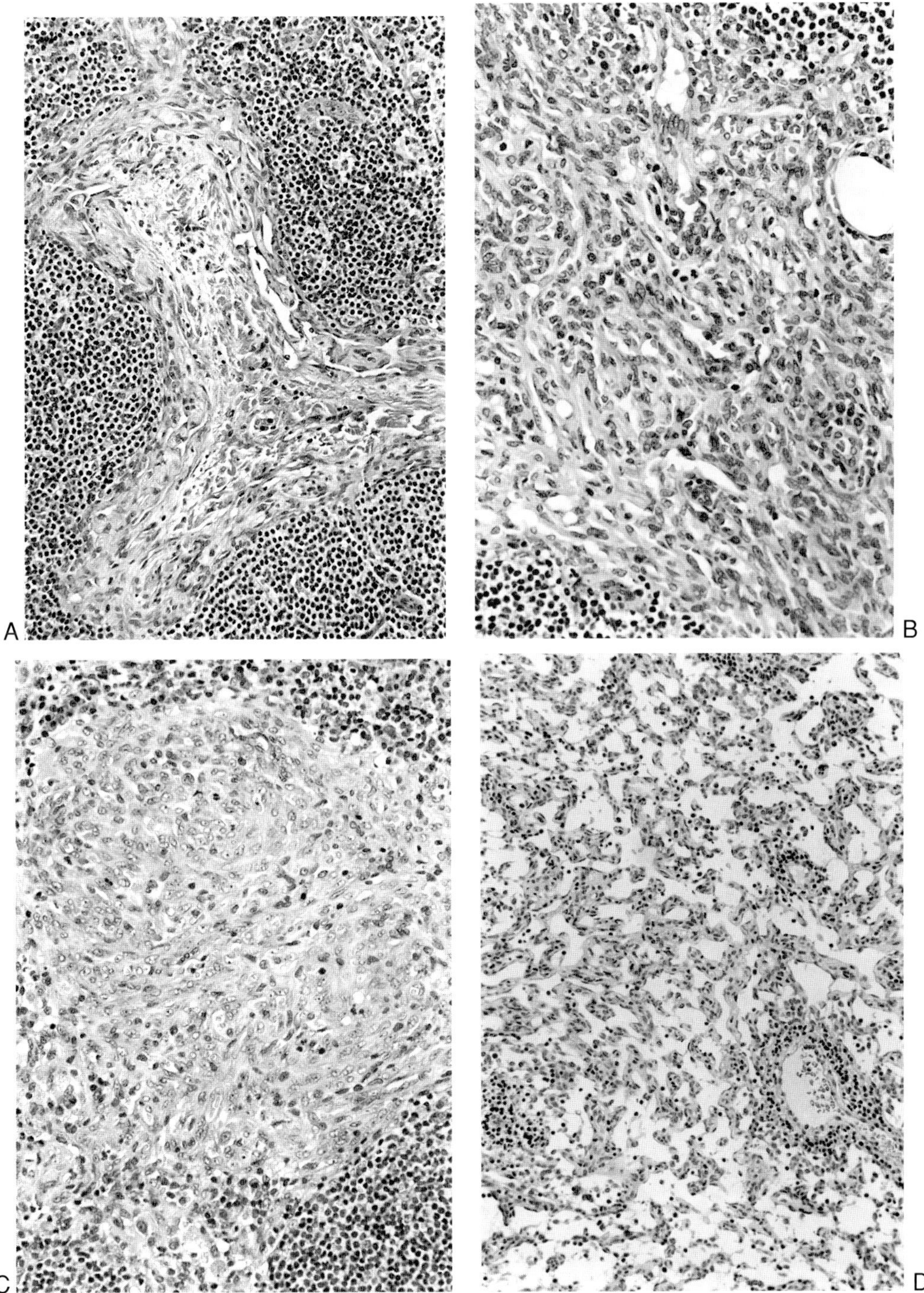

Fig. 2-61. The varied patterns of vascular transformation of sinuses. (**A**) The sinuses are fibrotic and contain irregular, branching vascular clefts. (**B**) Cellular example, in which branching vascular clefts are seen among bland-looking spindly cells. (**C**) Cellular (solid) example comprising plump cells. Few vascular clefts are seen. (**D**) Plexiform variant, characterized by irregularly dilated, labyrinth-like vascular spaces.

ized by striking spindle cell and vascular proliferations, resulting in formation of a single or multiple nodules, which often merge into areas showing typical features of VTS (Fig. 2-62).[14,239] The nodular foci are morphologically similar to the solid areas found in the usual form of VTS, with irregular branching vascular spaces being interspersed among spindly cells that form fascicles or whorls around the vascular spaces. Immunohistochemical studies show that a high proportion of the spindly cells are actin positive, and many surround the vascular spaces in a pericytic pattern.

Differential Diagnosis

VTS may be mistaken for Kaposi sarcoma, especially when it occurs in HIV-seropositive subjects.[232] The pattern of involvement is the key to distinction between the two entities: the vasoproliferation is confined to the sinuses in VTS, whereas Kaposi sarcoma commonly involves the nodal capsule and fibrous trabeculae. Sclerosis is much more prominent in VTS. The long, well-formed, criss-crossing spindle cell fascicles seen in well-developed Kaposi sarcoma are never a feature of VTS. The cellular form of VTS is characterized by irregular *branching* vascular spaces among spindly cells, contrasting with the short, nonbranching vascular slits in Kaposi sarcoma. Furthermore, ''maturation'' of the solid-appearing areas into better formed vascular spaces toward the nodal capsule is commonly observed in VTS (Fig. 2-60).

Nodal hemangioma and bacillary angiomatosis can be distinguished from VTS by the presence of solitary or multiple mass-forming vascular proliferations in the nodal parenchyma. Hemangioma is morphologically identical to its soft tissue counterpart. Bacillary angiomatosis is discussed in a subsequent section.

Nodal inflammatory pseudotumor also features proliferation of vessels and sclerosis, but it differs from VTS in showing selective involvement of the connective tissue framework, associated with prominent inflammatory cell infiltration and fibroblastic proliferation.

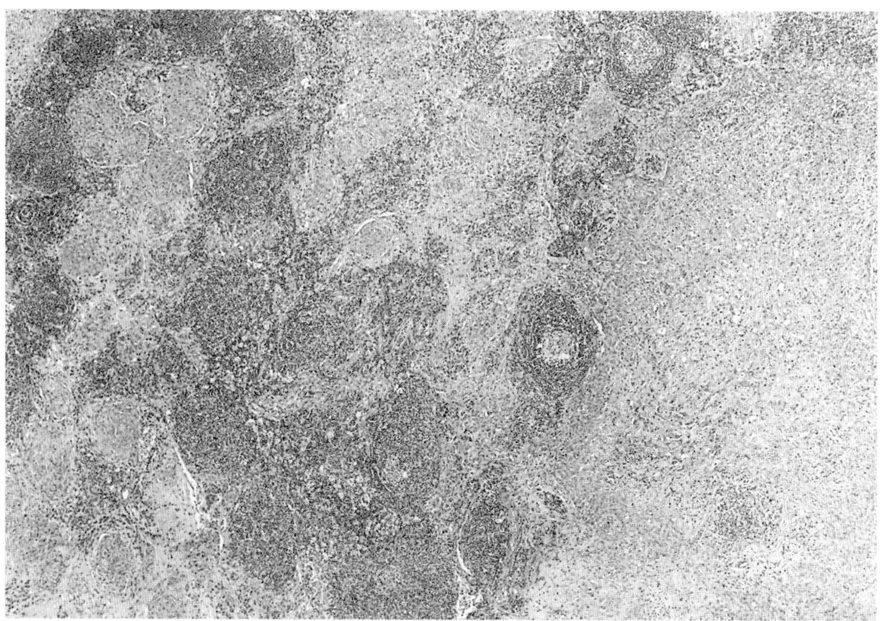

Fig. 2-62. Nodular spindle cell variant of vascular transformation of sinuses. A large nodule is seen in the right field. It merges into dilated sinuses in the left field. The vasoproliferation also forms smaller nodules within the sinuses.

NEWLY RECOGNIZED FORMS OF REACTIVE LYMPHADENOPATHY: A BRIEF TREATISE

HIV-ASSOCIATED LYMPHADENOPATHY

- Lymph node in HIV-seropositive patients appears to evolve through different stages.[5,240–246] Explosive follicular hyperplasia dominates the early phase (type A), followed by a phase in which explosive follicles are mixed with some hyaline-vascular follicles (type B). Later, the picture is characterized by hyaline-vascular follicles and paracortical vascular hyperplasia (type C). The terminal phase is characterized by lymphocyte depletion. It has been shown that the lymph node changes correlate with the prognosis (overall survival and progression to frank AIDS), with type A being the best and type C and lymphocyte depletion the worst.[5,244,246,247]
- The histologic features of explosive follicular hyperplasia (Figs. 2-22, 2-32, 2-33)[5,56,240–242,244,245,248–252] are as follows:
    - The crowded, large, irregular-shaped follicles look obviously benign by virtue of the cellular polarization and abundance of tingible-body macrophages
    - Follicular mantles are very thin or absent
    - Follicle lysis, characterized by hemorrhage, presence of clusters of degenerated cells, and invasion of small lymphocytes in the germinal centers, results from HIV infection of the follicular dendritic cells, causing disruption and weakening of the meshwork
    - The monocytoid B-cell reaction is prominent
    - Polykaryocytes are commonly found in germinal centers and paracortex
    - Plasma cells and occasionally neutrophils are increased in the paracortex; small epithelioid granulomas are sometimes seen

Although these findings are typical of HIV-associated lymphadenopathy, they are not pathognomonic and can be observed in patients with no evidence of HIV infection.[253,254] Thus when the above constellation of features is seen, the report can be worded as follows if serologic results or special studies are not available: "explosive follicular hyperplasia, with features suggestive of HIV-associated lymphadenopathy; recommend serologic studies."[255] The CD4/CD8 T-cell ratio in both the intrafollicular and interfollicular regions is much lower compared with the normal nodes or other reactive conditions.[243] HIV can be demonstrated in the follicular dendritic cells by ultrastructural studies, immunohistochemistry (p24 protein) and in situ hybridization.[240,241,243,256] These techniques can provide a firm diagnosis of HIV-associated lymphadenopathy in patients with unknown HIV status, but there may be legal problems in performing these HIV tests without obtaining patients' prior consent.

- Hypervascular follicular hyperplasia (also known as follicular involution with hypervascularity) is characterized by atrophic lymphoid follicles with centers being formed predominantly by follicular dendritic cells and penetrated by hyalinized venules, mimicking Castleman's disease (Fig. 2-63). The interfollicular zones are rich in high endothelial venules and plasma cells. With gradual loss of the follicles, the picture may mimic that of AILD.[240,244,246,257]
- Lymph nodes showing lymphocyte depletion usually do not cause nodal enlargement and are therefore much more frequently encountered in autopsy than surgical specimens. Lymphoid follicles are markedly decreased or absent, and the lymphocyte-depleted parenchyma often shows an increase in histiocytes (Fig. 2-64).[240–243]
- Having made a tentative diagnosis of HIV-associated lymphadenopathy, the pathologist should scrutinize the node for evidence of infection, lymphoma, and Kaposi sarcoma. In particular, the nodal capsule should be carefully evaluated for possible early Kaposi sarcoma. Presence of any of such features

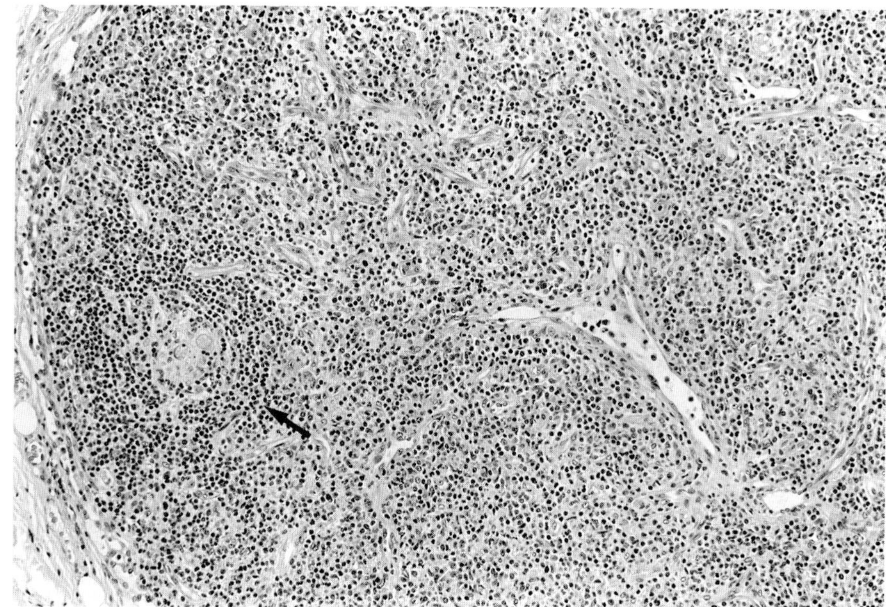

Fig. 2-63. HIV-associated lymphadenopathy, intermediate to late phase. There is some degree of lymphocyte depletion and vascular hyperplasia. A regressed germinal center is seen in the left field (*arrow*).

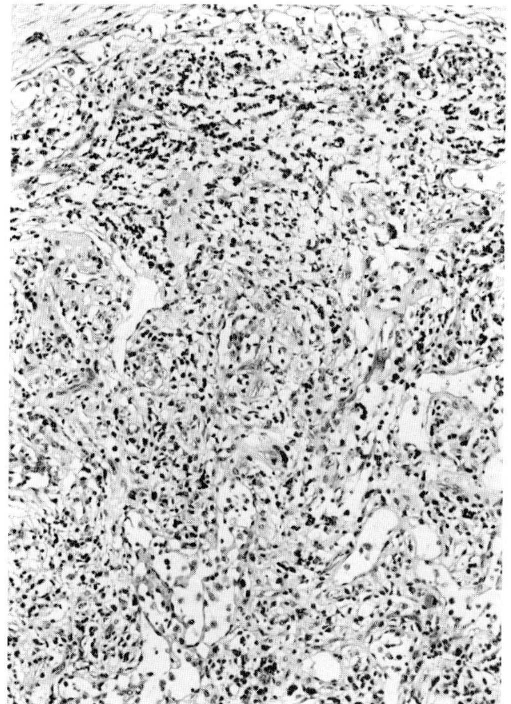

Fig. 2-64. HIV-associated lymphadenopathy. Marked lymphocyte depletion is evident, and the sinuses appear prominent.

will strengthen the diagnosis of HIV-associated lymphadenopathy.

Fine-Needle Aspiration-Associated Changes

- After fine needle aspiration, a reactive lymph node may undergo the following changes[14,258,259]:
  - Hemorrhage, often in the form of a linear tract; it may be associated with variable degrees of repair reaction, which can be so striking as to mimic Kaposi sarcoma.
  - Segmental infarction of lymph node, which is characterized by a wedge-shaped hypocellular focus with depletion of lymphocytes and/or fibrin deposition or hemorrhage (Fig. 2-65).[259,260] As a result, the sinuses and fibrous framework often appear prominent in this region. In some but not all cases, thrombosis of hilar veins may be seen. The segmental infarction is

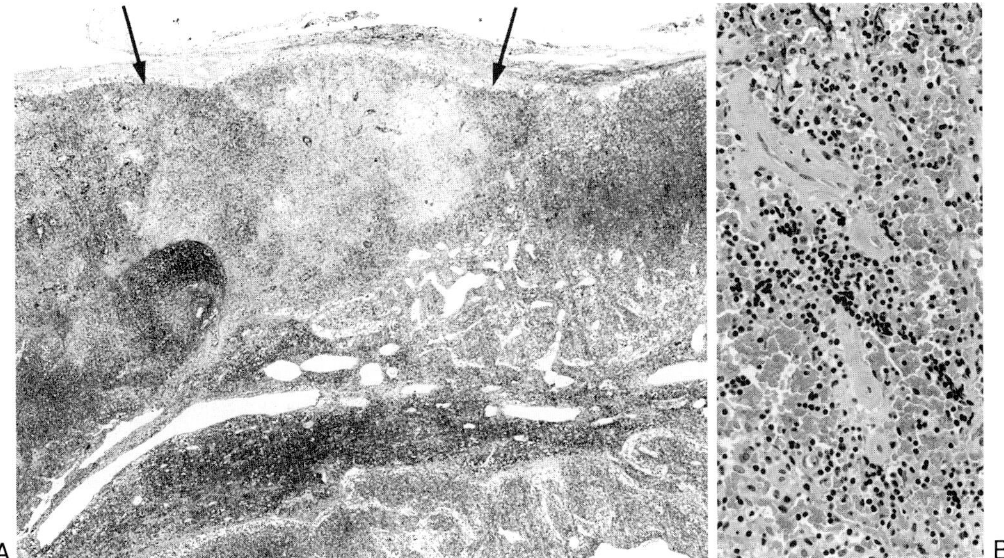

Fig. 2-65. Segmental infarction of lymph node after fine needle aspiration. (**A**) There is a wedge-shaped focus of hypocellularity (indicated between arrows). (**B**) The hypocellular area shows lymphocyte depletion and hemorrhage.

probably related to injury and/or thrombosis of hilar veins.

Mycobacterial Spindle Cell Pseudotumor

- Infection by *Mycobacterium,* especially *Mycobacterium avium intracellulare,* in an immunocompromised host (such as with AIDS) may produce a reaction pattern not unlike that sometimes seen in leprosy (the "histoid" pattern).[204–207,261]
- The lymph node is characterized by tumorous replacement by spindly cells (macrophages) that form short fascicles or storiform pattern (Fig. 2-66). This lesion may be mistaken for fibrous histiocytoma, inflammatory pseudotumor, or smooth muscle tumor. The spindly histiocytes may or may not show granularity in the cytoplasm (Figs. 2-66B, 2-67). Rarely, the cytoplasm contains delicate basophilic streaks, reminiscent of the "globi" seen in leprosy.[204] Ziehl-Neelsen stain reveals myriads of acid-fast bacilli within the spindly histiocytes, providing confirmation of the diagnosis (Fig. 2-67B). Touch preparations stained with Giemsa or Diff-Quik reveal histiocytes containing multiple rod-shaped negative images (representing the bacteria), permitting an intraoperative diagnosis to be made.[262]
- Surprisingly, the spindly histiocytes may (but not invariably) show immunoreactivity for desmin, increasing the probability of mistaking this lesion for a smooth muscle neoplasm.[207,262]

Bacterial Lymphadenitis Mimicking Lennert's Lymphoma

- Kaiserling et al.[263] have described a peculiar form of bacterial lymphadenitis with histologic features strongly mimicking Lennert's lymphoma. The patients present with lymphadenopathy and systemic symptoms.
- The lymph nodes show extensive infiltration by small clusters of epithelioid histiocytes

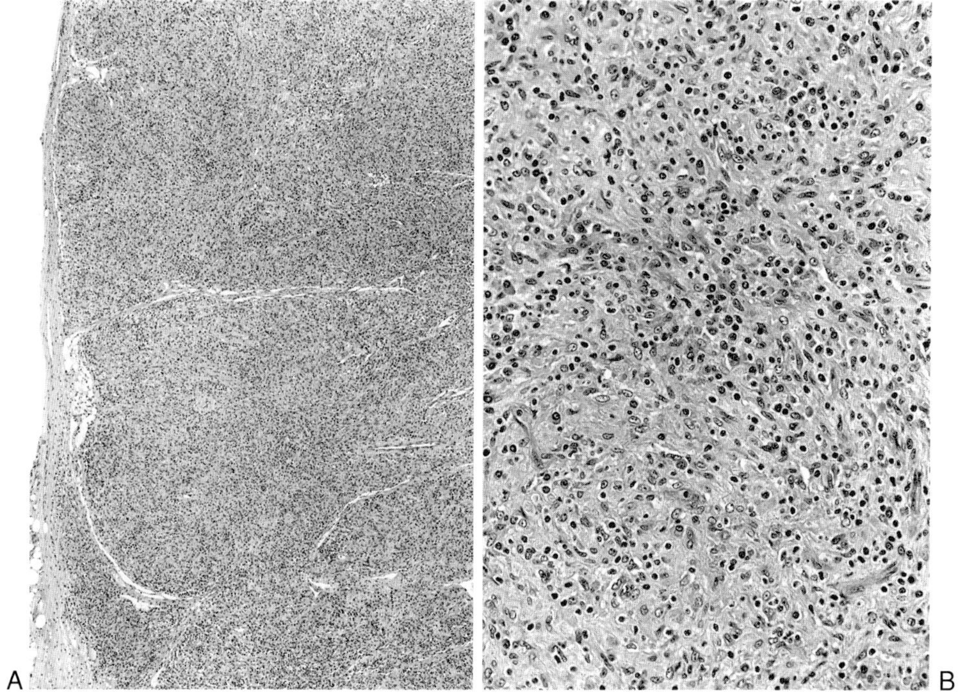

Fig. 2-66. Mycobacterial spindle cell pseudotumor. (**A**) There is extensive replacement of the nodal parenchyma by a fibro-inflammatory process. (**B**) The lesion comprises spindly cells, plasma cells, and small blood vessels.

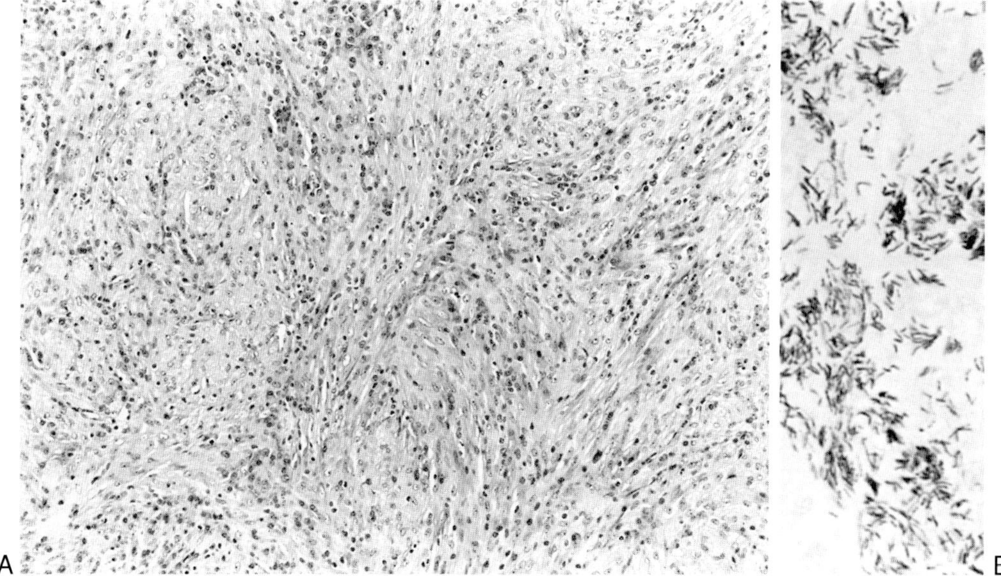

Fig. 2-67. Mycobacterial spindle cell pseudotumor. (**A**) This example shows spindly cells arranged in a vague storiform pattern. The spindly cells are shown on immunohistochemical staining to comprise mostly of histiocytes. (**B**) Numerous acid-fast bacilli can be demonstrated within the spindly cells by Ziehl-Neelsen stain.

without formation of discrete granulomas. The lymphocytes in between are mostly small lymphocytes mixed with some plasma cells. The bacteria cannot be demonstrated at the light microscopic level. On electron microscopy, there are some histiocytes packed with bacilli; the epithelioid histiocytes do not contain bacteria. This disease could represent a variant of Whipple's disease.

- Features that distinguish this peculiar form of lymphadenitis from Lennert's lymphoma are as follows:
  - Focal increase in reticulin fibers
  - Many more interspersed interdigitating reticulum cells, fibroblasts, and myofibroblasts
  - Demonstration of bacilli within histiocytes ultrastructurally

Pneumocystis Carinii Lymphadenitis

- *Pneumocystis carinii* is now considered a fungus rather than a protozoan.[264,265] With the frequent use of aerosolized Pentamidine for prophylaxis against pulmonary *P. carinii* infection in HIV-infected subjects, extrapulmonary pneumocystis infection is increasingly seen. This is because the drug is not absorbed into the circulation to produce a sufficient concentration for inhibition of the growth of *P. carinii* in extrapulmonary sites. Lymph node (especially mediastinal) is one of the most common sites of extrapulmonary involvement.[266–269]
- *P. carinii* lymphadenitis can give a false impression of extensive nodal necrosis on low magnification examination. However, careful analysis will reveal that the pink substance represents frothy exudate, with scattered lightly basophilic dots representing the organism (Fig. 2-68). There is usually no associated inflammation, although histiocytes can sometimes be found around the exudates. The exudate is period acid-Schiff positive, and a Grocott-Gomori methenamine silver stain shows myriads of *P. carinii*.[6]

Bacillary Angiomatosis

- Bacillary angiomatosis tends to occur in immunosuppressed patients (in particular those with AIDS). Lymph node may be involved

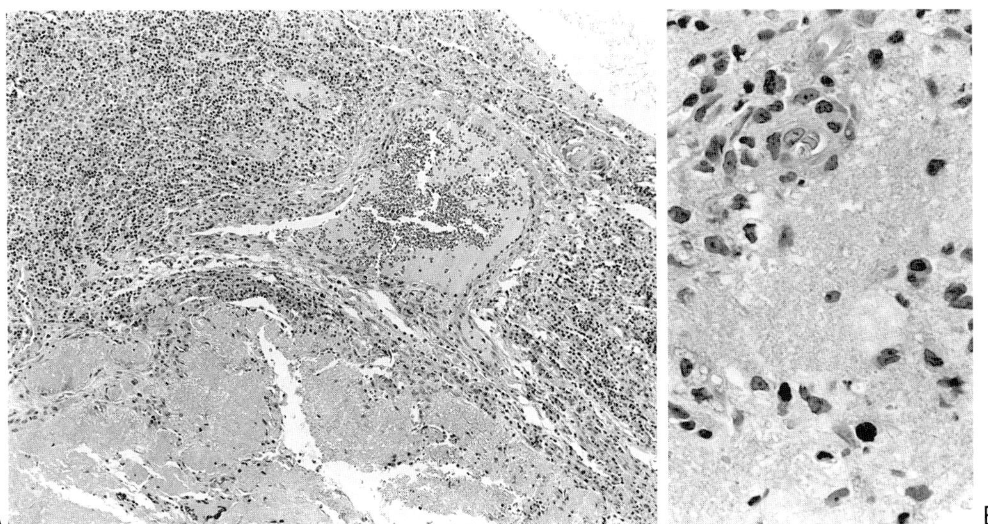

Fig. 2-68. *Pneumocystis carinii* lymphadenitis. (**A**) Pink-staining areas resembling necrosis are seen in the lower field. (**B**) They are in fact formed by frothy material with lightly basophilic dots. Special stains reveal myriads of organisms.

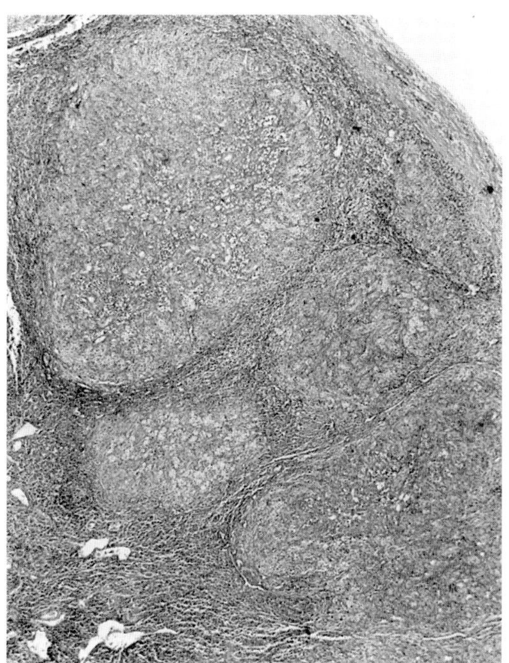

Fig. 2-69. Bacillary angiomatosis. The proliferated blood vessels typically form multiple nodules.

as the sole or one of many sites. It is a reactive vascular proliferation due to infection by *Bartonella* (*Rochalimaea*) *henselae* and rarely *B. quintana*.[14,193,194,270–283]

- The lymph node is usually involved in a multinodular pattern (Fig. 2-69). The diagnostic histologic triad is (1) proliferation of blood vessels lined by plump endothelium with pale cytoplasm; (2) interstitial amphophilic material (bacillary clumps); and (3) interstitial infiltration of neutrophils, often with leukocytoclasis (Fig. 2-70). The third feature may be absent in some cases (Fig. 2-71).[271] Some cases may show loculated edema or peliosis in the lymph node.[271,284]
- A firm diagnosis depends on demonstration of the distinctive clusters of bacilli in the interstitium, which can be achieved by one or more of the following methods:
  Warthin-Starry stain (Fig. 2-72)
  Giemsa stain[285]
  Toluidine blue-stained semithin sections
  Immunostaining with antibody against *B. henselae*[286]

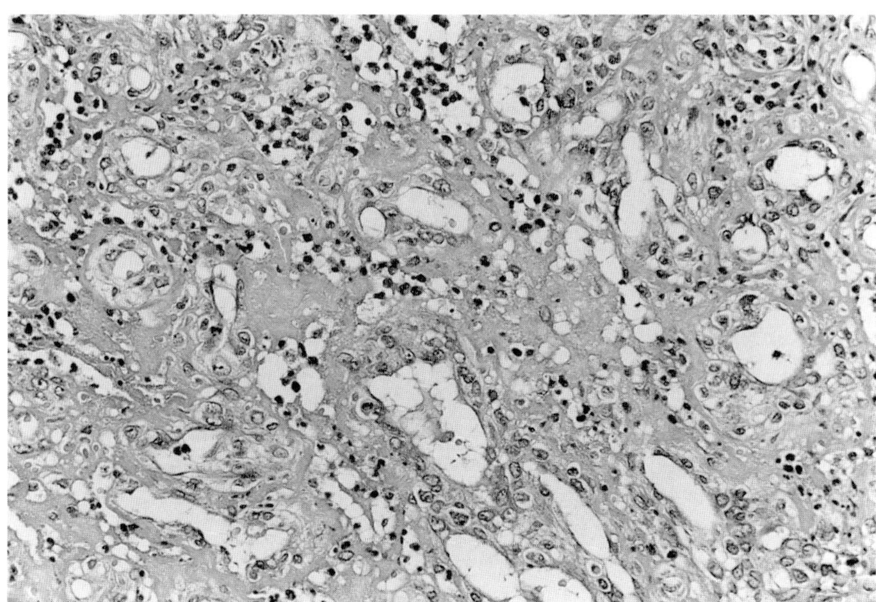

Fig. 2-70. Bacillary angiomatosis. This illustration depicts the classical triad of the condition: blood vessels lined by plump cells with pale cytoplasm, many neutrophils with karyorrhexis, and abundant interstitial amphophilic material (representing bacterial clumps).

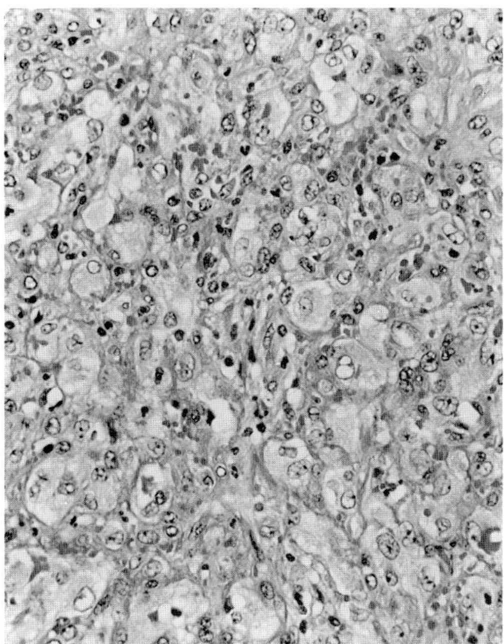

Fig. 2-71. Bacillary angiomatosis. A diagnosis is more difficult to make in this example, because neutrophils are absent and the blood vessels are barely canalized. The clues to diagnosis are the clinical setting for its occurrence (immunocompromised hosts) and the interstitial amphophilic material.

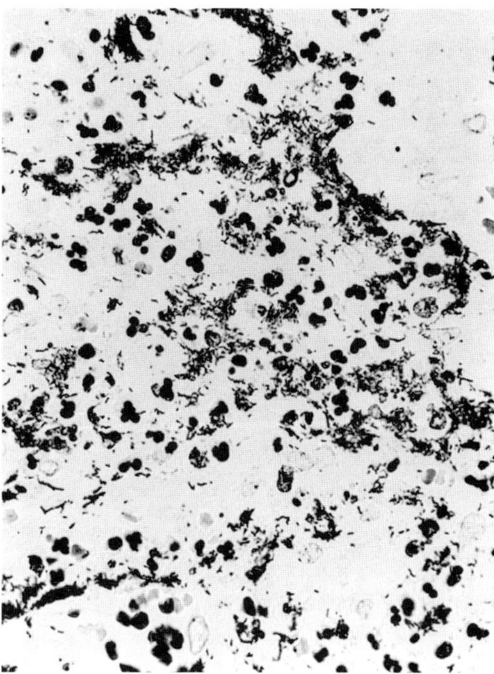

Fig. 2-72. Bacillary angiomatosis. The diagnosis is readily confirmed by Warthin-Starry stain, which demonstrates numerous short bacilli in the interstitial areas.

Hypha-Like Pseudofungus in Lymph Node

- An uncommon incidental finding in lymph node is the presence of fungal hyphae-like bodies in the sinuses. These bodies are amphophilic or golden brown and often exhibit septum-like structures and 45° to 90° branching (Fig. 2-73). Some can be ingested by multinucleated histiocytes. The histochemical staining pattern is as follows: Perls' stain positive (Fig. 2-73B), periodic acid-Schiff positive, von Kossa weak positive or negative, and Grocott-Gomori methenamine silver negative.[287,288] These fungus-like bodies are similar to Gamna-Gandy bodies of the spleen.
- According to our own experience and the cases reported in the literature, a biopsy or excision procedure has previously been performed in the drainage area of these nodes.[287,288] It is likely that red blood cells drained into the nodal sinuses break down, and the released hemosiderin impregnates and causes thickening of the reticulin fibers, after which calcium is deposited.
- Features that distinguish the pseudofungus from true fungus are lack of inflammatory reaction and lack of staining with Grocott-Gomori methenamine silver.

Silicone Lymphadenopathy

- Patients who have silicone breast implants or joint replacements may develop lymphadenopathy as a result of silicone draining into regional lymph nodes.[289–297] The lymph nodes may or may not be enlarged.
- Silicone lymphadenopathy is characterized by variable-sized, empty-looking rounded spaces, which are surrounded by histiocytes.

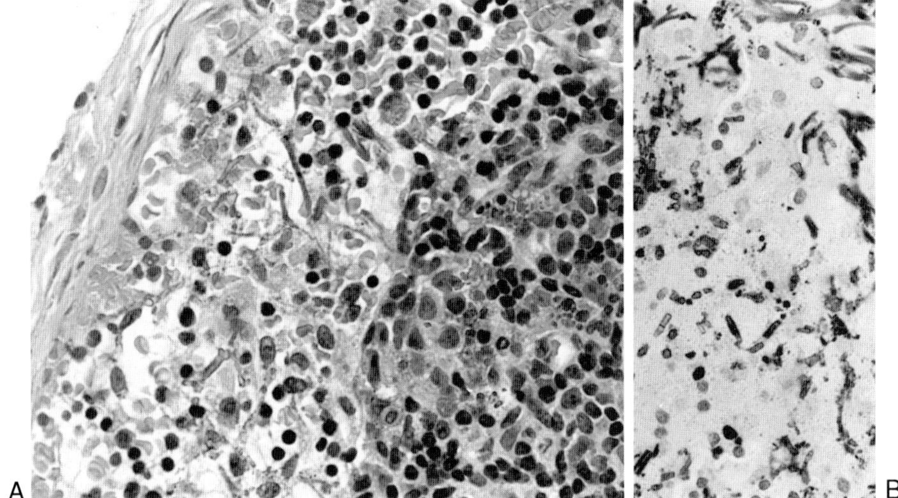

Fig. 2-73. Pseudofungus in an inguinal lymph node; this patient had a recent biopsy performed on a thigh tumor. In the subcapsular sinus, there are branching fungal hyphae-like structures. (**B**) These structures are strongly stained by Prussian blue reaction. There are even septum-like structures.

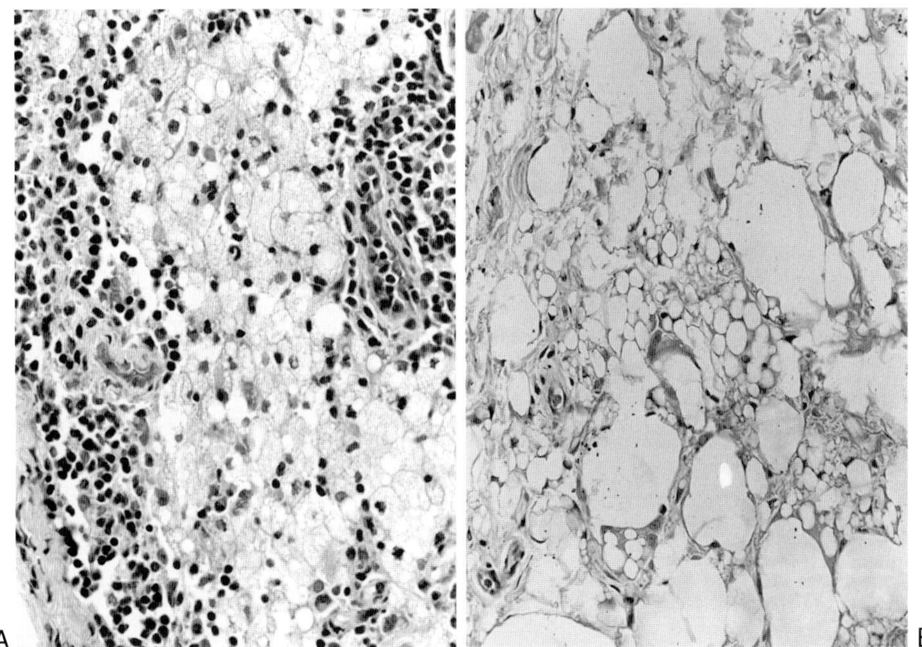

Fig. 2-74. Silicone lymphadenopathy. (**A**) This example is predominated by finely vacuolated histiocytes. (**B**) This example is predominated by extracellular silicone deposits (appearing as empty spaces) with some interspersed histiocytes. Some histiocytes also contain vacuoles.

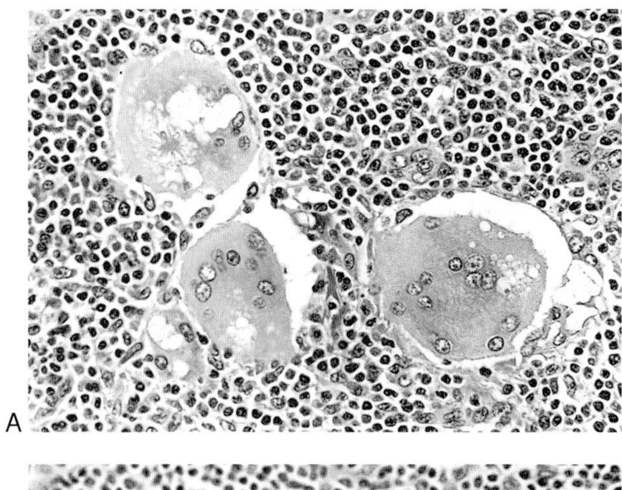

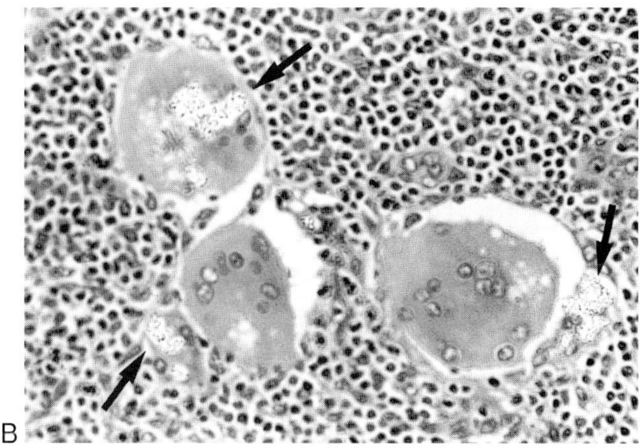

Fig. 2-75. Silicone lymphadenopathy. (**A**) In this example, the silicone occurs mostly within multinucleated histiocytes. An asteroid body is also seen in the histiocytes in the left upper field. (**B**) The refractile silicone material (*arrows*) is best seen on closing the diaphragm of the microscope.

Some cases may be predominated by mononuclear and multinucleated histiocytes containing multiple cytoplasmic vacuoles, and there can be confluent non-necrotizing granulomas (Fig. 2-74).[290,294,297] The spaces or vacuoles often appear empty because the silicone has been washed away during tissue processing, but at least some of the spaces and vacuoles can be shown to contain refractile, nonbirefringent, unstained material (best visualized by closing the condenser of the microscope) (Fig. 2-75). The major differential diagnoses are lymphangiogram effect, lepromatous leprosy, and hyperlipidemia (Fig. 2-76).

- The best ways to demonstrate silicone gel in tissue sections besides electron microscopy coupled with energy dispersive x-ray analysis include thick sections (more than 5 μm) for detection of nonstaining, refractile, nonbirefringent material; phase-contrast or dark-field microscopy; or adding stamp pad ink to the mounting medium (silicone totally lacking staining).[298,299]
- There are recent controversies as to whether use of silicone implant (breast) is associated with an increased risk of developing systemic autoimmune disease, although recent studies shed doubt on the existence of such an association.[300–302]
- There have been a few reports of silicone lymphadenopathy with concomitant malignant lymphoma.[303–305] It is unclear whether the lymphoma is coincidental or related to the silicone, or alternatively it may be related to the underlying autoimmune disease.

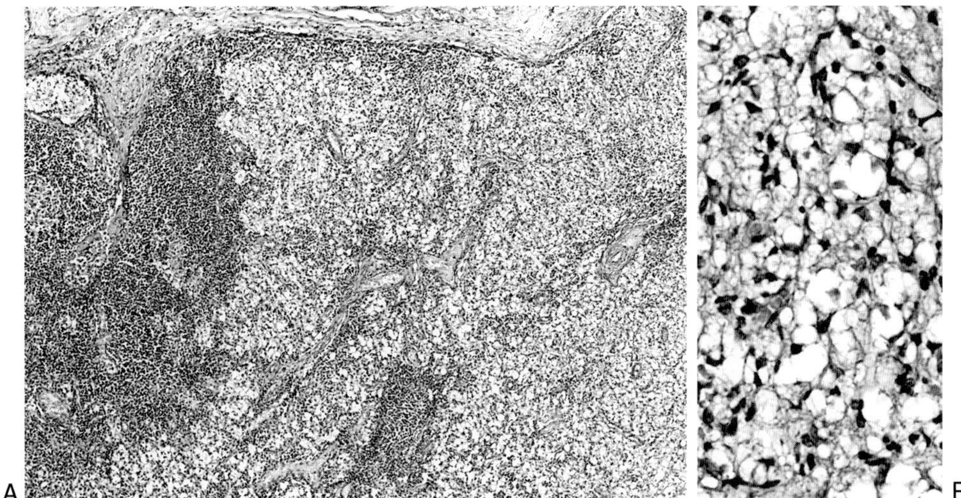

Fig. 2-76. Lepromatous leprosy. (**A**) There is marked replacement of the parenchyma by vacuolated cells. (**B**) The vacuolated cells are histiocytes, and some contain lightly basophilic material (globi).

Gold Lymphadenopathy

- Patients with rheumatoid arthritis are sometimes treated with long-term injection of gold, which can drain into the various tissues, including lymph node. The gold deposit can simulate microcalcifications on x-ray or can sometimes lead to lymphadenopathy.[306–308]
- Histologically, the gold particles are scattered in the parenchyma in the form of nonbirefringent, variable-shaped, thin plate-like crystalline structures or as dense black granules in clusters or discrete bodies. Some particles can occur within histiocytes. A firm diagnosis of gold lymphadenopathy can be made by x-ray microanalysis.[306,307] The background can show reactive follicular hyperplasia as typically observed in rheumatoid arthritis.

Polyvinylpyrrolidone Lymphadenopathy

- Polyvinylpyrrolidone (PVP) was previously widely used as a plasma expander and in various intravenous preparations, especially in areas of Asia. High molecular weight PVP introduced into the body persists in the reticuloendothelial system.[309,310] The lymph nodes are usually not enlarged, and the process is usually recognized incidentally in lymph nodes removed for other reasons.
- Deposits of PVP in the lymph node manifests morphologically as sinusoidal clusters of mononuclear and multinucleated histiocytes with abundant blue-gray, bubbly cytoplasm. Sometimes the nuclei are displaced to the periphery, resulting in a signet ring appearance (Fig. 2-77). The intracellular material characteristically stains with mucicarmine (hence the term *mucicarminophilic histiocytosis*), colloidal iron, Sirius red and Congo red, but not periodic acid-Schiff and Alcian blue. Extracellular oval or spherical brown particles of 1 to 15 μm diameter can be admixed with the histiocytes. There are few or no inflammatory cells. PVP lymphadenopathy can potentially be mistaken for metastatic adenocarcinoma, especially if further misled by the positive mucicarmine stain; it differs from the latter in showing no definite nuclear atypia, no cytokeratin immunoreactivity, and positive immunostaining with histiocytic markers.

Histiocytosis Related to Prosthesis, Such as Hip Replacement

- In the regional lymph nodes of patients who have undergone joint replacement, the sinuses are often packed with mononuclear and

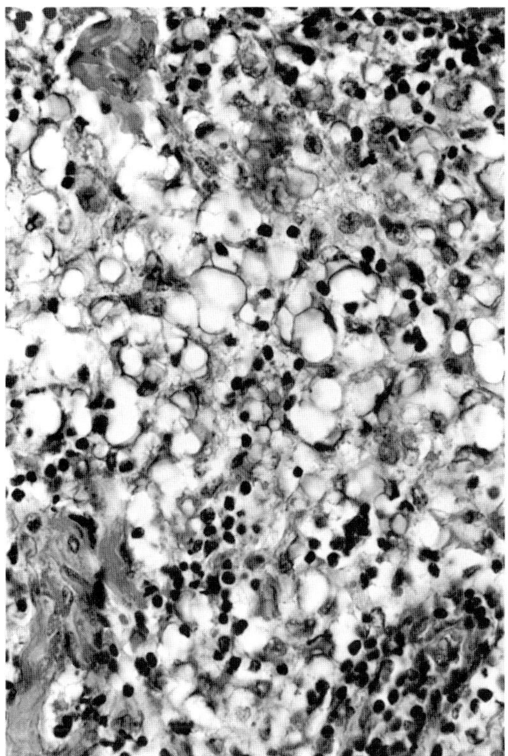

Fig. 2-77. PVP lymphadenopathy. The sinuses are packed with ''bubbly'' histiocytes containing blue-staining vacuoles. (Courtesy of Professor T. T. Kuo, Taiwan.)

multinucleated histiocytes as a florid reaction to debris derived from the prosthesis or cement. The appearances of the histiocytes are variable, depending on the nature of the foreign material. Lymph nodes showing such florid histiocytic reaction to prosthetic materials are increasingly encountered as incidental findings in pelvic lymph nodes removed as part of radical prostatectomy specimens.[311]

- Energy dispersive x-ray microanalysis shows presence of cobalt-chromium and titanium for those cases with foamy appearance and small black microparticles.[311]
- In other cases, the histiocytes have remarkably coarsely granular eosinophilic cytoplasm that is periodic acid Schiff positive (so-called granular histiocytic reaction).[312–314] They probably represent a reaction to polyester, polyethylene, or polyformaldehyde. In the cytoplasm, there might be occasional needle-shaped birefringent particles of polyethylene or birefringent black granules of metal.[313,314]
- It is most important not to mistake the prominent histiocytic reaction for metastatic carcinoma, granular cell tumor, or reticulohistiocytoma.[311]

Mantle Zone Hyperplasia

- Although not specifically singled out as a distinctive entity, mantle zone hyperplasia has been sporadically mentioned in the literature.[57,315,316] It appears to be uncommon and usually presents as a solitary, slightly enlarged lymph node in a young patient.[316] We have also observed lymph nodes adjacent to or draining a Castleman's disease lesion showing features of mantle zone hyperplasia.
- The reactive follicles have thick mantle zones that may exceed the diameter of the germinal centers. Some follicles may appear to be composed entirely of small lymphocytes because the small germinal centers may not be included in the plane of section (Fig. 2-78).
- In contrast to mantle cell lymphoma, the follicles are often confined to the cortex, there is no coalescence of the follicles, and the cells are small lymphocytes with dark round nuclei. Immunohistochemical studies to look for an aberrant immunophenotype (such as CD5 or CD43 expression) and monotypia may be required for the distinction.
- In contrast to hyaline-vascular Castleman's disease, hyalinized venules, striking interfollicular vascularity, and the ''single follicle, multiple germinal centers'' phenomenon are lacking.

Henoch-Schönlein Purpura Lymphadenitis

- Only recently have the lymph node changes in Henoch-Schönlein purpura been recorded.[317] The patients present with colicky abdominal pain and subsequently develop skin rash. In the mesenteric lymph

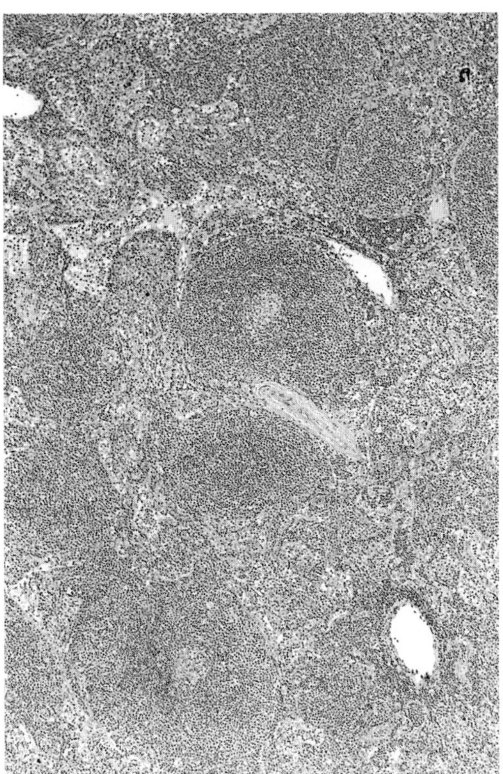

Fig. 2-78. Mantle zone hyperplasia. This node occurs adjacent to a mediastinal lesion of hyaline-vascular Castleman's disease. The mantle zones are broader than the germinal centers.

nodes, most germinal centers are replaced by histiocytes and follicular dendritic cells, while some are infiltrated by polymorphs. There are no extrafollicular granulomas. Some high endothelial venules show leukocytoclastic vasculitis, with endothelial degeneration, neutrophil infiltration, nuclear debris, and fibrin deposition.

REACTIVE LYMPHADENOPATHIES WITH NEW FINDINGS

Infectious Mononucleosis (EBV Infection)

- In infectious mononucleosis, the lymph node may show florid reactive follicular hyperplasia in the early phase. With time, there is striking paracortical proliferation of mitotically active large transformed cells (immunoblasts) that can form large clusters or diffuse sheets, leading to an erroneous diagnosis of large cell lymphoma. Frequently, the architecture is not totally effaced, with intact sinuses filled with activated lymphoid cells and some scattered reactive lymphoid follicles (which may exhibit necrosis) (Figs. 2-29, 2-30). The immunoblasts often show variations in size and degree of cytoplasmic basophilia; they can show a mild degree of atypia (Fig. 2-31). Single cell necrosis or patchy necrosis is common. Small lymphocytes, plasma cells, and plasmablasts are typically admixed, imparting a mottled appearance when the interspersed immunoblasts do not constitute the major component.[2,5,92,318,319]
- Reed-Sternberg-like cells (binucleated immunoblasts) can sometimes be found (Fig. 2-28), and they differ from the Reed-Sternberg cells of Hodgkin's disease in usually having basophilic rather than eosinophilic nucleoli and a prominent paranuclear pale hof.[10,92,320] In contrast to Hodgkin's disease, these giant cells occur in a background of many large activated cells, and they are almost always CD15 negative and Ki-B3 positive. The giant cells in both conditions are usually positive for CD30 and EBV LMP1.[88,321–324]
- As discussed in a previous section, EBV-associated infectious mononucleosis cannot be distinguished from other causes of reactive immunoblastic proliferation on morphologic grounds.
- The immunoblasts exhibit the following immunophenotype: B cells, 30 to 50 percent, T cells, 25 to 70 percent. Rarely, there may be coexpression of CD20 and CD43. They show variable expression of CD30 and EBV LMP1 and are negative for CD15.[79,88,321,323]
- In situ hybridization studies have shown that in EBV-associated infectious mononucleosis EBV DNA signals can be demonstrated in 10 to 20 percent of lymphoid cells in the involved regions, and EBER can be detected in more than 50 percent of the large lymphoid

cells but in less than 25 percent of the interfollicular small lymphocytes.[79,88,90,91,322] Among the EBER-positive cells, most are of B lineage, while a small fraction are of T lineage.[87,325] There is a concentration of EBV-positive cells around the necrotic foci.[88,90]

Cytomegalovirus Lymphadenitis

- The histologic picture of cytomegalovirus (CMV) lymphadenitis is highly variable.
- The subtle pattern (in immunocompetent host, presenting either as localized lymphadenopathy or CMV mononucleosis) is prominent reactive follicular hyperplasia and monocytoid B-cell reaction. The follicles may be deficient in mantles. There may be foci of necrosis within the monocytoid B-cell clusters. The interfollicular areas often show increased blood vessels and immunoblasts. Cells with CMV inclusions are very sparse (usually among the monocytoid B cells and occasionally in the paracortex) and may require careful examination of multiple levels for their detection.[326,327]
- The exuberant pattern (in immunocompromised host) includes many cells with recognizable CMV inclusions that efface the architecture of the lymph node, and there may be areas of necrosis.
- Although CMV may infect many cell types (including endothelium), CMV-infected lymphoid cells appear to be almost exclusively T cells, which can be of CD4+ or CD8+ phenotype.[328]
- CMV inclusion-containing cells can potentially be mistaken for Reed-Sternberg cells on morphologic grounds, while rare cases of Hodgkin's disease show localization of the neoplastic cells to the monocytoid B-cell clusters.[329,330] The mimicry is further strengthened on immunohistochemical staining, because the CMV-positive cells are often CD15 positive.[326] Confirmation of the diagnosis of CMV lymphadenitis can be readily obtained by immunohistochemical staining or in situ hybridization.

Herpes Simplex Lymphadenitis

- Herpes simplex lymphadenitis is uncommon and can occur in previously healthy subjects or immunocompromised hosts (especially those with lymphoproliferative disease). The lymphadenopathy can be localized or generalized and can be accompanied by fever and skin rash.
- The histologic features described for herpes simplex lymphadenitis are highly variable[331–338]:
  - A reported case shows paracortical hyperplasia with increased immunoblasts but no viral inclusions and is therefore indistinguishable from infectious mononucleosis.[334]
  - Some cases exhibit large areas of necrosis, which can be accompanied by suppuration, debris, abundant histiocytes or granulation tissue. The typical cytopathic effects of herpesvirus are seen in many cells: ''fractured'' nuclear membrane (chromatin margination), ground-glass nuclei, intranuclear eosinophilic inclusions with clear halos, and multinucleated forms.
  - Most cases show a combination of features, with tiny to large, discrete, infarct-like necrotic foci occurring in the background of diffuse or nodular paracortical hyperplasia. The paracortical immunoblasts are mostly of T lineage, and there can be intermingled eosinophils and histiocytes. Sinus histiocytosis may be prominent. Occasional viral inclusions are seen in cells around the necrotic foci or in immunoblast-like cells in the expanded paracortex.
- The diagnosis of herpes simplex infection can be confirmed by serology, immunohistochemistry, electron microscopy (nucleocapsids or empty capsids), Southern blot hybridization, or in situ hybridization.[331] The

immunoblasts with large viral inclusions can be potentially mistaken for the Reed-Sternberg cells of Hodgkin's disease.

Whipple's Lymphadenopathy

- Peripheral lymphadenopathy (such as in the neck, axilla, or groin) can sometimes be the first manifestation of Whipple's disease.[339,340] It is characterized by increased pale-staining and often finely vacuolated histiocytes (strongly periodic acid-Schiff positive) in the sinuses. There are typically interspersed lipid vacuoles.
- The organism responsible for Whipple's disease has been identified through molecular analysis: it is related to actinobacteria and has been named *Tropheryma whippeli*.[341] Rarely, the disease is caused by other bacteria, such as "Whipple's disease-associated bacterial organism" closely related to *Nocardioforms*.[342]
- The major differential diagnosis is *M. avium-intracellulare* infection, especially in HIV-seropositive subjects.

Toxoplasmic Lymphadenitis

- Toxoplasmic lymphadenitis is characterized by the morphologic triad of florid reactive follicular hyperplasia, monocytoid B-cell hyperplasia, and small aggregates of epithelioid histiocytes with encroachment on germinal centers.[343,344]
- It is exceptional to find the *Toxoplasma* organism in the lymph nodes.[345] By polymerase chain reaction, toxoplasmic genomes are only rarely detected in toxoplasmic lymphadenitis (one of nine cases), and in the positive case, only one of three tissue samples is positive.[346] These findings suggest an exceedingly low number of genomes or complete absence of the organism in most cases and that the nodal changes probably represent a reaction to products of the organisms previously present in the node or drained into the node rather than direct effects of contact with the organism.[346]

Anticonvulsant-Associated Lymphadenopathy

- A small proportion of patients on anticonvulsant therapy (in particular phenytoin/Dilantin and occasionally carbamazepine) may develop local or generalized lymphadenopathy, usually in less than 4 months (although the interval can be less than 1 week or up to many years). The lymph node enlargement can be accompanied by fever, rash, malaise, hepatosplenomegaly, and eosinophilia. The lymphadenopathy can show a spectrum of changes from florid reactive lymphoproliferations ("pseudolymphoma" or "atypical lymphoproliferative disease") to malignant lymphoma. There appears to be a slight increased risk for lymphoma (non-Hodgkin's or Hodgkin's type) with chronic phenytoin therapy.[347–354]
- The reactive nodes often resolve with withdrawal of the offending drug, but they may recur on reintroduction of the drug. Occurrence of the drug reaction may have an inherited predisposition.[355]
- The morphologic features of the benign lymphoproliferations are varied and can be indistinguishable from those of infectious mononucleosis except that the immunoblasts are usually CD30 negative[347,349]:
  - Florid paracortical immunoblastic proliferation associated with hyperplasia and disruption of germinal centers; eosinophils are present; occasionally there is obliterative vasculitis (Fig. 2-36)
  - Florid paracortical immunoblastic proliferation associated with atrophic germinal centers
  - Miscellaneous nonimmunoblastic lesions, such as nonspecific reactive follicular hyperplasia, dermatopathic lymphadenopathy, necrotizing lymphadenitis, and fibroxanthomatous le-

sion; these may represent coincidental changes in lymph node. The first pattern probably results from drug-induced hypersensitivity as evidenced by the early onset (short duration of use of the drug), while the second pattern probably represents a late effect of the drug

- Some cases reported as AILD have been associated with the use of phenytoin.[356–358] Such cases have a better prognosis than AILD in general, suggesting that they may merely represent AILD-like lesion.[354]

Angioimmunoblastic Lymphadenopathy

- This is a "vanishing" disease. The majority of cases so diagnosed in the past represent AILD-like T-cell lymphoma.[63]
- Now, a diagnosis of AILD should be made with great caution and viewed with a little skepticism. When the differential diagnosis is between AILD and AILD-like T-cell lymphoma, the former diagnosis should be reserved for cases showing[94]:
  - Hypocellularity
  - No significant irregular nuclear foldings in the lymphoid cells
  - Lack of clusters of clear cells (medium sized or large cells with small nucleoli) or clusters of immunoblasts with basophilic cytoplasm

Even defined in this way, some cases are shown on molecular analysis to contain clonal populations of T cells. It has been suggested that perhaps such cases should also be treated as for AILD-like T-cell lymphoma.[94]

Extramedullary Hemopoiesis

- Groups of hematopoietic cells can occur in lymph nodes in a variety of conditions, such as severe anemia of various types (including thalassemia) and agnogenic myeloid metaplasia. Megakaryocytes, if present, can potentially be mistaken for malignant cells because of their large polyploid nuclei; their identity can be confirmed by immunostaining for factor VIII-related antigen, CD31, or CD34. Erythroblasts can also be highlighted by immunostaining for glycophorin or hemoglobin. All these antibodies are applicable on routine paraffin sections.
- A recently documented cause for extramedullary hemopoiesis in lymph node is the use of granulocyte colony-stimulating factor.[359]

Reactive Follicular Hyperplasia

- Reactive follicular hyperplasia of the idiopathic type is seen mostly in children and young adults. Males are more commonly affected than females. The histologic features have been discussed in a previous section. The most typical presentation is that of a solitary, enlarged, nontender lymph node. The lymph nodes of the head and neck are most commonly affected, especially the submandibular and parotid region.[67,360]
- Reactive follicular hyperplasia has a different implication when it occurs in elderly subjects more than 60 years old, because this probably represents an imbalance of the immune system.[361] Thirty-one percent of cases either have concurrent lymphoma or subsequently develop lymphoma, especially those patients with multiple enlarged lymph nodes. The lymphoma may be of B lineage or T lineage. Thus lymph nodes from elderly patients showing reactive follicular hyperplasia should be scrutinized for lymphoma, which usually manifests as broadening of the interfollicular zones, presence of atypical lymphoid cells, and erosion of the mantle zones of the reactive lymphoid follicles. If the node shows no such sinister features, close follow-up and rebiopsy are required.

Rheumatoid Lymphadenopathy

- The histologic triad of lymphadenopathy associated with rheumatoid arthritis are well known: reactive follicular hyperplasia, interfollicular plasmacytosis, and neutrophils in sinuses (sometimes with the formation of microabscesses) (Fig. 2-12A). The nodal capsule can be thickened. In the perinodal tissue, there is frequently lymphocytic infiltration and possibly formation of lymphoid follicles. The changes are not pathognomonic and can be seen in other conditions, such as nonspecific reactive follicular hyperplasia, Sjögren syndrome, and Felty syndrome.[2,362,363] Of interest, this pattern of reactive follicular hyperplasia is uncommon in other collagen vascular diseases.[68]

- The appearances of the reactive lymphoid follicles in rheumatoid lymphadenopathy may deviate from those seen in the usual examples of reactive follicular hyperplasia in the following features[68]:

  Relatively low proliferative activity despite the large size of the follicles
  Fewer tingible-body macrophages
  Predominance of small cleaved cells (centrocytes)

Such features may invite an erroneous interpretation as follicular lymphoma.

- An uncommon pattern of reaction has recently been recognized: predominantly paracortical expansion by small lymphocytes with slightly contorted nuclei and scanty cytoplasm. The lymphoid follicles appear to be compressed by the expanded paracortex.[68,364] This pattern can mimic a low grade post-thymic T-cell lymphoma on morphologic grounds. The proliferated cells in the paracortex are mostly polytypic B cells that co-express CD5; this finding is of some interest because of the postulated role of CD5+ B cells in autoimmune diseases.[364]

Lymphadenopathy of Sjögren Syndrome

- Patients with Sjögren syndrome may show a spectrum of lymphoid proliferations in lymph node and in extranodal sites, including reactive lymphoid infiltrate, atypical lymphoid hyperplasia, and malignant lymphoma.[354,365–367]
- The most common nodal change is identical to that seen in rheumatoid arthritis, and there may be in addition monocytoid B-cell hyperplasia and focal dermatopathic changes.[354,367,368]
- The atypical lymphoid hyperplasias as described in the literature show different appearances. However, at least some cases show prominent collections of parafollicular pale (monocytoid) cells,[367,369] and we suspect that such cases represent partial nodal involvement by an occult low grade B-cell lymphoma of mucosa-associated lymphoid tissue type in the salivary gland.[370] Immunostaining for Ig light chains and molecular analysis are particularly helpful for detecting monoclonal populations in such lymphoid proliferations.
- The lymphomas that complicate Sjögren syndrome can occur in the salivary gland, lymph node, or other sites and are almost always of B lineage. The most common type is low grade B-cell lymphoma of mucosa-associated lymphoid tissue type (often reported in the literature as "monocytoid B-cell lymphoma" or "lymphoplasmacytic lymphoma") and diffuse B-large cell lymphoma.[365,367,370–372]
- Since patients with Sjögren syndrome have an increased risk for malignant lymphoma, lymphadenopathy should be investigated by prompt biopsy.[367]

Localized Castleman's Disease, Hyaline-Vascular Type

- Menke et al.[373] have found the mantle zone cells of Castleman's disease (both hyaline-vascular and plasma cell types) to exhibit an immunophenotype of KiB3− KiB5+. It is suggested that this aberrant phenotype may support a diagnosis of Castleman's disease in difficult cases.
- In hyaline-vascular Castleman's disease, the small germinal centers are usually predomi-

nated by follicular dendritic cells, which are mixed with small numbers of follicle center B cells. In some cases, scattered follicular dendritic cells may appear bizarre—enlarged, irregular nuclei with coarse chromatin (Fig. 2-79).[14,374] It is unclear whether these "dysplastic" cells are inconsequential (degenerative) or represent the forerunner of follicular dendritic cell tumors. The interfollicular zone is rich in high endothelial venules and small lymphocytes, and clusters of plasmacytoid monocytes are commonly found (Fig. 2-80). Occasional large bizarre cells with hyperchromatic nuclei and coarse chromatin can rarely be observed in the interfollicular zones; the significance of these cells is unknown, although they are probably degenerative in nature (Fig. 2-79). Sclerosis is common, occurring in the periphery, around the venules, or in the form of bands (Fig. 2-81).[2,375]

- Hyaline-vascular follicles per se are not pathognomonic of Castleman's disease; they have also been observed in HIV-associated lymphadenopathy, AILD, and as single follicles in otherwise nonspecific reactive lymphadenopathies.[2] Therefore, to qualify for a diagnosis of hyaline-vascular Castleman's disease, in addition to the predominance of hyaline-vascular follicles or follicles with multiple small germinal centers (Fig. 2-82), the interfollicular zones have to be rich in venules and small lymphocytes, although the percentage areas of follicular and interfollicular components are highly variable from case to case (Fig. 2-81).
- In immunohistochemical studies, the follicles consist mostly of polyclonal B cells, with the small lymphocytes in the thick mantle zones bearing IgM and IgD. They have an abnormal follicular dendritic cell network that is ex-

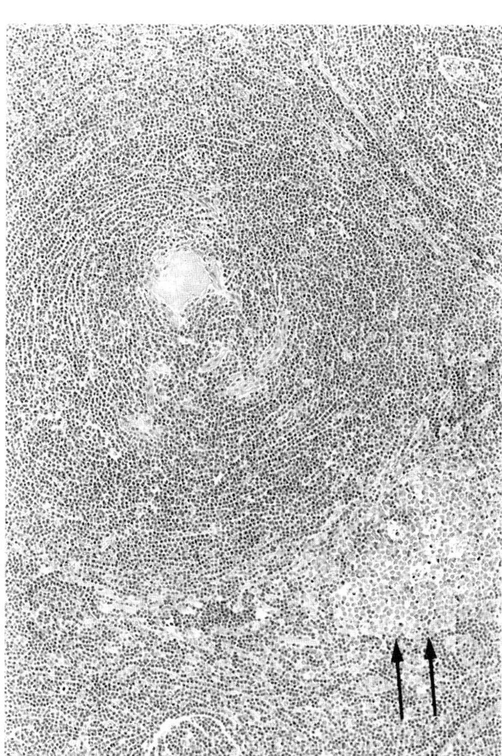

Fig. 2-80. Hyaline-vascular Castleman's disease. The follicle shows onion skin-like placement of small lymphocytes around the follicle, which is penetrated by a hyalinized venule. A cluster of plasmacytoid monocytes (*arrows*) is seen adjacent to the follicle.

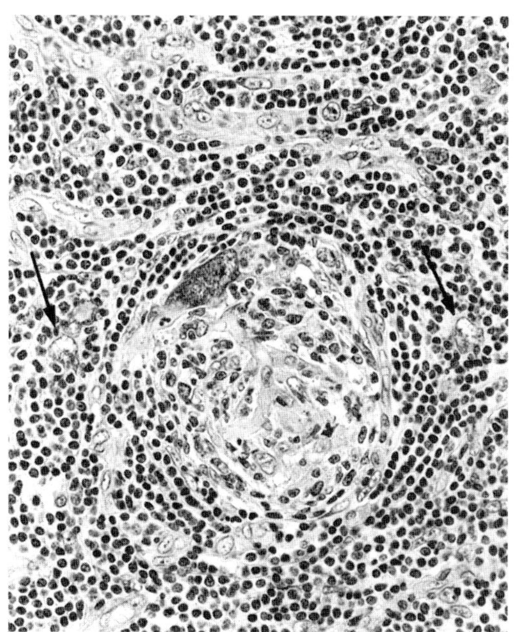

Fig. 2-79. Hyaline-vascular Castleman's disease with scattered atypical cells. A large bizarre cell in seen in the germinal center, and several large atypical cells are seen outside the follicle (*arrows*).

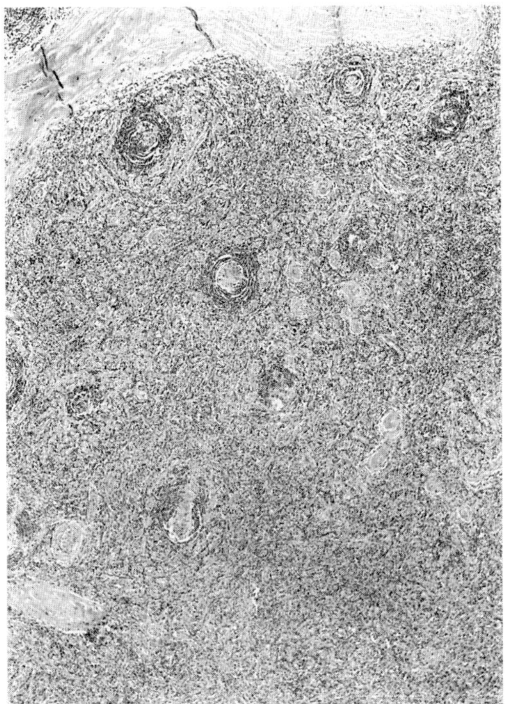

Fig. 2-81. Hyaline-vascular Castleman's disease. This case demonstrates that the interfollicular zones can be broad. Hyaline-vascular follicles are seen in the upper field. There is also a sclerotic band on top.

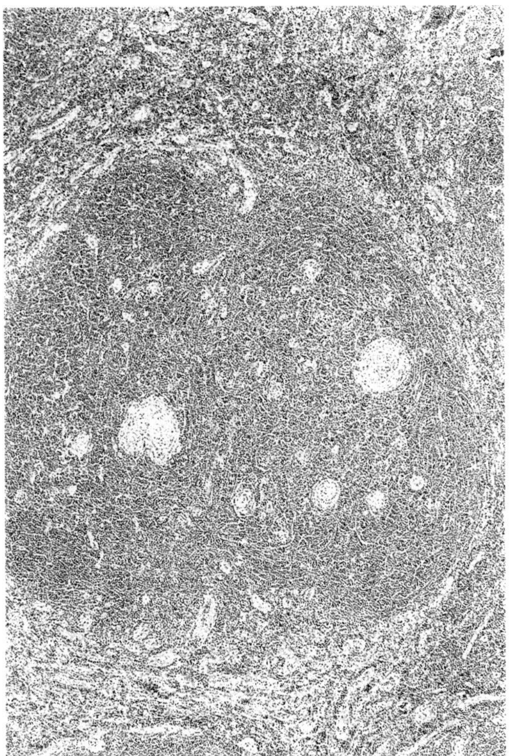

Fig. 2-82. Hyaline-vascular Castleman's disease. This large follicle contains multiple small germinal centers. This feature is virtually diagnostic of this entity although it is not invariably found. The interfollicular regions are rich in venules, a feature that is essential for diagnosis of this entity.

panded and disrupted or in the form of multiple tight concentric collections; this abnormal pattern is not observed in the plasma cell type of Castleman's disease.[376] In the centers of the follicles, the blood vessels stain with endothelial markers. The interfollicular zone is dominated by small lymphocytes with scarcely any immunoblasts; these cells are mostly mature T cells (more CD4+ than CD8+). Leu7 (CD57) positive cells are notably rare or absent.[377–380] The interfollicular venules stain with endothelial markers and markers of nodal high endothelial venules (HECA-452, MECA-79).[375]

- Genotypic studies reveal no rearrangements of the Ig or TCR genes and no viral genomes of EBV or CMV.[381,382]
- Danon et al.[375] have described a stroma-rich variant, characterized by an interfollicular or "stromal" zone comprising more than 75 percent of the lesion. Such cases tend to occur only in adults and mostly in an intra-abdominal or retroperitoneal location. The lesions tend to be larger (median diameter 7.5 cm) than the classic cases (4 to 5 cm). Histologically, the interfollicular zones are broadened and may be accompanied by formation of focal nodules. The nodules are often rich in blood vessels and spindly cells, which can form a storiform pattern. Their composition is highly variable and can include blood vessels, actin-positive myoid cells or fibroblastic reticulum cells, histiocytic reticulum cells (CD68+ dendritic cells), or follicular dendritic cells (Figs. 2-83, 2-84).[382a] It is not always easy to distinguish these "stromal proliferations" from a superimposed tumor.[382a]

- The localized hyaline-vascular form of Castleman's disease has been reported to be complicated or accompanied by the following neoplasms or hamartomas[14,383–385]:
    - Vascular neoplasm (the vascular nature of which has not been convincingly demonstrated in most reported cases), which can exhibit a spectrum of differentiation and behavior
    - Follicular dendritic cell tumor
    - Angiolipomatous hamartoma
- One case has been reported of histologic features of hyaline-vascular Castleman's disease occurring in the regional lymph nodes of a gastric stromal tumor.[386]

Localized Castleman's Disease, Plasma Cell Type

- While the hyaline-vascular type of Castleman's disease almost always occurs as a localized form, the plasma cell type can be solitary or more commonly multicentric.[387,388] At least some cases reported as "plasma cell type Castleman's disease" in the literature represent multicentric Castleman's disease.[389]
- Immunohistochemical studies indicate that the follicles have normal follicular dendritic cell networks.[376] The interfollicular plasma cells are found to be monotypic (almost always λ light chain restriction) in approximately 40 percent of the cases.[389,390] Yet even these cases do not exhibit a malignant behavior. It has been suggested that this represents the nodal counterpart of "benign monoclonal gammopathy."[390]
- Interleukin-6, a cytokine with pleiotropic effects on the immune system, may play a key role in the genesis of the plasma cell type of Castleman's disease. Almost all patients have raised serum interleukin-6. Within the lesion, immunoreactive interleukin-6 can be demonstrated in the germinal center B cells and immunoblastoid B cells around and outside the

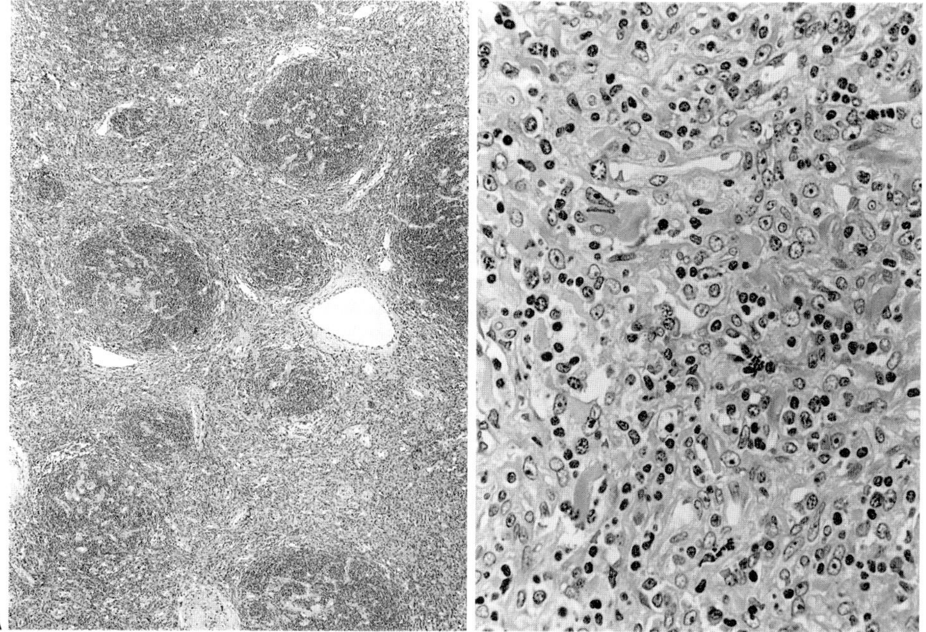

Fig. 2-83. Hyaline-vascular Castleman's disease with stromal proliferation. (**A**) The follicles are separated by a moderate amount of interfollicular tissue. (**B**) The interfollicular tissue is rich in plump cells with indistinct cell borders, oval nuclei, empty nucleoplasm, and small distinct nucleolus, characteristic of follicular dendritic cells.

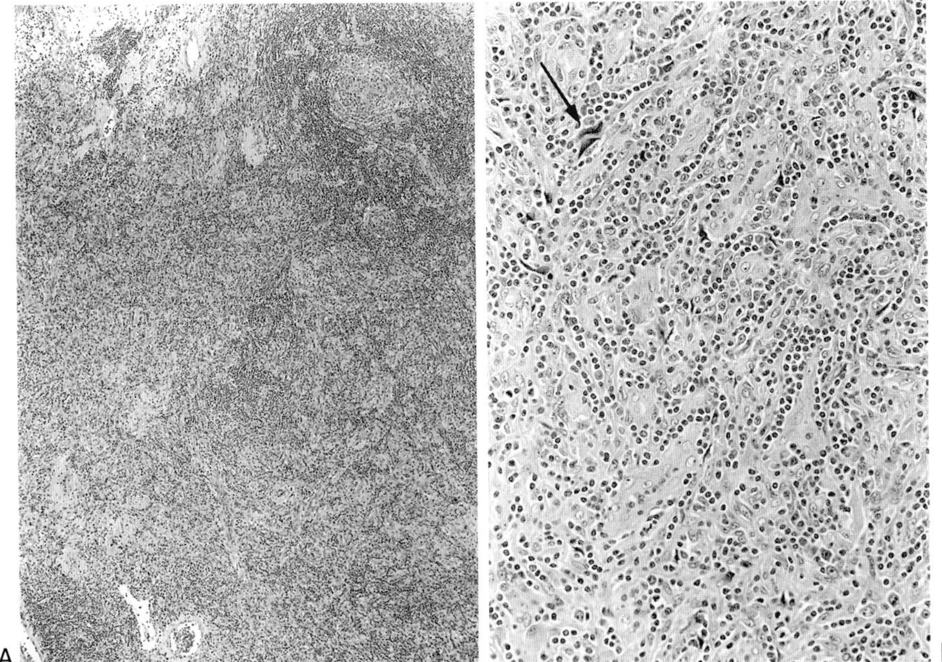

Fig. 2-84. Hyaline-vascular Castleman's disease with vascular overgrowth (stroma-rich variant). (**A**) There is marked expansion of the interfollicular zone. (**B**) There is profuse proliferation of small blood vessels, some of which are lined by cells with large hyperchromatic nuclei (*arrow*).

follicles.[391] Further evidence supporting the important role of interleukin-6 is the resolution of symptoms in a patient with the plasma cell type of Castleman's disease by treatment with monoclonal antibody against interleukin-6.[392]

- In some cases of plasma cell type Castleman's disease, the same lymph node or a subsequent lymph node biopsy may show Hodgkin's lymphoma. It is postulated that the Castleman's disease component may represent an abnormal immunologic response to the Hodgkin's disease (possibly mediated by excessive production of interleukin-6 by the Reed-Sternberg cells and histiocytes). Thus, the lymph node must be carefully scrutinized to exclude Hodgkin's disease before a diagnosis of plasma cell type Castleman's disease is rendered.[393–395]
- The histologic features of plasma cell type Castleman's disease are not pathognomonic, and hyaline-vascular follicles may or may not be found (Fig. 2-85). Similar features can be seen in HIV-associated lymphadenopathy, Wiskott-Aldrich syndrome, rheumatoid arthritis, ill-defined autoimmune syndromes, luetic lymphadenitis, lymph nodes draining carcinoma, lymphoma, or skin diseases, lipoid nephrosis, and peripheral vascular disease.[387,396] Thus the diagnosis should be made only when no cause is found and the clinical features are compatible.[387]

Castleman's Disease, Multicentric Type

- In comparison with the localized form of Castleman's disease, the multicentric (systemic) type generally occurs in an older age group.[397–400] The diagnostic criteria, as proposed by Frizzera,[401] are as follow[57,387]:

    Histologic features in the lymph node are those of plasma cell type Castleman's disease (although some hyaline-vascu-

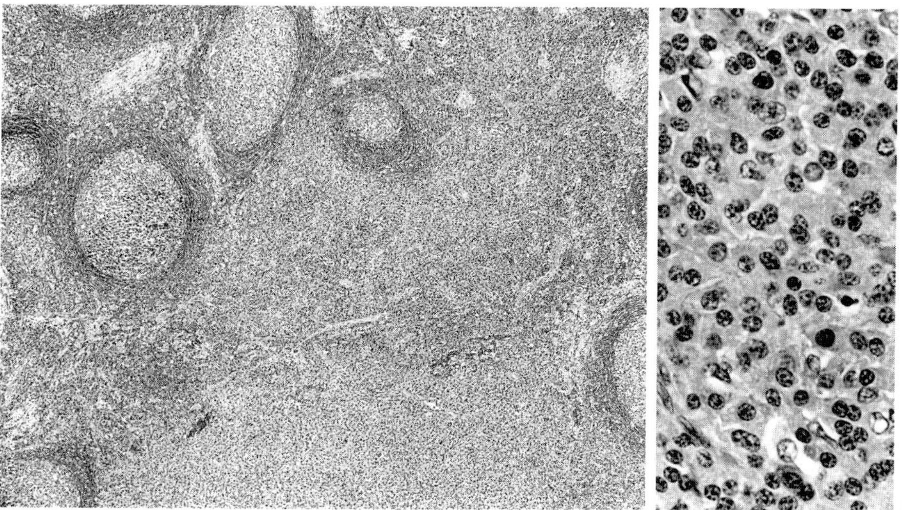

Fig. 2-85. Plasma cell type Castleman's disease. (**A**) The follicles do not look different from those seen in the usual reactive follicular hyperplasia. The interfollicular regions are expanded and appear violaceous on hematoxylin-eosin-stained sections. (**B**) Such areas are packed with mature plasma cells.

lar follicles can occur, especially in the burned out stage)

Clinical presentation is predominantly lymphadenopathic, with involvement of multiple peripheral nodes

Evidence of multisystem involvement, most notably bone marrow, liver, kidney, liver, skin, and nervous system, and systemic symptoms are very common

No known causes

- Although predominantly an adult disease, multicentric Castleman's disease can also occur in children.[402]
- Multicentric Castleman's disease appears to be related to the localized plasma cell type, but not the localized hyaline-vascular type, of Castleman's disease.[387,401,403]
- Immunohistochemical studies show that the follicles comprise B cells, and the mantle zone cells exhibit an IgM+ IgD+ phenotype. Surprisingly, one study reports that the mantle zone cells are CD5+, and this observation has been interpreted as suggesting a role for the CD5+ autoreactive B cells in pathogenesis.[389,404] The interfollicular plasma cells are either polytypic or monotypic.[381,389,390,405]
- Genotypic analysis shows that most cases exhibit rearrangements of the Ig genes and sometimes the TCR genes, although the rearranged bands may be weak, indicating presence of only a minor clonal population.[381,405–407] A recent study on a large number of cases, however, shows that Ig gene rearrangement is very rare and that the positive cases are associated with presence of frank lymphoma.[382] EBV or Kaposi sarcoma-associated herpesvirus can be detected in most cases.[381,408,409,409a]
- A small proportion of patients exhibit the clinical manifestations of POEMS syndrome, which includes polyneuropathy, organomegaly, endocrinopathy, M protein, and skin changes.[383,387,388,390,407]
- The multicentric form of Castleman's disease has been reported to be complicated by the following[383,397–399,407–413]:

    Malignant lymphoma
    Kaposi sarcoma
    Plasmacytoma
    Glomeruloid hemangioma

- The lymph node changes in patients with AIDS (HIV-associated lymphadenopathy) can be indistinguishable from those of multicentric Castleman's disease.[257]

Progressive Transformation of Germinal Centers

- Progressive transformation of germinal centers (PTGC) is a benign condition of unknown etiology. A possible histogenetic relationship with nodular lymphocyte predominance Hodgkin's disease (n-LPHD) has been suggested, that is, the two conditions may coexist, some patients with PTGC may eventually develop n-LPHD, and some patients with n-LPHD may develop PTGC on follow-up. Lymph nodes showing features of PTGC should therefore be scrutinized for evidence of coexisting n-LPHD.[414–419] Recent studies have shown that the risk of developing n-LPHD in a patient whose lymph node shows pure PTGC is in fact very low (0 to 5 percent).[416,420,421]
- A study from Germany also suggests a possible relationship between PTGC and classical Hodgkin's disease as well.[421]
- PTGC usually presents as solitary enlarged lymph node, most commonly in the neck, although it can also present with lymphadenopathy involving several sites. It occurs more commonly in young subjects, but no age is exempt. There is male predominance. PTGC may persist or recur (usually locally), especially in children.[416,421]
- Histologically, it is characterized by scattered large expansile follicles disposed in a background of usual-looking reactive follicles. These dark-staining ''transformed'' follicles, which are two to four times the size of the surrounding follicles, lack well-defined germinal centers or have irregular ''broken up'' germinal centers (Fig. 2-86). They are formed mostly by small lymphocytes, which are intermingled with isolated or small clusters of follicular center B cells (Fig. 2-87). Sometimes the large follicles are surrounded by wreaths of epithelioid histiocytes, a feature more commonly observed in PTGC in children.[416] There should be no polylobated lymphocytic and histiocytic (L&H) cells as characteristic of n-LPHD, although admittedly on occasion it can be difficult to distinguish large noncleaved cells (centroblasts) or follicular dendritic cells from L&H cells. In such borderline cases, a diagnosis of n-LPHD should be made only if there are at least some crowded or coalescent large nodules, and there should be more than a few convincing L&H cells.
- There is commonly a misunderstanding of the diagnostic criteria of PTGC, such as considering ''invasion'' of germinal centers by strands of mantle zone lymphocytes as being sufficient for the diagnosis (for example, illustration of this entity in a textbook on lymph node pathology).[5] Although such a feature could represent an early phase of PTGC, this is certainly not diagnostic of the condition.
- PTGC can also occur as part of the histologic picture of various forms of lymphadenopathy in which there is a component of reactive follicular hyperplasia.
- Immunohistochemical studies have shown the large lymphoid nodules of PTGC to comprise predominantly polytypic B cells with a mantle zone phenotype (IgM+ and IgD+) and meshworks of follicular dendritic cells.[415,422]
- The floral variant of follicular lymphoma can mimic PTGC by virtue of the thick mantles and ingrowth of small lymphocytes into the neoplastic follicles.[423] In contrast to PTGC, all the follicles are abnormal (often with dysplastic follicle cell center cells), and there are no reactive follicles in the background. Presence of atypical lymphoid cells between the follicles and in the perinodal tissues also supports a diagnosis of lymphoma over PTGC.

Lymph Node Infarction

- Lymph node may undergo spontaneous total or subtotal infarction. There may be variable degrees of histiocytic reaction and mesenchymal reaction in response to the infarct (Fig. 2-88). Infarction in reactive lymph nodes may be related to vascular thrombosis,

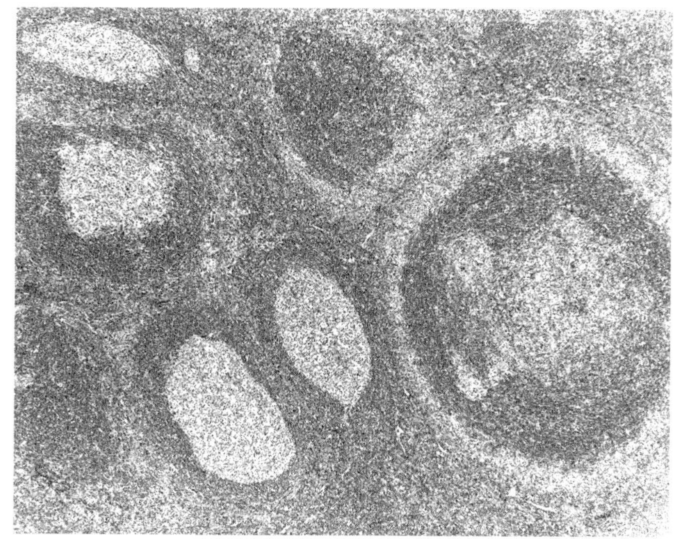

Fig. 2-86. Progressive transformation of germinal centers. A large, dark-staining follicle (right field) occurs among clearly reactive follicles.

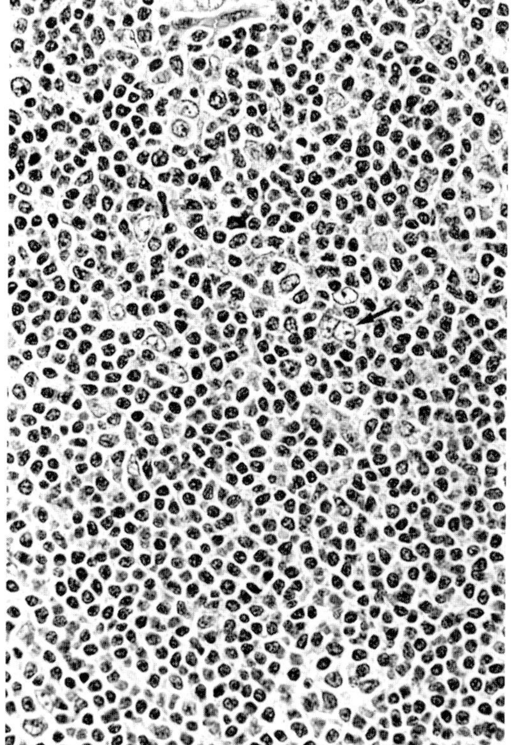

Fig. 2-87. Progressive transformation of germinal centers. The transformed follicle comprises predominantly small lymphocytes, with occasional interspersed large cells and follicular dendritic cells (*arrow*).

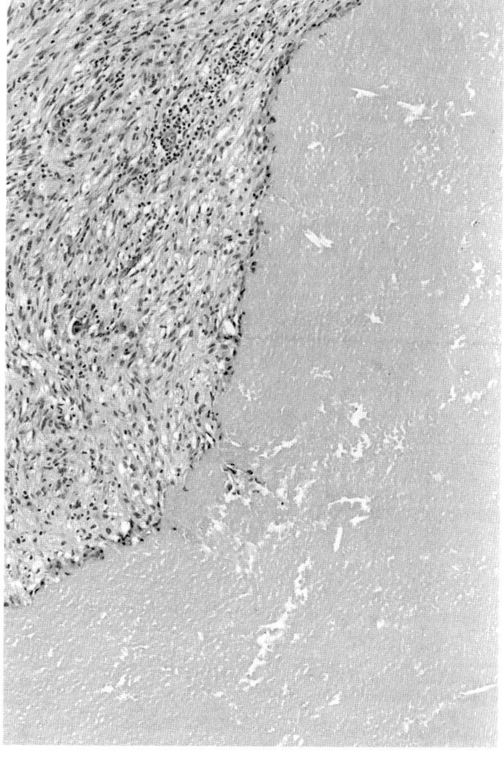

Fig. 2-88. Infarction of lymph node. The area of coagulative necrosis is surrounded by repair tissue.

mechanical pressure, active infection, or gold therapy.[424,425]

- The most significant implication of lymph node infarction is that it may be a harbinger of malignant lymphoma.[426] Thus it is important to exclude concomitant or underlying lymphoma and to follow-up for the possible development of lymphoma.
- Immunophenotyping on the paraffin sections of the infarcted tissue is still possible for suspected lymphoma,[427] and the demonstration of clonal Ig or TCR gene rearrangement in the infarcted lymph node should support a diagnosis of lymphoma.[428]
- A multicenter study has demonstrated that, among patients presenting with lymph node infarction, 27.5 percent are found to have malignant lymphoma at the time of diagnosis (in the same or at other nodes). Among patients without obvious evidence of lymphoma, 16.2 percent of cases are subsequently diagnosed as having lymphoma, all within 2 years. Given the short time interval between the lymph node infarct and the presentation of lymphoma, it is likely that such cases represent infarcted lymphoma. The risk is negligible after 2 years.[424]

Proteinaceous Lymphadenopathy

- The term *proteinaceous lymphadenopathy* has not been consistently applied in the literature, and some authors have included amyloid lymphadenopathy as a form of proteinaceous lymphadenopathy.[5] We prefer to reserve this term for nonamyloid type of proteinaceous deposits. Two types can be identified: (1) fibrillary appearance (nature unknown) on ultrastructural studies and (2) immunoglobulin type (with granular appearance on ultrastructural studies).[57]
- Patients with the fibrillary type of proteinaceous lymphadenopathy present with lymphadenopathy, hepatosplenomegaly, systemic symptoms, and polyclonal hypergammaglobulinemia.[429,430] Histologic examination of lymph node shows lymphocyte depletion and deposition of hyaline sclerotic material around the small and mid-sized blood vessels, often forming concentric rings. Therefore the descriptive term *angiocentric sclerosing lymphadenopathy* has also been applied to this condition. The hyaline-sclerotic material is Congo red negative. Similar deposits can be seen in other organs.
- The Ig type of proteinaceous lymphadenopathy is characterized by patchy, perivascular, or extensive deposition of homogeneous, noncongophilic material that shows a granular appearance on electron microscopy. The nature of the deposit (monoclonal light chain only, or complete immunoglobulin) can be confirmed by immunohistochemistry. The patients often have an underlying plasma cell dyscrasia or occasionally lymphoplasmacytoid lymphoma.[431–433]

REFERENCES

1. Chan JKC, Tsang WYW: Uncommon syndromes of reactive lymphadenopathy. Semin Oncol 20:648, 1993
2. Schnitzer B: Reactive lymphoid hyperplasias. P. 98. In Jaffe ES (ed): Surgical Pathology of the Lymph Nodes and Related Organs. 2nd Ed. Major Problems in Pathology. Vol. 16. WB Saunders, Philadelphia, 1995
3. Swerdlow SH: Biopsy Interpretation of Lymph Nodes. Biopsy Interpretation Series. Raven Press, New York, 1992
4. Stansfeld AG, d'Ardenne AJ: Lymph Node Biopsy Interpretation. 2nd Ed. Churchill Livingstone, Edinburgh, 1992
5. Ioachim HL: Lymph Node Pathology. 2nd Ed. JB Lippincott, Philadelphia, 1994
6. Symmers WStCP: Sarcoidosis and other varieties of granulomatous lymphadenitis of reactive cause. P. 495. In Henry K, Symmers WStC (eds): Thymus, Lymph Nodes, Spleen and Lymphatics. Systemic Pathology. 3rd Ed, Vol. 7. Churchill Livingstone, Edinburgh, 1992
7. Schnitzer B: Reactive lymphadenopathies. P. 427. In Knowles DM (ed): Neoplastic Hematopathology. Williams & Wilkins, Baltimore, 1992
8. Frizzera G: Atypical lymphoproliferative disorders. P. 459. In Knowles DM (ed): Neoplastic

Hematopathology. Williams & Wilkins, Baltimore, 1992

9. Burke JS: Reactive lymphadenopathies. Semin Diagn Pathol 5:312, 1988
10. Dorfman RF, Warnke RA: Lymphadenopathy simulating the malignant lymphomas. Hum Pathol 15:519, 1974
11. Rosai J: Ackerman's Surgical Pathology. p. 1661. 8th Ed: CV Mosby, St. Louis, 1996
12. Henry K: Lymph nodes. P. 141. In Henry K, Symmers WStC (eds): Thymus, Lymph Nodes, Spleen and Lymphatics. Systemic Pathology. 3rd Ed, Vol. 7. Churchill Livingstone, Edinburgh, 1992
13. Symmers WStC: Lymphadenitis caused by infection and infestation. P. 327. In Henry K, Symmers WStC (eds): Thymus, Lymph Nodes, Spleen and Lymphatics. Systemic Pathology. 3rd Ed, Vol. 7. Churchill Livingstone, Edinburgh, 1992
14. Tsang WYW, Chan JKC, Dorfman RF, Rosai J Vasoproliferative lesions of lymph nodes. Pathol Annu 29:63, 1994
15. Warnke RA, Weiss LM, Chan JKC, Cleary ML, Dorfman RF: Tumors of the Lymph Nodes and Spleen. Atlas of Tumor Pathology. 3rd series, Fascicle 14. Armed Forces Institute of Pathology, Washington DC, 1995
16. van der Volk P, Meijer CJLM: The histopathology of reactive lymph nodes. Am J Surg Pathol 11:866, 1987
17. van den Oord JJ, Facchetti F, Delabie J, de Wolf-Peeters C: T lymphocytes in non-neoplastic lymph nodes. P. 149. In Grundmann E, Vollmer E (eds): Reaction Patterns of the Lymph Node. Part 1: Cell Types and Functions. Current Topics in Pathology 84/1. Springer-Verlag, Berlin, 1990
18. De Wolf-Peeters C, Delabie J: Anatomy and histophysiology of lymphoid tissue. Semin Oncol 20:555, 1993
19. Kroese FGM, Timens W, Niewwenhuis P: Germinal center reaction and B lymphocytes: morphology and function. P. 103. In Grundmann E, Vollmer E (eds): Reaction Patterns of the Lymph Node. Part 1: Cell Types and Functions. Current Topics in Pathology 84/1. Springer-Verlag, Berlin, 1990
20. Doglioni C, Dell'Orto P, Zanetti G et al: Cytokeratin-immunoreactive cells of human lymph nodes and spleen in normal and pathological conditions, an immunocytochemical study. Virchows Arch [A] 416:479, 1990
21. van den Oord JJ, de Wolf-Peeters C, Desmet VJ et al: Nodular alteration of the paracortical area: an in situ immunohistochemical analysis of primary, secondary, and tertiary T-nodules. Am J Pathol 120:55, 1985
22. van den Oord JJ, de Wolf-Peeters C, Desmet VJ: The composite nodule, a structural and functional unit of the reactive human node. Am J Pathol 122:83, 1986
23. Gould E, Porto R, Albores-Saavedra J, Ibe MJ: Dermatopathic lymphadenitis, the spectrum and significance of its morphologic features. Arch Pathol Lab Med 112:1145, 1988
24. Sheibani K, Fritz R, Winberg C et al: Monocytoid cells in reactive follicular hyperplasia with and without histiocytic reaction: an immunohistochemical study of 21 cases including suspected cases of toxoplasmic lymphadenitis. Am J Clin Pathol 81:453, 1984
25. Stein H, Lennert K, Mason DY et al: Immature sinus histiocytosis: their identification as a novel B-cell population. Am J Pathol 117:44, 1984
26. Plank L, Hansmann ML, Fischer R: The cytological spectrum of the monocytoid B-cell reaction: recognition of its large cell type. Histopathology 23:425, 1993
27. Sohn CC, Sheibani K, Winberg CD, Rappaport H: Monocytoid B lymphocytes: their relation to the patterns of the acquired immunodeficiency syndrome and AIDS-related lymphadenopathy. Hum Pathol 16:979, 1985
28. van den Oord JJ, de Wolf-Peeters C, de Vos R, Desmet VJ: Immature sinus histiocytosis, light- and electron-microscopic features, immunohistologic phenotype, and relationship with marginal zone lymphocytes. Am J Pathol 118:266, 1985
29. Piris MA, Rivas C, Morente M et al: Immature sinus histiocytosis, a monocytoid B-lymphoid reaction. J Pathol 148:159, 1986
30. de Almeida PC, Harris NL, Bhan AK: Characterization of immature sinus histiocytes (monocytoid cells) in reactive lymph nodes by use of monoclonal antibodies. Hum Pathol 15:330, 1984
31. Sohn CC, Sheibani K, Winberg CD, Rappaport H: Monocytoid B lymphocytes: their relation to the patterns of the acquired immunodeficiency syndrome (AIDS) and AIDS-related lymphadenopathy. Hum Pathol 16:979, 1985

32. van den Oord JJ, Facchetti F, de Wolf-Peeters C: Reactivity of monocytoid B-cells with the B-cell panel of monoclonal antibodies, abstracted. Tissue Antigens 33:, 1989
33. Poppema S, Gilchrist M: Monocytoid B cells are bcl-2 protein negative in contrast to marginal zone cells and monocytoid B cell lymphoma, abstracted. Int J Surg Pathol 2:277, 1995
34. Nathwani BN, Mohrmann RL, Brynes RK et al: Monocytoid B-cell lymphomas: an assessment of diagnostic criteria and a perspective on histogenesis: Hum Pathol 23:1061, 1992
35. Plank L, Hell K, Hansmann ML et al: Reactive versus neoplastic monocytoid B-cell proliferations, in situ hybridization study of immunoglobulin light chain mRNA. Am J Clin Pathol 103:330, 1995
36. Facchetti F, de Wolf-Peeters C, van den Oord JJ et al: Plasmacytoid T cells: a cell population normally present in the reactive lymph node, an immunohistochemical and electronmicroscopic study. Hum Pathol 19:1085, 1988
37. Tsang WYW, Chan JKC, Ng CS: Kikuchi's lymphadenitis, a morphologic analysis of 75 cases with special reference to unusual features. Am J Surg Pathol 18:219, 1994
38. Facchetti F, de Wolf-Peeters C, van den Oord JJ et al: Plasmacytoid monocytes (so-called plasmacytoid T-cells) in Kikuchi's lymphadenitis. Am J Clin Pathol 92:42, 1989
39. Harris NL, Bhan AK: ''Plasmacytoid T cells'' in Castleman's disease, immunohistologic phenotype. Am J Surg Pathol 11:109, 1987
40. Horny HP, Feller AC, Horst HA, Lennert K: Immunocytology of plasmacytoid T cells: marker analysis indicates a unique phenotype of this enigmatic cell. Hum Pathol 18:28, 1986
41. Lennert K, Kaiserling E, Muller-Hermelink HK: T-associated plasma cells. Letter to the Editor. Lancet i:1031, 1975
42. Lennert K, Remmele W: Karyometrische Untersuchungen an Lymphknotenzellen des Menschen. I. Mitt. Germinoblasten, Lymphoblasten und Lymphozyten. Acta Hematol (Basel) 19:99, 1958
43. Vollenweider R, Lennert K: Plasmacytoid T-cell clusters in non-specific lymphadenitis. Virchows Arch [Cell Pathol] 44:1, 1983
44. de Vos R, de Wolf-Peeters C, Facchetti F, Desmet V: Plasmacytoid monocytes in epithelioid cell granulomas: ultrastructural and immunoelectron microscopic study. Ultrastruct Pathol 14:291, 1990
45. Facchetti F, de Wolf-Peeters C, de Vos R et al: Plasmacytoid monocytes (so-called plasmacytoid T cells) in granulomatous lymphadenitis. Hum Pathol 20:588, 1989
46. Beiske K, Munthe-Kaas A, Davies CDL et al: Single cell studies on the immunological marker profile of plasmacytoid T-zone cells. Lab Invest 56:381, 1987
47. Brubaker R, Swerdlow SH: Plasmacytoid T-cells in a reactive lymph node, detection by flow cytometry? Am J Clin Pathol 93:569, 1990
48. Facchetti F, de Wolf-Peeters C, Mason DY et al: Plasmacytoid T cells, immunohistochemical evidence for their monocyte/macrophage origin. Am J Pathol 133:15, 1988
49. Facchetti F, de Wolf-Peeters C, van de Oord JJ, Desmet VJ: Plasmacytoid T cells in a case of lymphocytic infiltration of skin, a component of the skin-associated lymphoid tissue? J Pathol 155:295, 1988
50. Takeshita M, Muller H, Mix D et al: Immuno- and enzymehistochemical characterization of ''plasmacytoid T-cells'' in formalin-fixed paraffin-embedded tissue of reactive lymph nodes. Pathol Res Pract 187:848, 1991
51. Toonstra J, van der Putte SCJ: Plasmacytoid monocytes in Jessner's lymphocytic infiltration of the skin, a valuable clue for the diagnosis. Am J Dermatopathol 13:321, 1991
52. Brado B, Moller P: The plasmacytoid T cell or plasmacytoid monocyte—a sessile lymphoid cell with unique immunophenotype and unknown function, still awaiting lineage affiliation. P. 179. In Grundmann E, Vollmer E (eds): Reaction Patterns of the Lymph Node. Part 1: Cell Types and Functions. Current Topics in Pathology 84/1. Springer-Verlag, Berlin, 1990
53. Kjeldsberg CR, Kim H: Polykaryocytes resembling Warthin-Finkeldey giant cells in reactive and neoplastic lymphoid disorders. Hum Pathol 12:267, 1981
54. Delsol G, Pradere M, Voigt JJ et al: Warthin-Finkeldey-like cells in benign and malignant lymphoid proliferations. Histopathology 6:451, 1982
55. Kamel OW, LeBrun DP, Gerry GJ et al: Warthin-Finkeldey polykaryocytes demonstrate a T-cell immunophenotype. Am J Clin Pathol 97: 179, 1992
56. Carbone A, Manconi R, Volpe R et al: Multinu-

cleated cells in the lymph nodes of HTLV-III seropositive intravenous drug abusers with generalized lymphadenopathy. Arch Pathol Lab Med 110:871, 1986

57. Frizzera G, Seo IS: Histopathology of non-malignant lymphadenopathies. P. 131. In Pangalis GA, Polliack A (eds): Benign and Malignant Lymphadenopathies, Clinical and Laboratory Diagnosis. Harwood Academic Publishers, Switzerland, 1993
58. Azadeh B: Localized Leishmania lymphadenitis: a light and electron microscopic study. Am J Trop Med Hyg 34:447, 1985
59. Azadeh B, Sells PG, Ejeckam GC, Rampling D: Localized Leishmania lymphadenitis, immunohistochemical studies. Am J Clin Pathol 102:11, 1994
60. Pangalis GA, Vassilakopoulos TP, Boussiotis VA, Fessas P: Clinical approach to lymphadenopathy. Semin Oncol 20:570, 1993
61. Woosley JT: Improved histology from inadequately fixed paraffin-embedded biopsy specimens. Am J Surg Pathol 13:246, 1989
62. Page DL, Nolen C, Womack JL: Histologic technique (Letter). Am J Surg Pathol 13:1072, 1989
63. Lennert K, Feller AO: Histopathology of Non-Hodgkin's Lymphomas (Based on the Updated Kiel Classification). 2nd Ed. Springer-Verlag, Berlin, 1992
64. Knowles DM: Immunophenotypic and immunogenotypic approaches useful in distinguishing benign and malignant lymphoid proliferations. Semin Oncol 20:583, 1993
65. Picker LJ, Weiss LM, Medeiros JL, Warnke RA: Immunophenotypic criteria for the diagnosis of non-Hodgkin's lymphoma. Am J Pathol 59:52, 1987
66. Chan JKC, Ng CS, Hui PK, Wong KF: Tumors of the lymphoreticular system (including thymus). P. 805. In Fletcher CDM (ed): Diagnostic Histopathology of Tumors. Churchill Livingstone, Edinburgh, 1995
67. Nathwani BN, Winberg CD, Diamond LW et al: Morphologic criteria for the differentiation of follicular lymphoma from florid reactive follicular hyperplasia: a study of 80 cases. Cancer 48:1794, 1981
68. Kondratowicz GM, Symmons DPM, Bacon PA et al: Rheumatoid lymphadenopathy: a morphological and immunohistochemical study. J Clin Pathol 43:106, 1990
69. Banks PM: When is a new diagnostic method established? Hum Pathol 24:1153, 1993
70. Browne G, Tobin B, Carney DN, Dervan PA: Aberrant MT2 positivity distinguishes follicular lymphoma from reactive follicular hyperplasia in B5 and formalin-fixed paraffin sections. Am J Clin Pathol 96:90, 1991
71. Crisan D, Anstett MJ: *bcl*-2 gene rearrangements in follicular lymphomas. Lab Med 24: 579, 1993
72. Gaulard P, d'Agay MF, Peuchmaur M et al: Expression of the *bcl*-2 gene product in follicular lymphoma. Am J Pathol 140:1089, 1992
73. Korsmeyer SJ: Bcl-2 initiates a new category of oncogenes: regulators of cell death. Blood 80: 869, 1992
74. Lee Wood B, Bacchi MM, Bacchi CE et al: Immunocytochemical differentiation of reactive hyperplasia from follicular lymphoma using monoclonal antibodies to cell surface and proliferation-related markers. Appl Immunohistochem 2:48, 1994
75. Norton AJ, Rivas C, Isaacson PG: A comparison between monoclonal antibody MT2 and immunoglobulin staining in the differential diagnosis of follicular lymphoid proliferation in routinely-fixed wax-embedded biopsies. Am J Pathol 134: 63, 1989
76. Segal GH, Scott M, Jorgensen T, Braylan RC: Standard polymerase chain reaction analysis does not detect t(14;18) in reactive lymphoid hyperplasia. Arch Pathol Lab Med 118:791, 1994
77. Utz GL, Swerdlow SH: Distinction of follicular hyperplasia from follicular lymphoma in B5-fixed tissues: comparison of MT2 and bcl-2 antibodies. Hum Pathol 24:1155, 1993
78. Weiss LM, Warnke RA, Sklar J, Cleary ML: Molecular analysis of the t(14;18) chromosomal translocation in malignant lymphomas. N Engl J Med 317:1185, 1987

78a. Ashton-Key M, Diss TO, Isaacson PG, Smith MEF: A comparative study of the value of immunohistochemistry and the polymerase chain reaction in the diagnosis of follicular lymphoma. Histopathology 27:501, 1995

79. Segal GH, Kjeldsberg CR, Smith GP, Perkins SL: CD30 antigen expression in florid immunoblastic proliferations: a clinicopathologic study of 14 cases. Am J Clin Pathol 102:292, 1994
80. Childs CC, Parham DM, Berard CW: Infectious mononucleosis: the spectrum of morphologic

changes simulating lymphoma in lymph nodes and tonsils. Am J Surg Pathol 11:122, 1987
81. Nathwani BN, Brynes RK: Reactive immunoblastic proliferations. Semin Diagn Pathol 5: 317, 1988
82. Hartsock RJ, Halling LW, King FM: Luetic lymphadenitis: a clinical and histologic study of 20 cases. Am J Clin Pathol 53:304, 1970
83. Evans N: Lymphadenopathy of secondary syphilis: its resemblance to giant follicular lymphadenopathy. Arch Pathol 37:175, 1944
84. Severson GS, Harrington DS, Johansson SL, McManus BM: Epithelioid germinal centers in overwhelming childhood infections, the aftermath of nonspecific destruction of follicular B cells by natural killer cells. Arch Pathol Lab Med 112:917, 1988
85. Howat AJ, Variend S: Nuclear fragmentation and epithelioid change of germinal centers in the lymphoid tissue of child deaths. Pediatr Pathol 5:125, 1986
86. Hartsock RJ: Postvaccinial lymphadenitis: hyperplasia of lymphoid tissue that simulates malignant lymphomas. Cancer 21:632, 1968
87. Anagnostopoulos I, Hummel M, Kreschel C, Stein H: Morphology, immunophenotype, and distribution of latently and/or productively Epstein-Barr virus-infected cells in acute infectious mononucleosis: implications for the interindividual infection route of Epstein-Barr virus. Blood 85:744, 1995
88. Reynolds DJ, Banks PM, Gulley ML: New characterization of infectious mononucleosis and a phenotypic comparison with Hodgkin's disease. Am J Pathol 146:379, 1995
89. Chang KL, Chen YY, Shibata D, Weiss LM: Description of an in situ hybridization methodology for detection of Epstein-Barr virus RNA in paraffin-embedded tissues, with a survey of normal and neoplastic tissues. Diagn Mol Pathol 1:246, 1992
90. Shin SS, Berry GJ, Weiss LM: Infectious mononucleosis, diagnosis by in situ hybridization in two cases with atypical features. Am J Surg Pathol 15:625, 1991
91. Weiss LM, Movahed LA: In situ demonstration of Epstein-Barr viral genomes in viral-associated B cell lymphoproliferations. Am J Pathol 134:651, 1989
92. Strickler JG, Fedeli F, Horwitz CA et al: Infectious mononucleosis in lymphoid tissue: histopathology, in situ hybridization, and differential diagnosis. Arch Pathol Lab Med 117:269, 1993
93. Schroder KR, Franssila KO: Atypical hyperplasia of lymph nodes, a follow-up study. Cancer 44:1155, 1979
94. Nathwani BN, Jaffe ES: Angioimmunoblastic lymphadenopathy (AILD) and AILD-like T-cell lymphomas. P. 390. In Jaffe ES (ed): Surgical Pathology of the Lymph Nodes and Related Organs. Major Problems in Pathology. Vol. 16. WB Saunders, Philadelphia, 1995
95. Koo CH, Nathwani BN, Winberg CD et al: Atypical lymphoplasmacytic and immunoblastic proliferation in lymph nodes of patients with autoimmune disease (autoimmune disease-associated lymphadenopathy). Medicine 63:274, 1984
96. Saltzstein SL: The fate of patients with nondiagnostic lymph node biopsies. Surgery 58:659, 1965
97. Sinclair S, Beckamn E, Ellman L: Biopsy of superficial enlarged lymph nodes. JAMA 228: 602, 1974
98. Kreyberg L, Iverson OH: Early diagnosis of malignant conditions in lymph nodes. Br J Cancer 13:26, 1958
99. Moore RD, Weisberger AS, Bowerfind ES: An evaluation of lymphadenopathy in systemic disease. Arch Intern Med 99:751, 1957
100. Williams ME, Lee JT, Innes DJ et al: Immunoglobulin gene rearrangement in abnormal lymph node hyperplasia. Am J Clin Pathol 96:746, 1991
101. Kung ITM, Ng WF, Yuen RWS, Chan JKC: Kikuchi's histiocytic necrotizing lymphadenitis, diagnosis by fine needle aspiration. Acta Cytol 34:323, 1990
102. Chan JKC, Saw D: Histiocytic necrotizing lymphadenitis (Kikuchi's disease): a clinicopathologic study of nine cases. Pathology 18:22, 1986
103. Dorfman RF: Histiocytic necrotizing lymphadenitis of Kikuchi and Fujimoto. Arch Pathol Lab Med 111:1026, 1987
104. Pileri S, Kikuchi M, Helborn D et al: Histiocytic necrotizing lymphadenitis without granulocytic infiltration. Virchows Arch [A] 395:257, 1982
105. Rivano MT, Falini B, Stein H et al: Histiocytic necrotizing lymphadenitis without granulocytic infiltration (Kikuchi's lymphadenitis): morphological and immunohistochemical study of eight cases. Histopathology 11:1013, 1987
106. Turner RR, Martin J, Dorfman RF: Necrotizing

lymphadenitis: a study of 30 cases. Am J Surg Pathol 7:115, 1983

107. Wakasa H, Takahashi H, Kimura N: Necrotizing lymphadenitis. Recent Adv Res 18:85, 1979
108. Kikuchi M, Takeshita M, Eimoto T et al: Histiocytic necrotizing lymphadenitis: clinicopathologic, immunologic, and HLA typing study. P. 251. In Hanaoka M, Kadin ME, Mikata A, Watanabe S (eds): Lymphoid Malignancy: Immunocytology and Cytogenetics. Field & Wood, New York, 1990
109. Dorfman RF, Berry GJ: Kikuchi's histiocytic necrotizing lymphadenitis: an analysis of 108 cases with emphasis on differential diagnosis. Semin Diagn Pathol 5:329, 1988
110. Asano S, Akaike Y, Muramatsu T et al: Necrotizing lymphadenitis: a clinicopathological and immunohistochemical study of four familial cases and five recurrent cases. Virchows Arch [A] 418:215, 1991
111. Smith KGC, Becker GJ, Busmanis I: Recurrent Kikuchi's disease. Lancet 340:124, 1992
112. Asano S, Akaike Y, Jinnouchi H et al: Necrotizing lymphadenitis: a review of clinicopathological, immunohistochemical and ultrastructural studies. Hematol Oncol 8:251, 1990
113. Imamura M, Ueno H, Matsuura A et al: An ultrastructural study of subacute necrotizing lymphadenitis. Am J Pathol 107:292, 1982
114. Fujimoto T, Shioda K, Sussman EB et al: Subacute necrotizing lymphadenitis: a clinicopathologic study. Acta Pathol Jpn 31:791, 1981
115. Kikuchi M, Takeshita M, Tashiro K et al: Immunohistological study of histiocytic necrotizing lymphadenitis. Virchows Arch [A] 409:299, 1986
116. Chamulak GA, Brynes R, Nathwani BN: Kikuchi-Fujimoto disease mimicking malignant lymphoma. Am J Surg Pathol 14:514, 1990
117. Chan JKC, Ng CS: Kikuchi's histiocytic necrotizing lymphadenitis in the regional lymph nodes of malignant fibrous histiocytoma, causal or coincidental? Histopathology 12:448, 1988
118. Suseelan AV, Augusty TS, Harilal KR: Necrotizing lymphadenitis: an analysis of seventeen cases. Ind J Pathol Microbiol 27:331, 1984
119. Ali MH, Horton LWL: Necrotizing lymphadenitis without granulocytic infiltration (Kikuchi's disease). J Clin Pathol 38:1252, 1985
120. Kuo TT: Kikuchi's disease (histiocytic necrotizing lymphadenitis), a clinicopathologic study of 79 cases with an analysis of histologic subtypes, immunohistology, and DNA ploidy. Am J Surg Pathol 19:798, 1995
121. Tanako Y, Saegusa M, Okudaira M: Pathologic analyses of non-overt necrotizing type Kikuchi and Fujimoto's disease. Acta Pathol Jpn 43:635, 1993
122. Kuo TT: Cutaneous manifestations of Kikuchi's histiocytic necrotizing lymphadenitis. Am J Surg Pathol 14:872, 1990
123. Sumiyoshi Y, Kikuchi M, Ohshima K et al: A case of histiocytic necrotizing lymphadenitis with bone marrow and skin involvement. Virchows Arch [A] 420:275, 1992
124. Kuo TT, Jung SM, Wu WJ: Kikuchi's disease of intraparotid lymph nodes presenting as a parotid gland tumor with extranodal involvement of salivary gland. Histopathology 28:185, 1996
125. McLoughlin J, Creagh T, Taylor A et al: Kikuchi's disease simulating acute appendicitis. Br J Surg 75:1206, 1988
126. Kapadia V, Robinson BA, Angus HB: Kikuchi's disease presenting as fever of unknown origin. Lancet ii:1519, 1989
127. Rudniki C, Kessler E, Zarfati M et al: Kikuchi's necrotizing lymphadenitis: a cause of fever of unknown origin and splenomegaly. Acta Hematol 79:99, 1988
128. Pileri SA, Sabattini E, Costigliola P et al: Kikuchi's lymphadenitis with HIV infection. AIDS 5:459, 1991
129. Pasquinucci S, Donisi PM, Cavinato F, Belussi F: Kikuchi's disease in a patient infected with AIDS. AIDS 5:235, 1991
130. Tsang WYW, Chan JKC: Fine needle aspiration cytologic diagnosis of Kikuchi's lymphadenitis: a report of 27 cases. Am J Clin Pathol 102:454, 1994
131. Hsueh EJ, Ko WS, Hwang WS, Yan LT: Fine-needle aspiration of histiocytic necrotizing lymphadenitis (Kikuchi's disease). Diagn Cytopathol 9:448, 1993
132. Ohshima K, Kikuchi M, Eguchi F et al: Analysis of Epstein-Barr viral genomes in lymphoid malignancy using Southern blotting, polymerase chain reaction and in situ hybridization. Virchow Arch [Cell Pathol] 59:383, 1990
133. Anagnostopoulos I, Hummel M, Korbjuhn P et al: Epstein-Barr virus in Kikuchi-Fujimoto disease. Lancet 341:893, 1993
134. Kikuchi M, Yoshizumi T, Nakamura H: Necrotizing lymphadenitis: possible acute toxoplas-

mic infection. Virchows Arch [A] 376:247, 1977

135. Eizuru Y, Minematsu T, Minamishima Y et al: Human herpesvirus 6 in lymph nodes. Lancet i: 40, 1989
136. Meyer O, Kahn MF, Grossin M et al: Parvovirus B19 infection can induce histiocytic necrotizing lymphadenitis (Kikuchi's disease) associated with systemeic lupus erythematosus. Lupus 1: 37, 41,1991
137. Sumiyoshi Y, Kikuchi M, Minematu T et al: Analysis of herpesvirus genomes in Kikuchi's disease. Virchows Arch [A] 424:437, 1994
138. Sumiyoshi Y, Kikuchi M, Ohshima K et al: Human herpesvirus-6 genomes in histiocytic necrotizing lymphadenitis (Kikuchi's disease) and other forms of lymphadenitis. Am J Clin Pathol 99:609, 1993
139. Chan JKC, Wong KC, Ng CS: A fatal case of multicentric Kikuchi's histiocytic necrotizing lymphadenitis. Cancer 63:1856, 1989
140. Lin SH, Ko WS, Lee HS, Hwang WS: Kikuchi's disease associated with lupus-like syndrome—a fatal case. J Rheumatol 19:1996, 1992
141. Chan JKC, Ng CS: Immunohistochemical studies on histiocytic necrotizing lymphadenitis. Pathology 19:104, 1987
142. Hansmann ML, Kikuchi M, Wacker HH et al: Immunohistochemical monitoring of plasmacytoid cells in lymph node sections of Kikuchi-Fujimoto disease by a new pan-macrophage antibody Ki-M1P. Hum Pathol 23:676, 1992
143. Asano S, Kanno H, Tominaga K et al: Necrotizing lymphadenitis: electron microscopical and immunohistochemical study. Acta Pathol Jpn 37:1071, 1987
144. Feller AC, Lennert K, Stein H et al: Immunohistology and aetiology of histiocytic necrotizing lymphadenitis, report of three instructive cases. Histopathology 7:825, 1983
145. Unger PD, Rappaport KM, Strauchen JA: Necrotizing lymphadenitis (Kikuchi's disease), report of four cases of an unusual pseudolymphomatous lesion and immunologic marker studies. Arch Pathol Lab Med 111:1031, 1987
146. Gourley I, Bell AL, Biggart D: Kikuchi's disease as a presenting feature of mixed connective tissue disease. Clin Rheumatol 14:104, 1995
147. Medeiros LJ, Kaynor B, Harris NL: Lupus lymphadenitis, report of a case with immunohistologic studies on frozen sections. Hum Pathol 20: 295, 1989
148. Fox RA, Rosahn PD: The lymph nodes in disseminated lupus erythematosus. Am J Pathol 19: 70, 1943
149. Giesker DW, Pastuszak WT, Forouhar FA et al: Lymph node biopsy for early diagnosis in Kawasaki disease. Am J Surg Pathol 6:493, 1982
150. Chan JKC, Hui PK, Ng CS et al: Epithelioid hemangioma (angiolymphoid hyperplasia with eosinophilia) and Kimura's disease in Chinese. Histopathology 15:557, 1989
151. Hui PK, Chan JKC, Ng CS et al: Lymphadenopathy of Kimura's disease. Am J Surg Pathol 13: 177, 1989
152. Googe PB, Harris NL, Mihms MC Jr: Kimura's disease and angiolymphoid hyperplasia with eosinophilia: two distinct histopathological entities. J Cutan Pathol 14:263, 1987
153. Kuo TT, Shih LY, Chan HL: Kimura's disease, involvement of regional lymph nodes and distinction from angiolymphoid hyperplasia with eosinophilia. Am J Surg Pathol 12:843, 1988
154. Ishikawa E, Tanaka H, Kakimoto S et al: A pathological study on eosinophilic lymphofolliculoid granuloma (Kimura's disease). Acta Pathol Jpn 13:767, 1981
155. Tham KT, Leung PC, Saw D, Gwi E: Kimura's disease with salivary gland involvement. Br J Surg 68:495, 1981
156. Kimura T, Yoshimura S, Ishikawa E: On the unusual granulation combined with hyperplastic changes of lymphatic tissue. Trans Soc Pathol Jpn 37:179, 1948
157. Atar S, Oberman AS, Ben-Izhak O, Flatau E: Recurrent nephrotic syndrome associated with Kimura's disease in a young non-Oriental male. Nephron 68:259, 1994
158. Konishi N, Tamura T, Kawai C, Shirai T: IgE-associated nephropathy in a patient with subcutaneous eosinophilic lymphoid granuloma (Kimura's disease). Virchows Arch [A] 392:127, 1981
159. Yamada A, Mitsuhashi K, Miyakawa Y et al: Membranous glomerulonephritis associated with eosinophilic lymphofolliculosis of the skin (Kimura's disease): report of a case and review of the literature. Clin Nephrol 18:211, 1982
160. Enokihara H, Koike T, Arimura H et al: IL-5 mRNA expression in blood lymphocytes from patients with Kimura's disease and parasite infection. Am J Hematol 47:69, 1994
161. Terada N, Konno A, Shirotori K et al: Mecha-

nism of eosinophil infiltration in the patient with subcutaneous angioblastic lymphoid hyperplasia with eosinophilia (Kimura's disease). Mechanism of eosinophil chemotaxis mediated by candida antigen and IL-5. Int Arch Allergy Immunol 104:18, 1994

162. Chan JKC, Frizzera G, Fletcher CDM, Rosai J: Primary vascular tumors of lymph nodes other than Kaposi's sarcoma, analysis of 39 cases and delineation of two new entities. Am J Surg Pathol 16:335, 1992
163. Kung ITM, Gibson JB, Bannatyne PM: Kimura's disease: a clinico-pathological study of 21 cases and its distinction from angiolymphoid hyperplasia with eosinophilia. Pathology 16:39, 1984
164. Rosai J, Gold J, Landy R: The histiocytoid hemangiomas. Hum Pathol 10:707, 1979
165. Suster S: Nodal angiolymphoid hyperplasia with eosinophilia. Am J Clin Pathol 88:236, 1987
166. Tsang WYW, Chan JKC: The family of epithelioid vascular tumors. Histol Histopathol 8:187, 1993
167. Chun SI, Ji HG: Kimura's disease and angiolymphoid hyperplasia with eosinophilia: clinical and histopathologic differences. J Am Acad Dermatol 27:954, 1992
168. Fetch JF, Weiss SW: Observations concerning the pathogenesis of epithelioid hemangioma (angiolymphoid hyperplasia). Mod Pathol 4: 449, 1991
169. Burg G: Collision dermatosis: angiolymphoid hyperplasia with eosinophilia developing within a congenital port wine nevus. Dermatology 187: 293, 1993
170. Fellbaum CH, Hansmann ML, Lennert K: Lymphadenitis mimicking Hodgkin's disease. Histopathology 12:153, 1988
171. Dorfman RF, Colby TV: The pathologist's role in management of patients with Hodgkin's disease. Cancer Treat Rep 66:675, 1982
172. Doggett RS, Colby TV, Dorfman RF: Interfollicular Hodgkin's disease. Am J Surg Pathol 7: 145, 1983
173. Facchetti F, Agostini C, Chilosi M et al: Suppurative granulomatous lymphadenitis. Immunohistochemical evidence for a B-cell-associated granuloma. Am J Surg Pathol 16:955, 1992
174. Van den Oord JJ, De Wolf-Peeters C, De Vos R, Desmet VJ: Cellular composition of suppurative granulomas: an immunohistochemical study of suppurative granulomatous lymphadenitis. Hum Pathol 16:1009, 1985

174a. Kojima M, Nakamura S, Kurabayashi Y et al: Suppurative lesions without prominent epithelioid cell response in abscess-forming granulomatous lymphadenitis. Pathol Res Pract 191:1072, 1995

175. Kojima M, Hosomura Y, Itoh H et al: Monocytoid B lymphocytes and epithelioid cell clusters in abscess-forming granulomatous lymphadenitis with special reference to cat scratch disease. Acta Pathol Jpn 41:363, 1991
176. Van den Oord JJ, de Wolf-Peeters C, Facchetti F, Desmet VJ: Cellular composition of hypersensitivity-type granulomas. Immunohistochemical analysis of tuberculous and sarcoidal lymphadenitis. Hum Pathol 15:559, 1984
177. Brincker H, Pederson NT: Immunohistologic separation of B cell-positive granulomas from B cell-negative granulomas in paraffin-embedded tissues with special reference to tumor-related sarcoid reactions. Acta Pathol Microbiol Immunol Scand 99:282, 1991
178. Kojima M, Nakamura S, Hosomura Y et al: Abscess-forming granulomatous lymphadenitis: histological typing of suppurative granulomas and clinicopathologic findings with special reference of cat scratch disease. Acta Pathol Jpn 43:11, 1993
179. Strano AJ: Cat-scratch fever. P. 85. In Binford CH, Connor DH (eds): Pathology of Tropical and Extraordinary Diseases. Armed Forces Institute of Pathology, Washington, DC, 1976
180. Strano AJ: Lymphogranuloma venereum. P. 91. In Binford CH, Connor DH (eds): Pathology of Tropical and Extraordinary Diseases. Armed Forces Institute of Pathology, Washington, DC, 1976
181. Lucas SB. Cat scratch disease. J Pathol 163:91, 1991
182. Margileth AM, Wear DJ, English CK: Systemic cat scratch disease: report of 23 patients with prolonged or recurrent severe bacterial infection. J Infect Dis 155:390, 1987
183. Naji AF, Carbonell F, Barker HJ: Cat scratch disease, a report of three new cases, review of the literature, and classification of the pathologic changes in the lymph nodes during various stages of the disease. Am J Clin Pathol 38:513, 1962
184. Tsubota YT, Nakamine H, Takenaka T et al: Atypical large plasma cells in lymph node gran-

ulomas in cat-scratch disease. Virchows Arch [A] 418:383, 1991

184a. Hadfield TL, Lamy Y, Wear DJ: Demonstration of *Chlamydia trachomatis* in inguinal lymphadenitis of lymphogranuloma venereum: a light microscopy, electron microscopy and polymerase chain reaction study. Mod Pathol 8:924, 1995

185. Kudo E, Sakaki A, Sumitomo M et al: Cat scratch disease, an epidemiological and ultrastructural study of lymphadenitis caused by Warthin-Starry positive bacteria. Virchows Arch [A] 412:563, 1988

186. Korbi S, Toccanier MF, Leyvraz G et al: Use of silver staining (Dieterle's stain) in the diagnosis of cat scratch disease. Histopathology 10: 1015, 1986

187. Wear DJ, Margileth AM, Hadfield TL et al: Cat scratch disease: a bacterial infection. Science 221:1043, 1983

188. Min KW, Reed JA, Welch DF, Slater LN: Morphologically variable bacilli of cat scratch disease are identified by immunocytochemical labeling with antibodies to *Rochalimaea henselae*. Am J Clin Pathol 101:607, 1994

189. English CK, Wear DJ, Margileth AM et al: Cat-scratch disease: isolation and culture of the bacterial agent. JAMA 259:1347, 1988

190. Miller-Catchpole R, Variakojis D, Vardiman JW et al: Cat scratch disease. Identification of bacteria in seven cases of lymphadenitis. Am J Surg Pathol 10:276, 1986

191. Osborne BM, Butler JJ, Mackay B: Ultrastructural observations in cat scratch disease. Am J Clin Pathol 87:739, 1987

192. Brenner DJ, Hollis DG, Moss CW et al: Proposal of *Afipia* gen. nov. with *Afipia felis* sp. nov., *Afipia clevelandensis* sp. nov., *Afipia broomeae* sp. nov., and three unnamed genospecies. J Clin Microbiol 29:2450, 1991

193. Brenner DJ, O'Connor SP, Winkler HH, Steigerwalt AG: Proposals to unify the genera *Bartonella* and *Rochalimaea,* with descriptions of *Bartonella quintana* comb. nov., *Bartonella vinsonii* comb. nov., *Bartonella henselae* comb. nov., *Bartonella elizabethae* comb. nov., and to remove the family Bartonellaceae from the order Rickettsiales. Int J Syst Bacteriol 43:777, 1993

194. Adal KA, Cockerell CJ, Petri WA: Cat scratch disease, bacillary angiomatosis, and other infections duet to *Rochalimaea.* N Engl J Med 330: 1509, 1994

195. Dolan MJ, Wong MT, Regnery RL et al: Syndrome of *Rochalimaea henselae* adenitis suggesting cat scratch disease. Ann Intern Med 118: 331, 1993

196. Regnery RL, Olson JG, Perkins BA, Bibb W: Serologic response to *Rochalimaea henselae* antigen in suspected cat scratch disease. Lancet 339:1443, 1992

197. Scott M, McCurley T, Vnencak-Jones C, et al: Cat scratch disease: detection of *Rochalimaea henselae* in paraffin embedded tissue by PCR and Southern blot techniques in 23 of 34 patients, abstracted. Mod Pathol 8:127A, 1995

198. Anderson B, Sims K, Regnery R et al: Detection of *Rochalimaea henselae* DNA in specimens from cat scratch disease patients by PCR. J Clin Microbiol 32:942, 1994

199. Alkan S, Morgan MB, Sandin RL et al: Dual role for *Afipia felis* and *Rochalimaea henselae* in cat-scratch disease. Lancet 345:385, 1995

200. Perrone T, de Wolf-Peeters C, Frizzera G: Inflammatory pseudotumor of lymph nodes. A distinctive pattern of nodal reaction. Am J Surg Pathol 23:351, 1988

201. Facchetti F, de Wolf-Peeters C, De Weber I, Frizzera G: Inflammatory pseudotumor of lymph nodes: immunohistochemical evidence for its fibrohistiocytic nature. Am J Pathol 137: 281, 1990

202. Davis RE, Warnke RA, Dorfman RF: Inflammatory pseudotumor of lymph nodes: additional observations and evidence for an inflammatory etiology. Am J Surg Pathol 15:744, 1991

203. Demper CA, Davis RE, Deresinski SC, Dorfman RF: Inflammatory pseudotumor of intra-abdominal lymph nodes manifesting as recurrent fever of unknown origin: a case report. Am J Med 90:519, 1991

204. Chen KTK: Mycobacterial spindle cell pseudotumor of lymph nodes. Am J Surg Pathol 16: 276, 1992

205. Wood C, Nickoloff BJ, Todes-Taylor NR: Pseudotumor resulting from atypical mycobacterial infection: a "histoid" variety of *Mycobacterium avium-intracellulare* complex infection. Am J Clin Pathol 83:524, 1985

206. Brandwein M, Choi HH, Strauchen J et al: Spindle cell reaction to nontuberculous mycobacteriosis in AIDS mimicking a spindle cell neoplasm: evidence for dual histiocytic and

fibroblast-like characteristics of spindle cells. Virchows Arch [A] 416:218, 1990

207. Umlas J, Federman M, Crawford C et al: Spindle cell pseudotumor due to *Mycobacterium avium-intracellulare* in patients with acquired immunodeficiency syndrome (AIDS). Positive staining of mycobacteria for cytoskeleton filaments. Am J Surg Pathol 15:1181, 1991
208. Myint MA, Medeiros LF, Sulaiman RA et al: Inflammatory pseudotumor of the ileum. A report of a multifocal, transmural lesion with regional lymph node involvement. Arch Pathol Lab Med 118:1138, 1994
209. McMahon RFT: Inflammatory pseudotumor of spleen. J Clin Pathol 41:734, 1988
210. Pettinato G, Manivel JC, De Rosa N, Dehner LP: Inflammatory myofibroblastic tumor (plasma cell granuloma): clincopathologic study of 20 cases with immunohistochemical and ultrastructural observation. Am J Clin Pathol 94:538, 1990
211. Coyne JD, Wilson G, Sandhu D, Young RH: Inflammatory pseudotumor of the urinary bladder. Histopathology 18:261, 1991
212. Tang TT, Segura AAD, Oechler HW et al: Inflammatory myofibrohistiocytic proliferation simulating sarcoma in children. Cancer 65:1626, 1990
213. Hammer J, Gradel E, Signer E et al: Plasma cell granuloma of the lung: associated laboratory findings and ultrastructural evidence of inflammatory origin. Pediatr Pulmonol 10:299, 1991
214. Hurt MA, Santa Cruz DJ: Cutaneous inflammatory pseudotumor: lesions resembling ''inflammatory pseudotumor'' or ''plasma cell granulomas'' of extracutaneous sites. Am J Surg Pathol 14:764, 1990
215. Bahadori M, Liebow AA: Plasma cell granuloma of the lung. Cancer 31:191, 1993
216. Spencer H: The pulmonary plasma cell/histiocytoma complex. Histopathology 8:903, 1984
217. Weidner N: Inflammatory (myofibroblastic) pseudotumor of the bladder, a review and differential diagnosis. Adv Anat Pathol 2:362, 1995
218. Nakanuma Y, Tsuneyama K, Masuda S, Tomioka T: Hepatic inflammatory pseudotumor associated with chronic cholangitis: report of three cases. Hum Pathol 25:86, 1994
219. Gough J, Chakrabarti S: Inflammatory pseudotumor of the liver in a patient with chronic sclerosing cholangitis. Am J Gastroenterol 88:1452, 1993
220. Kim I, Kim WS, Yeon KM, Chi JG: Inflammatory pseudotumor of the lung manifesting as a posterior mediastinal mass. Pediatr Radiol 22:467, 1992
221. Coffin CM, Watterson J, Preist JR, Dehner LP: Extrapulmonary inflammatory myofibroblastic tumor (inflammatory pseudotumor), a clinicopathologic and immunohistochemical study of 84 cases. Am J Surg Pathol 19:859, 1995
222. Meis JM, Enzinger FM: Inflammatory fibrosarcoma of the mesentery and retroperitoneum: a tumor closely simulating inflammatory pseudotumor. Am J Surg Pathol 15:1146, 1991
223. Fletcher CDM: Soft tissue tumors. P. 1043. In Fletcher CDM (ed): Diagnostic Histopathology of Tumors. Churchill Livingstone, Edinburgh, 1995
224. Treissman SP, Gillis DA, Lee CL et al: Omental-mesenteric inflammatory pseudotumor, cytogenetic demonstration of genetic changes and monoclonality in one tumor. Cancer 73:1433, 1994
225. Arber DA, Kamel OW, van de Rijn M et al: Frequent presence of the Epstein-Barr virus in inflammatory pseudotumor. Hum Pathol 26:1093, 1995
226. Shek TWH, Ho FCS, Ng IOL et al: Follicular dendritic cell tumor of the liver: evidence for an Epstein-Barr virus-related clonal proliferation of follicular dendritic cells. Am J Surg Pathol 20:313, 1996.

226a. Chan JKC: Inflammatory pseudotumor: a family of lesions of diverse nature and etiologies. Adv Anat Pathol 3:158, 1996

227. Haferkamp O, Rosenau W, Lennert K: Vascular transformation of lymph node sinuses due to venous congestion. Arch Pathol 92:81, 1971
228. Michal M, Koza V: Vascular transformation of lymph node sinuses—a diagnostic pitfall, histopathologic and immunohistochemical study. Pathol Res Pract 185:441, 1989
229. Chan JKC, Warnke RA, Dorfman RF: Vascular transformation of sinuses in lymph nodes, a study of its morphological spectrum and distinction from Kaposi's sarcoma. Am J Surg Pathol 15:732, 1991
230. Ostrowski ML, Siddiqui T, Barnes RE, Howton MJ: Vascular transformation of lymph node sinuses, a process displaying a spectrum of histologic features. Arch Pathol Lab Med 114:656, 1990
231. Scherrer C, Maurer R: La transformation vascu-

laire sinusienne du ganglion lymphatique, analyse morphologique et immunohistochimique de six cas. Ann Pathol (Paris) 5:231, 1985

232. Tenner-Racz K, Kruse R, Schmidt H, Racz P: Vascular sinus transformation in AIDS: a pathologic condition of lymph nodes resembling Kaposi's sarcoma, abstracted. Lab Invest 58: 92A, 1988
233. Fayemi AO, Toker C: Nodal angiomatosis. Arch Pathol Lab Med 99:170, 1975
234. Bedrosian SA, Goldman RL: Nodal angiomatosis: relationship to vascular transformation of lymph nodes. Arch Pathol Lab Med 108: 864, 1984
235. Lucke VM, Davies JD, Wood CM, Whitbread TJ: Plexiform vascularization of lymph nodes: an unusual but distinctive lymphadenopathy in cats. J Comp Pathol 97:109, 1987
236. Steinmann G, Foldi E, Foldi M et al: Morphologic findings in lymph nodes after occlusion of their efferent lymphatic vessels and veins. Lab Invest 47:43, 1982
237. Papadimitriou JC, Drachenberg CB: Vascular transformation of sinuses. Am J Surg Pathol 16: 730, 1992
238. Chan JKC, Warnke RA, Dorfman RF: Vascular transformation of sinuses. Am J Surg Pathol 16: 732, 1992
239. Cook PD, Czerniak B, Chan JKC et al: Nodular spindle cell vascular transformation of lymph nodes: a benign process occurring predominantly in retroperitoneal lymph nodes draining carcinomas that can simulate Kaposi's sarcoma or metastatic tumor. Am J Surg Pathol 19:1010, 1995
240. Diebold J, Audouin J, Le Tourneau L et al: Lymph node reaction patterns in patients with AIDS or AIDS-related complex. P. 189. In Grundmann E, Vollmer E (eds): Reaction Patterns of the Lymph Node. Part 2: Reactions Associated with Neoplasia and Immune Deficient States. Current Topics in Pathology 84/2. Springer-Verlag, Berlin, 1991
241. Said JW: AIDS-related lymphadenopathies. Semin Diagn Pathol 5:365, 1988
242. Ewing EP, Chandler FW, Spira TJ et al: Primary lymph node pathology in AIDS and AIDS-related lymphadenopathy. Arch Pathol Lab Med 109:977, 1985
243. Racz P, Tenner-Racz K, Kahl C et al: Spectrum of morphologic changes of lymph nodes from patients with AIDS or AIDS-related complexes. Prog Allergy 37:81, 1986
244. Ioachim HL, Cronin W, Roy M, Maya M: Persistent lymphadenopathies in people at high risk for HIV infection, clinicopathologic correlations and long-term follow-up in 79 cases. Am J Clin 93:208, 1990
245. Burke AP, Anderson D, Mannan P et al: Systemic lymphadenopathic histology in human immunodeficiency virus 1-seropositive drug addicts without apparent acquired immunodeficiency syndrome. Hum Pathol 25248, 1994
246. Chadburn A, Metroka C, Mouradian J: Progressive lymph node histology and its prognostic value in patients with acquired immunodeficiency syndrome and AIDS-related complex. Hum Pathol 20:579, 1989
247. Fernandez R, Mouradian J, Metroka C, Davis J: The prognostic value of histopathology in persistent generalized lymphadenopathy in homosexual men. N Engl J Med 309:185, 1983
248. Wood GS, Garcia CF, Dorfman RF, Warnke RA: The immunohistology of follicle lysis in lymph node biopsies from homosexual men. Blood 66:1092, 1985
249. Meyer PR, Yanagihara ET, Parker JW, Lukes RJ: A distinctive follicular hyperplasia in the acquired immune deficiency syndrome (AIDS) and the AIDS related complex. Hematol Oncol 2:319, 1984
250. Turner RR, Meyer PR, Taylor CR et al: Immunohistology of persistent generalized lymphadenopathy, evidence for progressive lymph node abnormalities in some patients. Am J Clin Pathol 88:10, 1987
251. Burns BF, Wood GS, Dorfman RF: The varied histopathology of lymphadenopathy in the homosexual male. Am J Surg Pathol 9:287, 1985
252. Piris MA, Rivas C, Morente M et al: Persistent and generalized lymphadenopathy: a lesion of follicular dendritic cells? An immunohistologic and ultrastructural study. Am J Clin Pathol 87: 716, 1987
253. Stanley MW, Frizzera G: Diagnostic specificity of histologic features in lymph node biopsy specimens at risk for the acquired immunodeficiency syndrome. Hum Pathol 17:1231, 1986
254. O'Murchada MT, Wolf BC, Neiman RS: The histologic features of hyperplastic lymphadenopathy in AIDS-related complex are non specific. Am J Surg Pathol 11:94, 1987
255. Butler JJ, Osborne BM: Lymph node enlarge-

ment in patients with unsuspected human immunodeficiency virus infections. Hum Pathol 19: 849, 1988

256. Biberfeld P, Chayt KJ, Marselle LM et al: HTLV-III expression in infected lymph nodes and relevance to pathogenesis of lymphadenopathy. Am J Pathol 125:436, 1986
257. Lowenthal DA, Filippa DA, Richardson ME et al: Generalized lymphadenopathy with morphologic features of Castleman's disease in an HIV-positive man. Cancer 60:2454, 1987
258. Chan JKC, Tang SK, Tsang WYW et al: Histologic changes induced by fine needle aspiration. Adv Anat Pathol 3:71, 1996
259. Tsang WYW, Chan JKC: Spectrum of morphologic changes in lymph nodes attributable to fine needle aspiration. Hum Pathol 23:562, 1992
260. Davies JD, Webb AJ: Segmental lymph node infarction after fine needle aspiration. J Clin Pathol 35:855, 1982
261. Wade HW: The histoid variety of lepromatous leprosy. Int J Lepr 31:129, 1963
262. Wolf DA, Wu CD, Medeiros LJ: Mycobacterial pseudotumors of lymph node, a report of two cases diagnosed at the time of intraoperative consultation using touch imprint preparations. Arch Pathol Lab Med 119:811, 1995
263. Kaiserling E, Patsouris E, Muller-Hermelink HK et al: Bacterial lymphadenitis with the picture of a lymphoepithelioid cell lymphoma—Lennert's lymphoma. Histopathology 14:161, 1989
264. Edman JC, Kovacs JA, Masur H et al: Ribosomal RNA sequence shows *Pneumocystis carinii* to be a member of the fungi. Nature 334: 519, 1988
265. Stringer JR: The identity of *Pneumocystis carinii:* not a single protozoan, but a diverse group of exotic fungus. Infect Agent Dis 2:109, 1993
266. Sun T: Current topics in protozoal diseases. Am J Clin Pathol 102:16, 1994
267. Raviglime MC: Extrapulmonary pneumocystosis, the first 50 cases. Rev Infect Dis 12: 1127, 1990
268. Gal AA, Koss MN, Strigle S, Angritt P: *Pneumocystis carinii* infection in the acquired immune deficiency syndrome. Semin Diagn Pathol 6:287, 1989
269. DeRoux SJ, Adsay NV, Ioachim HL: Disseminated pneumocystosis without pulmonary involvement during prophylactic aerosolized pentamidine therapy in a patient with the acquired immunodeficiency syndrome. Arch Pathol Lab Med 115:1137, 1991
270. Angritt P: Case for diagnosis—May 1988. Milit Med 153:M26, 1988
271. Chan JKC, Lewin KJ, Lombard CM et al: The histopathology of bacillary angiomatosis of lymph nodes. Am J Surg Pathol 15:430, 1991
272. Cockerell CJ, Webster GF, Whitlow MA, Friedman-Kien AE: Epithelioid angiomatosis: a distinct vascular disorder in patients with the acquired immunodeficiency syndrome or AIDS-related complex. Lancet 2:654, 1987
273. Cockerell CJ, LeBoit PE: Bacillary angiomatosis: a newly characterized, pseudoneoplastic, infectious, cutaneous vascular disorder. J Am Acad Dermatol 22:501, 1990
274. Kemper CA, Lombard CM, Deresinski SC, Tompkins LS: Visceral bacillary epithelioid angiomatosis: possible manifestations of disseminated cat scratch disease in the immunocompromised host: a report of two cases. Am J Med 89:216, 1990
275. Koehler JE, Quinn FD, Berger TG et al: Isolation of Rochalimaea species from cutaneous and osseous lesions of bacillary angiomatosis. N Engl J Med 327:1625–1631, 1992
276. LeBoit PE, Berger TC, Egbert BM et al: Epithelioid hemangioma-like vascular proliferation in AIDS: manifestations of cat-scratch disease bacillus infection? Lancet 2:960, 1988
277. LeBoit PE, Berger TG, Egbert BM et al: Bacillary angiomatosis, the histopathology and differential diagnosis of a pseudoneoplastic infection in patients with human immunodeficiency virus disease. Am J Surg Pathol 13:909, 1989
278. LeBoit PE: The expanding spectrum of a new disease, bacillary angiomatosis. Arch Dermatol 126:808, 1990
279. Perkocha LA, Ferrell L, Yen TSB et al: Extracutaneous manifestations of bacillary angiomatosis, abstracted. Mod Pathol 4:88A, 1991
280. Regnery R, Anderson BE, Clarridge JE et al: Characterization of a novel *Rochalimaea species, R. henselae* sp. nov., isolated from blood of a febrile, human immunodeficiency virus-positive patient. J Clin Microbiol 30:265, 1992
281. Relman DA, Loutit JS, Schmidt TM et al: The agent of bacillary angiomatosis, an approach to the identification of uncultured pathogens. N Engl J Med 323:1573, 1990
282. Tsang WYW, Chan JKC: Bacillary angiomatosis: a "new" disease with a broadening

clinicopathologic spectrum. Histol Histopathol 7:143, 1992

283. Welch DF, Pickett DA, Slater LN et al: *Rochalimaea henselae* sp. nov., a cause of septicemia, bacillary angiomatosis and parenchymal bacillary peliosis. J Clin Microbiol 30:275, 1992
284. Leong SS, Cazen RA, Yu GSM et al: Abdominal visceral peliosis associated with bacillary angiomatosis, ultrastructural evidence of endothelial destruction by bacilli. Arch Pathol Lab Med 116:866, 1992
285. Tsang WYW, Chan JKC: Giemsa stain for histological diagnosis of bacillary angiomatosis. Histopathology 21:299, 1992
286. Reed JA, Brigati DJ, Flynn SD et al: Immunocytochemical identification of *Rochalimaea henselae* in bacillary (epithelioid) angiomatosis, parenchymal bacillary peliosis, and persistent fever with bacteremia. Am J Surg Pathol 16: 650, 1992
287. Teague MD, Tham KT: Hyphalike pseudofungus in a lymph node. Arch Pathol Lab Med 118: 95, 96, 1994
288. Connelly J, Ro JY, Cartwright J: Pseudofungi in a lymph node: a case report with energy dispersive x-ray elemental analysis. Arch Pathol Lab Med 115:1166, 1991
289. Hausner RJ, Schoen FJ, Mendez-Fernandez MA et al: Migration of silicone gel to axillary lymph nodes after prosthetic mammoplasty. Arch Pathol Lab Med 105:371, 1981
290. Truong LD, Cartwright J, Goodman D, Woznicki D: Silicone lymphadenopathy associated with augmentation mammoplasty, morphologic features of nine ncases. Am J Surg Pathol 12: 484, 491, 1988
291. Corrin B: Silicone lymphadenopathy. J Clin Pathol 35:901, 1982
292. Harvey T, Leahy M: Silicone lymphadenopathy: a complication of silicone elastomer finger joint prostheses. J Rheum 11:104, 1984
293. Lin RP, DiLeonardo M, Jacoby RA: Silicone lymphadenopathy, a case report and review of the literature. Am J Dermatopathol 15:82, 1993
294. Rogers LA, Longtine JA, Garnick MB, Pinkus GS: Silicone lymphadenopathy in a long distance runner: complication of a silastic prosthesis. Hum Pathol 19:1237, 1988
295. Travis WD, Balogh K, Abraham JL: Silicone granulomas: report of three cases and review of the literature. Hum Pathol 16:19, 1985
296. Kircher T: Silicone lymphadenopathy, a complication of silicone elastomer finger joint prosthesis. Hum Pathol 3:240, 1980
297. Paplanus SH, Payne CM: Axillary lymphadenopathy 17 years after silicone implants: study with x-ray microanalysis. J Hand Surg 13:411, 1988
298. Roggli VL, McDonald JW, Shelburne JD: The detection of silicone within tissues. Arch Pathol Lab Med 118:963, 1994
299. Raso DS, Greene WB, Vesely JJ, Willingham MC: Light microscopy techniques for the demonstration of silicone gel. Arch Pathol Lab Med 118:984, 1994
300. Kessler DA: The basis of the FDA's decision on breast implants. N Engl J Med 326:1713, 1992
301. Sanchez-Guerroero J, Colditz GA, Karlson WE, et al: Silicone breast implants and the risk of connective-tissue diseases and symptoms. N Engl J Med 332:1666, 1995
302. Gabriel SE, Fallon WM, Kurland LT et al: Risk of connective tissue diseases and other disorders after breast implantation. N Engl J Med 330: 1697, 1994
303. Benjamin E, Ahmed A, Rashio ATMF, Wright DH: Silicone lymphadenopathy: a report of two cases, one with concomitant malignant lymphoma. Diagn Histopathol 5:133, 1982
304. Digby JM: Malignant lymphoma with intranodal silicone rubber particles following metacarpophalangeal joint replacements. Hand 14:326, 1982
305. Murakata LA, Ruagwala AF: Silicone lymphadenopathy with concomitant malignant lymphoma. J Rheumatol 16:1481, 1989
306. Carter TR: Intramammary lymph node gold deposits simulating microcalcifications on mammogram. Hum Pathol 19:992, 1988
307. Rollins SD, Craig JP: Gold-associated lymphadenopathy in a patient with rheumatoid arthritis. Arch Pathol Lab Med 115:175, 1991
308. Bruwer A, Nelson GW, Spark RP: Punctate intranodal gold deposits simulating microcalcifications on mammograms. Radiology 163:87, 1987
309. Kuo TT, Hsueh S: Mucicarminophilic histiocytosis, a polyvinylpyrrolidone storage disease simulating signet-ring cell carcinoma. Am J Surg Pathol 8:419, 1984
310. Enzinger FM, Weiss SW: Soft Tissue Tumors. 3rd Ed. p. 317. CV Mosby, St. Louis, 1995
311. Albores-Saavedra J, Vuitch F, Delgado R et al:

Sinus histiocytosis of pelvic lymph nodes after hip replacement, a histiocytic proliferation induced by cobalt-chromium and titanium. Am J Surg Pathol 18:83, 1994

312. Judkins AR, Sickel JZ, Hicks DG et al: Granular histiocytosis of pelvic lymph nodes following total hip arthroplasty, abstracted. Mod Pathol 9: 7A, 1995
313. O'Connell JX, Rosenberg AE: Histiocytic lymphadenitis associated with a large joint prosthesis. Am J Clin Pathol 99:314, 1993
314. Gray MH, Talbert ML, Talbert WM et al: Changes seen in lymph nodes draining sites of large joint prosthesis. Am J Surg Pathol 13: 1050, 1989
315. Nathwani BN: Diagnostic significance of morphologic patterns in lymph node proliferations. P. 407. In Knowles DM (ed): Neoplastic Hematopathology. Williams & Wilkins, Baltimore, 1992
316. Weisenburger DD, Duggan MJ, Perry DA et al: Non-Hodgkin's lymphomas of mantle zone origin. Pathol Annu 26:139, 1991
317. Akosa AB, Ali MH: Lymph node pathology in Henoch-Schonlein purpura. Histopathology 15: 297, 1989
318. Gowing NFC: Infectious mononucleosis: histopathologic aspects. Pathol Annu 10:1, 1975
319. Frizzera G: The clinicopathological expressions of Epstein-Barr virus infection in lymphoid tissues. Virchows Arch [B] 53:1, 1987
320. Tindle BH, Parker JW, Lukes RJ: ''Reed-Sternberg cells'' in infectious mononucleosis. Am J Clin Pathol 58:607, 1972
321. Isaacson PG, Schmid C, Pan LX et al: Epstein-Barr virus latent membrane protein expression by Hodgkin and Reed-Sternberg-like cells in acute infectious mononucleosis. J Pathol 167: 267, 1992
322. Hudnall SD, Conway J, Lazarides A et al: Epstein Barr virus positive Reed-Sternberg-like cells in infectious mononucleosis associated lymphadenopathy, abstracted. Mod Pathol 8: 113A, 1995
323. Abbondanzo SL, Sato N, Straus SE, Jaffe ES: Acute infectious mononucleosis: CD30 (Ki-1) antigen expression and histologic correlations. Am J Clin Pathol 93:698, 1990
324. Fellbaum C, Hansmann ML, Parwaresch MR, Lennert K: Monoclonal antibodies Ki-B3 and Leu-M1 discriminate giant cells of infectious mononucleosis and of Hodgkin's disease. Hum Pathol 19:1168, 1988
325. Niedobitek G, Herbst H, Young LS et al: Patterns of Epstein-Barr virus infection in non-neoplastic lymphoid tissue. Blood 79:2520, 1992
326. Rushin JM, Riordan GP, Heaton RB et al: Cytomegalovirus-infected cells express Leu-M1 antigen: a possible source of diagnostic error. Am J Pathol 136:989, 1990
327. Vago JF, Titman WE, Swerdlow SH: CMV-associated lymphadenopathy in the ''normal'' host: a histopathologic and immunophenotypic description, abstracted. Lab Invest 60:100A, 1989
328. Younes M, Podesta A, Buckley P: Infection of T but not B lymphocytes by cytomegalovirus in lymph node, an immunophenotypic study. Am J Surg Pathol 15:75, 1991
329. Mohrmann RL, Nathwani BN, Brynes RK, Sheibani K: Hodgkin's disease occurring in monocytoid B-cell clusters. Am J Clin Pathol 95:802, 1991
330. Rushin JM, Cotelingam JD, Heaton RB: Hodgkin's disease in monocytoid B-cell clusters and cytomegalovirus lymphadenitis (Letter, and reply by Nathwani BN, Brynes RK). Am J Clin Pathol 97:158, 1992
331. Gaffey MJ, Ben-Ezra JM, Weiss LM: Herpes simplex lymphadenitis. Am J Clin Pathol 95: 709, 1991
332. Audouin J, Tourneau AL, Albert JP, Diebold J: Herpes simplex lymphadenitis mimicking tumoral relapse in a patient with Hodgkin's disease in remission. Virchows Arch [A] 408:313, 1985
333. Taxy JB, Tillawi I, Goldman PM: Herpes simplex lymphadenitis: an unusual presentation with necrosis and viral particles. Arch Pathol Lab Med 109:1043, 1985
334. Lapsley M, Kettle P, Sloan JM: Herpes simplex lymphadenitis: a case report and review of the published work. J Clin Pathol 37:1119, 1984
335. Howat AJ, Campbell AR, Stewart DJ: Generalized lymphadenopathy due to herpes simplex virus type I. Histopathology 19:563, 1991
336. Epstein JI, Ambinder RF, Kuhajda FP et al: Localized herpes simplex lymphadenitis. Am J Clin Pathol 86:444, 1986
337. Tamaru J, Atsuo M, Horie H et al: Herpes simplex lymphadenitis, report of two cases with review of the literature. Am J Surg Pathol 14:571, 1990

338. Miliauskas JR, Leong ASY: Localized herpes simplex lymphadenitis: report of three cases and review of the literature. Histopathology 19:355, 1991
339. Chears WC, Smith AG, Ruffin JM: Diagnosis of Whipple's disease by peripheral lymph node biopsy: report of a case. Am J Med 27:351, 1959
340. Mansbach CM, Shelburne JD, Stevens RD, Dobbins WO: Lymph node bacilliform bodies resembling those of Whipple's disease in a patient without intestinal involvement. Ann Intern Med 89:64, 1978
341. Relman DA, Schmidt TM, MacDermott RP, Falkow S: Identification of the uncultured bacillus of Whipple's disease. N Engl J Med 327: 293, 1992
342. Harmsen D, Heesemann J, Brabletz T et al: Heterogeneity among Whipple's disease-associated bacteria. Lancet 343:1288, 1994
343. Stansfeld AG: The histologic diagnosis of toxoplasmic lymphadenitis. J Clin Pathol 14:565, 1961
344. Dorfman RF, Remington JS: Value of lymph node biopsy in the diagnosis of acute acquired toxoplasmosis. N Engl J Med 289:878, 1973
345. Aisner SC, Aisner J, Moravec C, Arnett EN: Acquired toxoplasmic lymphadenitis with demonstration of the cyst form. Am J Clin Pathol 79:125, 1983
346. Weiss LM, Chen YY, Berry GJ et al: Infrequent detection of *Toxoplasma gondii* genome in toxoplasmic lymphadenitis: a polymerase chain reaction study. Hum Pathol 23:154, 1992
347. Abbondanzo SL, Irye NS, Frizzera G: Dilantin-associated lymphadenopathy: spectrum of histopathologic patterns. Am J Surg Pathol 19:675, 1995
348. Katzin WE, Julius CJ, Tubbs RR, McHenry MC: Lymphoproliferative disorders associated with carbamazepine. Arch Pathol Lab Med 114: 1244, 1990
349. Saltzstein SL, Ackerman LV: Lymphadenopathy induced by anticonvulsant drugs and mimicking clinically and pathologically malignant lymphomas. Cancer 12:164, 1959
350. Yates P, Stockdill G, McIntyre M: Hypersensitivity to carbamazepine presenting as pseudolymphoma. J Clin Pathol 39:1224, 1986
351. Abratt RP, Sealy R, Uys CJ et al: Lymphadenopathy associated with diphenylhydantoin therapy. Clin Oncol 8:351, 1982
352. Gams RA, Neal JA, Conrad FG: Hydantoin-induced pseudopseudolymphoma. Ann Intern Med 69:557, 1968
353. Hyman GA, Sommers SC: The development of Hodgkin's disease and lymphoma during anticonvulsant therapy. Blood 28:416, 1966
354. Segal GH, Clough JD, Tubbs RR: Autoimmune and iatrogenic causes of lymphadenopathy. Semin Oncol 20:611, 1993
355. Gennis MA, Vemuri R, Burns EA et al: Familial occurrence of hypersensitivity to phenytoin. Am J Med 91:631, 1991
356. Frizzera G, Moran EM, Rappaport H: Angioimmunoblastic lymphadenopathy, diagnosis and clinical course. Am J Med 59:803, 1975
357. Lukes RJ, Tindle BH: Immunoblastic lymphadenopathy, a hyperimmune entity resembling Hodgkin's disease. N Engl J Med 292:1, 1975
358. Tsung SH, Lin JL: Angioimmunoblastic lymphadenopathy in a patient taking diphenylhydantoin. Ann Clin Lab Sci 11:542, 1981
359. Redmond J, Kantor RS, Auerbach HE et al: Extramedullary hematopoiesis during therapy with granulocyte colony-stimulating factor. Arch Pathol Lab Med 118:1014, 1994
360. Osborne BM, Butler JJ, Variakojis D, Kott M: Reactive lymph node hyperplasia with giant follicles. Am J Clin Pathol 78:493, 1982
361. Osborne BM, Butler JJ: Clinical implications of nodal reactive follicular hyperplasia in the elderly patients with enlarged lymph nodes. Mod Pathol 4:24, 1991
362. Motulsky AG, Weinberg S, Saphir O, Rosenberg E: Lymph nodes in rheumatoid arthritis. Arch Intern Med 90:660, 1952
363. Nosanchuk JS, Schnitzer B: Follicular hyperplasia in lymph nodes from patients with rheumatoid arthritis, a clinicopathologic study. Cancer 24:343, 1969
364. Wong SY, Sewell HF: CD5 positive B cells in peripheral blood and lymph nodes in rheumatoid arthritis. J Clin Pathol 44:85, 1991
365. Anderson L, Talal N: The spectrum of benign to malignant lymphoproliferation in Sjogren's syndrome. Clin Exp Immunol 9:199, 1971
366. Kassan SS, Thomas TL, Moutsopoulos HM et al: Increased risk of lymphoma in sicca syndrome. Ann Intern Med 89:888, 1978
367. McCurley TL, Collins RD, Ball E, Collins RD: Nodal and extranodal lymphoproliferative disorders in Sjogren's syndrome: a clinical and immunopathologic study. Hum Pathol 21:482, 1995

368. Talal N, Schnitzer B: Lymphadenopathy and Sjogren's syndrome. Clin Rheum Dis 3:421, 1977
369. Swerdlow SH, Sukpanichnant S, Glick AD, Collins RD: Reactive states in lymph nodes resembling lymphomas or progressing to lymphomas: a selective review. Mod Pathol 6:378, 1993
370. Isaacson PG, Norton AJ: Extranodal Lymphomas. Churchill Livingstone, Edinburgh, 1994
371. Shin SS, Sheibani K, Fishleder AJ et al: Monocytoid B cell lymphoma in patients with Sjogren's syndrome: a clinicopathologic study of 13 patients. Hum Pathol 22:422, 1991
372. Hyjek E, Smith WJ, Isaacson PG: Primary B-cell lymphoma of salivary gland and its relationship to myoepithelial sialadenitis. Hum Pathol 19:766, 1988
373. Menke D, Tiemann M, Cameriano J et al: Diagnosis of Castleman's disease by paraffin section immunohistochemistry: identification of an aberrant mantle zone immunophenotype and mantle zone restricted disease, abstracted. Mod Pathol 9:116A, 1995
374. Ruco LP, Gearing AJH, Pigott R et al: Expression of ICAM-1, VCAM-1 and ELAM-1 in angiofollicular lymph node hyperplasia (Castleman's disease): evidence for dysplasia of follicular dendritic reticulum cells. Histopathology 19:523, 1991
375. Danon AD, Krishnan J, Frizzera G: Morpho-immunophenotypic diversity of Castleman's disease, hyaline-vascular type: with emphasis on a stroma-rich variant and a new pathogenetic hypothesis. Virchows Arch [A] 423:369, 1993
376. Nguyen DT, Diamond LW, Hansmann ML et al: Castleman's disease, differences in follicular dendritic network in hyaline vascular and plasma cell variants. Histopathology 24:437, 1994
377. Nagai K, Sato I, Shimoyama N: Pathohistological and immunohistochemical studies on Castleman's disease of the lymph node. Virchows Arch [A] 409:287, 1986
378. Martin JME, Bell B, Ruether BA: Giant lymph node hyperplasia (Castleman's disease) of hyaline vascular type, clinical heterogeneity with immunohistologic uniformity. Am J Clin Pathol 84:439, 1985
379. Carbone A, Manconi R, Volpe R et al: Immunohistochemical, enzyme histochemical and immunologic features of giant lymph node hyperplasia of hyaline vascular type. Cancer 58:908, 1986
380. Harris NL, Bhan AK: Immunohistology of Castleman's disease: a monoclonal antibody study, abstracted. Lab Invest 52:28A, 1985
381. Hanson CA, Frizzera G, Patton DF et al: Clonal rearrangement for immunoglobulin and T-cell receptor genes in systemic Castleman's disease: association with Epstein-Barr virus. Am J Pathol 131:84, 1988
382. Soulier J, Grollet L, Oksenhendler et al: Molecular analysis of clonality in Castleman's disease. Blood 86:1131, 1995
382a. Lin O, Rosai J, Frizzera G: Angiomyoid and dendritic cell proliferative lesions in Castleman's disease of hyaline-vascular type (HV CD): a study of nine cases, abstracted. Mod Pathol 9:116A, 1996
383. Chan JKC, Tsang WYW, Ng CS: Follicular dendritic cell tumor and vascular neoplasm complicating hyaline-vascular Castleman's disease. Am J Surg Pathol 18:517, 1994
384. Madero S, Onate JM, Garzon A: Giant lymph node hyperplasia in an angiolipomatous mediastinal mass. Arch Pathol Lab Med 110:853, 1986
385. Gerald W, Kostianovsky M, Rosai J: Development of vascular neoplasia in Castleman's disease: report of seven cases. Am J Surg Pathol 14:603, 1990
386. McMurry NK, Katikaneni PR, Demian SDE, Lechago J: Gastric stromal tumor associated with regional angiofollicular lymph node hyperplasia (Castleman's disease). Surg Pathol 4:167, 1991
387. Frizzera G: Castleman's disease and related disorders. Semin Diagn Pathol 5:346, 1988
388. Menke DM, Camoriano JK, Banks PM: Angiofollicular lymph node hyperplasia: a comparison of unicentric, multicentric, hyaline vascular, and plasma cell types of disease by morphometric and clinical analysis. Mod Pathol 5:525, 1992
389. Hall PA, Donaghy M, Cotter FE et al: An immunohistochemical and genotypic study of the plasma cell form of Castleman's disease. Histopathology 14:333, 1989
390. Radaszkiewicz T, Hansmann ML, Lennert K: Monoclonality and polyclonality of plasma cells in Castleman's disease of the plasma cell variant. Histopathology 14:11, 1969
391. Hsu SM, Waldron JA, Xie SS, Barlogie B:

Expression of interleukin-6 in Castleman's disease. Hum Pathol 24:833, 1993

392. Beck JT, Hsu SM, Wijdenes J et al: Alleviation of systemic manifestations of Castleman's disease by monoclonal interleukin-6 antibody. N Engl J Med 330:602, 1994
393. Zarate-Osorno A, Medeiros LJ, Danon AD, Neiman RS: Hodgkin's disease with coexistent Castleman-like histologic features, a report of three cases. Arch Pathol Lab Med 118:270, 1994
394. Maheswaran PR, Ramsay AD, Norton AJ, Roche WR: Hodgkin's disease presenting with the histological features of Castleman's disease. Histopathology 18:249, 1991
395. Molinie V, Diebold J, Perie G: Hodgkin's disease associated with localized or multicentric Castleman's disease. Arch Pathol Lab Med 119: 201, 1995
396. Frizzera G: Castleman's disease: more questions than answers. Hum Pathol 16:202, 1985
397. Kessler E: Multicentric giant lymph node hyperplasia, a report of seven cases. Cancer 56:2446, 1985
398. Frizzera G, Peterson BA, Bayrd ED, Goldman A: A systemic lymphoproliferative disorder with morphologic features of Castleman's disease: clinical findings and clinicopathologic correlations in 15 patients. J Clin Oncol 3:1202, 1985
399. Weisenburger DD, Nathwani BN, Winberg CD, Rappaport H: Multicentric angiofollicular lymph node hyperplasia: a clinicopathologic study of 16 cases. Hum Pathol 16:162, 1985
400. Frizzera G, Massarelli G, Banks PM, Rosai J: A systemic lymphoproliferative disorder with morphologic features of Castleman's disease: pathological findings in 15 patients. Am J Surg Pathol 7:211, 1983
401. Frizzera G: Systemic Castleman's disease, abstracted. Am J Surg Pathol 15:192, 1991
402. Smir BN, Weisenburger DD: Multicentric angiofollicular lymph node hyperplasia in children, abstracted. Mod Pathol 9:120A, 1995
403. Gaba AR, Stein RS, Sweet DL et al: Multicentric giant lymph node hyperplasia. Am J Clin Pathol 69:86, 1978
404. Isaacson PG: Castleman's disease. Histopathology 14:429, 1989
405. Ohyashiki JH, Ohyashiki K, Kawakubo K et al: Molecular genetic, cytogenetic, and immunophenotypic analyses of Castleman's disease of the plasma cell type. Am J Clin Pathol 101:290, 1994
406. Nagai M, Irino S, Uda H et al: Molecular genetic and immunohistochemical analyses of a case of multicentric Castleman's disease. Jpn J Clin Oncol 18:149, 1988
407. Peterson BA, Frizzera G: Multicentric Castleman's disease. Semin Oncol 20:636, 1993
408. Soulier J, Grollet L, Oksenhendler E et al: Kaposi's sarcoma-associated herpesvirus-like DNA sequences in multicentric Castleman's disease. Blood 86:1276, 1995
409. Cesarman E, Knowles DM: Herpes-like DNA sequences, AIDS-related tumors, and Castleman's disease. N Engl J Med 333:799, 1995

409a. Chadburn A, Nador RG, Cesarman E et al: Kaposi's sarcoma associated herpesvirus sequences in non-HIV-associated lymphoproliferative lesions, abstracted. Mod Pathol 9:109A, 1996

410. Chen KTK: Multicentric Castleman's disease and Kaposi's sarcoma. Am J Surg Pathol 8:287, 1984
411. Dickson D, Ben-Ezra JM, Reed J et al: Multicentric giant lymph node hyperplasia, Kaposi's sarcoma, and lymphoma. Arch Pathol Lab Med 109:1013, 1985
412. Chan JKC, Fletcher CDM, Hicklin GA, Rosai J: Glomeruloid hemangioma, a distinctive cutaneous lesion of multicentric Castleman's disease associated with POEMS syndrome. Am J Surg Pathol 14:1036, 1990
413. Gould JS, Diss T, Isaacson PG: Multicentric Castleman's disease in association with a solitary plasmacytoma: a case report. Histopathology 17:135, 1990
414. Poppema S, Kaiserling E, Lennert K: Hodgkin's disease with lymphocytic predominance, nodular type (nodular paragranuloma) and progressively transformed germinal centres—a cytohistological study. Histopathology 3:295, 1979
415. Poppema S, Kaiserling E, Lennert K: Nodular paragranuloma and progressively transformed germinal centers, ultrastructural and immunohistologic findings. Virchows Arch [B] 31:211, 1979
416. Osborne BM, Butler JJ, Gresik MV: Progressive transformation of germinal centers: comparison of 23 pediatric patients to the adult population. Mod Pathol 5:135, 1992
417. Osborne BM, Butler JJ: Clinical implications of

progressive transformation of germinal centers. Am J Surg Pathol 8:725, 1984

418. Burns BF, Colby TV, Dorfman RF: Differential diagnostic features of nodular L&H Hodgkin's disease, including progressive transformation of germinal centers. Am J Surg Pathol 8:725, 1984
419. Crossley B, Heryet A, Gatter KC: Does nodular lymphocyte predominant Hodgkin's disease arise from progressively transformed germinal centers? A case report with an unusually prolonged history. Histopathology 11:621, 1987
420. Ferry JA, Zukerberg LR, Harris NL: Florid progressive transformation of germinal centers, a syndrome affecting young men, without early progression to nodular lymphocyte predominance Hodgkin's disease. Am J Surg Pathol 16: 252, 1992
421. Hansmann ML, Fellbaum C, Hui PK, Moubayed P: Progressive transformation of germinal centres with and without association to Hodgkin's disease. Am J Clin Pathol 93:219, 1990
422. van den Oord JJ, de Wolf-Peeters C, Desmet VJ: Immunohistochemical analysis of progressively transformed follicle centers. Am J Clin Pathol 83:560, 1985
423. Goates JJ, Kamel OW, LeBrun DP et al: Floral variant of follicular lymphoma: immunological and molecular studies support a neoplastic process. Am J Surg Pathol 18:37, 1994
424. Maurer R, Schmid U, Davies JD et al: Lymph node infarction and malignant lymphoma: a multicenter survey of European, English and American cases. Histopathology 10:571, 1986
425. Rothschild B, Marshall H: Lymphadenopathy and lymph node infarction in the course of gold therapy. Am J Med 80:537, 1986
426. Cleary KR, Osborne BM, Butler JJ: Lymph node infarction foreshadowing malignant lymphoma. Am J Surg Pathol 6:435, 1982
427. Norton AJ, Ramsay AD, Isaacson PG: Antigen preservation in infarcted lymphoid tissue, a novel approach to the infarcted lymph node using monoclonal antibodies effective in routinely processed tissue. Am J Surg Pathol 12: 759, 1988
428. Laszewski MJ, Belding PJ, Feddersen RM et al: Clonal immunoglobulin gene rearrangement in the infarcted lymph node syndrome. Am J Clin Pathol 96:116, 1991
429. Osborne BM, Butler JJ, Mackay B: Proteinaceous lymphadenopathy with hypergammaglobulinemia. Am J Surg Pathol 3:137, 1979
430. Michaeli J, Niesvizky R, Siegel D et al: Proteinaceous (angiocentric sclerosing) lymphadenopathy: a polyclonal systemic, nonamyloid deposition disorder. Blood 86:1159, 1995
431. Banerjee D, Mills DM, Hearn SA et al: Proteinaceous lymphadenopathy due to monoclonal nonamyloid immunoglobulin deposit disease. Arch Pathol Lab Med 114:34, 1990
432. Buxbaum JN, Chuba JV, Hellman GC et al: Monoclonal immunoglobulin deposition disease: light chain and light and heavy chain deposition diseases and their relation to light chain amyloidosis, clinical features, immunopathology, and molecular analysis. Ann Intern Med 112:455, 1990
433. Ramos FJ, Gomez-Martino JR, Fernandez-Rojo FP, Suarez D: Proteinaceous lymphadenopathy and the kidney. Arch Pathol Lab Med 116:8, 1992

3

Classical Hodgkin's Disease

John G. Strickler, Lawrence J. Burgart, and Lawrence M. Weiss

Hodgkin's disease is a lymphoid malignancy composed of Reed-Sternberg cells and variants in a characteristic mixed inflammatory background. The pathologic and clinical features of the disease, first described by Thomas Hodgkin in 1832,[1] are well known and widely recognized by pathologists and clinicians. Nevertheless, our knowledge and understanding of Hodgkin's disease has been enhanced by recent pathologic and clinical studies, which suggest that Hodgkin's disease is a heterogeneous syndrome rather than a single disease.[2] In particular, lymphocyte predominant Hodgkin's disease has pathologic and clinical features distinct and increasingly divergent from the "classical" subtypes of Hodgkin's disease[3] and therefore is discussed in a separate chapter. The current chapter reviews classical Hodgkin's disease, including recent histologic, immunologic, molecular, cytogenetic, viral, and clinical studies.

HISTOPATHOLOGIC FEATURES

Definition of Classical Hodgkin's Disease

Reed-Sternberg (RS) cells and variants (Hodgkin's cells) are the neoplastic cells of Hodgkin's disease. Classical (diagnostic) RS cells are an important component in confidently identifying primary Hodgkin's disease. RS cell variants are very useful in recognizing and subtyping Hodgkin's disease and are universally present when classical RS cells are identified. We believe that a diagnosis of Hodgkin's disease may be rendered on the basis of RS variants, even in the absence of classical RS cells, when the overall histologic findings are typical of Hodgkin's disease or with support by immunohistochemical studies.

The characteristic mixed inflammatory background is the second essential component for the histologic diagnosis of Hodgkin's disease. The background cells account for the vast majority of the cell population in Hodgkin's disease, and RS cells and variants typically comprise less than 5 percent of the lesion. Cells resembling RS cells and variants may be found in non-Hodgkin's lymphomas and in reactive lymph nodes (especially infectious mononucleosis), demonstrating the importance of having both the appropriate neoplastic cytology and reactive milieu.

A confident diagnosis of Hodgkin's disease is therefore based on identification of RS cells and variants in an appropriate mixed inflammatory background. While routine histopathology will often allow for fulfillment of these two criteria, immunophenotypic analysis of the RS cells, RS variants, and the inflammatory background is commonly performed to verify the diagnosis.

Reed-Sternberg Cells and Variants

Classical RS cells are large cells that are lobulated, binucleated, or multinucleated (Fig. 3-1). Each nucleus or nuclear lobe contains a single nucleolus, which is characteristically large (greater than one-third the diameter of the entire

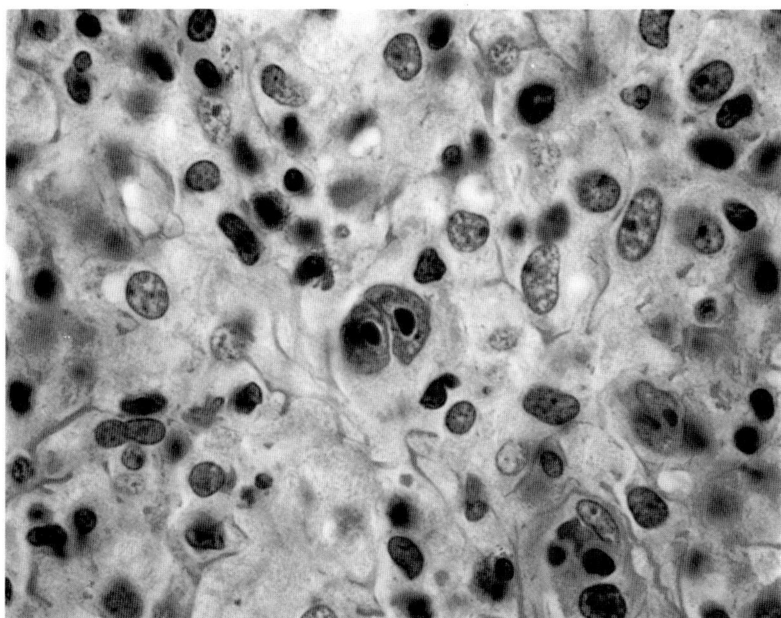

Fig. 3-1. Classical RS cells are binucleated, and each nucleus contains a macronucleolus surrounded by a clear halo. The RS cell is surrounded by a mixed inflammatory infiltrate. (H&E.)

nucleus), centrally located, eosinophilic, and surrounded by a halo. As suggested by the morphologic features, the nucleolus often has the appearance of a nuclear inclusion. The cytoplasm of RS cells is abundant and eosinophilic or amphophilic.

RS cell variants (''Hodgkin's cells'') may have various histologic features, which often include multinucleated or multilobulated nuclei (Fig. 3-2). Mononuclear RS cell variants are large cells that have a single large nucleus and a prominent eosinophilic nucleolus (Fig. 3-3). Mummified RS cell variants (''zombie'' cells) are partially degenerating cells characterized by pyknotic nuclei and eosinophilic cytoplasm (Fig. 3-4). Lacunar cells are RS cell variants in clear ''lacunar'' spaces, which are cytoplasmic retraction artifacts caused by formalin fixation (Fig. 3-5). In other fixatives, lacunar cells have abundant pale cytoplasm and prominent cytoplasmic membranes. The nuclei of lacunar cells are typically polylobated (multilobated) and lack the huge nucleoli of classic RS cells.

RS cells and variants are distinguished from immunoblasts by their morphologic features. The nucleoli of immunoblasts are smaller, multiple, peripherally located, basophilic, and often accompanied by clumped chromatin. The cytoplasm of immunoblasts (basophilic, plasmacytoid) is also distinctive. Furthermore, immunoblasts are typically found in association with large transformed lymphocytes, which are rare in Hodgkin's disease.

The origin of RS cells have been widely debated. Various authors have identified these cells as derivatives of macrophages/histiocytes, interdigitating reticulum cells, dendritic reticulum cells, granulocytes, monocytes, and other cell types. Recent evidence (discussed below) suggests that many RS cells are of lymphoid (usually B-cell) origin.[4–8]

BACKGROUND CELLS

Lymphocytes consist predominantly of small lymphocytes with round regular (to mildly irregular) nuclei, sometimes associated with plasma cells (Fig. 3-6). Large transformed cells and immunoblasts may be present but are infrequent.

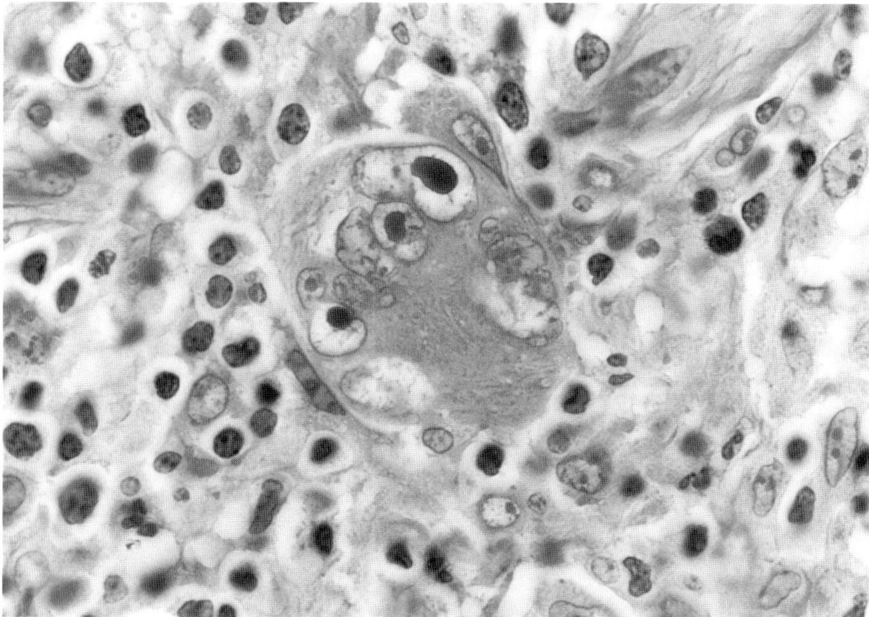

Fig. 3-2. Multinucleated RS cells show eosinophilic macronucleoli in each nucleus. (H&E.)

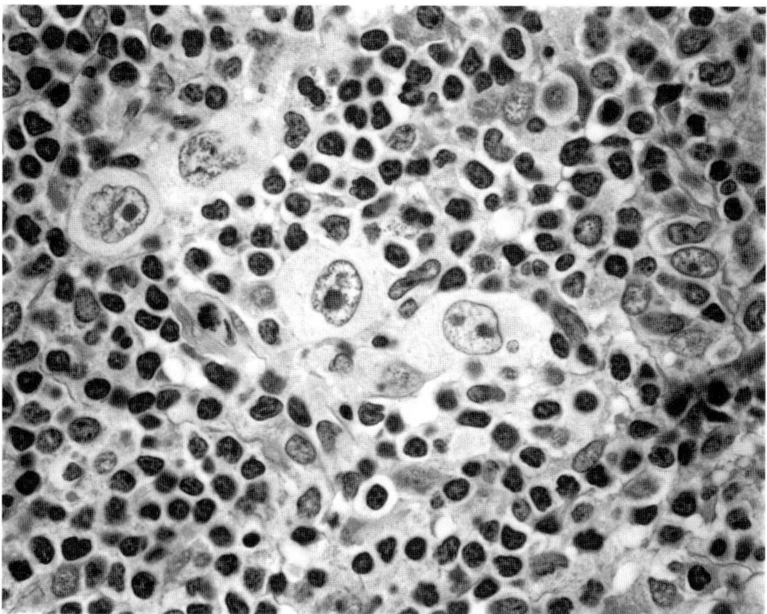

Fig. 3-3. Mononuclear RS cell variants, characterized by large vesicular nuclei with prominent eosinophilic macronucleoli, are located in a background of lymphocytes, eosinophils, and histiocytes. Note the dichotomy between the RS cell variants and the small lymphocytes. (H&E.)

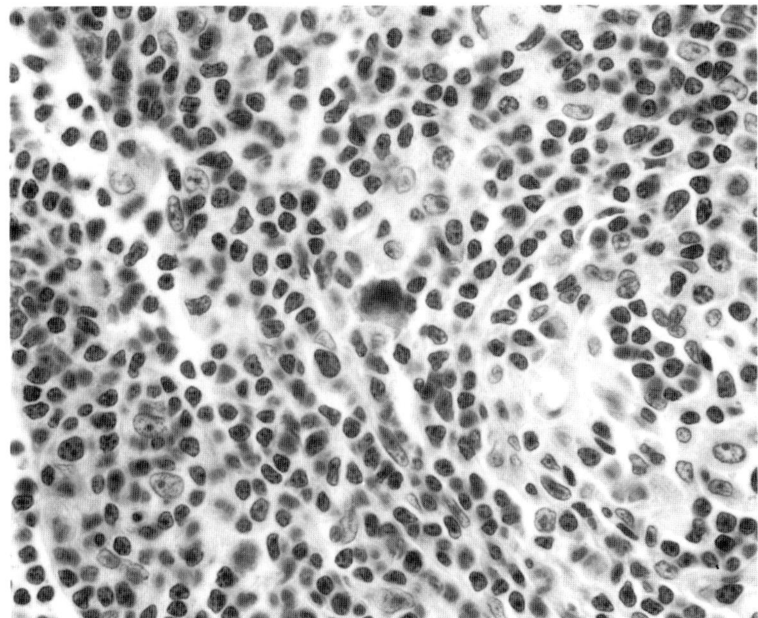

Fig. 3-4. A mummified RS variant, characterized by a pyknotic nucleus and eosinophilic homogenized cytoplasm, located in a background of small lymphocytes. (H&E.)

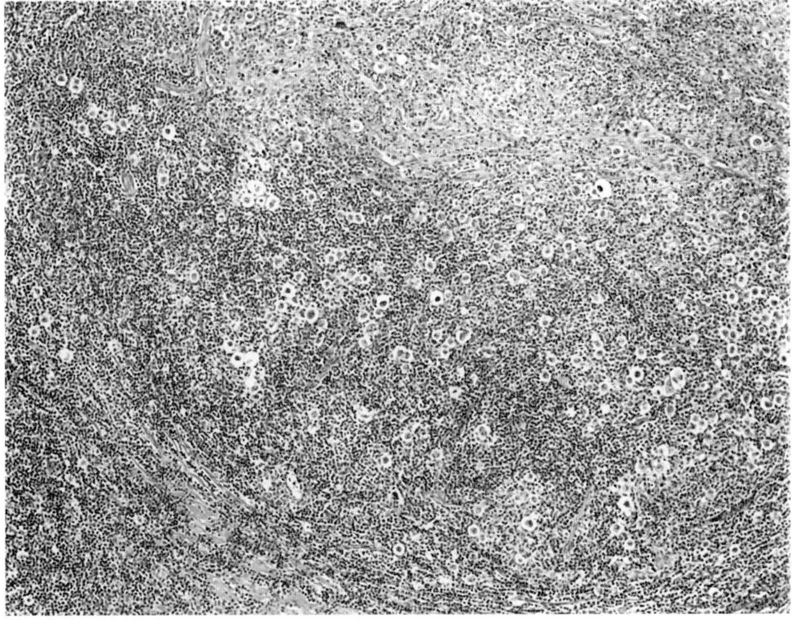

Fig. 3-5. Lacunar RS cell variants are typical of NSHD fixed in formalin. (H&E.)

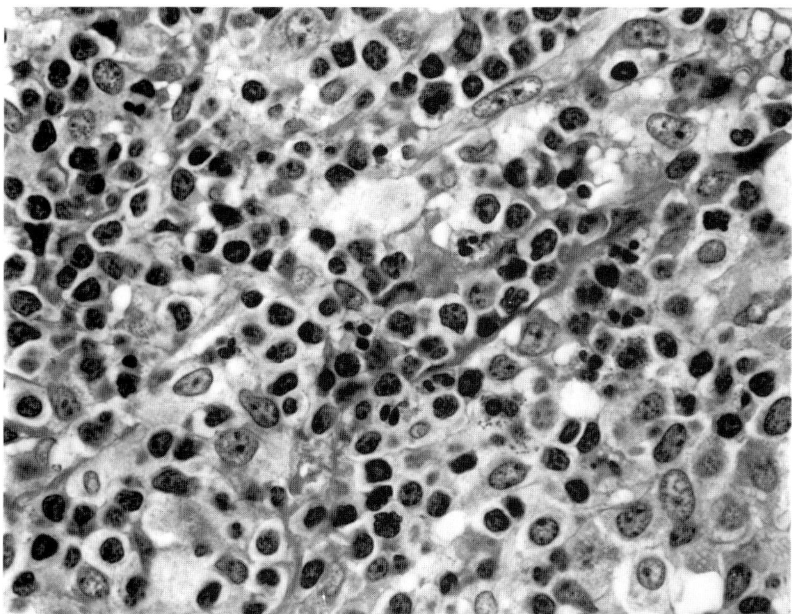

Fig. 3-6. The characteristic admixture of inflammatory cells in Hodgkin's disease includes neutrophils, bilobed eosinophils, lymphocytes with slight nuclear irregularities, and histiocytes with large oval nuclei. (H&E.)

The lymphocytes are predominantly T cells with a variable CD4:CD8 ratio, although CD4+ lymphocytes (T-helper cells) typically predominate.[9–13] A small population of polyclonal B cells also may be present, and the B cells may form monocytoid clusters.[14,15] When a spectrum of atypical lymphocytes is present ranging from large to middle size, the diagnosis of Hodgkin's disease should be seriously questioned, since Hodgkin's disease typically demonstrates dichotomous large cell (neoplastic) and small cell (reactive) populations (Fig. 3-3).

Granulocytes in Hodgkin's disease include both eosinophils and neutrophils (Fig. 3-6). The number of eosinophils is widely variable, but usually present, and eosinophilic microabscesses tend to form when eosinophils are numerous. The presence of neutrophils may correlate with "B" symptoms.

Fibroblasts are usually difficult to detect in the background cell population of typical cases of Hodgkin's disease. However, fibroblasts may be numerous, particularly in the "fibroblastic variant" of the nodular sclerosing subtype, or when Hodgkin's disease involves bone marrow.

Histiocytes in variable numbers are present in the background cell population. Foamy histiocytes may be numerous, creating the appearance of xanthogranulomatous inflammation or a lipid-storage disease.[16] Numerous epithelioid histiocytes, which may or may not form granulomas (see below), may also be identified (Fig. 3-7). Histiocytosis X (Langerhans cell granulomatosis) may be an incidental finding in Hodgkin's disease.[17]

Follicular dendritic cells may be present, although immunologic studies may be required for their identification. These cells typically form expanded and disrupted cell networks, admixed with RS cells and variants.[18,19]

Other Histologic Features

Fibrosis is very common in Hodgkin's disease and may take the form of thick collagen bands or fine sclerosis. The exact form of the fibrosis is important in the classification of Hodgkin's disease.

Granulomas, which are usually non-necrotiz-

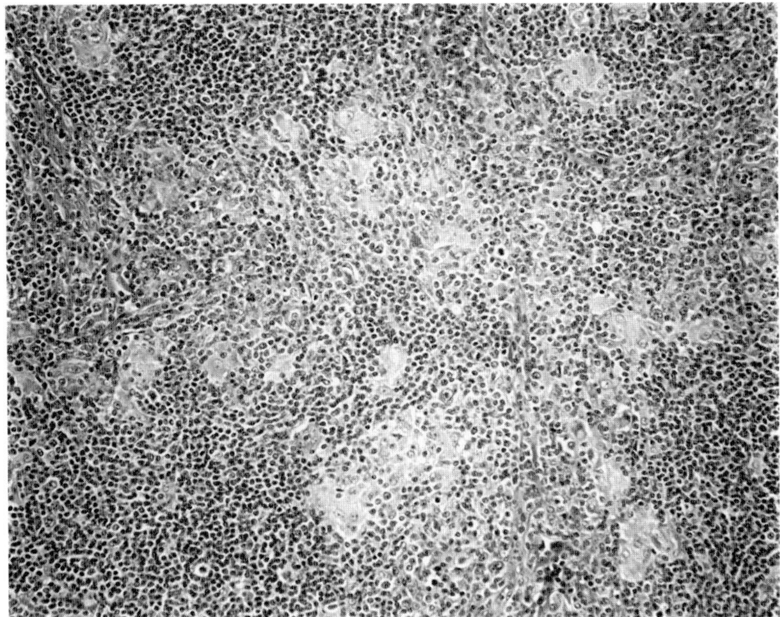

Fig. 3-7. Epithelioid histiocytes are a common finding in Hodgkin's disease, although various non-Hodgkin's lymphomas also contain epithelioid cell clusters. (H&E.)

ing ("sarcoid-like"), are commonly found in tissues involved by Hodgkin's disease.[20] In addition, uninvolved tissue specimens from patients with Hodgkin's disease may contain isolated sarcoid-like granulomas, which should not be interpreted as evidence of Hodgkin's disease or influence the pathologic stage.[21] "Sarcoid-like" granulomas are usually not associated with clinical evidence of sarcoidosis.

Necrosis is a common finding in Hodgkin's disease and is especially characteristic of the nodular sclerosing subtype. The necrotic areas may contain many neutrophils and/or eosinophils, and they are typically surrounded by histiocytes and numerous RS cells and variants.

Castleman's disease-like changes (usually resembling the plasma cell type) are occasionally associated with Hodgkin's disease, either in the same node or subsequent node biopsy.[22,23] The Castleman's disease-like changes are thought be a nonspecific immune response to the Hodgkin's disease rather than a separate disease, and they may be related interleukin-6 secretion by RS cells. The Hodgkin's disease typically has an interfollicular distribution.

Florid reactive follicular hyperplasia may occur in lymph nodes involved by Hodgkin's disease. The Hodgkin's disease is typically located in interfollicular areas but may have an intrafollicular distribution, as demonstrated by immunohistochemical staining for follicular dendritic cells.[19] The interfollicular Hodgkin's disease may be overshadowed by the florid reactive follicular hyperplasia and may therefore be difficult to recognize, especially when there is no significant effacement of the lymph node architecture.[24]

Unusual histologic findings include infiltration of the lymph node capsule, which should suggest the possibility of an alternative diagnosis. Furthermore, vascular invasion is not typical of Hodgkin's disease[25] but is commonly associated with disseminated and extranodal disease, especially at autopsy.[26–29]

Extranodal Hodgkin's Disease

Primary extranodal Hodgkin's disease is very unusual[30] except in patients with HIV infections. Furthermore, many extranodal lymphoid infiltrates with histologic features resembling Hodgkin's disease, when carefully studied by immunologic or genetic techniques, are non-Hodgkin's lymphomas or reactive infiltrates. Therefore, a primary diagnosis of extranodal Hodgkin's disease should be made with caution. Histologic criteria for this diagnosis (RS cells and variants in an appropriate cellular background) are identical to those of nodal Hodgkin's disease. Architectural effacement of the extranodal tissue, which can usually be appreciated grossly, provides additional support for the histologic diagnosis. However, a confident diagnosis of primary extranodal Hodgkin's disease usually requires immunohistochemical confirmation.

Secondary extranodal involvement by Hodgkin's disease (previously established by lymph node biopsy) occurs more frequently than primary extranodal disease. In this clinical setting, an unequivocal diagnosis of Hodgkin's disease can be established by identifying RS cell variants (with or without diagnostic RS cells) in an appropriate cellular background.[31] Histologic features that are suggestive of secondary extranodal involvement by Hodgkin's disease include an appropriate cellular background and cells suggestive of RS cells variants; these findings should prompt serial sections and immunohistochemical studies in an attempt to confirm the diagnosis. However, nonspecific lymphoid infiltrates without RS cell variants are not suggestive of Hodgkin's disease, since they are a common finding in liver biopsies and other uninvolved tissue specimens from patients with Hodgkin's disease.[32]

Thymic involvement is commonly associated with mediastinal Hodgkin's disease, and it may be difficult to determine whether the Hodgkin's disease is primary in the thymus or mediastinal lymph nodes. Thymic involvement associated with a granulomatous reaction has been referred to as "granulomatous thymoma."[33] Secondary cystic changes are often present in the thymus, and persistence of thymic cysts after successful treatment may cause the radiographic appearance of "residual" Hodgkin's disease.

Splenic involvement by Hodgkin's disease (25 to 40 percent at staging laparotomy) is characterized by discrete nodules, usually visible on gross examination, which first arise in the white pulp.[34] Each nodule typically consists of coalescing microscopic foci of Hodgkin's disease. The number of nodules should be carefully documented, since the presence of five or more nodules is important for up-staging and adequately treating patients with Hodgkin's disease.[35] Since involvement can be quite focal, the spleen should be breadloafed at 3 mm intervals.[35] Although Hodgkin's disease is typically associated with splenomegaly, focal involvement may occur in spleens of normal weight and size. Sections of any gross lesions should be examined microscopically, since the gross appearance of Hodgkin's disease may be difficult to distinguish from localized reactive lymphoid hyperplasia (Fig. 3-8).[36] The splenic hilar lymph nodes also should be examined for microscopic evidence of Hodgkin's disease.

Liver involvement by Hodgkin's disease is located in and around portal triads, especially when the involvement is focal (Fig. 3-9).[37,38] Extensive liver involvement is characterized by white nodules centered in portal regions, which are visible grossly and radiographically.

Bone marrow involvement is present in less than 15 percent of patients and is characterized by focal fibrosis, associated with RS cells and variants in an appropriate cellular background.[39,40] Focal fibrosis should prompt a careful search for RS cells and variants by serial sections, immunohistochemical stains, or additional biopsy specimens (Fig. 3-10). The surrounding bone marrow commonly shows nonspecific reactions, including myeloid hyperplasia and increased plasma cells.[41]

Pulmonary involvement by Hodgkin's disease occurs in up to 50 percent of patients, often resulting from contiguous spread from the mediastinum. Pulmonary Hodgkin's disease typically forms one or more nodules or masses, whereas secondary involvement by non-Hodgkin's lymphoma is often diffuse. Primary presentations in the lung have been reported with demographics similar to nodal Hodgkin's (Fig. 3-11). Prog-

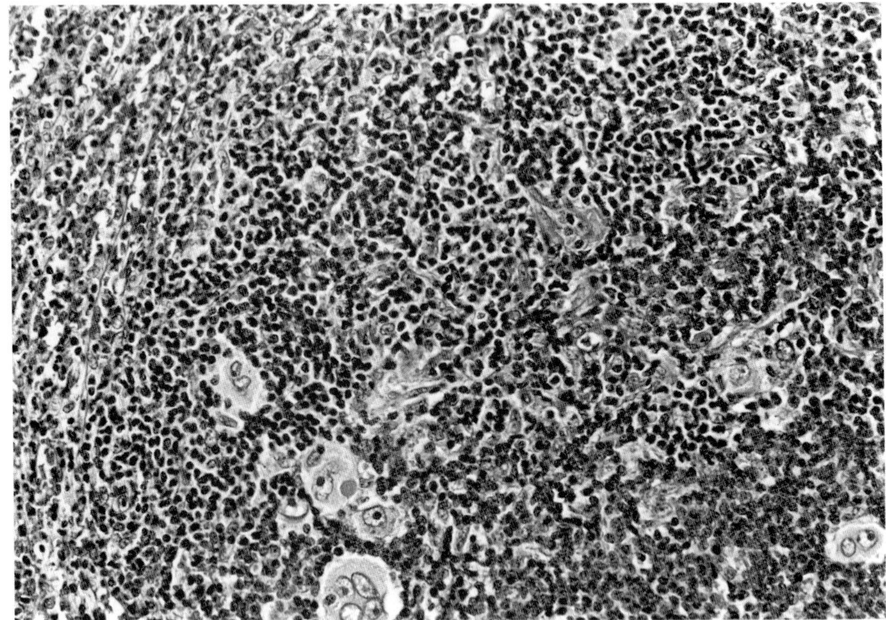

Fig. 3-8. Splenic Hodgkin's disease forms nodules, which may be difficult to differentiate (by gross examination) from reactive lymphoid hyperplasia. (H&E.)

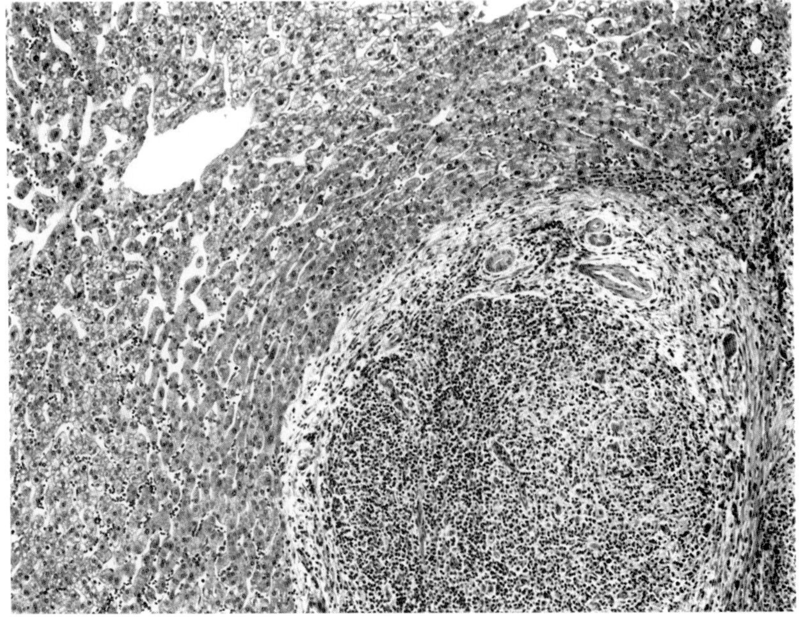

Fig. 3-9. Hepatic Hodgkin's disease characteristically forms portocentric nodules, and RS cells and variants are visible even at low power in this instance. (H&E.)

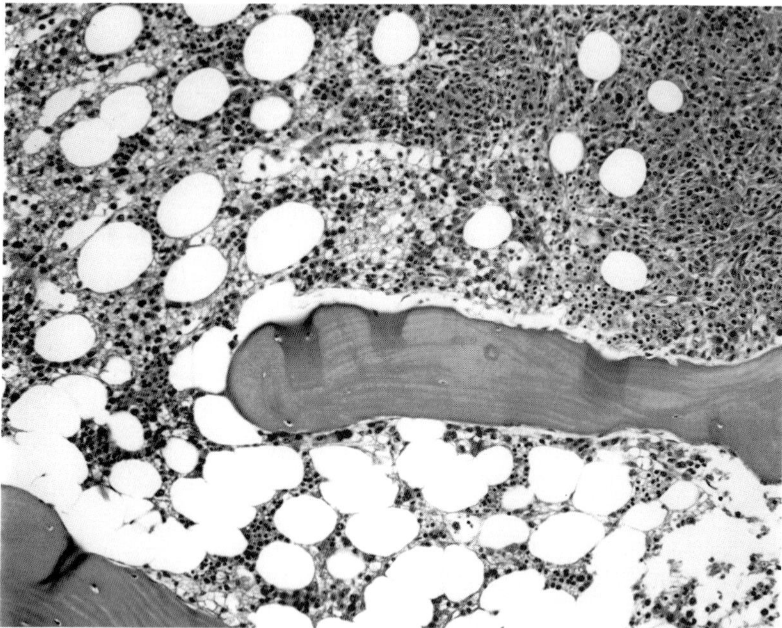

Fig. 3-10. This bone marrow biopsy shows an area of fibrosis (upper right), which should prompt a careful search for RS cells and variants (including serial sections or immunohistochemistry if necessary). (H&E.)

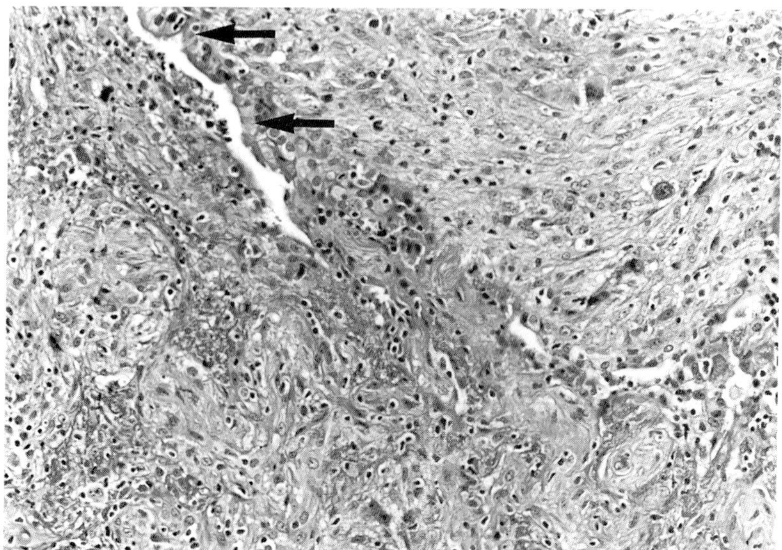

Fig. 3-11. Pulmonary Hodgkin's disease is commonly peribronchial (*arrows* indicate residual bronchial epithelium), and the fibrohistiocytic response may obscure the RS cells and variants. (H&E.)

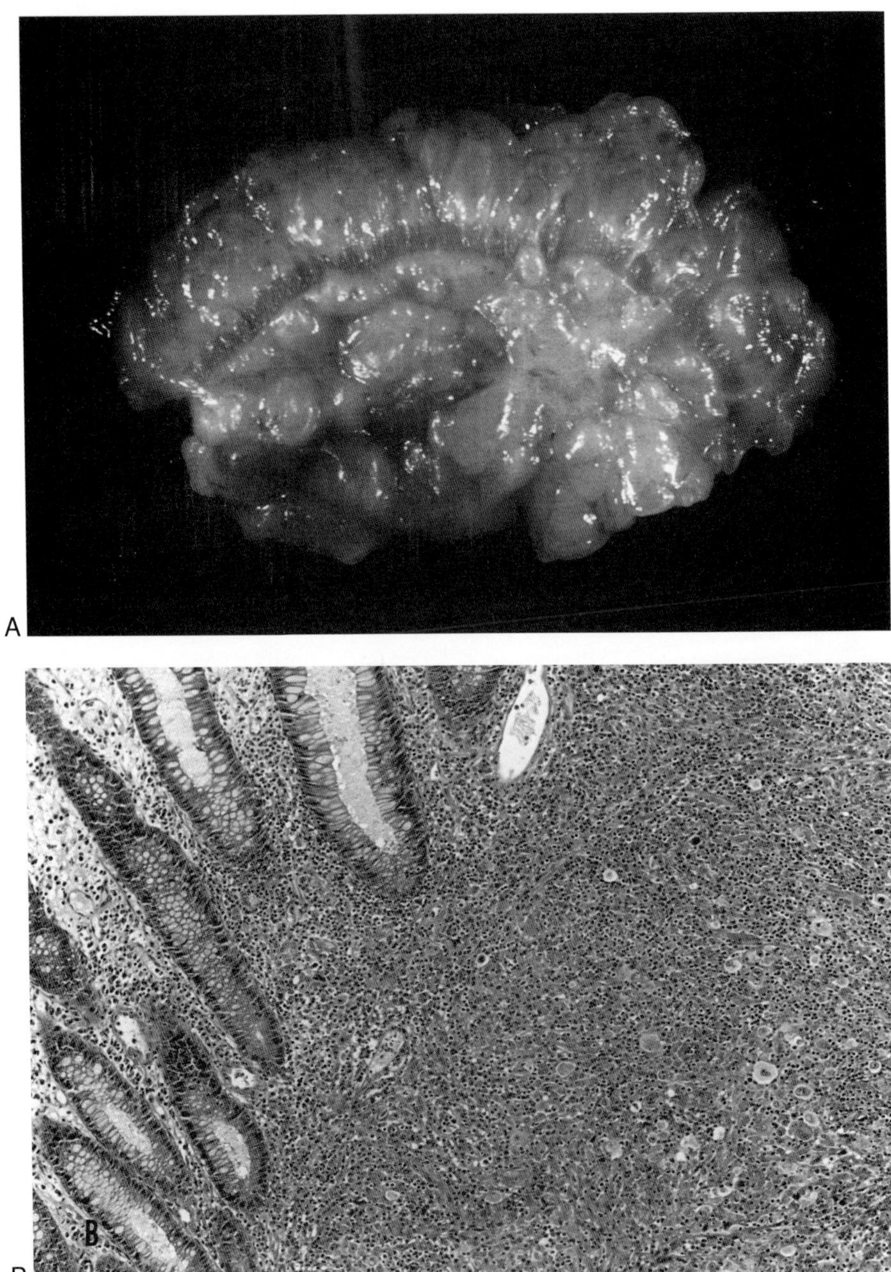

Fig. 3-12. Gastrointestinal (colon in this example) Hodgkin's disease forms large mural nodules. (**A**) Cross section of colon wall demonstrates mural nodules. Note muscularis propria for orientation. (**B**) Photomicrograph shows typical histologic features of Hodgkin's disease. (H&E.)

nosis is adversely affected by bilaterality and multilobe involvement.[42–44]

Gastrointestinal tract involvement by Hodgkin's disease is uncommon, especially as the primary site of disease.[45,46] Reported sites of involvement include the stomach, small bowel, and colon, where immunohistochemical studies are essential for distinguishing Hodgkin's disease from intestinal non-Hodgkin's lymphomas. As with other sites, involvement of the gastrointestinal tract is typically tumefactive and causes obstructive symptoms (Fig. 3-12). Mucosal damage and luminal constriction may mimic Crohn's disease.

Cutaneous involvement by Hodgkin's disease is uncommon. Secondary cutaneous involvement usually occurs by direct extension from lymph nodes or by retrograde lymphatic spread. Primary Hodgkin's disease is extremely rare but has been reported.[47,48] However, this diagnosis should be made with caution, since cutaneous lesions containing RS-like cells are likely to be lymphomatoid papulosis or anaplastic large cell lymphoma, which may be closely related entities.[49]

Other extranodal sites, including intracranial,[50,51] breast,[52] and Waldeyer's ring,[53,54] may be involved by Hodgkin's disease. However, these sites of involvement are rare, especially as the primary site of involvement.

Recurrent Hodgkin's Disease

Recurrent Hodgkin's disease in untreated sites (sites not exposed to prior radiation therapy) usually has histologic features similar to the initial Hodgkin's disease.[55,56] The initial and recurrence specimens tend to have the same histologic subtypes and other distinctive histologic patterns (such as extensive necrosis). However, recurrent Hodgkin's disease may show changes indicative of histologic progression, especially at autopsy, which include loss of nodularity and/or sclerosis, vascular invasion, involvement of extranodal and/or noncontiguous sites, loss of lymphocytes or eosinophils, and increased numbers of histiocytes and RS cell variants. Therefore, recurrent Hodgkin's disease may progress to lymphocyte depleted patterns, and sheets of

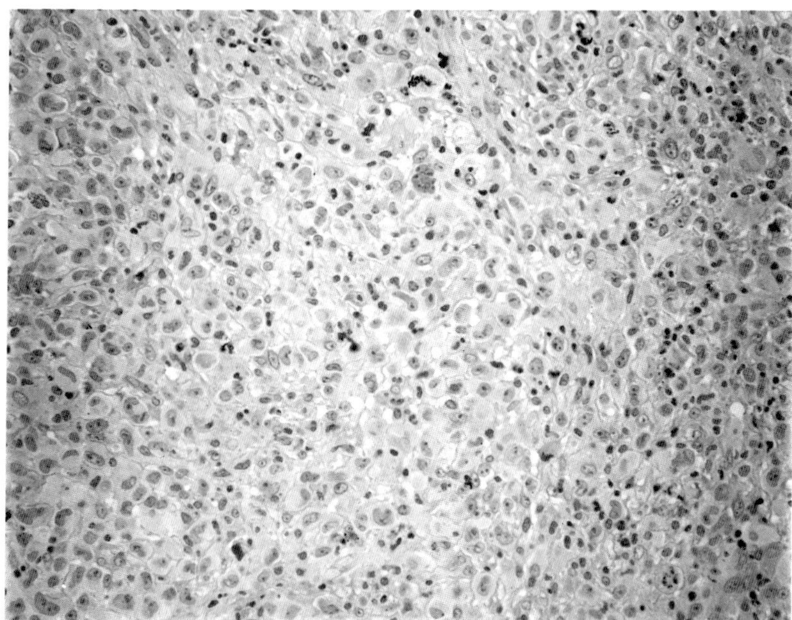

Fig. 3-13. Recurrent Hodgkin's disease in untreated sites shows numerous RS cell variants, resembling the lymphocyte depleted subtype. (H&E.)

RS cell variants may simulate non-Hodgkin's lymphoma (Fig. 3-13).[26,57]

Recurrent Hodgkin's disease in treated sites (previously irradiated sites) usually has histologic features different from those of the original biopsy specimen, such as a marked increase in pleomorphic RS cell variants and a marked decrease in the number of small lymphocytes.[58] Residual Hodgkin's disease in treated sites must be distinguished from focal hyalinized acellular scars, which represent sites of successfully treated disease. Biopsy may be required to make this distinction, since both may appear as persistent nonresolving masses after treatment.[57,59]

HISTOPATHOLOGIC CLASSIFICATION

The histopathologic classification of classical Hodgkin's disease is based on the Rye modification of the Lukes-Butler classification.[60,61] This classification is best applied to lymph node specimens at the time of initial diagnosis. Nodular sclerosing Hodgkin's disease is the most common subtype (40 to 70 percent of cases); if features of this subtype are present, even focally, this classification takes precedence over other subtypes.[31] Other subtypes include mixed cellularity Hodgkin's disease (15 to 50 percent), lymphocyte depletion Hodgkin's disease (less than 5 percent), and unclassifiable Hodgkin's disease (less than 15 percent).[62] In developing countries, the mixed cellularity and lymphocyte depletion subtypes are more common than in the United States. Lymphocyte predominant Hodgkin's disease is discussed in a separate chapter.

Nodular Sclerosis Hodgkin's Disease

Nodular sclerosis Hodgkin's disease (NSHD) has two defining characteristics: lacunar cells (a RS cell variant) and dense birefringent fibrous bands (Fig. 3-14). The sclerotic collagen bands, which are often associated with thickening of the capsule, subdivide the lymph node into cellular nodules. Other characteristic (but not invariable) findings in NSHD include prominent necrosis with numerous granulocytes. NSHD is sometimes subdivided, based on the number of RS cells and variants, into lymphocyte-predominant, mixed cellularity, and lymphocyte-depleted subtypes.[60,61,63]

The cellular phase of NSHD consists of Hodgkin's disease with numerous lacunar cells (often in nodules), which are not associated with fibrotic bands. This variant is usually classified with NSHD, since subsequent biopsies from these patients may demonstrate typical NSHD.[55,64] However, others prefer to classify these cases with the mixed cellularity group, since this diagnosis may be more reproducible.[65]

The syncytial variant of NSHD is characterized by numerous RS cells and variants (Fig. 3-15). These cells may form sheets and/or cohesive clusters, often surrounding necrotic foci.[66] In large biopsy specimens, "syncytial" areas may be located adjacent to areas showing features of typical NSHD. In small biopsy specimens, immunohistochemical studies are strongly recommended, since the histologic features of the "syncytial" areas may closely resemble those of large cell lymphoma, metastatic carcinoma, and melanoma (discussed below).

The fibroblastic variant of Hodgkin's disease (usually NSHD) contains areas with numerous fibroblasts, which may not be associated with deposition of thick collagen (Fig. 3-16).[67] The proliferation of fibroblasts may obscure the RS cell variants, and immunohistochemical studies may be necessary for their identification. The histologic features (at least in some areas) may resemble those of malignant fibrous histiocytoma or other sarcoma.

The obliterative total sclerosis variant consists of nodules that have been obliterated by fibrous tissue and sclerosis. Since the nodules consist predominantly of fibrous tissue (nonbirefringent), they contain few lymphocytes or RS cell variants. The connective tissue between the nod-

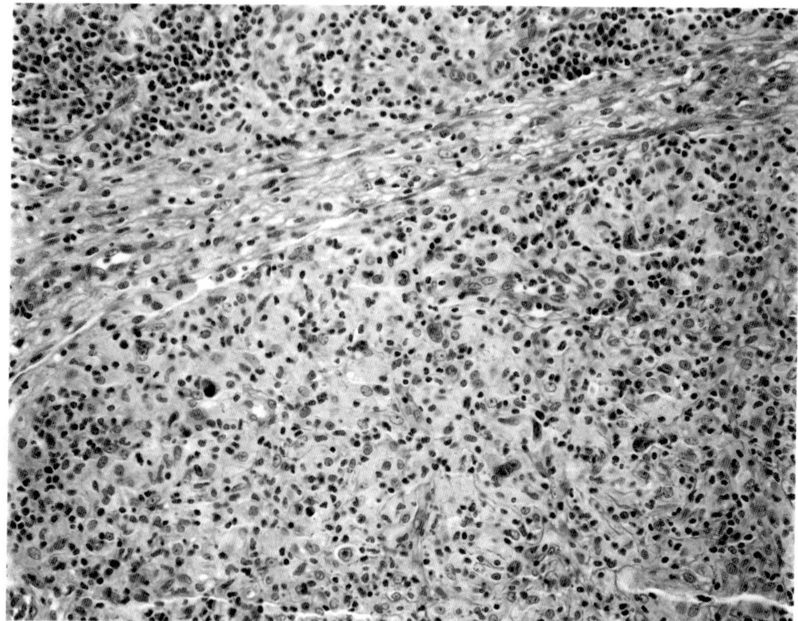

Fig. 3-14. Nodular sclerosing Hodgkin's disease shows fibrotic bands. This tissue was prepared with a mercury-based fixative; therefore, lacunar cells are not present. (H&E.)

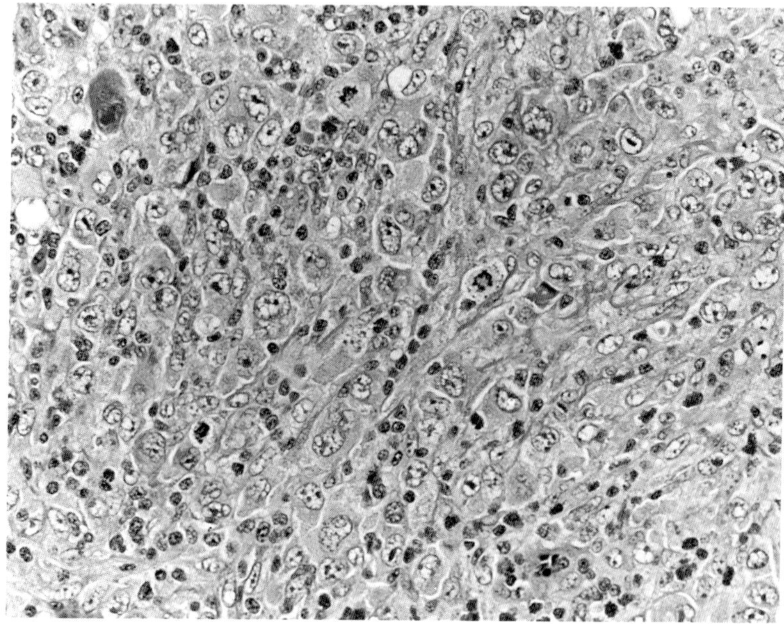

Fig. 3-15. The syncytial variant of NSHD may simulate large cell lymphoma, carcinoma, or melanoma. (H&E.)

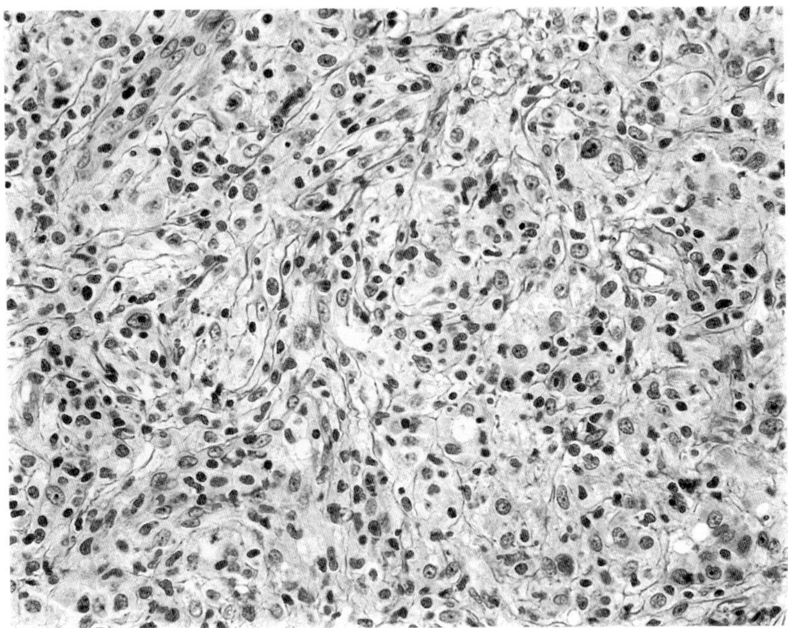

Fig. 3-16. The fibroblastic variant of NSHD shows numerous fibroblasts, fine fibrosis, and scattered RS cell variants. (H&E.)

ules is collagenous and birefringent.[60,61] While such a pattern may suggest the diagnosis of Hodgkin's disease, the diagnostic criteria of RS cells in the appropriate milieu must be fulfilled somewhere within the lesion.

NSHD has been histologically divided into two grades by the British National Lymphoma Investigation. Grade II NSHD is defined as meeting one or more of the following criteria: (1) more than 25 percent of the cellular nodules are lymphocyte depleted (reticular variant), (2) more than 80 percent of the nodules are lymphocyte depleted (fibrohistiocytic variant), or (3) more than 25 percent of the nodules (without lymphocyte depletion) contain numerous anaplastic RS cell variants.[68] NSHD (grade II) therefore includes most (if not all) cases of NSHD of the ''lymphocyte-depleted,'' ''syncytial,'' and ''fibroblastic'' variants. Grade I NSHD lacks these three features and accounts for 65 to 90 percent of NSHD cases. The possible clinical importance of grading is discussed below.

Mixed Cellularity Hodgkin's Disease

RS cells and variants are easily identifiable, since they are intermediate in number (5 to 15 per high power field) between the lymphocyte predominance and lymphocyte depletion types.[63] RS cell variants in mixed cellularity Hodgkin's disease include mononuclear variants, multinucleated variants, and mummified cells. Mixed cellularity Hodgkin's disease usually effaces the lymph node architecture, although partial involvement (usually interfollicular) may occur. The lymph node capsule is usually intact, and necrosis is typically absent.

Background cells in mixed cellularity Hodgkin's disease vary widely but typically consist of a mixed population of lymphocytes, eosinophils, plasma cells, neutrophils, and histiocytes (Fig. 3-6). Numerous epithelioid histiocytes may occur in cohesive clusters,[69] and these cases must be distinguished from nodular lymphocyte predominant Hodgkin's disease (with epithelioid histiocytes), Lennert's lymphoma (peripheral T-cell lymphoma with numerous epithelioid histiocytes), lymphoplasmacytoid lymphomas with numerous epithelioid histiocytes, and T-cell-rich B-cell lymphoma with numerous histiocytes

Lymphocyte Depletion Hodgkin's Disease

Lymphocyte depletion Hodgkin's disease (LDHD) consists of numerous RS cells and variants in a sparse background population of small reactive lymphocytes, which lack significant nuclear atypia or evidence of transformation to large lymphoid cells. Two subcategories are recognized by Lukes and Butler.[61] The diffuse fibrosis variant is characterized by reticulin fibrosis that tends to envelop individual cells, relatively low cellularity, and rare diagnostic RS cells (Fig. 3-17). The reticular variant is characterized by RS cells and variants with bizarre and/or highly pleomorphic features, which are difficult if not impossible to distinguish from anaplastic large cell lymphoma cells.

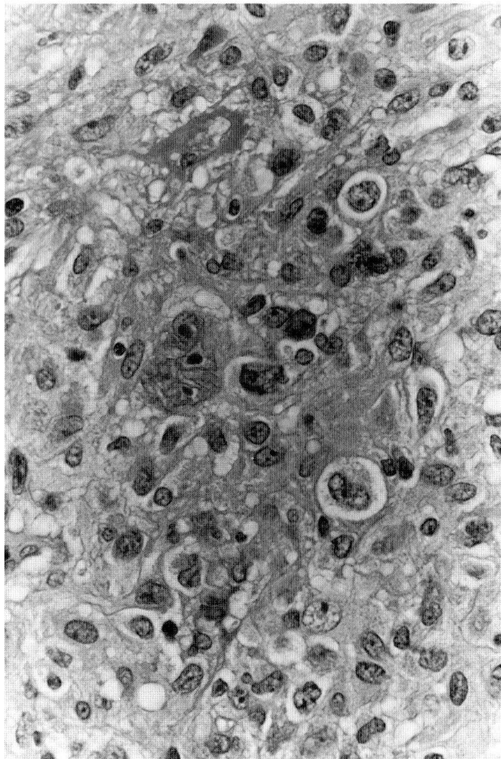

Fig. 3-17. Lymphocyte depletion, diffuse fibrosis type. One diagnostic RS cell and several mononuclear variants are present. (H&E.)

LDHD has always been a rare subtype of Hodgkin's disease, comprising less than 5 percent of cases. The prevalence of LDHD has decreased even further in recent years, since various studies have cast doubt on many cases diagnosed prior to 1985.[70–73] Therefore, an unequivocal diagnosis of LDHD in the 1990s is made with caution, since immunologic and/or molecular studies are required to exclude anaplastic large cell lymphoma, peripheral T-cell lymphoma, T-cell rich B-cell large cell lymphoma, and metastatic carcinoma.[70] Furthermore, a careful histologic search for broad collagen bands is necessary, since this finding mandates the classification of NSHD (with numerous RS cell variants) rather than LDHD. Nevertheless, even when stringent criteria for LDHD are applied, rare but legitimate cases of LDHD still exist.

Unclassifiable Hodgkin's Disease

Unclassifiable cases do not fit into one of the above subtypes. Lukes[65] and Lukes and Butler[61] proposed that these cases be grouped with the mixed cellularity subtype, which serves as a "waste basket" and/or diagnosis of exclusion. However, many pathologists now use a separate unclassifiable category for these cases, which results in a more uniform definition of mixed cellularity Hodgkin's disease. Common reasons for the unclassifiable designation include small sample size, primary extranodal presentation, and treatment effects.

Interfollicular Hodgkin's disease, associated with florid follicular hyperplasia, usually is assigned to the unclassifiable category, since these cases represent focal lymph node involvement by Hodgkin's disease of various subtypes. Some authors prefer to classify these cases with the mixed cellularity group, although focal involvement by nodular sclerosing Hodgkin's disease also may have an interfollicular pattern.[24] Furthermore, biopsy of other involved lymph nodes may show features of one of the classic subtypes.

Lymphocyte-rich classical Hodgkin's disease contains infrequent RS cells and variants with "classical" morphologic and immunophenotypic features. Since the background cell population consists of a diffuse population of small lymphocytes, these cases may be confused with the diffuse type of lymphocyte predominant Hodgkin's disease. Nevertheless, the morphologic and immunophenotypic features of the RS cells and variants, as well as the clinical features of these cases, appear to be those of classical Hodgkin's disease.[74]

Follicular Hodgkin's disease presents as a follicular lesion, characterized by classic RS cells and variants (including lacunar cells) located within expanded follicles. Mantle zone B cells surround the RS cells, and the germinal centers are atrophic, eccentrically placed, and do not contain RS cells. Follicular dendritic cell meshworks (detected by immunohistochemistry) surround the RS cells and variants, suggesting that the Hodgkin's disease involves preexisting follicles.[4]

IMMUNOHISTOCHEMICAL STUDIES

Diagnostic Panel

A panel of antibodies that is useful for diagnostic purposes includes antibodies to CD15 (Leu-M1), CD30 (Ber-H2), and CD45 (LCA).[75–77] RS cells and variants have a characteristic immunophenotype (CD15+, CD30+, CD45−), but this phenotype supports Hodgkin's disease only if the histologic findings are compatible. Furthermore, Hodgkin's disease with typical histologic features may lack CD15+ and/or CD30+ cells, although the vast majority of cases express one of these antigens. In addition, the immunophenotype of RS cells and variants in simultaneous or consecutive biopsy specimens from the same patient may not remain constant.[78] Although Hodgkin's disease often is confidently diagnosed by histologic criteria alone,[79] immunohistochemical studies are often essential when atypical clinical or histologic features are present.[70,80] A primary diagnosis of mixed cellularity or lymphocyte depleted Hodgkin's disease should almost always be accompanied by immunophenotypic confirmation.

Paraffin section immunohistochemistry is the best technique for demonstrating the characteristic immunophenotype (CD15+, CD30+, CD45−) of RS cells and variants in classical Hodgkin's disease. Frozen section immunohistochemical studies are more difficult to interpret, since assessing the reactivity of RS cells and variants is hampered by the relative lack the morphologic detail in frozen sections. Immunohistochemical studies using plastic embedded tissue or other specialized methods may increase sensitivity but are not practical for routine use. Flow cytometric studies do not help to confirm a diagnosis of Hodgkin's disease, since RS cells and variants are difficult to isolate and evaluate, but these studies are useful for excluding differential entities such as B-cell lymphomas.

CD15 expression by RS cells and variants is identified in 85 to 90 percent of classical Hodgkin's disease, as summarized in a recent review (Fig. 3-18).[81] The most characteristic reactivity pattern is paranuclear (juxtanuclear, "Golgi"), although membranous and cytoplasmic patterns also may be observed. Although paranuclear CD15 expression by RS-like cells supports the diagnosis of Hodgkin's disease, CD15 positivity has been identified in 4 percent of B-cell and 21 percent of T-cell non-Hodgkin's lymphomas,[81] and one series reported CD15 reactivity in 67 percent of peripheral T-cell lymphomas.[82] Peripheral T-cell lymphomas usually show weak cytoplasmic reactivity, which can usually (but not always) be distinguished from the paranuclear pattern of RS cells and variants.[83–85] CD15 expression also has been identified in carcinomas,[82,85,86] reactive histiocytes,[83] and cytomegalovirus-infected cells.[87]

CD30 expression by RS cells and variants is present in 89 percent of classical Hodgkin's disease, as indicated in a recent review.[88] Antibodies to CD30 (Ber-H2 in paraffin sections and Ki-1 in frozen sections) typically produce both

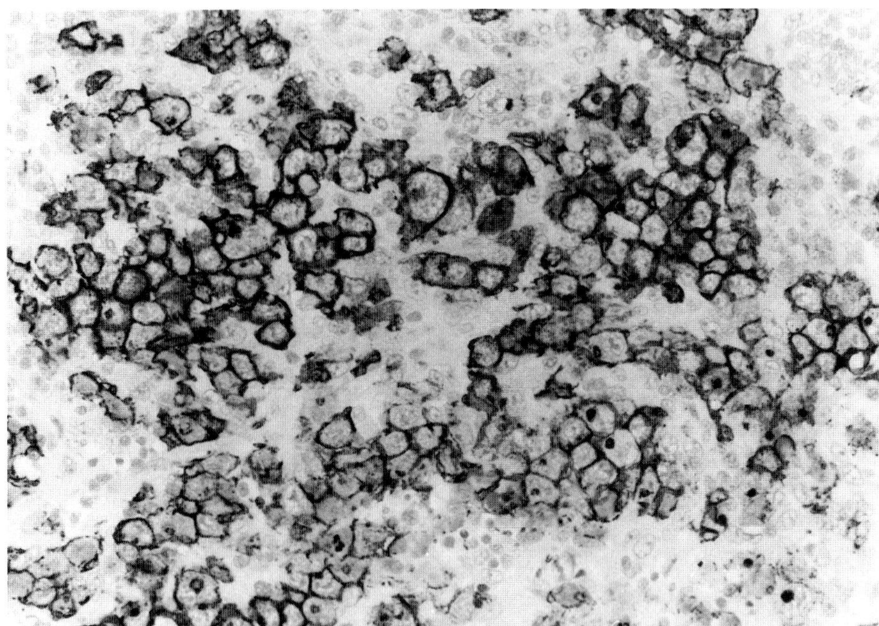

Fig. 3-18. CD15 (Leu-M1) reactivity in the RS cell variants in this example of NSHD (with syncytial areas) shows juxtanuclear and membranous patterns. CD15 (immunohistochemistry).

paranuclear and membrane reactivity. The percentage of positive cases, as well as the number of CD30+ RS cells and variants, is dependent on variables of fixation and other methodology. CD30 expression is not specific for Hodgkin's disease, since CD30+ neoplastic cells are characteristic of anaplastic large cell lymphoma and are present in a minority of other non-Hodgkin's lymphomas. Other CD30+ cells include reactive immunoblasts, plasma cells, histiocytes, some carcinomas, and germ cell tumors (mainly embryonal carcinomas).[89–92]

CD45 expression is detectable in RS cells and variants in approximately 7 percent of classical Hodgkin's disease in paraffin sections and in most cases in frozen sections.[93] The absence of CD45 expression by paraffin section immunohistochemistry, coupled with CD15 and/or CD30 expression by RS cells and variants, provides strong support for Hodgkin's disease.[94] Although the presence of CD45 expression does not exclude Hodgkin's disease, alternative diagnoses should be strongly considered when the CD45+ cells also fail to react with antibodies to CD15 or CD30.

Other Antigens

Proliferation antigens are typically present on RS cells and variants, indicating that they are mitotically active. For example, Ki-67 staining of RS cell variants (using frozen section immunohistochemical techniques) indicate that these cells have a high proliferative rate.[95,96] Paraffin section immunohistochemical studies support these findings, since antibodies to proliferating cell nuclear antigen react with RS cell variants.[96–100] These cells also react with antibodies to P34, the protein product of the cell cycle control *cdc*-2 gene.[101]

The p53 antibodies react with the nuclei of RS cells and variants in up to 90 percent of classical Hodgkin's disease. The most frequent staining pattern is characterized by a few strongly positive cells, although the number of p53-reactive cells varies from 10 to 60 percent.[102–105] Recent polymerase chain reaction (PCR) studies have demonstrated *p53* gene mutations in single RS cells.[106,107] There is no correlation between p53 reactivity and Epstein-Barr virus (EBV) infection of RS cells and variants, and the p53-positive RS cells often co-express MDM2, a p53-binding protein.[108] The background cells do not react with p53 antibodies.[109]

Lectin reactivity is characteristic of RS cells and variants. Peanut agglutinin antibodies react with approximately 60 percent of Hodgkin's disease but not with most non-Hodgkin's lymphoma.[110–112] *Bauhinia purpurea* reactivity also has been reported in Hodgkin's disease and in some anaplastic large cell lymphomas.[113,114]

Other antigens that may be expressed by RS cells and variants include CD21 (C3d receptor, EBV receptor), CD25 (Tac, interleukin-2 receptor), CD71 (transferrin receptor), and vimentin.[19,115] RS cells and variants react with antibodies to HLA class II but not HLA class I.[11] Restin, an intermediate filament-associated protein, is another antigen expressed by RS cells and variants.[116] B-lineage and T-lineage markers have also been reported to react with RS cells and variants in Hodgkin's disease (see below).

LYMPHOID ANTIGENS AND GENES

"Typical" Hodgkin's Disease

Most cases of classical Hodgkin's disease do not show any evidence of lymphoid differentiation, even when numerous RS cells and variants are present.[117] The RS cells and variants do not express B-lineage or T-lineage antigens, either in paraffin-embedded or frozen tissue. Furthermore, most unselected cases of Hodgkin's disease do not show evidence of clonal rearrangements of the immunoglobulin or T-cell receptor genes by conventional Southern blot analysis.[118]

B-lineage Hodgkin's Disease

B-lineage Hodgkin's disease refers to cases of classical Hodgkin's disease with evidence of B-cell differentiation, including B-lineage antigens on RS cells and variants and/or immunoglobulin gene rearrangements in tissues from these cases. These studies (see below) suggest that at least 20 percent of classical Hodgkin's disease contains "B-lineage" RS cells and variants, indicating that a subset of classical Hodgkin's disease are B-cell lymphomas.

Immunohistochemical studies have provided convincing evidence that the RS cells and variants in approximately 20 to 30 percent (and up to 87 percent) of classical Hodgkin's disease react with at least one B-lineage marker.[119] These studies have carefully excluded lymphocyte predominant Hodgkin's disease, which almost always contains B-lineage RS cell variants. CD20 expression in classical RS cells and variants (best demonstrated by L-26 reactivity in paraffin-embedded tissue) has been reported in up to 60 percent of cases, and these cells also may express various other B-lineage antigens, including CD19, CD22, CD40, CD74, CD79a, and BLA.36.[119–132] B-lineage Hodgkin's disease characteristically contains only a few RS cells and variants with strong expression of B-lineage markers, while remaining RS cell variants show weak or negative expression. It should be noted B-lineage antigen expression (including CD20) is not entirely specific for B cells.[133] RS cells and variants also may contain polyclonal immunoglobulins, more likely from passive uptake rather than active synthesis.[134,135]

Southern blot hybridization studies have identified small immunoglobulin rearrangement bands in approximately 10 to 20 percent of classical Hodgkin's disease, and the clonal bands tend to occur in cases of Hodgkin's disease with a B-cell phenotype.[136–141] The presence and/or intensity of clonal rearrangement bands in Hodgkin's disease tends to correlate with the number of RS cells and variants, suggesting that negative results in some studies may be due to problems with sensitivity of the Southern blot technique.[142–145] However, other studies have failed to show a correlation between clonal rearrangement bands and the number of RS variants.[141,146] Clonal rearrangements of the immunoglobulin light chain genes are less frequent than heavy chain rearrangements, although light chain gene rearrangements may occur without heavy chain rearrangements.[144]

PCR studies provide additional evidence for B-cell clonality in classical Hodgkin's disease. When RS cells and variants express B-lineage antigens, most (50 to 67 percent) cases contain detectable clonal variable-diversity-joining (VDJ) rearrangements of the IgH gene.[7,8,147] However, single cell PCR studies for heavy chain V (V_H) gene rearrangements have yielded conflicting results. Most studies suggest that the RS cell population may be polyclonal, monoclonal, or a mixed population of polyclonal and monoclonal cells.[148,149] However, one study utilizing single cell methodology failed to reveal clonal IgH gene rearrangements in the RS cells of 13 cases of Hodgkin's disease of all types.[150]

T-Lineage Hodgkin's Disease

T-lineage Hodgkin's disease refers to cases of classical Hodgkin's disease in which the RS cell variants express T-lineage antigens and/or show T-cell receptor gene rearrangements. Although most authors agree that T-lineage Hodgkin's disease is rare (and possibly nonexistent), a few studies report that a significant proportion of Hodgkin's disease may contain RS cells expressing T-lineage antigens. Additional evidence for T-lineage Hodgkin's disease is provided by reports of Hodgkin's disease developing in patients with mycosis fungoides and lymphomatoid papulosis, although such a correlation might reflect a subtle defect in cellularity immunity.[151–153]

Immunohistochemical studies (especially in frozen sections) are not ideal for evaluating T-lineage antigen expression by RS cells, because of the surrounding reactive T-cell population. Nevertheless, these and other techniques have been used to demonstrate one or more T-lineage markers in up to 40 percent of Hodgkin's disease. RS cells and variants may express various T-lineage antigens, including CD1, CD2, CD3, CD4, CD5, CD8, CD43, CD45RO, and the T-cell receptor (β chain) antigen.[8,47,120,122,154–162] However, these studies do not provide unequivocal evidence that RS cells have a T lineage, since many of these antigens are not lineage specific, and the possibility of passive antigen absorption is difficult to exclude.

Southern blot hybridization studies have demonstrated faint clonal T-cell receptor (TCR) rearrangement bands in a few cases (less than 10 percent) of Hodgkin's disease. The TCRβ chain gene is occasionally clonally rearranged, and the TCRγ chain is more commonly rearranged (up to 70 percent in one study).[137,138,146,163–166] However, these studies do not prove the existence of true "T-lineage" Hodgkin's disease, since the histologic distinction between Hodgkin's disease and peripheral T cell lymphomas may have been difficult in some of these studies, since the significance of non-germline bands with TCRγ probes is controversial and since there is no direct evidence that the RS cells themselves have the clonal TCR rearrangements.[167,168]

ANCILLARY STUDIES

Cytogenetics

Cytogenetic analysis of Hodgkin's disease has been limited in some studies by the infrequency of RS cells and variants as well as the low prevalence of mitotic figures.[169] However, a number of investigators have successfully grown neoplastic cells and demonstrated complex karyotypes in approximately 35 to 45 percent of cases. Using FICTION (fluorescence immunophenotyping and interphase cytogenetic analysis) techniques, all cases of Hodgkin's disease have RS cells with numerical chromosome aberrations.[170] The karyotypes usually feature multiple nonrandom structural and numerical abnormalities and aneuploidy (especially hyperdiploidy).[171] Numerical abnormalities most commonly involve chromosomes 1, 2, 5, 9, 12, 15, 21, 22, and X.[171,172] Consistent structural alterations have not been identified, but nonrandom abnormalities may occur in bands 3q26–28, 4q32–34, 6q11–21, 6q24, 7q31–35, 8q22–24, 11q23, 12q13, 12q23–24, 12p11–13, 13p11–13, and 14q32.[172–176] Structural abnormalities tend to occur close to sites of proto-oncogenes and/or breakpoints that are important in other hematologic neoplasms. For example, structural abnormalities in band 14q32 (the site of the immunoglobulin heavy chain gene) occur in Hodgkin's disease and B-cell lymphomas. However, the t(14:18) translocation (typical of follicular lymphoma) is infrequent in Hodgkin's disease.[175]

BCL-2 Studies

The *bcl*-2 rearrangements, which juxtapose the *bcl*-2 gene on chromosome 18 with the immunoglobulin heavy chain gene on chromosome 14, imply the presence of t(14:18). However, the presence and significance of *bcl*-2 rearrangements in Hodgkin's disease is controversial. One PCR study reported this rearrangement in 32 percent of Hodgkin's disease,[177] and other authors have reported similar findings.[178,179] A more recent study shows that the *bcl*-2 rearrangement occurs in 6 percent of Hodgkin's disease and is limited to patients with a prior history of follicular lymphoma.[180] Other studies have found no evidence of *bcl*-2 rearrangements in Hodgkin's disease, either by Southern blot or PCR analysis.[181–186] Technical factors are the most likely explanation for these discrepant *bcl*-2 findings. Specifically, authors who report a high incidence of *bcl*-2 rearrangements may have used a very sensitive PCR technique, capable of detecting *bcl*-2 rearrangements in the background reactive lymphocytes rather than RS cells.[175] This interpretation is supported by PCR studies that have detected *bcl*-2 rearrangements in non-neoplastic lymphoid tissue and blood.[187,188]

Bcl-2 protein overexpression has been demonstrated in RS cells and variants in classical Hodgkin's disease.[103,180] This expression may be more common is NSHD (51 of 86 cases) than in mixed cellularity Hodgkin's disease (4 of 16 cases).[189] However, bcl-2 staining of RS cells does not correlate with t(14:18), *bcl*-2 rearrangements, EBV-reactivity, or clinical findings.[190–193]

Other Oncogenes

While *bcl*-2 has gained the greatest attention at the genomic and mRNA levels, other oncogenes have also been investigated in recent years. Methods of analysis include continuous cell lines developed from neoplastic Hodgkin's disease cells[194] and single cell analysis of RS cells.[107] Early data suggest that c-*myc* and c-*fes*/*tps* (a cytoplasmic tyrosine kinase) are expressed in most RS cells/variants. c-*kit* is a transmembrane oncogenic protein present in subsets of normal B and T lymphocytes. Neoplastic transcription and expression of c-*kit* has recently been shown to be limited to Hodgkin's disease and CD30+ ALCL.[195] Numerous other oncogenes, including n-*ras*, c-*sis*, and c-*mas*, have not been shown to be significantly expressed in Hodgkin's disease.[196] The evolving oncogene profile will enhance our understanding of the pathogenesis and heterogenicity of Hodgkin's disease.

Epstein-Barr Virus

Clinical and epidemiologic studies have repeatedly demonstrated an association between EBV and Hodgkin's disease. For example, infectious mononucleosis is associated with a fourfold increased risk of subsequent Hodgkin's disease.[197,198] Furthermore, patients who develop Hodgkin's disease tend to have high titers of antibodies against EBV capsid (VCA) antigens,[199] and this association is strongest in samples taken more than 3 years prior to diagnosis.[200]

Immunohistochemical and molecular studies have demonstrated EBV genomes and proteins in RS cells and variants (Figs. 3-19 and 3-20). In situ hybridization studies (especially using EBER probes) provide the most convincing evidence for EBV-positive RS cells, which usually co-express CD15 and CD30.[201–203] These cells react with antibodies to latent membrane protein and EBV nuclear antigen 1 (EBNA-1) but not with antibodies to EBNA-2,[204–208] consistent with EBV latency pattern II. Southern blot hybridization studies (using terminal repeat probes) have demonstrated monoclonality in the

EBV-positive cells, suggesting that EBV infection occurs prior to clonal cellular proliferation.[209–211] If EBV-positive RS cells are present in the initial biopsy, concurrent or subsequent specimens also contain EBV-positive RS cells, and the same EBV strain persists in early and late relapses.[212,213]

The incidence of cases containing EBV-positive RS cells in Hodgkin's disease ranges from 15 to 100 percent, depending on assay techniques, histology, and clinical findings.[214] PCR and Southern blot hybridization studies do not distinguish EBV-positive RS cells from EBV-positive reactive lymphocytes.[117,215–219] In situ hybridization studies (with EBER probes) show that 40 to 50 percent of unselected Hodgkin's disease contains EBV-positive RS cells.[186,202,203,220] EBV is more common in the mixed cellularity subtype (50 to 80 percent) than in nodular

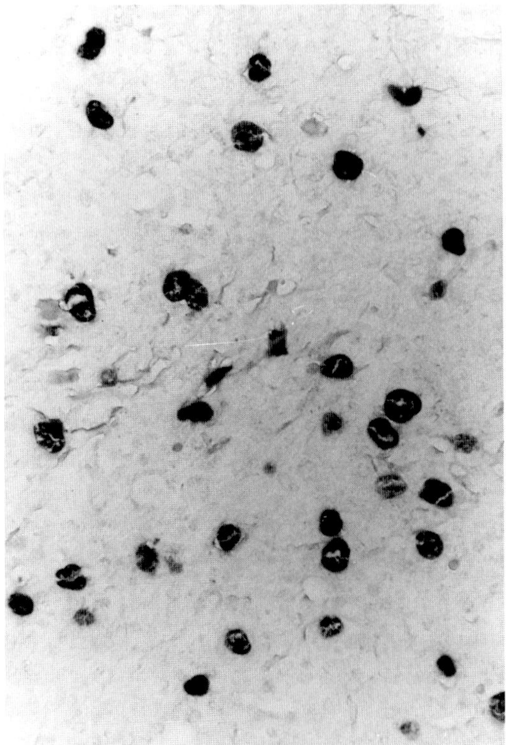

Fig. 3-19. EBV-positive Hodgkin's disease. This in situ hybridization study for EBV-encoded RNA (EBER) demonstrates nuclear positivity in the RS cells. In situ hybridization with no counterstain.

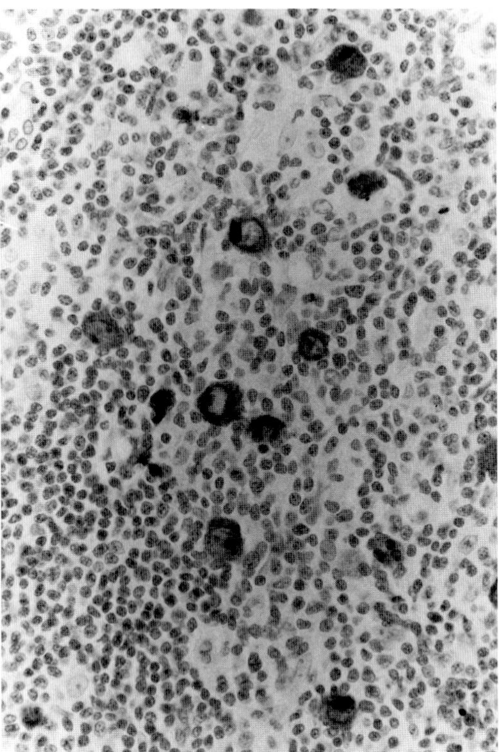

Fig. 3-20. EBV-positive Hodgkin's disease. The RS cells and variants are positive for LMP. LMP-1 (immunohistochemistry).

sclerosing subtype (10 to 30 percent).[201,202,221–223] Furthermore, the incidence of EBV positivity in Hodgkin's disease is 65 percent in Oriental patients[224] and approaches 100 percent in HIV-positive patients[225,226] and Central and South American patients.[227,228] In addition, Hodgkin's disease in patients younger than 15 years or older than 50 years is more likely to be EBV positive than Hodgkin's disease in young adults.[222,229] EBV-infected small lymphocytes may comprise a component of the background cells whether or not EBV is detected in RS cells and variants.[202,230,231]

The pathogenetic role of EBV in Hodgkin's disease is poorly understood, although the monoclonality of EBV-positive RS cells suggests an important role for EBV. However, typical cases of Hodgkin's disease may not contain EBV-positive RS cells or variants, even when highly sensitive molecular techniques are utilized to study these cases. Therefore, factors other than EBV must be involved in the pathogenesis of Hodgkin's disease.

Human herpesvirus-6 is the only other virus that has been associated with Hodgkin's disease to date.[232] However, preliminary studies have not determined whether this virus is located in small lymphocytes or in the RS cells and variants. Furthermore, it is unclear whether human herpesvirus-6 occurs more frequently in Hodgkin's disease than in reactive lymph nodes.

Cytokines

Cytokine production by RS cells and variants may be responsible for the histologic appearance, host response, and clinical symptoms of Hodgkin's disease. Identification of cytokines and/or cytokine receptors in RS cell variants suggests that these cells recruit the host response cells, including lymphocytes, eosinophils, and fibrosis. Cytokine production by the background lymphocyte population may mediate other features of Hodgkin's disease.

There is no unique pattern of cytokine expression in Hodgkin's disease, as indicated in recent reviews by Hsu et al.[233] and Haluska et al.[234] However, cytokines implicated in the development of Hodgkin's disease include various interleukins (IL-1, IL-2, IL-3, IL-4, IL-5, IL-6, IL-9, and IL-12), colony-stimulating factors, tumor necrosis factor, lymphotoxin, transforming growth factor-β, and others. For example, IL-5 production by RS cells and variants may be responsible for the blood and tissue eosinophilia in patients with Hodgkin's disease.[235] In addition, transforming growth factor-β production by RS cells may promote fibrosis, necrosis, syncytial aggregates of lacunar cells, and granulomas.[236]

DIFFERENTIAL DIAGNOSIS

Lymphocyte Predominant Hodgkin's Disease

Lymphocyte predominant Hodgkin's disease (LPHD), discussed in detail in the next chapter, has distinctive pathologic and clinical features. Nodular LPHD is the predominant subtype, since many "diffuse LPHD" cases are examples of nodular LPHD with diffuse areas, lymphocyte-rich classical Hodgkin's disease, or T-cell-rich B-cell lymphoma. The background cells of LPHD consist of a mixture of lymphocytes and/or histiocytes, which sometimes form granulomas near the periphery of the nodular areas. The RS cell variants in LPHD are referred to as *L&H cells* or *popcorn cells,* and classical RS cells are difficult (if not impossible) to find. The RS cells and variants in LPHD (L&H cells) show consistent and uniform reactivity with antibodies to CD45 (LCA) and CD20 (L-26), indicating a B-cell phenotype. These cells show variable (often weak or negative) reactivity with antibodies to CD15 (Leu-M1) but more often react with antibodies to CD30 (Ber-H2).

The distinction between LPHD and classical Hodgkin's disease is based on histologic and immunophenotypic criteria. Classical RS cells and variants, especially when present in large numbers, exclude the possibility of LPHD. Fibrotic bands are characteristic of NSHD but are rare in LPHD. The immunophenotype of classical RS cell variants (CD15+, CD30+, CD45−, CD20−/+) also differs from the immunophenotype of L&H RS cell variants (CD15−/+, CD30+/−, CD45+, CD20+). Furthermore, J chain antibodies react with the RS cell variants of nodular LPHD but not with classical RS cell variants.[237] The distinct phenotypes of LPHD and classical Hodgkin's disease are maintained, even when they occur in the same patient.[238]

Small Lymphocytic Lymphoma

Small lymphocytic lymphoma, with or without plasmacytoid features, consists of numerous small lymphoma cells that may mimic the background cells of Hodgkin's disease, either of the lymphocyte predominant or lymphocyte rich classical types. Other similarities include numerous epithelioid histiocytes[239] and large cells with RS-like features. However, unlike Hodgkin's disease, the RS-like cells of small lymphocytic lymphoma are prolymphocytes and paraimmunoblasts, which tend to form proliferation centers. Immunologic demonstration of monoclonality, often with CD5 co-expression, is diagnostic of small lymphocytic lymphoma. The clinical features of small lymphocytic lymphoma (old age, bone marrow involvement, and association with chronic lymphocytic leukemia) provide further evidence against Hodgkin's disease.

Large Cell Lymphoma (B-Cell Phenotype)

Large cell lymphoma (B-cell phenotype) may be confused with Hodgkin's disease, especially in small biopsy specimens from the mediastinum and retroperitoneum.[240–242] Follicular center cell lymphomas in these locations tend to become sclerotic and lose their tight follicular growth pattern, retaining their mixture of small and large cells. T-cell-rich B-cell large cell lymphomas are especially difficult to distinguish from Hodgkin's disease, since both lymphomas consist of a minor population of large neoplastic cells in a background of numerous reactive T cells.[243,244] B-cell immunoblastic lymphoma with numerous RS-like lymphoma cells also may mimic Hodgkin's disease. In addition, NSHD may have "syncytial" areas that are histologically indistinguishable from large cell lymphoma.

Immunohistochemical studies in paraffin-embedded tissue are useful when making this distinction. RS cells and variants typically express CD15 (Leu-M1) and CD30 (Ber-H2), and these cells do not typically express CD45 (LCA), B-lineage markers (such as CD20) or T-lineage markers (such as CD3). In contrast, large cell lymphoma (B-cell phenotype) typically reacts with antibodies to LCA (CD45) and with B-lineage markers (such as CD20), but not with antibodies to CD15, CD30, or CD3. Use of an antibody panel is recommended, since individual antibodies may be misleading. For example, large lymphoma cells may express CD15 (less than 5 percent of cases), and RS cells may express CD20 (as previously discussed).

Immunohistochemical and/or molecular studies of fresh (snap frozen) tissue are occasionally required to distinguish large cell lymphoma (B-cell phenotype) from Hodgkin's disease. In frozen section immunohistochemical studies, expression of B-lineage markers (CD19, CD20, and CD22) is characteristic of B-cell lymphomas but unusual in Hodgkin's disease, and monoclonal immunoglobulin expression is diagnostic of large cell lymphoma. Clonal immunoglobulin gene rearrangements (especially large bands) are further evidence against Hodgkin's disease.

Anaplastic Large Cell Lymphoma

Anaplastic large cell lymphoma (ALCL) has histologic features that closely resemble those in Hodgkin's disease, since both lymphomas contain neoplastic cells with RS-like features in a background of reactive cells.[125,245–249] This differential diagnosis is typically resolved by assimilating various histologic, immunophenotypic, cytogenetic, and clinical features. Histologic features favoring ALCL include involvement of lymph node sinuses by anaplastic cells, which may have multiple wreath-like nuclei, and a predominance of large anaplastic cells with a minimal mixed inflammatory infiltrate. Immunohistochemical findings (paraffin-embedded tissue) that favor ALCL over Hodgkin's disease include expression of CD45 (LCA), EMA, T-lineage markers (CD3, CD43, CD45RO), and a novel antigen detected by the CBF.78 antibody,[250] whereas absence of these markers and presence of CD15 (Leu-M1) expression favor Hodgkin's disease. BNH-9 reacts with 26 percent of ALCL and may be the most specific marker for ALCL.[251] BLA.36 expression cannot be used to distinguish Hodgkin's disease from ALCL.[252] Cytogenetic data are rarely available at the time of diagnosis, but the t(2:5) translocation strongly supports ALCL.[253] The molecular counterpart of the t(2:5) translocation is the *npm-alk* chimeric transcript (detected by reverse transcriptase PCR), which is present in ALCL cases with t(2:5) and usually absent in most series of Hodgkin's disease[254–258] except one.[259] Clinical features that are more common in ALCL than in Hodgkin's disease include presentation in children and location in the skin or inguinal regions.[260]

ALCL is believed by some to form a morphologic and immunologic continuum with cases of Hodgkin's disease containing numerous RS cells and variants. Evidence for this overlap is based on their continuous spectrum of nuclear profiles, immunophenotypes, and immunogenotypes.[261] Furthermore, Hodgkin's disease has been reported to evolve into ALCL, and ALCL may evolve into Hodgkin's disease.[262] Cases that are "borderline" or "intermediate" between anaplastic large cell lymphoma and Hodgkin's disease may be divided into two types: "borderline ALCL" (Hodgkin's-related ALCL) and "borderline Hodgkin's disease" (including NSHD grade II and LDHD). The lack of precise histologic or immunologic criteria for separating these borderline cases contributes to the apparent overlap of ALCL and Hodgkin's disease, and treatment of these borderline cases with large cell lymphoma regimens has been recommended.[263] Nevertheless, the majority of cases in each category do not present a diagnostic dilemma after careful consideration of the histologic and immunophenotypic data.

Peripheral T-Cell Lymphoma

The histologic distinction between peripheral T cell lymphomas (other than ALCL) and Hodgkin's disease may be difficult, since both lymphomas contain a mixed population of background cells (eosinophils, plasma cells, epithelioid histiocytes), bands of sclerosis, and large neoplastic cells with prominent nucleoli.[264–267] However, the neoplastic cells in peripheral T-cell lymphomas have a spectrum of cell sizes (small, medium, and large lymphoma cells), in contrast to Hodgkin's disease, which consists of dimorphic populations of cells (small lymphocytes and RS cell variants). Furthermore, the small lymphoma cells in peripheral T-cell lymphoma have angular "atypical" nuclei, whereas the small lymphocytes of Hodgkin's disease are usually indistinguishable from normal lymphocytes, although this distinction can be painfully subjective. Other histologic clues favoring peripheral T-cell lymphoma include vascular proliferation, capsular invasion, and numerous mitotic figures.[268,269] These histologic features, when present in patients with typical clinical features (old age at diagnosis, presence of generalized lymphadenopathy, "B" symptoms), usually permit an accurate diagnosis.

Immunohistochemical studies also help to distinguish Hodgkin's disease from peripheral T-cell lymphoma, especially when panels of antibodies are used.[75,270] In paraffin-embedded tissue, reactivity with antibodies to CD45 (LCA) and T lineage markers (CD3, CD43, CD45 RO) favors peripheral T-cell lymphoma over Hodgkin's disease. Reactivity with antibodies to CD15 (Leu-M1) favors Hodgkin's disease, since most peripheral T-cell lymphomas are negative or show rare cells with fine granular reactivity.[81,83] However, a few authors report CD15 expression in a significant number of peripheral T-cell lymphomas, and the staining pattern of the neoplastic T cells may resemble the staining pattern of RS cells and variants.[82,84,85] CD30 expression (present in 90 percent of Hodgkin's disease and 20 percent of peripheral T-cell lymphomas), as well as CD40 expression (present in 70 percent of Hodgkin's disease and 13 percent of non-Hodgkin's lymphomas), also may help in the differential diagnosis.[88,127] In frozen section immunohistochemical studies, an aberrant T-cell phenotype strongly favors peripheral T-cell lymphoma over Hodgkin's disease.[271]

Molecular genetic studies also may help to distinguish peripheral T-cell lymphoma from Hodgkin's disease, since the presence of a large T-cell receptor gene rearrangement band favors T-cell lymphoma. However, these studies may not be definitive, since small clonal rearrangement bands have been identified in Hodgkin's disease and since some T-cell lymphomas may lack T-cell receptor gene rearrangements.

Metastatic Neoplasms

Metastatic carcinoma (especially nasopharyngeal carcinoma) and metastatic melanoma can mimic Hodgkin's disease, since both may contain single neoplastic cells in a background of small lymphocytes (Fig. 3-21).[272] Furthermore, the syncytial variant of NSHD may show sheets and clusters of RS cells and variants, which may closely resemble metastatic tumor cells. However, metastatic neoplasms tend to form cell clusters in lymph node sinuses, which is an unusual distribution for Hodgkin's disease. Furthermore, metastatic neoplasms often show characteristic cytologic features, including nuclear pseudoinclusions (melanoma), signet ring cells (adenocarcinoma), and spindle cells (squamous cell carcinoma).[273] Immunohistochemical studies in paraffin-embedded tissue may be required to establish an unequivocal diagnosis of carcinoma (keratin positive) or melanoma (S100 and HMB-45 positive). CD15 (Leu-M1) should not be used to distinguish Hodgkin's disease from carcinoma, since adenocarcinomas and other nonhematopoietic tumors may express this antigen.[82]

Reactive Lymph Nodes

Viral lymphadenitis, especially infectious mononucleosis, may be difficult to distinguish from Hodgkin's disease, since both may contain RS-like cells that express CD30.[274–276] Architectural clues that favor viral lymphadenitis include marked paracortical hyperplasia (with intact lymph node architecture), reactive follicular hyperplasia, and patent sinuses (often containing monocytoid B cells). The paracortical immunoblasts in viral lymphadenitis may resemble RS cells, but their large number, even distribution, and association with a maturational sequence of transformed lymphocytes and plasma cells help to exclude Hodgkin's disease.[277,278] CD15 is not expressed by the RS-like cells of infectious mononucleosis[279] but may be expressed by cyto-

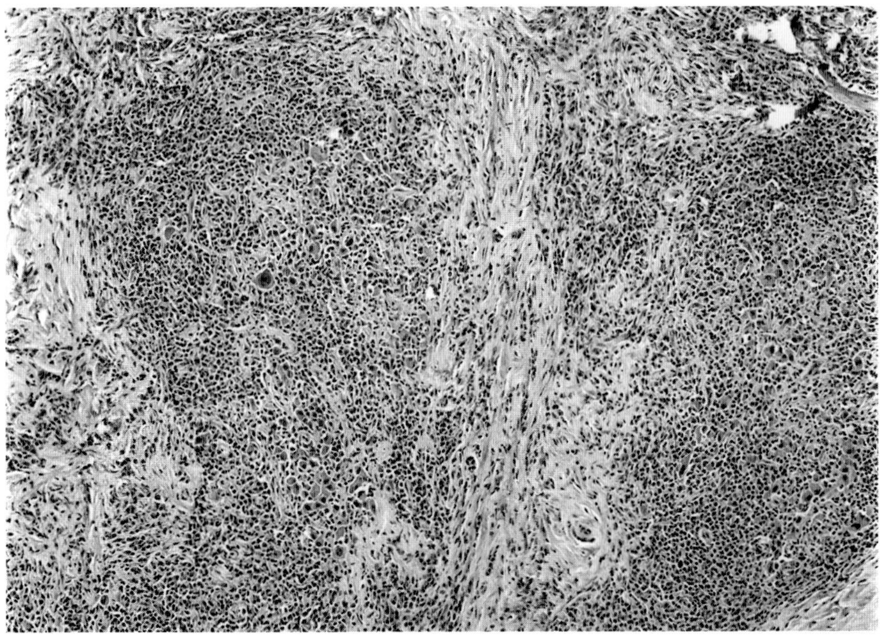

Fig. 3-21. Metastatic carcinoma may have histologic features that closely resemble NSHD, since both may show nodules (surrounded by fibrotic bands) and dichotomous cell populations. The large cells in this photomicrograph were cytokeratin positive, and the patient was subsequently found to have a primary nasopharyngeal carcinoma. (H&E.)

megalovirus-infected cells.[87] Therefore, establishing a confident diagnosis of viral lymphadenitis requires maintaining a high index of suspicion and confirming the diagnosis by clinical studies. For example, a tonsillar biopsy from a young patient is much more likely to be infectious mononucleosis than Hodgkin's disease (which is rare in this location), and this possibility should be further evaluated by serologic studies and peripheral blood smears (searching for atypical lymphocytes).

Necrotizing granulomatous lymphadenitis (including cat scratch and similar diseases) can mimic Hodgkin's disease, since both contain focal necrosis surrounded by large cells. This distinction is based on careful examination of the cytologic features at the edges of the necrosis. In necrotizing granulomatous lymphadenitis, the stellate necrosis is surrounded by epithelioid histiocytes. In contrast, the necrotic foci of Hodgkin's disease are surrounded by RS cells and variants, associated with epithelioid histiocytes.[280] While immunophenotypic studies could be helpful in this situation, they are rarely needed.

CLINICAL FEATURES

Epidemiology

The incidence of Hodgkin's disease in the United States was 2.5 per 100,000 population from 1973 to 1977,[281] and this incidence appears to be unchanged in recent years. In 1993, 7,900 new cases of Hodgkin's disease were reported, which represented approximately 15 percent of the lymphomas diagnosed that year.[282] The incidence of Hodgkin's disease shows marked geographic variations and is more common in the United States than in other parts of the world.[283]

The sex and age of these patients varies with the histologic subtype and geographic distribution. The overall male to female ratio is 1.5:1, and the male predominance persists for all subtypes except for NSHD.[284] Hodgkin's disease occurs in three age periods[283,285]: childhood (0 to 14 age group), young adults (14 to 40 age group), and older adults (55 to 74 age group). In most economically developed countries, Hodgkin's disease tends to have a bimodal age distribution, with most cases occurring in young adults or older adults. In Third World countries, the childhood and older adult forms of Hodgkin's disease are relatively more common than the young adult form.[286]

Environmental and genetic factors have been reported to increase the risk of Hodgkin's disease, although some of the data are conflicting. Risk factors include small sibship size, higher social class, more education, relatives with Hodgkin's disease, employment in wood-related industries, and certain HLA types.[283,287–289] Monozygotic twins of patients with Hodgkin's disease have a greatly increased risk, whereas dizygotic twins are not at increased risk.[290] Reports of Hodgkin's disease occurring in clusters may be nothing more than chance occurrences.

Clinical Presentation

Asymptomatic patients present with enlarged lymph nodes, and these slow-growing masses occasionally reach considerable size before their detection. Occasionally, enlarged lymph nodes are first detected by routine radiographic examination, especially of the mediastinum and retroperitoneum.

Constitutional symptoms (25 to 40 percent of patients) may occur with localized or advanced disease.[53] "B" symptoms, which tend to correlate with necrosis and neutrophils, include unexplained fever (above 38°C) during the previous month, recurrent drenching night sweats during the previous month (from nocturnal fever defervescence), and unexplained weight loss (more than 10 percent of body weight) during the previous 6 months.[291,292] Two other characteristic symptoms of Hodgkin's disease are generalized pruritus (often severe) and pain in involved nodes after alcohol consumption. Symptoms of specific organ system involvement include bone pain (due to bone involvement), neurologic disturbances (due to spinal cord compression), or ascites or edema (due to compression of the inferior vena cava). Superior vena caval syndrome is occasionally associated with mediastinal

Hodgkin's disease but is much more common with mediastinal non-Hodgkin's lymphomas.

Immunologic deficiencies occur in patients with Hodgkin's disease and may persist even after successful treatment.[293,294] Most defects involve cell-mediated immunity due to inhibition of T-lymphocyte function. The blood shows lymphopenia and decreased numbers of circulating CD4+ cells.[295–298] These immunologic deficiencies result in an increased susceptibility for certain infections (bacterial, fungal, and viral) and a decreased capacity for delayed hypersensitivity reactions. The functions of B lymphocytes do not appear to be impaired.

Histologic subtype shows some correlation with clinical presentation. For example, NSHD tends to occur in young adult females and involve the mediastinum, supraclavicular nodes, and cervical nodes.[53,284] LDHD tends to present with constitutional symptoms, spare peripheral lymph nodes, involve subdiaphragmatic areas (abdominal organs, retroperitoneal nodes), have advanced stages, and spread to bone marrow.[71,299] LDHD and MCHD tend to occur more frequent in elderly patients, Third World patients, and patients of lower socioeconomic status in the United States.[286,300] However, none of these subtypes appears to be a distinct clinicopathologic entity.[284,301]

HIV-infected patients, especially intravenous drug abusers, appear to have an increased risk of Hodgkin's disease in most studies.[302–305] Distinctive findings of Hodgkin's disease in these patients include frequent extranodal involvement (lung, skin, liver, bone marrow), atypical patterns of dissemination (such as bone marrow disease without splenic involvement), frequent subdiaphragmatic disease, tendency for high stage disease, high incidence of B symptoms, and high incidence of mixed cellularity and lymphocyte-depleted subtypes.[306–310] HIV-infected patients also tend to respond poorly to therapy for Hodgkin's disease,[311,312] although a recent study demonstrates that cures are possible.[313]

Patterns of Dissemination

Sites of involvement by Hodgkin's disease include nodal and extranodal locations. Lymph node involvement is especially common in cervical, supraclavicular, mediastinal, and axillary regions.[314] Infrequent sites of involvement (especially as the primary site) include Waldeyer's ring, mesenteric nodes, hypogastric nodes, midline presacral nodes, and epitrochlear nodes.[53] Extranodal involvement (including spleen, liver, skin, and bone) usually occurs secondary to lymph node involvement.

Lymphatic dissemination of Hodgkin's disease occurs in a contiguous and highly predictable pattern. For example, Hodgkin's disease in axillary lymph nodes spreads first to ipsilateral infraclavicular and low cervical nodes. Another characteristic sequence of spread is from supraclavicular nodes to mediastinal nodes to pulmonary hilar nodes to lungs. Hodgkin's disease in the supraclavicular, infraclavicular, and lower cervical nodes tends to spread to lumbar paraaortic lymph nodes and then to splenic hilar nodes and spleen. Splenic involvement almost always precedes liver and bone marrow involvement. In addition to lymphatic spread, Hodgkin's disease may directly extend from lymph nodes to adjacent tissues such as skin and skeletal muscle. These predictable patterns of dissemination are the rationale for curative radiation therapy.[53,315]

Hematogenous dissemination of Hodgkin's disease is unusual in low stage disease but tends to occur in late stages of progressive disease, resulting in wide dissemination, which is typical of Hodgkin's disease at autopsy. In addition to confluent nodular masses in the usual sites (major lymph node groups, spleen, liver, bone marrow), disseminated disease can massively involve organs such as skeletal muscle, adrenals, lungs, pancreas, and bladder.[57]

Stage

The Cotswald staging classification (Table 3-1), which is a modification of the Ann Arbor classification, is the currently accepted staging system.[291,292] Clinical staging requires extensive evaluation by history, physical examination, plain chest radiography, computed tomography

Table 3-1. The Cotswolds Staging Classification of Hodgkin's Disease

Classification	Description
Stage I	Involvement of a single lymph node region or lymphoid structure
Stage II	Involvement of two or more lymph node regions on the same side of the diaphragm (the mediastinum is considered a single site, whereas hilar lymph nodes are considered bilaterally)
Stage III	Involvement of lymph node regions or structures on both sides of the diaphragm
Stage III-1	With or without involvement of splenic hilar, celiac, or portal nodes
Stage III-2	With involvement of para-aortic, iliac, and mesenteric nodes
Stage IV	Involvement of one or more extranodal sites in addition to a site for which the designation "E" has been used
Designations applicable to any disease stage	
A	No symptoms
B	Fever (temperature >38°C), drenching night sweats, unexplained loss of >10% of body weight within the preceding 6 months
X	Bulky disease (a widening of the mediastinum by more than ⅓ or the presence of a nodal mass with a maximal dimension >10 cm)
E	Involvement of a single extranodal site that is contiguous or proximal to the known nodal site
CS	Clinical stage
PS	Pathologic stage (as determined by laparotomy)

(Modified from Lister et al.,[291,292] with permission.)

scans (chest, abdomen), and lymphangiography. Special procedures include magnetic resonance imaging, gallium scan, bone scan, and liver/spleen scan. Pathologic staging procedures include the initial diagnostic biopsy, bilateral bone marrow biopsies, and biopsy of any clinically suspicious lesion.

Staging laparotomy includes splenectomy, liver biopsy, and abdominal lymph node biopsies. This procedure detects unsuspected disease below the diaphragm (usually in the spleen) in 25 to 40 percent of patients.[316] Although pathologic staging was commonly performed in past years, this procedure does not improve survival and is associated with late complications such as infections and acute leukemia.[317] Currently, staging laparotomy is performed only when radiation therapy is the treatment of choice and when detection of intra-abdominal disease would alter the choice of therapy. Therefore, formal staging laporatomy is not performed when clinical features (such as a large mediastinal mass or high clinical stage) mandate systemic chemotherapy or when clinical features are associated with low probability (less than 10 percent) of abdominal involvement (e.g., clinical stage IA female patients with NSHD).[318–320]

Treatment

Classical Hodgkin's disease is treated with curative intent using radiation therapy or chemotherapy, and stage is the most important factor in choosing the treatment modality. Radiation therapy and chemotherapy are best used alone, except in patients with massive mediastinal disease, for whom combinations of radiation therapy and chemotherapy are superior.[321] Bone marrow transplantation has cured patients in relapse following chemotherapy. When the pathologic distinction between Hodgkin's disease and non-Hodgkin's lymphoma cannot be resolved with certainty, patients are typically treated for large cell lymphoma, since these protocols effectively treat both large cell lymphoma and Hodgkin's disease.

Radiation therapy is the usual treatment for patients with pathologic stage I and IIA disease (and possibly stage III-1A patients). Patients who are candidates for curative radiation therapy should not have a large mediastinal mass or disease located below the diaphragm (although less than five splenic nodules are allowed). Relapses after radiation therapy usually occur within 3 years and can be successfully treated with chemotherapy, with no adverse effect on overall survival.[322–324]

Combination chemotherapy is used to treat patients with IIB, III-2A, and IV disease. Intensity of the chemotherapy dose is the most important factor to influence the outcome.[325] The most common regimens are MOPP (mechlorethamine, vincristine, procarbazine, and prednisone) and ABVD (doxorubicin, bleomycin, vinblastine, dacarbazine). Relapse after chemotherapy is treated with additional chemotherapy or bone marrow transplantation.[317,324]

Bone marrow transplantation is used as salvage therapy for patients with relapsed or resistant Hodgkin's disease following high dose chemotherapy and radiation therapy. These therapeutic regimens have cured patients with poor prognostic features, such as relapse after two or more chemotherapy regimens or remissions lasting less than 12 months.[326–328] Many hematologists now recommend autologous bone marrow transplantation for patients in first relapse after any chemotherapeutic regimen, irrespective of the duration of remission, to avoid the development of drug resistance and end organ damage from repeated attempts at salvage therapy.[329]

Prognosis

The 5 year survival rate of untreated patients with Hodgkin's disease is less than 5 percent.[324] Using current treatment protocols, approximately 70 percent of patients with Hodgkin's disease are cured,[321] and survival rates of 80 to 90 percent at 15 years are common. The most important adverse prognostic factor is high stage, which is a function of other adverse factors such as multiple (five or more) splenic nodules, multiple sites of extranodal involvement, and large mediastinal masses. Clinical features associated with diminished prognosis include decreased hematocrit, elevated lactate dehydrogenase, increased erythrocyte sedimentation rate,[330] increased β_2-microglobulin,[331] and elevated serum levels of soluble CD25 and CD30.[332–336] The diminished prognosis of older patients with Hodgkin's disease may be due to deaths from other causes.[337]

Several histologic features may correlate with prognosis, but their prognostic and therapeutic importance has decreased in recent years.[67] For example, the favorable prognosis of NSHD, when compared with mixed cellularity Hodgkin's disease and LDHD, is probably not independent of stage and other prognostic factors.[301] In addition, the poor prognosis of LDHD is at least partially explained by its difficult distinction from non-Hodgkin's lymphoma.[72] Favorable histologic findings have been reported to include granulomas in uninvolved tissues[20] and extensive networks of follicular dendritic cells in involved tissues,[338] although their prognostic significance with current treatment is debatable. Histologic features that do not appear to correlate with prognosis include Castleman's disease-like changes, interfollicular lymph node involvement,[24] and numbers of RS cells in recurrent disease.[58] Furthermore, EBV and CD20 expression of RS cells and variants do not correlate with clinical features, response to treatment, or disease-free survival.[339–341]

The prognostic significance of histologic grading of NSHD is controversial. Recent studies suggest that grade II NSHD (histologic criteria discussed above), which includes the syncytial and fibroblastic variants, has a worse prognosis than grade I NSHD, mainly due to failure of salvage therapy after first relapse.[62,66,68,342,343] However, other recent studies have found no differences in overall survival or survival after relapse.[344–346] Important considerations in evaluating this issue include statistical aberrations (due to chance alone), difficulties in applying the published grading criteria, incorporation of staging data, and aggressiveness of treatment regimens. Grading does not influence treatment decisions, at least in most centers in the United States, and the practice of grading has not become routine in most pathology practices.

Treatment complications significantly affect prognosis, although newer chemotherapy protocols have reduced their significance. Treatment effects include pneumococcal sepsis (postsplenectomy), infertility, amenorrhea, cardiomyopathy (doxorubicin), pneumonitis (radiation), and pulmonary fibrosis. However, the most significant long-term complication is the risk for developing secondary cancers, which approaches 20 percent at 20 years. The most common secondary malignancy is carcinoma (70 percent), and others include sarcoma,[347] acute myelogenous leukemia, myelodysplastic syndromes, and non-Hodgkin's lymphoma.[348–352] Patients who have received chemotherapy (especially multiple doses) are at highest risk for developing a second malignancy.

HODGKIN'S DISEASE AND NON-HODGKIN'S LYMPHOMA IN THE SAME PATIENT

Significance

Classical Hodgkin's disease and non-Hodgkin's lymphoma occur in the same patient more frequently than would be predicted by chance alone.[353] This association provides further evidence for a common lymphoid origin for Hodgkin's disease and non-Hodgkin's lymphoma.[354] Furthermore, classical Hodgkin's disease may be clonally related to the non-Hodgkin's lymphomas, although this possibility remains somewhat theoretical.[353]

Hodgkin's Disease May Evolve Into or Coexist With Non-Hodgkin's Lymphoma

Patients with Hodgkin's disease (usually NSHD) may subsequently develop non-Hodgkin's lymphoma, usually many years following successful treatment and often in extranodal sites (especially abdominal). The non-Hodgkin's lymphomas are usually follicular lymphomas, large cell lymphomas, small noncleaved cell lymphomas, or "monomorphic" lymphomas. Most have a B-cell phenotype, although T-cell lymphomas have been reported.[355–359] The increased actuarial risk (4 percent at 10 years) may be related to late complications of therapy, underlying immunodeficiencies in patients with Hodgkin's disease, or morphologic transformation of Hodgkin's disease into monomorphic or pleomorphic lymphomas. Although most of the non-Hodgkin's lymphomas are EBV negative, other clinicopathologic features resemble those of lymphoproliferative disorders in patients with immune deficiencies such as HIV infection.[354,360,361]

Hodgkin's disease and non-Hodgkin's lymphoma may be detected simultaneously at different sites in the same patient. The clinical and pathologic findings are similar to secondary non-Hodgkin's lymphomas in patients with Hodgkin's disease, as described above.

Composite lymphomas, consisting of classical Hodgkin's disease and non-Hodgkin's lymphoma in the same anatomic site, have also been reported.[362] Histologic subtypes of the non-Hodgkin's component include follicular lymphoma and large cell lymphoma, usually with a B-cell phenotype. The RS cells and variants have the phenotype (CD15+ CD30+ CD45−) of classical Hodgkin's disease. Double staining techniques show that EBV may be present (33 percent of cases) in both the RS cell variants and the neoplastic B cells, suggesting the possibility of a common origin from an EBV-infected lymphoid cell.[262,354]

Chronic Lymphocytic Leukemia May Evolve Into or Resemble Hodgkin's Disease

RS cells and variants (or histologic mimics) may be found in chronic lymphocyte leukemia (or small lymphocytic lymphoma) in three different circumstances, each with different implications. First, chronic lymphocyte leukemia may evolve into large cell lymphoma with numerous RS-like cells. These large cells have a B-cell phenotype (CD15− CD30− CD20+) rather than a Hodgkin's disease phenotype (CD15+ CD30+ CD20−), and they usually are EBV negative. The features are those of "Richter's transformation" of chronic lymphocytic leukemia.[363]

Second, chronic lymphocyte leukemia may coexist with or evolve into classical Hodgkin's disease. The preexisting chronic lymphocyte leukemia has pathologic and clinical features that are indistinguishable from typical chronic lymphocyte leukemia. The subsequent Hodgkin's disease may be NSHD or mixed cellularity Hodgkin's disease and may contain EBV-positive RS cells and variants with a classical (CD15+ CD30+ CD45−) phenotype.[364] These cases have been described as the "Hodgkin's disease variant of Richter syndrome," although the prognosis has not been as dismal as true large cell transformation.[365–367]

Third, chronic lymphocytic leukemia may contain scattered RS cells and variants. The background chronic lymphocytic leukemia cells have immunophenotypic features of usual chronic lymphocytic leukemia, including expression of B-lineage markers (CD20 and CD22), CD5 coexpression, and monoclonal surface immunoglobulins. The scattered RS cells and variants have a typical Hodgkin's phenotype (CD15+ CD30+) and usually contain EBV RNA. Expression of CD20 and other B-cell antigens may be identified but is difficult to evaluate because of the numerous surrounding B cells.[354] The pathologic features are indicative of a "composite" lymphoma (Hodgkin's disease and chronic lymphocytic leukemia), and some patients later develop systemic Hodgkin's disease.[368,369]

Non-Hodgkin's Lymphoma May Evolve Into Hodgkin's Disease

B-cell lymphoma may evolve into Hodgkin's disease, which is the most common secondary malignancy in non-Hodgkin's lymphoma patients.[370] The B-cell lymphomas are typically follicular lymphomas or large cell lymphomas. The subsequent Hodgkin's disease (NSHD or mixed cellularity) has the phenotype (CD15+ CD30+ CD45−) of classical Hodgkin's disease and has a poor prognosis.[371,372]

T-cell lymphomas also may be associated with Hodgkin's disease. This association may be more common than reported, since the distinction between Hodgkin's disease and peripheral T-cell lymphoma in the same patient is difficult to make with certainty.[354] Peripheral T-cell lymphomas that coexist with or evolve into Hodgkin's disease include mycosis fungoides, anaplastic large cell lymphoma, and adult T-cell lymphoma/leukemia.[354,371,373–376] A single report describes mycosis fungoides, Hodgkin's disease, and anaplastic large cell lymphoma arising sequentially in one patient, all being derived from a single T-cell clone.[151] While intriguing, this report makes it difficult to preclude the possibility of peripheral T-cell lymphoma mimicking Hodgkin's disease at one point in time.

SUMMARY

Classical Hodgkin's disease has characteristic histologic and immunophenotypic features that form the basis for its distinction from non-Hodgkin's lymphomas and other neoplasms. However, recent evidence suggests that Hodgkin's disease and non-Hodgkin's lymphomas are closely related and may share a common lymphoid origin. Nevertheless, classical Hodgkin's disease has unique clinical findings, including treatment sensitivity and good prognosis, which continue to justify its separation from non-Hodgkin's lymphoma.

ACKNOWLEDGMENTS

The authors thank Kelly J. Hain for her secretarial expertise and assistance.

REFERENCES

1. Hodgkin T: On some morbid appearances of the absorbent glands and spleen. Med-Chir Trans 17:68, 1832
2. Rosenberg SA: Hodgkin's disease: challenges for the future. Cancer Res 49:767, 1989
3. Mason DY, Banks PM, Chan J et al: Nodular lymphocyte predominance Hodgkin's disease: a

distinct clinicopathological entity. Am J Surg Pathol 18:526, 1994
4. Ashton-Key M, Thorpe PA, Allen JP, Isaacson PG: Follicular Hodgkin's disease. Am J Surg Pathol 19:1294, 1995
5. Bucsky P: Hodgkin's disease: the Reed-Sternberg cell. Blut 55:413, 1987
6. Diehl V, von Kalle C, Fonatsch C et al: The cell of origin in Hodgkin's disease. Semin Oncol 17: 660, 1990
7. Kamel OW, Chang PP, Hsu FJ et al: Clonal VDJ recombination of the immunoglobulin heavy chain gene by PCR in classical Hodgkin's disease. Am J Clin Pathol 194:419, 1995
8. Orazi A, Jiang B, Lee C-H et al: Correlation between presence of clonal rearrangements of immunoglobulin heavy chain genes and B-cell antigen expression in Hodgkin's disease. Am J Clin Pathol 104:413, 1995
9. Abdulaziz Z, Mason DY, Stein H et al: An immunohistological study of the cellular constituents of Hodgkin's disease using a monoclonal antibody panel. Histopathology 8:1, 1984
10. Pinkus GS, Barbuto D, Said JW, Churchill WH: Lymphocyte subpopulations of lymph nodes and spleens in Hodgkin's disease. Cancer 42: 1270, 1978
11. Poppema S, Visser L: Absence of HLC class I expression by Reed-Sternberg cells. Am J Pathol 145:37, 1994
12. Romagnani S, Del Prete GF, Maggi E et al: Displacement of T lymphocytes with the "helper/inducer" phenotype from peripheral blood to lymphoid organs in untreated patients with Hodgkin's disease. Scand J Haematol 31:305, 1983
13. Valente G, Ferrara P, Stramignoni A: Lymphocyte populations of nonscleronodular Hodgkin's disease subtypes in different stages of lymphocyte depletion: an immunophenotypic and quantitative study. Virchows Arch [B] 58:289, 1990
14. Mohrmann RL, Nathwani BN, Brynes RK, Sheibani K: Hodgkin's disease occurring in monocytoid B-cell clusters. Am J Clin Pathol 95:802, 1991
15. Plank L, Hansmann M-L, Fisher R: Monocytoid B-cells occurring in Hodgkin's disease. Virchows Arch 424:321, 1994
16. Variakojis D, Strum SB, Rappaport H: The foamy macrophages in Hodgkin's disease. Arch Pathol 93:453, 1972
17. Burns BF, Colby TV, Dorfman RF: Langerhans' cell granulomatosis (histiocytosis X) associated with malignant lymphomas. Am J Surg Pathol 7:529, 1983
18. Alavaikko MJ, Hansmann M-L, Nebendahl C et al: Follicular dendritic cells in Hodgkin's disease. Am J Clin Pathol 95:194, 1991
19. Delsol G, Meggetto F, Brousset P et al: Relation of follicular dendritic reticulum cells to Reed-Sternberg cells of Hodgkin's disease with emphasis on the expression of CD21 antigen. Am J Pathol 142:1729, 1993
20. Sacks EL, Donaldson SS, Gordon J, Dorfman RF: Epithelioid granulomas associated with Hodgkin's disease: clinical correlations in 55 previously untreated patients. Cancer 41:562, 1978
21. Kadin ME, Donaldson SS, Dorfman RF: Isolated granulomas in Hodgkin's disease. N Engl J Med 283:859, 1970
22. Maheswaran PR, Ramsay AD, Norton AJ, Roche WR: Hodgkin's disease presenting with the histological features of Castleman's disease. Histopathology 18:249, 1991
23. Zarate-Osorno A, Medeiros LJ, Danon AD, Neiman RS: Hodgkin's disease with coexistent Castleman-like histologic features: a report of three cases. Arch Pathol Lab Med 118:270, 1994
24. Doggett RS, Colby TV, Dorfman RF: Interfollicular Hodgkin's disease. Am J Surg Pathol 7: 145, 1983
25. Lamoureux KB, Jaffe ES, Berard CW, Johnson RE: Lack of identifiable vascular invasion in patients with extranodal dissemination of Hodgkin's disease. Cancer 31:824, 1973
26. Grogan TM, Berard CW, Steinhorn SC et al: Changing patterns of Hodgkin's disease at autopsy: a 25-year experience at the National Cancer Institute, 1953–1978. Cancer Treat Rep 66: 653, 1982
27. Naeim F, Waisman J, Coulson WF: Hodgkin's disease: the significance of vascular invasion. Cancer 34:655, 1974
28. Strum SB, Allen LW, Rappaport H: Vascular invasion in Hodgkin's disease: its relationship to involvement of the spleen and other extranodal sites. Cancer 28:1329, 1971
29. Strum SB, Hutchison GB, Park JK, Rappaport H: Further observations on the biologic significance of vascular invasion in Hodgkin's disease. Cancer 27:1, 1971
30. Wood NL, Coltman CA: Localized primary ex-

tranodal Hodgkin's disease. Ann Intern Med 78: 113, 1973
31. Rappaport H, Berard CW, Butler JJ et al: Report of the committee on histopathological criteria contributing to staging of Hodgkin's disease. Cancer Res 31:1864, 1971
32. Leslie KO, Colby TV: Hepatic parenchymal lymphoid aggregates in Hodgkin's disease. Hum Pathol 15:808, 1984
33. Katz A, Lattes R: Granulomatous thymoma or Hodgkin's disease of the thymus? A clinical and histological study and a re-evaluation. Cancer 23:1, 1969
34. Dorfman RF, Colby TV: The pathologist's role in management of patients with Hodgkin's disease. Cancer Treat Rep 66:675, 1982
35. Hoppe RT, Rosenberg SA, Kaplan HS, Cox RS: Prognostic factors in pathological stage IIIA Hodgkin's disease. Cancer 46:1240, 1980
36. Burke JS, Osborne BM: Localized reactive lymphoid hyperplasia of the spleen simulating malignant lymphoma: a report of seven cases. Am J Surg Pathol 7:373, 1983
37. Bagley CM, Roth JA, Thomas LB, DeVita VT: Liver biopsy in Hodgkin's disease: clinicopathologic correlations in 127 patients. Ann Intern Med 76:219, 1972
38. Dich NH, Goodman ZD, Klein MA: Hepatic involvement in Hodgkin's disease: clues to histologic diagnosis. Cancer 64:2121, 1989
39. Bartl R, Frisch B, Burkhardt R et al: Assessment of bone marrow histology in Hodgkin's disease: correlation with clinical factors. Br J Haematol 51:345, 1982
40. O'Carroll DI, McKenna RW, Brunning RD: Bone marrow manifestations of Hodgkin's disease. Cancer 38:1717, 1976
41. Te Velde J, Den Ottolander GJ, Spaander PJ et al: The bone marrow in Hodgkin's disease: the non-involved marrow. Histopathology 2:31, 1978
42. Kern WH, Crepeau AG, Jones JC: Primary Hodgkin's disease of the lung: report of 4 cases and review of the literature. Cancer 14:1151, 1961
43. Radin AI: Primary pulmonary Hodgkin's disease. Cancer 65:550, 1990
44. Yousem SA, Weiss LM, Colby TV: Primary pulmonary Hodgkin's disease: a clinicopathologic study of 15 cases. Cancer 57:1217, 1986
45. Devaney K, Jaffe ES: The surgical pathology of gastrointestinal Hodgkin's disease. Am J Clin Pathol 95:794, 1991
46. Söderström K-O, Joensuu H: Primary Hodgkin's disease of the stomach. Am J Clin Pathol 89:806, 1988
47. Sioutos N, Kerl H, Murphy SB, Kadin ME: Primary cutaneous Hodgkin's disease: unique clinical, morphologic, and immunophenotypic findings. Am J Dermatopathol 16:2, 1994
48. Smith JL, Butler JJ: Skin involvement in Hodgkin's disease. Cancer 45:354, 1980
49. Kaudewitz P, Stein H, Dallenbach F et al: Primary and secondary cutaneous Ki-1+ (CD30+) anaplastic large cell lymphomas: morphologic, immunohistologic, and clinical characteristics. Am J Pathol 135:359, 1989
50. Ashby MA, Barber PC, Holmes AE et al: Primary intracranial Hodgkin's disease: a case report and discussion. Am J Surg Pathol 12:294, 1988
51. Sapozink MD, Kaplan HS: Intracranial Hodgkin's disease: a report of 12 cases and review of the literature. Cancer 52:1301, 1983
52. Meis JM, Butler JJ, Osborne BM: Hodgkin's disease involving the breast and chest wall. Cancer 57:1859, 1986
53. Kaplan H: Patterns of Anatomic Distribution. Hodgkin's Disease. 2nd Ed. Harvard University Press, Cambridge, 1980
54. Todd GB, Michaels L: Hodgkin's disease involving Waldeyer's lymphoid ring. Cancer 34: 1769, 1974
55. Colby TV, Warnke RA: The histology of the initial relapse of Hodgkin's disease. Cancer 45: 289, 1980
56. Strum SB, Rappaport H: Consistency of histologic subtypes in Hodgkin's disease in simultaneous and sequential biopsy specimens. Natl Cancer Inst Monogr 36:1973
57. Colby TV, Hoppe RT, Warnke RA: Hodgkin's disease at autopsy: 1972–1977. Cancer 47: 1852, 1981
58. Dolginow D, Colby TV: Recurrent Hodgkin's disease in treated sites. Cancer 48:1124, 1981
59. Chen JL, Osborne BM, Butler JJ: Residual fibrous masses in treated Hodgkin's disease. Cancer 60:407, 1987
60. Lukes RJ, Butler JJ, Hicks EB: Natural history of Hodgkin's disease as related to its pathologic picture. Cancer 19:317, 1966
61. Lukes RJ, Butler JJ: The pathology and nomen-

clature of Hodgkin's disease. Cancer Res 26: 1063, 1966
62. Georgii A, Fischer R, Hübner K et al: Classification of Hodgkin's disease biopsies by a panel of four histopathologists. Report of 1,140 patients from the German National Trial. Leuk Lymphoma 9:365, 1993
63. Mann RB, Jaffe ES, Berard CW: Malignant lymphomas—a conceptual understanding of morphologic diversity: a review. Am J Pathol 94:105, 1979
64. Strum SB, Rappaport H: Interrelations of the histologic types of Hodgkin's disease. Arch Pathol 91:127, 1971
65. Lukes RJ: Criteria for involvement of lymph node, bone marrow, spleen, and liver in Hodgkin's disease. Cancer Res 31:1755, 1971
66. Ben-Yehuda-Salz D, Ben-Yehuda A, Polliak A et al: Syncytial variant of nodular sclerosing Hodgkin's disease: a new clinicopathologic entity. Cancer 65:1167, 1990
67. Colby TV, Hoppe RT, Warnke RA: Hodgkin's disease: a clinicopathologic study of 659 cases. Cancer 49:1848, 1981
68. MacLennan KA, Bennett MH, Tu A et al: Relationship of histopathologic features to survival and relapse in nodular sclerosing Hodgkin's disease: a study of 1,659 patients. Cancer 64:1686, 1989
69. Patsouris E, Noël H, Lennert K: Cytohistologic and immunohistochemical findings in Hodgkin's disease, mixed cellularity type, with a high content of epithelioid cells. Am J Surg Pathol 13:1014, 1989
70. Butler JJ: The histologic diagnosis of Hodgkin's disease. Semin Diagn Pathol 9:252, 1992
71. Greer JP, Kinney MC, Cousar JB et al: Lymphocyte-depleted Hodgkin's disease: clinicopathologic review of 25 patients. Am J Med 81:208, 1986
72. Kant JA, Hubbard SM, Longo DL et al: The pathologic and clinical heterogeneity of lymphocyte-depleted Hodgkin's disease. J Clin Oncol 4:284, 1986
73. Kinney MC, Greer JP, Collins RD: Assessment of lymphocyte depleted Hodgkin's disease, reticular variant (LDHD-R) by monoclonal antibodies reactive in paraffin sections, abstracted. Mod Pathol 4:75A, 1991
74. Harris NL, Jaffe ES, Stein H et al: A revised European-American classification of lymphoid neoplasms: a proposal from the international lymphoma study group. Blood 84:1361, 1994
75. Chittal SM, Caverivière P, Schwarting R et al: Monoclonal antibodies in the diagnosis of Hodgkin's disease: the search for a rational panel. Am J Surg Pathol 12:9, 1988
76. Medeiros LJ, Weiss LM, Warnke RA, Dorfman RF: Utility of combining antigranulocyte with antileukocyte antibodies in differentiating Hodgkin's disease from non-Hodgkin's lymphoma. Cancer 62:2475, 1988
77. Said JW: The immunohistochemistry of Hodgkin's disease. Semin Diagn Pathol 9:265, 1992
78. Chu W-S, Abbondanzo SL, Frizzera G: Inconsistency of the immunophenotype of Reed-Sternberg cells in simultaneous and consecutive specimens from the same patients: a paraffin section evaluation in 56 patients. Am J Pathol 141:11, 1992
79. Banks PM: The pathology of Hodgkin's disease. Semin Oncol 17:683, 1990
80. Blaustein JC, Lewkon L: Recurrent ''syncytial variant'' of Hodgkin's disease: an immunohistologic diagnosis. Hum Pathol 18:746, 1987
81. Arber DA, Weiss LM: CD15: a review. Appl Immunohistochem 1:17, 1993
82. Sheibani K, Battifora H, Burke JS, Rappaport H: Leu-M1 antigen in human neoplasms: an immunohistologic study of 400 cases. Am J Surg Pathol 10:227, 1986
83. Pinkus GS, Thomas P, Said JW: Leu-M1—a marker for Reed-Sternberg cells in Hodgkin's disease: an immunoperoxidase study of paraffin-embedded tissues. Am J Pathol 119:244, 1985
84. Strauchen JA, Breakstone B: Leu M1 antigen: comparitive expression in Hodgkin's disease and T-cell lymphoma. Hematol Oncol 5:107, 1987
85. Wieczorek R, Burke JS, Knowles DM: Leu-M1 antigen expression in T-cell neoplasia. Am J Pathol 121:374, 1985
86. Pinkus GS, Said JW: Leu-M1 immunoreactivity in nonhematopoietic neoplasms and myeloproliferative disorders: an immunoperoxidase study of paraffin sections. Am J Clin Pathol 85:278, 1986
87. Rushin JM, Riordan GP, Heaton RB et al: Cytomegalovirus-infected cells express Leu-M1 antigen: a potential source of diagnostic error. Am J Pathol 136:989, 1990

88. Chang KL, Arber DA, Weiss LM: CD30: a review. Appl Immunohistochem 1:244, 1993
89. Andreesen R, Brugger W, Löhr GW, Bross KJ: Human macrophages can express the Hodgkin's cell-associated antigen Ki-1 (CD30). Am J Pathol 134:187, 1989
90. Ferreiro JA: Ber-H2 expression in testicular germ cell tumors. Hum Pathol 25:522, 1994
91. Pallesen G, Hamilton-Dutoit SJ: Ki-1 (CD30) antigen is regularly expressed by tumor cells of embryonal carcinoma. Am J Pathol 133:446, 1988
92. Schwarting R, Gerdes J, Durkop H et al: Ber-H2: a new anti-Ki-1 (CD30) monoclonal antibody directed at a formol-resistant epitope. Blood 74:1678, 1989
93. Weiss LM, Arber DA, Chang KL: CD45: a review. Appl Immunohistochem 1:166, 1993
94. Strauchen J: Leucocyte common antigen in the differential diagnosis of Hodgkin's disease. Hematol Oncol 7:149, 1989
95. Gerdes J, van Baarlen J, Pileri S et al: Tumor cell growth fraction in Hodgkin's disease. Am J Pathol 129:390, 1987
96. Sabattini E, Gerdes J, Gherlinzoni F et al: Comparison between the monoclonal antibodies Ki-67 and PC10 in 125 malignant lymphomas. J Pathol 169:397, 1993
97. Freeman J, Kellock DB, Yu CC-W et al: Proliferating cell nuclear nuclear antigen (PCNA) and nucleolar organiser regions in Hodgkin's disease: correlation with morphology. J Clin Pathol 46:446, 1993
98. Hell K, Lorenzen J, Hansmann ML et al: Expression of the proliferating cell nuclear antigen in the different types of Hodgkin's disease. Am J Clin Pathol 99:598, 1993
99. Schmid C, Sweeney E, Isaacson PG: Proliferating cell nuclear antigen (PCNA) expression in Hodgkin's disease. J Pathol 168:1, 1992
100. Tsenga A, Korkolopoulou P, Patsouris E et al: Proliferating cell nuclear antigen, Ki-67, c-myc p62 oncoprotein, and nucleolar organizer regions in Hodgkin's disease. Appl Immunohistochem 2:191, 1994
101. Gupta RK, Lister TA, Bodmer JG: Proliferation of Reed-Sternberg cells and variants in Hodgkin's disease. Ann Oncol 5(Suppl 1):S117, 1994
102. Doglioni C, Pelosio P, Mombello A et al: Immunohistochemical evidence of abnormal expression of the antioncogene-encoded p53 phosphoprotein in Hodgkin's disease and CD30+ anaplastic lymphomas. Hematol Pathol 5:67, 1991
103. Doussis IA, Pezzella F, Lane DP et al: An immunocytochemical study of p53 and bcl-2 protein expression in Hodgkin's disease. Am J Clin Pathol 99:663, 1993
104. Gupta RK, Norton AJ, Thompson IW et al: p53 expression in Reed-Sternberg cells of Hodgkin's disease. Br J Cancer 66:649, 1992
105. Lauritzen AF, Hou-Jensen K, Ralfkiaer E: p53 protein expression in Hodgkin's disease. APMIS 101:689, 1993
106. Gupta RK, Patel K, Bodmer WF, Bodmer JG: Mutation of p53 in primary biopsy material and cell lines from Hodgkin disease. Proc Natl Acad Sci USA 90:2817, 1993
107. Trümper LH, Brady G, Bagg A et al: Single-cell analysis of Hodgkin and Reed-Sternberg cells: molecular heterogeneity of gene expression and p53 mutations. Blood 81:3097, 1993
108. Chilosi M, Doglioni C, Menestrina F et al: Abnormal expression of the p53-binding protein MDM2 in Hodgkin's disease. Blood 84:4295, 1994
109. Inamura J, Miyoshi I, Koeffler HP: p53 in hematologic malignancies. Blood 84:2412, 1994
110. Hsu S-M, Jaffe ES: Leu M1 and peanut agglutinin stain the neoplastic cells of Hodgkin's disease. Am J Clin Pathol 82:29, 1984
111. Möller P: Peanut lectin: a useful tool for detecting Hodgkin cells in paraffin sections. Virchows Arch [Pathol Anat] 396:313, 1982
112. Ree HJ, Neiman RS, Martin AW et al: Paraffin section markers for Reed-Sternberg cells: a comparative study of peanut agglutinin, Leu-M1, LN-2, and Ber-H2. Cancer 63:2030, 1989
113. Chang KL, Curtis CM, Momose H et al: Sensitivity and specificity of *Bauhinia purpurea* as a paraffin section marker for the Reed-Sternberg cells of Hodgkin's disease. Appl Immunohistochem 1:208, 1993
114. Sarker AB, Akagi T, Jeon HJ et al: *Bauhinia purpurea*—a new paraffin marker for Reed-Sternberg cells of Hodgkin's disease: a comparison with Leu-M1 (CD15), LN2 (CD74), peanut agglutinin, and Ber-H2 (CD30). Am J Pathol 141:19, 1992
115. Tamaru J, Mikata A, Azuma K, Takagi T: Reciprocal/dichotomic expression of vimentin and B cell differentiation antigens in Reed-Sternberg's cells. Virchows Arch [A Pathol Anat] 416:213, 1990

116. Delabie J, Shipman R, Bruggen J et al: Expression of the novel intermediate filament-associated protein restin in Hodgkin's disease and anaplastic large-cell lymphoma. Blood 80:2891, 1992
117. Knecht H, Odermatt BF, Bachmann E et al: Frequent detection of Epstein-Barr virus DNA by the polymerase chain reaction in lymph node biopsies from patients with Hodgkin's disease without genomic evidence of B- of T-cell clonality. Blood 78:760, 1991
118. Angel CA, Pringle JH, Naylor J et al: Analysis of antigen receptor genes in Hodgkin's disease. J Clin Pathol 46:337, 1993
119. Schmid C, Pan L, Diss T, Isaacson PG: Expression of B-cell antigens by Hodgkin's and Reed-Sternberg cells. Am J Pathol 139:701, 1991
120. Agnarsson BA, Kadin ME: The immunophenotype of Reed-Sternberg cells: a study of 50 cases of Hodgkin's disease using fixed frozen tissues. Cancer 63:2083, 1989
121. Angel C, Warford A, Campbell AC et al: The immunohistology of Hodgkin's disease—Reed-Sternberg cells and their variants. J Pathol 153: 21, 1987
122. Casey TT, Olson SJ, Cousar JB, Collins RD: Immunophenotypes of Reed-Sternberg cells: a study of 19 cases of Hodgkin's disease in plastic-embedded sections. Blood 74:2624, 1989
123. Carbone A, Gloghini A, Gattei V et al: Expression of functional CD40 antigen on Reed-Sternberg cells and Hodgkin's disease cell lines. Blood 85:780, 1995
124. Della Croce DR, Imam A, Brynes RK et al: Anti-BLA.36 monoclonal antibody shows reactivity with Hodgkin's cells and B lymphocytes in frozen and paraffin-embedded tissues. Hematol Oncol 9:103, 1991
125. Hall PA, D'Ardenne AJ, Stansfeld AG: Paraffin section immunohistochemistry. II. Hodgkin's disease and large cell anaplastic (Ki1) lymphoma. Histopathology 13:161, 1988
126. Korkolopoulou P, Cordell J, Jones M et al: The expression of the B-cell marker mb-1 (CD79a) in Hodgkin's disease. Histopathology 24:511, 1994
127. O'Grady JT, Stewart S, Lowrey J et al: CD40 expression in Hodgkin's disease. Am J Pathol 144:21, 1994
128. Pinkus GS, Said JW: Hodgkin's disease, lymphocyte predominance type, nodular-further evidence for a B cell derivation: L & H variants of Reed-Sternberg cells express L26, a pan B cell marker. Am J Pathol 133:211, 1988
129. Sherrod AE, Felder B, Levy JN et al: Immunohistologic identification of phenotypic antigens associated with Hodgkin and Reed-Sternberg cells. A paraffin section study. Cancer 57:2135, 1986
130. Siebert JD, McClure SP, Banks PM, Gulley ML: Hodgkin's disease, mixed cellularity type, with a B-cell immunophenotype: report of a case and literature review. Arch Pathol Lab Med 119: 474, 1995
131. Strauchen JA, Dimitriu-Bona A: Immunopathology of Hodgkin's disease. Characterization of Reed-Sternberg cells with monoclonal antibodies. Am J Pathol 123:293, 1986
132. Zukerberg LR, Collins AB, Ferry JA, Harris NL: Coexpression of CD15 and CD20 by Reed-Sternberg cells in Hodgkin's disease. Am J Pathol 139:475, 1991
133. Quintanilla-Martinez L, Preffer F, Rubin D et al: CD20 + T-cell lymphoma: neoplastic transformation of a normal T-cell subset. Am J Clin Pathol 102:483, 1994
134. Kadin ME, Stites DP, Levy R, Warnke R: Exogenous immunoglobulin and the macrophage origin of Reed-Sternberg cells in Hodgkin's disease. N Engl J Med 299:1208, 1978
135. Ruprai AK, Pringle JH, Angel CA et al: Localization of immunoglobulin light chain mRNA expression in Hodgkin's disease by in situ hybridization. J Pathol 164:37, 1991
136. Brinker MGL, Poppema S, Buys CHCM et al: Clonal immunoglobulin gene rearrangements in tissues involved by Hodgkin's disease. Blood 70:186, 1987
137. Griesser H, Feller AC, Mak TW, Lennert K: Clonal rearrangements of T-cell receptor and immunoglobulin genes and immunophenotypic antigen expression in different subclasses of Hodgkin's disease. Int J Cancer 40:157, 1987
138. Herbst H, Tippelmann G, Anagnostopoulos I et al: Immunoglobulin and T-cell receptor gene rearrangements in Hodgkin's disease and Ki-1-positive anaplastic large cell lymphoma: dissociation between phenotype and genotype. Leuk Res 13:1989
139. Hu EHL, Ellison D, Zovich D et al: Molecular analysis of Hodgkin's disease with abundant Reed-Sternberg cells. Hematol Pathol 4:27, 1990
140. O'Connor NTJ, Crick JA, Gatter KC et al: Cell

lineage in Hodgkin's disease. Lancet 1:158, 1987
141. Raghavachar A, Binder T, Bartram CR: Immunoglobulin and T-cell receptor gene rearrangements in Hodgkin's disease. Cancer Res 48: 3591, 1988
142. Cossman J, Sundeen J, Uppenkamp M et al: Rearranging antigen-receptor genes in enriched Reed-Sternberg cell fractions of Hodgkin's disease. Hematol Oncol 6:205, 1988
143. Sundeen J, Lipford E, Uppenkamp J et al: Rearranged antigen receptor genes in Hodgkin's disease. Blood 70:96, 1987
144. Weiss LM, Strickler JG, Hu E et al: Immunoglobulin gene rearrangements in Hodgkin's disease. Hum Pathol 17:1009, 1986
145. Weiss L, Warnke RA, Sklar J: Clonal antigen receptor gene rearrangements and Epstein-Barr viral DNA in tissues of Hodgkin's disease. Hematol Oncol 6:233, 1988
146. Knowles D, Neri A, Pelicci PG et al: Immunoglobulin and T-cell receptor β-chain gene rearrangement analysis of Hodgkin's disease: implications for lineage determination and differential diagnosis. Proc Natl Acad Sci USA 83:7942, 1986
147. Tamaru J, Hummel M, Zemlin M et al: Hodgkin's disease with a B-cell phenotype often shows a VDJ rearrangement and somatic mutations in the V_H genes. Blood 84:708, 1994
148. Hummel M, Ziemann K, Lammert H et al: Hodgkin's disease with monoclonal and polyclonal populations of Reed-Sternberg cells. N Engl J Med 333:901, 1995
149. Küppers R, Rajewsky K, Zhao M et al: Hodgkin disease: Hodgkin and Reed-Sternberg cells picked from histological sections show clonal immunoglobulin gene rearrangements and appear to be derived from B cells at various stages of development. Proc Natl Acad Sci USA 91: 10962, 1994
150. Roth J, Daus H, Trumper L et al: Detection of immunoglobulin heavy-chain gene rearrangement at the single-cell level in malignant lymphomas: no rearrangement is found in Hodgkin and Reed-Sternberg cells. Int J Cancer 57:799, 1994
151. Davis TH, Morton CC, Miller-Cassman R et al: Hodgkin's disease, lymphomatoid papulosis, and cutaneous T-cell lymphoma derived from a common T-cell clone. N Engl J Med 326:1115, 1992
152. Kadin ME: Common activated helper-T-cell origin for lymphomatoid papulosis, mycosis fungoides, and some types of Hodgkin's disease. Lancet 2:864, 1985
153. Willemze R, Scheffer E, Van Vloten WA, Meijer CJLM: Lymphomatoid papulosis and Hodgkin's disease: are they related? Arch Dermatol Res 275:159, 1983
154. Cibull ML, Stein H, Gatter KC, Mason DY: The expression of CD3 antigen in Hodgkin's disease. Histopathology 15:597, 1989
155. Clark JR, Williams ME, Swerdlow SH: Detection of B- and T-cells in paraffin-embedded tissue sections: diagnostic utility of commercially obtained 4KB5 and UCHL-1. Am J Clin Pathol 93:58, 1990
156. Dallenbach FE, Stein H: Expression of T-cell-receptor β chain in Reed-Sternberg cells. Lancet 2:828, 1989
157. Enblad G, Sundstrom C, Glimerlius B: Immunohistochemical characteristics of Hodgkin and Reed-Sternberg cells in relation to age and clinical outcome. Histopathology 22:535, 1993
158. Falini B, Stein H, Pileri S et al: Expression of lymphoid-associated antigens on Hodgkin's and Reed-Sternberg cells of Hodgkin's disease: an immunocytochemical study on lymph node cytospins using monoclonal antibodies. Histopathology 11:1229, 1987
159. Kadin ME, Muramoto L, Said J: Expression of T-cell antigens on Reed-Sternberg cells in a subset of patients with nodular sclerosing and mixed cellularity Hodgkin's disease. Am J Pathol 130:345, 1988
160. Oka K, Mori N, Kojima M: Anti-Leu-3a antibody reactivity with Reed-Sternberg cells of Hodgkin's disease. Arch Pathol Lab Med 112: 139, 1988
161. Strickler JG, Weiss LM, Copenhaver CM et al: Monoclonal antibodies reactive in routinely processed tissue sections of malignant lymphoma, with emphasis on T-cell lymphomas. Hum Pathol 18:808, 1987
162. Wieczorek R, Buck D, Bindl J, Knowles DM: Monoclonal antibody Leu-22 (L60) permits the demonstration of some neoplastic T cells in routinely fixed and paraffin-embedded tissue sections. Hum Pathol 19:1434, 1988
163. Drexler HG, Jones DB, Diehl V, Minowada J: Is the Hodgkin cell a T- or B-lymphocyte? Recent evidence from geno- and immunophenotypic

analysis and in-vitro cell lines. Hematol Oncol 7:95, 1989

164. Griesser H, Feller A, Lennert K et al: Rearrangement of the β chain of the T cell antigen receptor and immunoglobulin genes in lymphoproliferative disorders. J Clin Invest 78:1179, 1986
165. Griesser H, Mak TW: Immunogenotyping in Hodgkin's disease. Hematol Oncol 6:239, 1988
166. Roth MS, Schnitzer B, Bingham EL et al: Rearrangement of immunoglobulin and T-cell receptor genes in Hodgkin's disease. Am J Pathol 131:331, 1988
167. Daus H, Trümper L, Roth J et al: Hodgkin and Reed-Sternberg cells do not carry T-cell receptor g gene rearrangements: evidence from single-cell polymerase chain reaction examination. Blood 85:1590, 1995
168. Jacobson JO, Wilkes BM, Harris NL: Polyclonal rearrangement of the T-cell antigen receptor genes in Hodgkin's disease: implications for diagnosis. Mod Pathol 4:172, 1991
169. Rowley JD: Chromosomes in Hodgkin's disease. Cancer Treat Rep 66:639, 1982
170. Weber-Matthiesen K, Deerberg J, Poetsch M et al: Numerical chromosome aberrations are present within the CD30+ Hodgkin and Reed-Sternberg cells in 100% of analyzed cases of Hodgkin's disease. Blood 86:1464, 1995
171. Thangavelu M, LeBeau MM: Chromosomal abnormalities in Hodgkin's disease. Hematol Oncol Clin North Am 3:221, 1989
172. Schouten HC, Sanger WG, Duggan M et al: Chromosomal abnormalities in Hodgkin's disease. Blood 73:2149, 1989
173. Cabanillas F: A review and interpretation of cytogenetic abnormalities identified in Hodgkin's disease. Hematol Oncol 6:271, 1988
174. Cabanillas F, Pathak S, Trujillo J et al: Cytogenetic features of Hodgkin's disease suggest possible origin from a lymphocyte. Blood 71:1615, 1988
175. Poppema S, Kaleta J, Hepperle B: Chromosomal abnormalities in patients with Hodgkin's disease: evidence for frequent involvement of the 14q chromosomal region but infrequent bcl-2 gene rearrangement in Reed-Sternberg cells. J Natl Cancer Inst 84:1789, 1992
176. Tilly H, Bastard C, Delastre T et al: Cytogenetic studies in untreated Hodgkin's disease. Blood 77:1298, 1991
177. Stetler-Stevenson M, Crush-Stanton S, Cossman J: Involvement of the *bcl*-2 gene in Hodgkin's disease. J Natl Cancer Inst 82:855, 1990
178. Gupta RK, Whelan JS, Lister TA et al: Direct sequence analysis of the t(14;18) chromosomal translocation in Hodgkin's disease. Blood 79: 2084, 1992
179. Reid AH, Cunningham RE, Frizzera G, O'Leary TJ: bcl-2 rearrangement in Hodgkin's disease: results of polymerase chain reaction, flow cytometry, and sequencing on formalin-fixed, paraffin-embedded tissue. Am J Pathol 142:395, 1993
180. Lebrun DP, Ngan BY, Weiss LM et al: The bcl-2 oncogene in Hodgkin's disease arising in the setting of follicular non-Hodgkin's lymphoma. Blood 83:223, 1994
181. Athan E, Chadburn A, Knowles D: The bcl-2 gene translocation is undetectable in Hodgkin's disease by Southern blot hybridization and polymerase chain reaction. Am J Pathol 141:193, 1992
182. Koduru PRK, Susin M, Schulman P et al: Phenotypic and genotypic characterization of Hodgkin's disease. Am J Hematol 44:117, 1993
183. Louie DC, Kant JA, Brooks JJ, Reed JC: Absence of t(14;18) major and minor breakpoints and of *bcl*-2 protein overproduction in Reed-Sternberg cells of Hodgkin's disease. Am J Pathol 139:1231, 1991
184. Said JW, Sassoon AF, Shintaku IP et al: Absence of *bcl*-2 major breakpoint region and J_H gene rearrangement in lymphocyte predominance Hodgkin's disease: results of Southern blot analysis and polymerase chain reaction. Am J Pathol 138:261, 1991
185. Shibata D, Hu E, Weiss LM et al: Detection of specific t(14;18) chromosomal translocations in fixed tissues. Hum Pathol 21:199, 1990
186. Weiss LM, Chang KL: Molecular biologic studies of Hodgkin's disease. Semin Diagn Pathol 9:272, 1992
187. Limpens J, de Jong D, van Krieken JHJM et al: *bcl*-2/J_H rearrangements in benign lymphoid tissues with follicular hyperplasia. Oncogene 6: 2271, 1991
188. Limpens J, Stad R, Vos C et al: Lymphoma-associated translocation t(14;18) in blood B cells of normal individuals. Blood 85:2528, 1995
189. Lones MA, Pinkus GA, Shintaku P, Said JW: bcl-2 oncogene protein is preferentially expressed in Reed-Sternberg cells in Hodgkin's

disease of the nodular sclerosis subtype. Am J Clin Pathol 102:464, 1994

190. Bhagat SK, Medeiros LJ, Weiss LM et al: bcl-2 expression in Hodgkin's disease: correlation with the t(14;18) translocation and Epstein-Barr virus. Am J Clin Pathol 99:604, 1993
191. Jiwa NM, Kanavaros P, van der Valk P et al: Expression of c-*myc* and *bcl*-2 oncogene products in Reed-Sternberg cells independent of presence of Epstein-Barr virus. J Clin Pathol 46: 211, 1993
192. Khan G, Gupta RK, Coates PJ, Slavin G: Epstein-Barr virus infection and bcl-2 proto-oncogene expression: separate events in the pathogenesis of Hodgkin's disease? Am J Pathol 143: 1270, 1993
193. Lorenzen J, Hansmann ML, Pezzella F et al: Expression of the bcl-2 oncogene product and chromosomal translocation t(14;18) in Hodgkin's disease. Hum Pathol 23:1205, 1992
194. Drexler HG: Recent results on the biology of Hodgkin and Reed-Sternberg cells. II. Continuous cell lines. Leuk Lymphoma 9:1, 1993
195. Pinto A, Gloghini A, Gattei V et al: Expression of the c-kit receptor in human lymphomas is restricted to Hodgkin's disease and CD30+ anaplastic large cell lymphomas. Blood 83:785, 1994
196. Jones DB, Cossman J, Hansmann ML: Oncogenes in Hodgkin's disease. Ann Oncol 3(Suppl 4):9, 1992
197. Kvåle G, Høiby EA, Pederson E: Hodgkin's disease in patients with previous infectious mononucleosis. Int J Cancer 23:593, 1979
198. Muñoz N, Davidson RJL, Witthoff B et al: Infectious mononucleosis and Hodgkin's disease. Int J Cancer 22:10, 1978
199. Evans AS, Gutensohn NM: A population-based case-control study of EBV and other viral antibodies among persons with Hodgkin's disease and their siblings. Int J Cancer 34:149, 1984
200. Mueller N, Evans A, Harris NA et al: Hodgkin's disease and Epstein-Barr virus: altered antibody pattern before diagnosis. N Engl J Med 320:689, 1989
201. Brousset P, Chittal S, Schlaifer D et al: Detection of Epstein-Barr virus messenger RNA in Reed-Sternberg cells of Hodgkin's disease by in situ hybridization with biotinylated probes on specially processed modified acetone methyl benzoate xylene (ModAMeX) sections. Blood 77:1781, 1991
202. Weiss LM, Chen YY, Liu X, Shibata D: Epstein-Barr virus and Hodgkin's disease: a correlative in situ hybridization and polymerase chain reaction study. Am J Pathol 139:1259, 1991
203. Herbst H, Steinbrecher E, Niedobitek G et al: Distribution and phenotype of Epstein-Barr virus-harboring cells in Hodgkin's disease. Blood 80:484, 1992
204. Deacon EM, Pallesen G, Niedobitek G et al: Epstein-Barr virus and Hodgkin's disease: transcriptional analysis of virus latency in the malignant cells. J Exp Med 177:339, 1993
205. Grässer FA, Murray PG, Kremmer E et al: Monoclonal antibodies directed against the Epstein-Barr virus-encoded nuclear antigen 1 (EBNA1): immunohistologic detection of EBNA1 in the malignant cells of Hodgkin's disease. Blood 84:3792, 1994
206. Herbst H, Dallenbach F, Hummel M et al: Epstein-Barr virus latent membrane protein expression in Hodgkin and Reed-Sternberg cells. Proc Natl Acad Sci USA 88:4766, 1991
207. Pallesen G, Hamilton-Dutoit SJ, Rowe M, Young LS: Expression of Epstein-Barr virus latent gene products in tumour cells of Hodgkin's disease. Lancet 337:320, 1991
208. Poppema S, van Imhoff G, Torensma R, Smit J: Lymphadenopathy morphologically consistent with Hodgkin's disease associated with Epstein-Barr virus infection. Am J Clin Pathol 84: 385, 1985
209. Weiss LM, Mohaved LA, Warnke RA, Sklar J: Detection of Epstein-Barr viral genomes in Reed-Sternberg cells of Hodgkin's disease. N Engl J Med 320:502, 1989
210. Weiss LM, Strickler JG, Warnke RA et al: Epstein-Barr viral DNA in tissues of Hodgkin's disease. Am J Pathol 129:86, 1987
211. Anagnostopoulos I, Herbst H, Niedobitek G, Stein H: Demonstration of monoclonal EBV genomes in Hodgkin's disease and Ki-1 positive anaplastic large cell lymphoma by combined Southern blot and in situ hybridization. Blood 74:810, 1989
212. Brousset P, Schlaifer D, Meggetto F et al: Persistence of the same viral strain in early and late relapses of Epstein-Barr virus-associated Hodgkin's disease. Blood 84:2447, 1994
213. Vasef MA, Kamel OW, Chen Y-Y et al: Detection of Epstein-Barr virus in multiple sites involved by Hodgkin's disease. Am J Pathol 147: 1408, 1995

214. Armstrong AA, Weiss LM, Gallagher A et al: Criteria for the definition of Epstein-Barr virus association in Hodgkin's disease. Leukemia 6: 869, 1992
215. Brocksmith D, Angel C, Pringle JH, Lauder I: Epstein-Barr viral DNA in Hodgkin's disease: amplification and detection using polymerase chain reaction. J Pathol 165:11, 1991
216. Herbst H, Niedobitek G, Kneba M et al: High incidence of Epstein-Barr virus genomes in Hodgkin's disease. Am J Pathol 137:13, 1990
217. Masih A, Weisenburger D, Duggan M et al: Epstein-Barr viral genome in lymph nodes from patients with Hodgkin's disease may not be specific to Reed-Sternberg cells. Am J Pathol 139: 37, 1991
218. Shibata D, Hansmann ML, Weiss LM, Nathwani BN: Epstein-Barr virus infection and Hodgkin's disease: a study of fixed tissues using the polymerase chain reaction. Hum Pathol 22: 1262, 1991
219. Wright CF, Reid AH, Tsai MM et al: Detection of Epstein-Barr virus sequences in Hodgkin's disease by the polymerase chain reaction. Am J Pathol 139:393, 1991
220. Hamilton-Dutoit SJ, Pallesen G: Detection of Epstein-Barr virus small RNAs in routine paraffin sections using non-isotopic RNA/RNA in situ hybridization. Histopathology 25:101, 1994
221. Carbone A, Gloghini A, Zanette I et al: Coexpression of Epstein-Barr virus latent membrane protein and vimentin in "aggressive" histological subtypes in Hodgkin's disease. Virchows Arch [A Pathol Anat] 422:39, 1993
222. Jarrett RF: Viral involvement in Hodgkin's disease. Int J Cell Cloning 10:315, 1992
223. Khan G, Norton AJ, Slavin G: Epstein-Barr virus in Hodgkin's disease. Relation to age and subtype. Cancer 71:3124, 1993
224. Chan JKC, Yip TTC, Tsang WYW et al: Detection of Epstein-Barr virus in Hodgkin's disease occurring in an Oriental population. Hum Pathol 26:314, 1995
225. Herndier BG, Sanchez HC, Chang KL et al: High prevalence of Epstein-Barr virus in the Reed-Sternberg cells of HIV-associated Hodgkin's disease. Am J Pathol 142:1073, 1993
226. Uccini S, Monardo F, Stoppacciaro A et al: High frequency of Epstein-Barr virus genome detection in Hodgkin's disease of HIV-positive patients. Int J Cancer 46:581, 1990
227. Chang KL, Albujar PF, Chen YY et al: High prevalence of Epstein-Barr virus in the Reed-Sternberg cells of Hodgkin's disease occurring in Peru. Blood 81:496, 1993
228. Ambinder RF, Browning PJ, Lorenzana I et al: Epstein-Barr virus and childhood Hodgkin's disease in Honduras and the United States. Blood 81:496, 1993
229. Jarrett RF, Gallagher A, Jones DB et al: Detection of Epstein-Barr virus genomes in Hodgkin's disease: relation to age. J Clin Pathol 44: 844, 1991
230. Hummel M, Anagnostopoulos I, Dallenbach F et al: EBV infection patterns in Hodgkin's disease and normal lymphoid tissue: expression and cellular localization of EBV gene products. Br J Haematol 82:689, 1992
231. Khan G, Coates PJ, Gupta RK et al: Presence of Epstein-Barr virus in Hodgkin's disease is not exclusive to Reed-Sternberg cells. Am J Pathol 140:757, 1992
232. Torelli G, Marasca R, Luppi M et al: Human herpesvirus-6 in human lymphomas: identification of specific sequences in Hodgkin's lymphomas by polymerase chain reaction. Blood 77:2251, 1991
233. Hsu S-M, Waldron Jr JW, Hsu P-L, Hough Jr AJ: Cytokines in malignant lymphomas: review and prospective evaluation. Hum Pathol 24: 1040, 1993
234. Haluska FG, Brufsky AM, Canellos GP: The cellular biology of the Reed-Sternberg cell. Blood 84:1005, 1994
235. Samoszuk M, Nansen L: Detection of interleukin-5 messenger RNA in Reed-Sternberg cells of Hodgkin's disease with eosinophilia. Blood 75:13, 1990
236. Kadin ME, Agnarsson BA, Ellingsworth LR, Newcom SR: Immunohistochemical evidence of a role for transforming growth factor beta in the pathogenesis of nodular sclerosing Hodgkin's disease. Am J Pathol 136:1209, 1990
237. Poppema S: The diversity of the immunohistological staining pattern of Sternberg-Reed cells. J Histochem Cytochem 28:788, 1980
238. Gelb AB, Dorfman RF, Warnke RA: Coexistence of nodular lymphocyte predominance Hodgkin's disease and Hodgkin's disease of the usual type. Am J Surg Pathol 17:364, 1993
239. Patsouris E, Noël H, Lennert K: Lymphoplasmacytic/lymphoplasmacytoid immunocytoma with a high content of epithelioid cells: histo-

logic and immunohistochemical findings. Am J Surg Pathol 14:660, 1990

240. Perrone T, Frizzera G, Rosai J: Mediastinal diffuse large-cell lymphoma with sclerosis: a clinicopathologic study of 60 cases. Am J Surg Pathol 10:176, 1986
241. Strickler JG, Kurtin PJ: Mediastinal lymphoma. Semin Diagn Pathol 8:2, 1991
242. Warnke RA: The distinction of Hodgkin's disease from B cell lymphoma. Semin Diagn Pathol 9:284, 1992
243. Macon WR, Williams ME, Greer JP et al: T-cell-rich B-cell lymphomas. A clinicopathologic study of 19 cases. Am J Surg Pathol 16:351, 1992
244. Osborne BM, Butler JJ, Pugh WC: The value of immunophenotyping on paraffin sections in the identification of T-cell rich B-cell large-cell lymphoma: lineage confirmed by J_H rearrangement. Am J Surg Pathol 14:933, 1990
245. Agnarsson BA, Kadin ME: Ki-1 positive large cell lymphoma: a morphologic and immunologic study of 19 cases. Am J Surg Pathol 12: 264, 1988
246. Chott A, Kaserer K, Augustin I et al: Ki-1 positive large cell lymphoma. A clinicopathologic study of 41 cases. Am J Surg Pathol 14:439, 1990
247. Frizzera G: The distinction of Hodgkin's disease from anaplastic large cell lymphoma. Semin Diagn Pathol 9:291, 1992
248. Penny RJ, Blaustein JC, Longtine JA, Pinkus GS: Ki-1 positive large cell lymphomas, a heterogenous group of neoplasms. Morphologic, immunophenotypic, genotypic, and clinical features of 24 cases. Cancer 68:362, 1991
249. Pileri S, Falini B, Delsol G et al: Lymphohistiocytic T-cell lymphoma (anaplastic large cell lymphoma CD30+/Ki-1+ with a high content of reactive histocytes). Histopathology 16:383, 1990
250. Al Saati T, Tkaczuk J, Krissansen G et al: A novel antigen detected by the CBF.78 antibody further distinguishes anaplastic large cell lymphoma from Hodgkin's disease. Blood 86:2741, 1995
251. Larson RS, Collins RD, Macon WR, Kinney MC: Differentiation of anaplastic large cell lymphoma (ALCL) from Hodgkin's disease (HD) by a monoclonal antibody (mAb) panel reactive in paraffin. Mod Pathol 7:113A, 1994
252. Cohen PL, Butmarc J, Kadin ME: Expression of Hodgkin's disease associated antigen BLA.36 in anaplastic large cell lymphomas and lymphomatoid papulosis primarily of T-cell origin. Am J Clin Pathol 104:50, 1995
253. Bitter MA, Franklin WA, Larson RA et al: Morphology in Ki-1 (CD30)-positive non-Hodgkin's lymphoma is correlated with clinical features and the presence of a unique chromosomal abnormality, t(2;5) (p23;q35). Am J Surg Pathol 14:305, 1990
254. Downing JR, Shurtleff SA, Zielenska M et al: Molecular detection of the (2;5) translocation of non-Hodgkin's lymphoma by reverse transcriptase-polymerase chain reaction. Blood 85: 3416, 1995
255. Elmberger PG, Lozano MD, Weisenburger DD et al: Transcripts of the npm-alk fusion gene in anaplastic large cell lymphoma, Hodgkin's disease, and reactive lymphoid lesions. Blood 86:3517, 1995
256. Herbst H, Anagnostopoulos J, Heinze B et al: *ALK* gene products in anaplastic large cell lymphomas and Hodgkin's disease. Blood 86:1694, 1995
257. Wellmann A, Otsuki T, Vogelbruch M et al: Analysis of the t(2;5) (p23;q35) translocation by reverse transcription-polymerase chain reaction in CD30+ anaplastic large-cell lymphomas, in other non-Hodgkin's lymphoma's of T-cell phenotype, and in Hodgkin's disease. Blood 86: 2321, 1995
258. Weiss LM, Lopategui JR, Sun L-H et al: Absence of the t(2;5) in Hodgkin's disease. Blood 85:2845, 1995
259. Orscheschek K, Merz H, Hell J et al: Large-cell anaplastic lymphoma-specific translocation (t[2;5] [p23;q35]) in Hodgkin's disease: indication of a common pathogenesis? Lancet 345:87, 1995
260. Greer J, Kinney MC, Collins RD et al: Clinical features of 31 patients with Ki-1 anaplastic large cell lymphoma. J Clin Oncol 9:539, 1991
261. Leoncini L, Del Vecchio MT, Kraft R et al: Hodgkin's disease and CD30-positive anaplastic large cell lymphomas—a continuous spectrum of malignant disorders: a quantitative morphometric and immunohistologic study. Am J Pathol 137:1047, 1990
262. Harris NL: The relationship between Hodgkin's disease and non-Hodgkin's lymphoma. Semin Diagn Pathol 9:304, 1992
263. Pileri S, Bocchia M, Baroni CD et al: Anaplastic

large cell lymphoma (CD30+/Ki-1+): results of a prospective clinico-pathological study of 69 cases. Br J Haematol 86:513, 1994
264. Patsouris E, Noël H, Lennert K: Histologic and immunohistologic findings in lymphoepithelioid cell lymphoma (Lennert's lymphoma). Am J Surg Pathol 12:341, 1988
265. Patsouris E, Noël H, Lennert K: Angioimmunoblastic lymphadenopathy—type of T-cell lymphoma with a high content of epithelioid cells. Histopathology and comparison with lymphoepithelioid cell lymphoma. Am J Surg Pathol 13: 262, 1989
266. Waldron JA, Leech JH, Glick AD et al: Malignant lymphoma of peripheral T-lymphocyte origin: immunologic, pathologic, and clinical features in six patients. Cancer 40:1604, 1977
267. Weis JW, Winter MW, Phyliky RL, Banks PM: Peripheral T-cell lymphomas: histologic, immunohistologic and clinical characterization. Mayo Clin Proc 61:411, 1986
268. Nguyen D, Nathwani BN, Ellison DJ, Hackett C: Differential diagnosis between T-cell lymphoma and Hodgkin's disease: the value of mitotic counts and pericapsular infiltration. Hematol Pathol 3:63, 1989
269. Osborne BM, Uthman MO, Butler JJ, McLaughlin P: Differentiation of T-cell lymphoma from Hodgkin's disease: mitotic rate and S-phase analysis. Am J Clin Pathol 93:227, 1990
270. Banks PM: The distinction of Hodgkin's disease from T-cell lymphoma. Semin Diagn Pathol 9: 279, 1992
271. Weiss LM, Crabtree GS, Rouse RV, Warnke RA: Morphologic and immunologic characterization of 50 peripheral T-cell lymphomas. Am J Pathol 118:316, 1985
272. Giffler RF, Gillespie JJ, Ayala AG, Newland JR: Lymphoepithelioma in cervical lymph nodes of children and young adults. Am J Surg Pathol 1:293, 1977
273. Bacchi CE, Dorfman RF, Hoppe RT et al: Metastatic carcinoma in lymph nodes simulating "syncytial variant" of nodular sclerosing Hodgkin's disease. Am J Clin Pathol 96:589, 1991
274. Abbandanzo SL, Sato N, Straus SE, Jaffe ES: Acute infectious mononucleosis. CD30 (Ki-1) antigen expression and histologic correlations. Am J Clin Pathol 93:698, 1990
275. Lukes RJ, Tindle BH, Parker JW: Reed-Sternberg-like cells in infectious mononucleosis. Lancet 2:1003, 1969
276. Tindle BH, Parker JW, Lukes RJ: "Reed-Sternberg cells" in infectious mononucleosis? Am J Clin Pathol 58:607, 1972
277. Childs CC, Parham DM, Berard CW: Infectious mononucleosis: the spectrum of morphologic changes simulating lymphoma in lymph nodes and tonsils. Am J Surg Pathol 11:122, 1987
278. Strickler JG, Fedeli F, Horwitz CA et al: Infectious mononucleosis in lymphoid tissue. Histopathology, in situ hybridization, and differential diagnosis. Arch Pathol Lab Med 117:269, 1993
279. Fellbaum C, Hansmann ML, Parwaresch MR, Lennert K: Monoclonal antibodies Ki-B3 and Leu-M1 discriminate giant cells of infectious mononucleosis and Hodgkin's disease. Hum Pathol 19:1168, 1988
280. Strickler JG, Warnke RA, Weiss LM: Necrosis in lymph nodes. Pathol Annu Part 2 22:253, 1987
281. Young JL, Percy C, Asire AJ: Cancer incidence and mortality in the United States. Natl Cancer Inst Monogr 57:72, 1981
282. Boring CC, Squires TS, Tong T: Cancer statistics, 1993. Ca Cancer J Clin 43:7, 1993
283. Grufferman S, Delzell E: Epidemiology of Hodgkin's disease. Epidemiol Rev 6:76, 1984
284. Berard CW, Thomas LB, Axtell LM et al: The relationship of histopathological subtype to clinical stage of Hodgkin's disease at diagnosis. Cancer Res 31:1776, 1971
285. MacMahon B: Epidemiology of Hodgkin's disease. Cancer Res 26:1189, 1966
286. Correa P, O'Conor GT: Epidemiologic patterns of Hodgkin's disease. Int J Cancer 8:192, 1971
287. Gutensohn N, Cole P: Epidemiology of Hodgkin's disease. Semin Oncol 7:92, 1980
288. Gutensohn N, Cole P: Childhood social environment and Hodgkin's disease. N Engl J Med 304: 135, 1981
289. Marshall WH, Barnard JM, Buehler SK et al: HLA in familial Hodgkin's disease: results and new hypothesis. Int J Cancer 19:450, 1977
290. Mack TM, Cozen W, Shibata DK et al: Concordance for Hodgkin's disease in identical twins suggesting genetic susceptibility to the young-adult form of the disease. N Engl J Med 332: 413, 1995
291. Lister TA, Crowther D, Sutcliffe SB et al: Report of a committee convened to discuss the evaluation and staging of patients with Hodg-

kin's disease: Cotswolds meeting. J Clin Oncol 7:1630, 1989
292. Lister TA, Crowther D: Staging for Hodgkin's disease. Semin Oncol 17:696, 1990
293. Fisher RI, De Vita VT, Bostick F et al: Persistent immunologic abnormalities in long-term survivors of advanced Hodgkin's disease. Ann Intern Med 92:595, 1980
294. Levy R, Kaplan HS: Impaired lymphocyte function in untreated Hodgkin's disease. N Engl J Med 290:181, 1974
295. Kaplan HS: Hodgkin's disease: unfolding concepts concerning its nature, management and prognosis. Cancer 45:2439, 1980
296. Lauria F, Foa R, Gobbi M et al: Increased proportion of suppressor/cytotoxic (OKT8 +) cells in patients with Hodgkin's disease in long-lasting remission. Cancer 52:1385, 1983
297. Liberati AM, Ballatori E, Fizzoti M et al: Immunologic profile in patients with Hodgkin's disease in complete remission. Cancer 59:1906, 1987
298. Tullgren O, Grimfors G, Holm G et al: Lymphocyte abnormalities predicting a poor prognosis in Hodgkin's disease: a long-term follow-up. Cancer 68:768, 1991
299. Neiman RS, Rosen PJ, Lukes RJ: Lymphocyte-depletion Hodgkin's disease: a clinicopathologic entity. N Engl J Med 288:751, 1973
300. Hu E, Hufford S, Lukes R et al: Third-World Hodgkin's disease at Los Angeles County—University of Southern California Medical Center. J Clin Oncol 6:1285, 1988
301. Bearman RM, Pangalis GA, Rappaport H: Hodgkin's disease, lymphocyte depletion type: a clinicopathologic study of 39 patients. Cancer 41:293, 1978
302. Ahmed T, Wormser GP, Stahl RE et al: Malignant lymphomas in a population at risk for acquired immune deficiency syndrome. Cancer 60:719, 1987
303. Hessol NA, Katz MH, Kiu JY et al: Increased incidence of Hodgkin disease in homosexual men with HIV infection. Ann Intern Med 117: 309, 1992
304. Roithmann S, Tourani J-M, Andrieu J-M: Hodgkin's disease in HIV-infected intravenous drug abusers. N Engl J Med 323:275, 1990
305. Tirelli U, Vaccher E, Rezza G et al: Hodgkin disease and infection with the human immunodeficiency virus (HIV) in Italy. Ann Intern Med 108:309, 1988
306. Pelstring RS, Zellmer RB, Sulak LA et al: Hodgkin's disease in association with human immunodeficiency virus infection: pathologic and immunologic features. Cancer 67:1865, 1991
307. Rubio R: Hodgkin's disease associated with human immunodeficiency virus infection: a clinical study of 46 cases (for the cooperative study group of malignancies with HIV infection of Madrid). Cancer 73:2400, 1994
308. Ree HJ, Strauchen JA, Khan AA et al: Human immunodeficiency virus-associated Hodgkin's disease: clinico-pathologic studies of 24 cases and preponderance of mixed cellularity type characterized by the occurrence of fibrohistiocytoid stromal cells. Cancer 67:1614, 1991
309. Schoeppel SL, Hoppe RT, Dorfman RF et al: Hodgkin's disease in homosexual men with generalized lymphadenopathy. Ann Intern Med 102:68, 1985
310. Unger PD, Strauchen JA: Hodgkin's disease in AIDS complex patients: report of four cases and tissue immunologic marker studies. Cancer 58: 821, 1986
311. Knowles DM, Chamulak GA, Subar M et al: Lymphoid neoplasia associated with the acquired immunodeficiency syndrome (AIDS): The New York University Medical Center experience with 105 patients (1981–1986). Ann Intern Med 108:744, 1988
312. Serrano M, Bellas C, Campo E et al: Hodgkin's disease in patients with antibodies to human immunodeficiency virus: a study of 22 patients. Cancer 65:2248, 1990
313. Tirelli U, Errante D, Dolcetti R et al: Hodgkin's disease and human immunodeficiency virus infection: clinicopathologic and virologic features of 114 patients from the Italian cooperative group on AIDS and tumors. J Clin Oncol 13: 1758, 1995
314. Mauch PM, Kalish LA, Kadin M et al: Patterns of presentation of Hodgkin disease: implications for etiology and pathogenesis. Cancer 71:2062, 1993
315. Rosenberg SA, Kaplan HS: Evidence for an orderly progression in the spread of Hodgkin's disease. Cancer Res 26:1225, 1966
316. Gamble JF, Fuller LM, Martin RG et al: Influence of staging celiotomy in localized presentations of Hodgkin's disease. Cancer 35:817, 1975
317. Urba WJ, Longo DL: Hodgkin's disease. N Engl J Med 326:678, 1992
318. Leibenhaut MH, Hoppe RT, Efron B et al: Prog-

nostic indicators of laparotomy findings in clinical stage I–II supradiaphragmatic Hodgkin's disease. J Clin Oncol 7:81, 1989
319. Mauch P, Larson D, Osteen R et al: Prognostic factors for positive surgical staging in patients with Hodgkin's disease. J Clin Oncol 8:257, 1990
320. Rosenberg SA: Exploratory laparotomy and splenectomy for Hodgkin's disease: a commentary. J Clin Oncol 6:574, 1988
321. DeVita VT, Hubbard SM, Longo DL: Treatment of Hodgkin's disease. J Natl Cancer Inst Monogr 10:19, 1990
322. Healey EA, Tarbell NJ, Kalish LA et al: Prognostic factors for patients with Hodgkin disease in first relapse. Cancer 71:2613, 1993
323. Mauch P, Tarbell N, Weinstein H et al: Stage IA and IIA supradiaphragmatic Hodgkin's disease: prognostic factors in surgically staged patients treated with mantle and para-aortic irradiation. J Clin Oncol 6:1576, 1988
324. Weinshel EL, Peterson BA: Hodgkin's disease. Ca Cancer J Clin 43:327, 1993
325. Longo DL: The use of chemotherapy in the treatment of Hodgkin's disease. Semin Oncol 17:716, 1990
326. Anderson JE, Litzow MR, Appelbaum FR et al: Allogeneic, syngeneic, and autologous marrow transplantation for Hodgkin's disease: the 21-year Seattle experience. J Clin Oncol 11:2342, 1993
327. Jones RJ, Piantadosi S, Mann RB et al: High-dose cytotoxic therapy and bone marrow transplantation for relapsed Hodgkin's disease. J Clin Oncol 8:527, 1990
328. Linch DC, Winfield D, Goldstone AH et al: Dose intensification with autologous bone-marrow transplantation in relapsed and resistant Hodgkin's disease: results of a BNLI randomised trial. Lancet 341:1051, 1993
329. Nademanee A, O'Donnell MR, Snyder DS et al: High-dose chemotherapy with or without total body irradiation followed by autologous bone marrow and/or peripheral blood stem cell transplantation for patients with relapsed and refractory Hodgkin's disease: results in 85 patients with analysis of prognostic factors. Blood 85: 1381, 1995
330. Straus DJ, Gaynor JJ, Myers J et al: Prognostic factors among 185 adults with newly diagnosed advanced Hodgkin's disease treated with alternating potentially noncross-resistant chemotherapy and intermediate-dose radiation therapy. J Clin Oncol 8:1173, 1990
331. Dimopoulos MA, Cabanillas F, Lee JJ et al: Prognostic role of serum β_2-microglobulin in Hodgkin's disease. J Clin Oncol 11:1108, 1993
332. Gause A, Roschansky V, Tschiersch A et al: Low serum interleukin-2 levels correlate with a good prognosis in patients with Hodgkin's lymphoma. Ann Oncol 2:43, 1991
333. Gause A, Pohl C, Tschiersch A et al: Clinical significance of soluble CD30 antigen in the sera of patients with untreated Hodgkin's disease. Blood 77:1983, 1991
334. Pizzolo G, Chilosi M, Vinante F et al: Soluble interleukin-2 receptors in the serum of patients with Hodgkin's disease. Br J Cancer 55:427, 1987
335. Pizzolo G, Vinante F, Chilosi M et al: Serum levels of soluble CD30 molecule (Ki-1 antigen) in Hodgkin's disease: relationship with disease activity and clinical stage. Br J Haematol 75: 282, 1990
336. Pui C-H, Ip SH, Thompson E et al: High serum interleukin-2 receptor levels correlate with a poor prognosis in children with Hodgkin's disease. Leukemia 3:481, 1989
337. Guinee VF, Giacco GG, Durand M et al: The prognosis of Hodgkin's disease in older adults. J Clin Oncol 9:947, 1991
338. Alavaikko MJ, Blanco G, Aine R et al: Follicular dendritic cells have prognostic relevance in Hodgkin's disease. Am J Clin Pathol 101:761, 1994
339. Claviez A, Tiemann M, Peters J et al: The impact of EBV, proliferation rate, and bcl-2 expression in Hodgkin's disease in childhood. Ann Hematol 68:61, 1994
340. Fellbaum C, Hansmann M-L, Niedermeyer H et al: Influence of Epstein-Barr virus genomes on patient survival in Hodgkin's disease. Am J Clin Pathol 98:319, 1992
341. Molot RJ, Mendenhall NP, Barre DM, Braylan RC: The clinical relevance of L26, a B-cell-specific antibody, in Hodgkin's disease. Am J Clin Oncol 17:185, 1994
342. Ferry JA, Linggood RM, Convery KM et al: Hodgkin's disease, nodular sclerosis type: implications of histologic subclassification. Cancer 71:457, 1993
343. Wijlhuizen TJ, Vrints LW, Jairam R et al: Grades of nodular sclerosis (NSI-NSII) in

Hodgkin's disease: are they of independent prognostic value? Cancer 63:1150, 1989

344. d'Amore ESG, Lee CKK, Aeppli DM: Lack of prognostic value of histopathologic parameters in Hodgkin's disease, nodular sclerosis type: a study of 123 patients with limited stage disease who had undergone laparotomy and were treated with radiation therapy. Arch Pathol Lab Med 116:856, 1992
345. Hess JL, Bodis S, Pinkus G et al: Histopathologic grading of nodular sclerosis Hodgkin's disease: lack of prognostic significance in 254 surgically staged patients. Cancer 74:708, 1994
346. Masih AS, Weisenburger DD, Vose JM et al: Histologic grade does not predict prognosis in optimally treated, advanced-stage nodular sclerosing Hodgkin's disease. Cancer 69:228, 1992
347. Suster S: Transformation of Hodgkin's disease into malignant fibrous histiocytoma. Cancer 57: 264, 1986
348. Cimino G, Papa G, Tura S et al: Second primary cancer following Hodgkin's disease: updated results of an Italian multicentric study. J Clin Oncol 9:432, 1991
349. Swerdlow AJ, Douglas AJ, Hudson GV et al: Risk of second primary cancers after Hodgkin's disease by type of treatment: analysis of 2846 patients in the British National Lymphoma Investigation. BMJ 304:1137, 1992
350. Tucker MA, Coleman CN, Cox RS et al: Risk of second cancers after treatment for Hodgkin's disease. N Engl J Med 318:76, 1988
351. Valagussa P, Santoro A, Fossati-Bellani F et al: Second acute leukemia and other malignancies following treatment for Hodgkin's disease. J Clin Oncol 4:830, 1986
352. van Rijswijk REN, Verbeek J, Haanen C et al: Major complications and causes of death in patients treated for Hodgkin's disease. J Clin Oncol 5:1624, 1987
353. Jaffe ES, Zarate-Osorno A, Medeiros LJ: The interrelationship of Hodgkin's disease and non-Hodgkin's lymphomas—lessions learned from composite and sequential malignancies. Semin Diagn Pathol 9:297, 1992
354. Jaffe ES, Zarate-Osorno A, Kingma DW et al: The interrelationship between Hodgkin's disease and non-Hodgkin's lymphomas. Ann Oncol 5(Suppl 1):S7, 1994
355. Bennett MH, MacLennon KA, Hudson G, Hudson B: Non-Hodgkin's lymphoma arising in patients treated for Hodgkin's disease in the BNLI: a 20-year experience. Ann Oncol 2(Suppl 2):83, 1991
356. Büchner SA: Sézary syndrome after successful treatment of Hodgkin's disease. Arch Dermatol 117:50, 1981
357. Casey TT, Cousar JB, Mangum M et al: Monomorphic lymphomas arising in patients with Hodgkin's disease: correlation of morphologic, immunophenotypic, and molecular genetic findings in 12 cases. Am J Pathol 136:81, 1990
358. Dick FR, Maca RD, Hankenson R: Hodgkin's disease terminating in a T-cell immunoblastic leukemia. Cancer 42:1325, 1978
359. Gowitt GT, Chan WC, Brynes RK, Heffner LT: T-cell lymphoma following Hodgkin's disease. Cancer 56:1191, 1985
360. Krikorian JG, Burke JS, Rosenberg SA, Kaplan HS: Occurrence of non-Hodgkin's lymphoma after therapy for Hodgkin's disease. N Engl J Med 300:452, 1979
361. Zarate-Osorno A, Medeiros LJ, Longo DL, Jaffe ES: Non-Hodgkin's lymphomas arising in patients successfully treated for Hodgkin's disease: a clinical, histologic, and immunophenotypic study of 14 cases. Am J Surg Pathol 16: 885, 1992
362. Gonzalez CL, Medeiros LJ, Jaffe ES: Composite lymphoma: a clinicopathologic analysis of nine patients with Hodgkin's disease and B-cell non-Hodgkin's lymphoma. Am J Clin Pathol 96:81, 1991
363. Richter MN: Generalized reticular cell sarcoma of lymph nodes associated with lymphatic leukemia. Am J Pathol 4:285, 1928
364. Rubin D, Hudnall SD, Aisenberg A et al: Richter's transformation of chronic lymphocytic leukemia with Hodgkin's-like cells is associated with Epstein-Barr virus infections. Mod Pathol 7:91, 1994
365. Brecher M, Banks PM: Hodgkin's disease variant of Richter's syndrome: report of eight cases. Am J Clin Pathol 93:333, 1990
366. Choi H, Keller RH: Coexistance of chronic lymphocytic leukemia and Hodgkin's disease. Cancer 48:48, 1981
367. Weisenberg E, Anastasi J, Adeyanju M et al: Hodgkin's disease associated with chronic lymphocytic leukemia. Eight additional cases, including two of the nodular lymphocyte predominant type. Am J Clin Pathol 103:479, 1995
368. Momose H, Jaffe ES, Shin SS et al: Chronic lymphocytic leukemia/small lymphocytic lym-

phoma with Reed-Sternberg-like cells and possible transformation to Hodgkin's disease: mediation by Epstein-Barr virus. Am J Surg Pathol 16:859, 1992

369. Williams J, Schned A, Cotelingam JD, Jaffe ES: Chronic lymphocytic leukemia with coexistent Hodgkin's disease: implications for the origin of the Reed-Sternberg cell. Am J Surg Pathol 15:33, 1991
370. Travis LB, Curtis RE, Boice JD et al: Second cancers following non-Hodgkin's lymphoma. Cancer 67:2002, 1991
371. Travis LB, Gonzalez CL, Hankey BF, Jaffe ES: Hodgkin's disease following non-Hodgkin's lymphoma. Cancer 69:2337, 1992
372. Zarate-Osorno A, Medeiros LJ, Kingma DW et al: Hodgkin's disease following non-Hodgkin's lymphoma: a clinicopathologic and immunophenotypic study of nine cases. Am J Surg Pathol 17:123, 1993
373. Chan WC, Griem ML, Grozea PN et al: Mycosis fungoides and Hodgkin's disease occurring in the same patient. Report of three cases. Cancer 44:1408, 1979
374. Donald D, Green JA, White M: Mycosis fungoides associated with nodular sclerosing Hodgkin's disease: a case report. Cancer 46:2505, 1980
375. Hawkins KA, Schinella R, Schwartz M et al: Simultaneous occurrence of mycosis fungoides and Hodgkin's disease: clinical and histologic correlations in three cases with ultrastructural studies in two. Am J Hematol 14:355, 1983
376. Simrell CR, Boccia RV, Longo DL, Jaffe ES: Coexisting Hodgkin's disease and mycosis fungoides: immunohistochemical proof of its existence. Arch Pathol Lab Med 110:1029, 1986

4

Nodular Lymphocyte Predominance Type of Hodgkin's Disease

Sibrand Poppema

DEVELOPMENT OF THE TERMINOLOGY

In the classification of Hodgkin's disease as published by Jackson and Parker[1] in 1947, three subtypes were identified, termed *Hodgkin's paragranuloma, Hodgkin's granuloma,* and *Hodgkin's sarcoma.* Hodgkin's paragranuloma was characterized by obliteration of the normal lymph node architecture by an abundance of small lymphocytes among which Reed-Sternberg (RS) cells were present as single cells or in small groups. Neither necrosis nor fibrosis was present, and plasma cells and eosinophils were absent or inconspicuous. Jackson had previously described such cases under the name *early Hodgkin's disease,* but, because of the often very long duration of the disease (up to 39 years) with no change in the histologic picture, he subsequently coined the term *Hodgkin's paragranuloma,* meaning a condition closely related to Hodgkin's granuloma. In a study of follicular lymphomas, Rappaport et al.[2] described a nodular variant of paragranuloma.

In the classification of Hodgkin's disease as proposed by Lukes and Butler[3] in 1966, six subgroups were identified, including lymphohistiocytic nodular subtype and lymphohistiocytic diffuse subtype. In the nodular lymphohistiocytic cases, a nodular growth pattern with a predominance of small lymphocytes and varying numbers of benign appearing histiocytes could be identified in addition to so-called L&H (lymphocytic and histiocytic) RS cells. It was stated that typical RS cells could and should be found, be it in low numbers.

In the diffuse lymphohistiocytic cases the cellular proliferation was essentially the same as in the nodular type. Some cases had a very high content of histiocytes. At the Rye Symposium on "Obstacles to the Control of Hodgkin's Disease," the histologic grading of Hodgkin's disease was discussed. It was decided that for general use it would be better to reduce the six subclasses of Lukes and Butler to four, combining the lymphohistiocytic nodular and diffuse types to lymphocyte predominance. This so-called Rye classification[4] subsequently became generally accepted for subclassification of Hodgkin's disease.

Lennert and Mohri[5] introduced a more differentiated classification system for Hodgkin's disease. This included four subtypes of lymphocyte predominance: nodular paragranuloma; diffuse paragranuloma; lymphocyte predominance, others; and partial involvement. The key feature of this classification was the distinction between nodular and diffuse paragranuloma and the "other" lymphocyte predominance cases. These other lymphocyte predominance cases did not show the L&H type RS cells, but instead did have typical RS cells or lacunar cells, and they contained more eosinophils, plasma cells, and more pronounced fibrosis than paragranuloma.

In 1979, we published a series of three papers on the histology, immunophenotype, and epidemiology of the nodular and diffuse lymphocyte predominance subtype of Hodgkin's disease, indicating that nodular lymphocyte predominance Hodgkin's disease (NLPHD) is a separate entity.[6–8] In these papers also the association between progressively transformed germinal centers and NLPHD was established as well as the first documented cases of transition to a large cell lymphoma. Further, it was shown that NLPHD and its diffuse variant (nodular paragranuloma and diffuse paragranuloma) did not transform to other subtypes in contrast to the category of lymphocyte predominance, other, that has few but typical RS cells and will transform to mixed cellularity in subsequent biopsies.

In the past decade, NLPHD (i.e., nodular paragranuloma) has been resurrected in recognition of a large number of studies confirming the striking differences in histogenesis and immunophenotype between this type of Hodgkin's disease and the other subtypes. This distinction was recently recognized in a proposal by the European and American Lymphoma Study Group in the so-called REAL classification.[9]

HISTOLOGY OF NODULAR LYMPHOCYTE PREDOMINANCE HODGKIN'S DISEASE

Complete obliteration of the lymph node architecture is usually present. In some cases a compressed rim of normal lymphoid tissue with reactive follicles is present in the periphery of the node, usually sharply demarcated from the tumor tissue. Between the nodules, small areas of diffuse lymphoid tissue are found. The nodular character of the process is generally easily appreciated in routine H&E slides, but in some cases a reticulin stain aids in recognition of the nodularity by virtue of the compression of reticulin fibers in the interfollicular area. The nodules vary in size, but are mostly large and oval (Fig. 4-1). In some cases, part of the process or even the vast majority has a diffuse growth pattern. This strongly suggests a relation between the nodular type and a diffuse variant.

The predominant cell population in the nodules is small lymphocytes. The presence of histiocytes and L&H type RS cells leads to a ''moth-eaten'' appearance. The number of epithelioid histiocytes varies, and in some cases they are the most conspicuous type of cell. This finding lead to the original term *lymphocytic and histiocytic type of Hodgkin's disease*. Scattered dendritic reticulum cell nuclei can be identified; in some cases multinucleated, Warthin-Finkeldey type giant cells are seen. These are multinucleated dendritic reticulum cell variants. The cellular composition of the nodules may vary within the same lymph node: nodules with a predominance of lymphocytes can be seen together with nodules showing a large proportion of epithelioid histiocytes. While occasionally only a small number of L&H type RS cells are present, usually they are found with little difficulty. In rare cases they form large clusters and are the most conspicuous cell type within some nodules. The compressed internodular areas contain small lymphocytes and high endothelial venules. Plasma cells and eosinophils are characteristically scarce or absent. In some cases, groups of epithelioid cells similar to those in toxoplasmosis can be found in the internodular areas, sometimes in a circular pattern around the nodules.

In some cases of NLPHD with classical features, both histomorphologic and immunophenotypic, there is a nodular sclerotic stromal reaction. Because a documented history of long-term nodal enlargement was available in some of these, it is possible that this represents a very chronic phase tissue reaction to the NLPHD.

MORPHOLOGICAL CHARACTERISTICS OF L&H TYPE RS CELLS

L&H type RS cells are large cells. Their nuclei are clearly larger than those of large noncleaved cells (Fig. 4-2). Due to their complex lobation my colleagues and I likened them to elephant's feet, although the term *popcorn cells* has been more widely applied (Fig. 4-2). The nucleoli are medium sized and appear relatively smaller than those of typical RS cells. The cytoplasm of L&H type RS cells is relatively sparse (Fig. 4-3). In Giemsa-stained tissue sections and

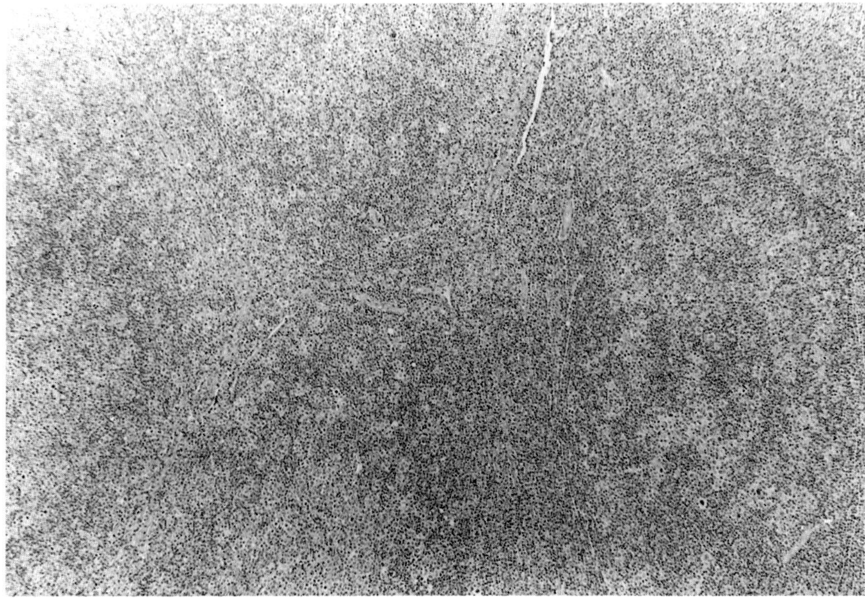

Fig. 4-1. Low magnification (objective ×2.5) of case of NLPHD. Note the presence of vague nodules with a so called moth-eaten aspect of the nodules as a result of the presence of L&H cells and some histiocytes between a majority of small lymphocytes.

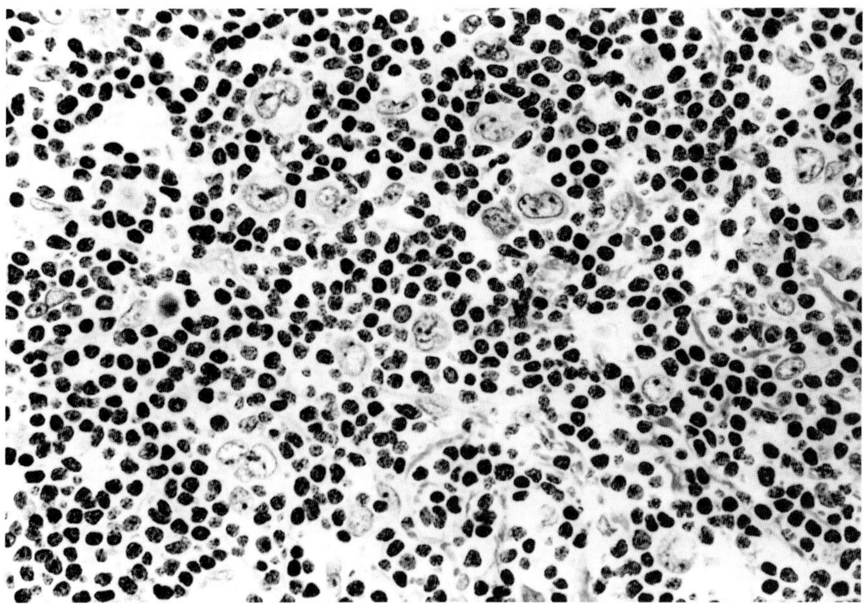

Fig. 4-2. Higher magnification (objective ×25) of a nodule of NLPHD. Note the presence of lobated nuclei with relatively small nucleoli and a small rim of cytoplasm in the L&H type R-S cells.

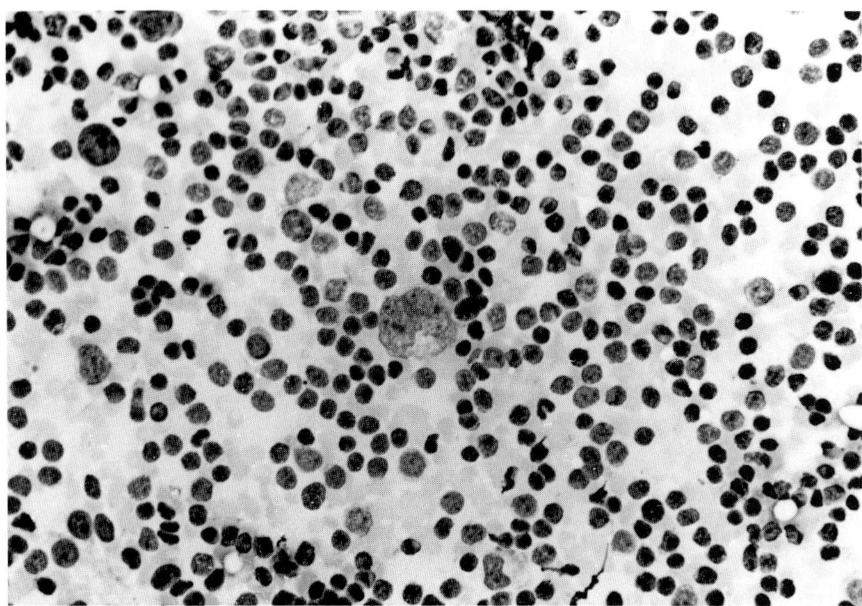

Fig. 4-3. Higher magnification (objective ×25) of inprint of the same lymph node showing lobated L&H type R-S cell with small rim of cytoplasm.

in Wright-stained imprints or smears the cytoplasm stains moderately or darkly basophilic, whereas the cytoplasm of typical RS cells is only lightly basophilic and that of lacunar cells is abundant and lightly stained. There may be a considerable number of mitoses in the L&H type RS cells. At the ultrastructural level, rough endoplasmic reticulum and a prominent Golgi area can be identified.

IMMUNOPHENOTYPE AND GENOTYPE OF THE L&H TYPE RS CELLS

Immunostains for proliferation associated nuclear proteins such as Ki-67 or PCNA-cyclin are positive in the L&H cells, indicating that they are in cycle. In contrast to the immunophenotyping studies of RS cells in general, the findings in L&H type RS cells have been very consistent. The original demonstration[10] that they produce J chain in contrast to other types of RS cells has recently been confirmed.[11] Since J chain is not present in serum, the demonstration of J chain in the L&H cells is definitive proof of the B-cell origin of L&H cells.

Many groups have found consistent staining for pan-B-cell markers such as CD20 and CD22 in frozen sections and MB1, MB2, KiB3, and L26 in paraffin tissue sections of NLPHD cases[12–16] (Fig. 4-4). This differs from RS cells in other subtypes that stain for B-cell markers in only a minority of cases and generally only in a proportion of the cells.[17,18] The staining for L26 that recognizes a cytoplasmic precursor of CD20 clearly exceeds that of membrane CD20 in many cases. We have recently found that such a dissociation of L26 and membrane CD20 staining can be found in some Epstein-Barr virus transformed lymphoblastoid cell lines (S. Poppema, unpublished data).

L&H type cells also stain for CD40, CD70, CD80, CD86, CDw75, HLA class II, and CD74 (the invariant chain of HLA class II).[19,20] All of these are also expressed on normal germinal center blasts, with the exception of CD70, which is the receptor for CD27. Frequently, a proportion of the L&H type Reed-Sternberg cells also reacts with antibodies against epithelial membrane antigen.[11,12,21] With respect to CD30 (Ki-1, Ber-H2) staining, variable results have been obtained.[22,23] At most, L&H type RS cells show

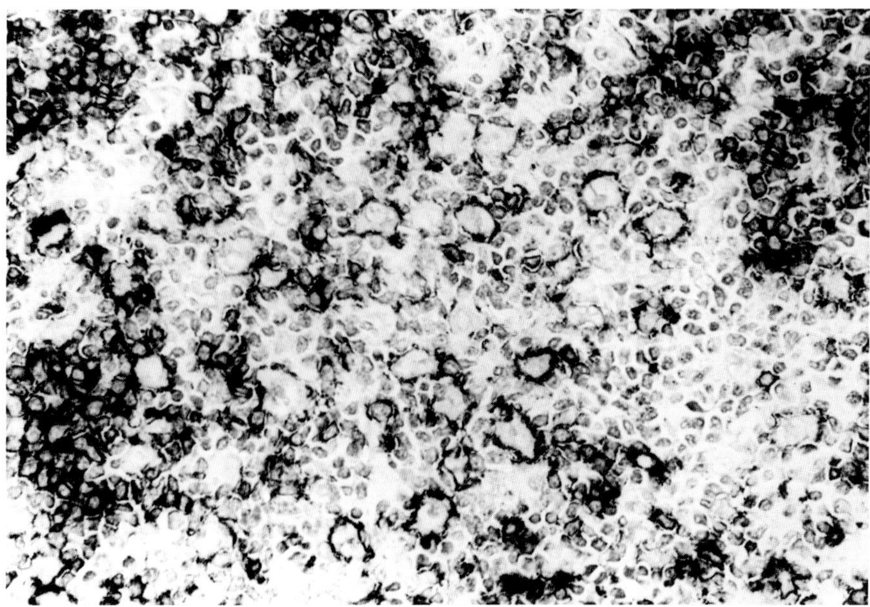

Fig. 4-4. Immunoperoxidase stain on formalin fixed paraffin section of NLPHD stained for L26 (CD20). Note strongly stained large L&H cells surrounded by negative small lymphocytes and some small aggregates of B lymphocytes in a nodule of this relatively T cell rich NLPHD case (objective ×25).

weak staining in frozen tissue sections. Similarly, staining for CD15 (Leu M1) has been reported varyingly, though most studies conclude that L&H type RS cells are negative.[24,25] The immunotypes for L&H cells are as follows:

CD20 +, CD75 +
J chain +
CD40 +, CD70 +
CD80 +, CD86 +
Class II +, CD74 +
CD45 +, EMA +
CD15 −, CD30 −

L&H type RS cells have been found to stain with antileukocyte common antigen (LCA, CD45) antibodies, specifically with CD45RB and CD45RA reagents, whereas other RS cells generally are not reactive with anti-LCA reagents.[25] This is interesting since it indicates that RS cells generally lack the dominant lymphoid tyrosine phosphatase, which has been found to be necessary for T-cell differentiation and activation and for B-cell activation.

The results indicate that L&H type RS cells are of B-cell origin. Clonality of the L&H cell population has been difficult to demonstrate. This is an important question, since this in combination with chromosomal alterations would provide a clue toward the question as to whether NLPHD is a (low grade) B-cell lymphoma or should be considered a premalignant condition. Attempts to demonstrate clonality immunohistochemically by light chain restriction have generally been unsuccessful. In our original study we found that the cells in one nodule were predominantly of one light chain class; however, cells positive for both κ and λ were found.[7] A complicating factor is the presence of endocytosed IgG in addition to IgG produced by the L&H cells. A recent study reported clonal staining in a majority of the 19 cases studied with paraffin tissue section.[26]

Studies using in situ hybridization to detect κ or λ mRNA have lead to conflicting results.[27–29] A recent paper[29] reported that 80 percent of the cases studied had monotypic light chain, with virtually all cases being κ positive. This is consistent with immunohistologic findings showing a predominance of κ. However, the study also showed the small lymphocytic component to be κ positive in half of the cases. This is inconsistent with light chain typing on frozen tissue and suggests that the κ probe in this study may have outperformed the λ probe. Southern blot analysis of NLPHD tissue does not show clonal Ig gene rearrangement.[30] The use of a polymerase chain reaction (PCR) procedure for the analysis of immunoglobulin heavy chain gene rearrangements has been reported as showing frequent clonal VDJ rearrangement with somatic mutations in the V_H genes.[31] Single cell analysis by PCR for the Ig gene was reported as clonal in one paper but was not confirmed in another study.[32,33] A problem of single cell analysis is the small number of cells analyzed, which when taken from one region of the node may show one clone and when taken from multiple regions may show multiple clones. The ideal method would entail the preparation of a probe based on the sequence of one identified clone and testing by in situ hybridization on tissue sections to analyze which proportion of L&H cells, and perhaps other cells, belongs to this clone. Subsequently, cells negative for this probe could be analyzed, and the procedure could be repeated until the majority of L&H cells were accounted for. In addition, the clonal relation between NLPHD, progressively transformed germinal centers (PTGCs), and large cell lymphoma could be established by such a procedure.

In conclusion, it is likely that at least some cases of NLPHD contain one or a limited number of B-cell clones, most likely the L&H cells. Cytogenetic studies in a small number of cases have shown the presence of clonal cytogenetic abnormalities, indicating the presence of an abnormal clone in NLPHD, similar to findings in other types of Hodgkin's disease. One has to realize, however, that these abnormalities are not necessarily exclusively in the L&H cells or present in all the L&H cells. Surprisingly, there appears to be an overrepresentation of κ positive L&H cells in individual cases and of κ positive cases overall. In some cases this may develop into a clonal tumor, the so-called large cell lymphomas developing in approximately 5 percent of patients with NLPHD. PTGCs are most likely a polyclonal precursor lesion. The natural history of NLPHD then might consist of a polyclonal stage, the progressively transformed germinal centers, an oligoclonal stage, NLPHD, and a monoclonal stage, the large cell B-cell lymphoma (see below).

IMMUNOPHENOTYPE OF THE B LYMPHOCYTES

In most cases the majority of lymphocytes in the nodules consist of small B lymphocytes. This was originally demonstrated by erythrocyte antibody complement rosetting and by their reactivity for immunoglobulin.[34] The accumulation of small B lymphocytes in PTGCs and in NLPHD nodules can result from increased migration through high endothelial venules or from retainment or a combination of these factors. The size of follicles normally is determined by a balance between the entry and exit of the recirculating follicular B-cell population and the degree of transformation to follicular center blasts and the amount of apoptosis. The small mantle zone lymphocytes have a lifespan of several weeks (more than 3 weeks), and new cells are continuously produced in the bone marrow. The lymphocytes are of polyclonal origin (i.e., they stain partly for κ and partly for λ light chains) and by gene rearrangement show no clonally rearranged bands. In addition, the majority expresses membrane IgM and IgD, similar to normal mantle zone B lymphocytes.[35,36] These lymphocytes otherwise also have the immunophenotype of mantle zone primary B lymphocytes, are Ki-B3 positive, and are MT3 negative.[37] The expression of CD23 is relatively strong, which has also been noted in progressively transformed germinal centers.[38] Interleukin-4 (IL-4) is known to upregulate CD23 on B cells[39] and also to induce immunoglobulin producing B cells to switch isotype to IgG1 or IgE in mice and IgE in human.[40] The immunophenotype of small B cells in NLPHD/PTGC are as follows:

Polyclonal
CD20 +
IgM +, IgD +
CD5 −, CD43 −
CD10 −
CD23 +
KiB3 +, MT3 −

IMMUNOPHENOTYPE OF THE T CELLS

The number of T cells in the nodules is highly variable, ranging from a minority to a vast majority of cells directly surrounding the L&H cells (Fig. 4-5). They have a distinctive T-cell immunophenotype, being CD2 +, CD3 +, CD4 +, and CD57 +.[12,36,41,42] The complete immunophenotype of T cells in NLPHD/PTGC as follows:

Polyclonal
CD2 +, CD3 +, TCR$\alpha\beta$+
CD4 +, CD8 −
CD45R0 +, CD45RB^{dim}
CD69 +, CD26 −
CD57 (leu7) +
CD40L −

This T-cell subset is normally present only in germinal centers of secondary follicles.[44] The CD57/CD4 T cells are an intriguing T-cell subpopulation. They are exclusively present in germinal centers and within these are mostly confined to the light zones, where cleaved cells and cells with plasmacellular differentiation predominate. They are not found in the earliest phases of germinal center reactions when proliferating small noncleaved cells predominate. They are also not the population of T cells that can be identified in a rim-like pattern at the border of germinal center and mantle zone. The localization of the CD57 + cells suggests that these T cells are involved in B-cell differentiation rather than B-cell proliferation. The staining intensity for CD57 varies, and it appears that it represents an activation antigen on germinal center T cells. In accordance with this, germinal center T cells and the T cells in PTGC and NLPHD also strongly express CD69 as an early activation marker, but not HLA class II, CD25, or CD71. In a semiquantitative study we have demonstrated that the T cells directly surrounding L&H cells in NLPHD are CD57 positive,

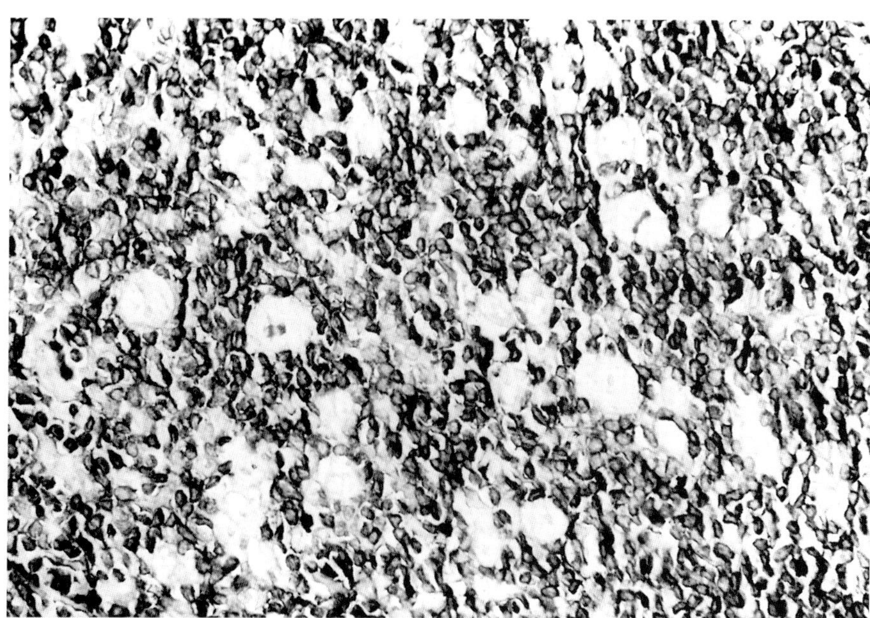

Fig. 4-5. Immunoperoxidase stain on formalin fixed paraffin section of NLPHD stained for CD3. Note majority of positive staining small lymphocytes surrounding the negative L&H cells. (Same case as Fig. 4-4.)

whereas those in other subtypes are negative. This finding appears to be another useful criterion in the differential diagnosis of NLPHD from other types of Hodgkin's disease.[16] The function of CD57+ cells is largely unknown. They do not have natural killer cell function in vitro.[44] Bowen et al.[45] studied isolated CD57+ cells in vitro and found that they did not produce IL-2, IL-4, interferon-α, or interferon-γ. Recently, it was demonstrated that unstimulated, CD57+ CD4+ T cells isolated from tonsils consistently express mRNA for IL-4, whereas CD57− CD4+ cells generally do not.[46] IL-4 is known to induce CD23[39] and also to induce B cells to switch isotype to IgG1 or IgE in mice and IgE in humans.[40] It is likely that these cells play a role in the regulation of B cell differentiation in the light zone of germinal centers.

In the nodules of NLPHD, CD57/CD4 T cells surround the L&H type RS cells, but they are also increased in PTGCs, and we have seen increased numbers in the mantle zones of reactive follicles in a case with PTGCs. This suggests that the CD57/CD4 cells may play a primary role in the development of the lesions. The relatively high expression of CD23 on the B lymphocytes in NLPHD and in progressively transformed germinal centers is of interest in view of the known ability of IL-4 to induce CD23. A subpopulation of T helper cells present in follicles can interact with B cells through a receptor termed T-BAM,[47] now known to be the CD40 ligand and increase the CD23 expression. However, we have not been able to identify CD40 ligand positive T cells in the nodules of NLPHD or in PTGC.

DENDRITIC RETICULUM CELLS

The dendritic reticulum cells are CD21+, CD35+, DRC+, but CD23− and therefore resemble the dendritic reticulum cells as seen in mantle zones and not those in germinal centers. They also do not carry immunoglobulin complexes. The major interaction between dendritic reticulum cells and B cells appears to be mediated by the LFA-1 (CD11a/CD18) and ICAM-1 (CD54) pathway.[48]

RELATION TO PROGRESSIVELY TRANSFORMED GERMINAL CENTERS

PTGCs can be found in nonspecific reactive lymphadenitis and are characterized by their large size and high content of small lymphocytes compared with primary and secondary follicles.[8,49] Some large noncleaved cells and cleaved cells can be found among the small lymphocytes, and these are sometimes arranged in clusters. In addition, dendritic reticulum cells and multinucleated Warthin-Finkeldey type giant cells can be seen. There are transitions between hyperplastic secondary follicles and PTGC. Distinguishing characteristics of PTGCs are as follows:

Larger than normal follicle
Absence of germinal center cells
Increase of small B lymphocytes
IgM+, IgD+, CD23+, KiB3+, MT3−, CD5−, CD43−
Increase of CD4+, CD57+ T cells
Decrease of CD40L+ T cells
Dendritic reticulum cells without Ig complexes
DRC+, CD21+, CD23−, as in mantle zones

Immunophenotypic studies of PTGC show polyclonal IgM, IgD positive lymphocytes, dendritic reticulum cells, and CD57+ T cells. In fact, the only difference between PTGC and the nodules of NLPHD is the absence of L&H type RS cells.

In the original report on the association between the presence of PTGC and NLPHD, five cases that had PTGC and nodular paragranuloma in lymph node biopsies that were performed at various times over 2 to 20 years were presented.[6] All possible combinations were encountered, with PTGC preceding or following NLPHD or occurring in separate lymph nodes at the same time. Since then, many other studies have confirmed this association.[50–53] PTGC are most often found in the second decade with a predominance of male patients. In a series of 66 cases of hyperplasia with PTGC it was found that the number of PTGC per slide was 1 to 3 in 53 percent, 4 to 7 in 25.8 percent, 8 to 12 in 16.7 percent, and over 11 in only 4.5 percent. The remaining follicles were hyperplastic. In 27 percent groups of epithelioid histiocytes were present. In this series 11 patients who had PTGC were found to have NLPHD, three before, four simultaneous, and four after the diagnosis of NLPHD.[53] However, no study has convincingly shown that the presence of a few progressively transformed germinal centers in a case of reactive nonspecific hyperplasia actually carries an increased risk for the development of NLPHD. Osborne and Butler[54] followed 50 patients with progressive transformation of germinal centers. Ten of these had coincidental or prior NLPHD, eight had prior Hodgkin's disease of other subtype, and one developed myeloma. The remaining 31 had no evidence of malignant disease at all, although the median follow-up was only 4 years (range 1 month to 20 years).

The extremely long natural history of some cases of NLPHD should be kept in mind before dismissing the possibility of such an association. Moreover, cases in which one cannot make a diagnosis of Hodgkin's disease only because of the absence of (L&H type) RS cells have a high incidence of NLPHD in subsequent biopsies. The frequent association and the structural similarity between PTGC and the nodules of NLPHD suggest either that PTGC are a precursor of NLPHD or that both may be manifestations of a similar abnormal B-cell reaction.

We have identified two patients with NLPHD who had progressive hypogammaglobulinemia during their disease; additionally we found PTGC in the lymph nodes of a patient with documented acquired hypogammaglobulinemia.[55] Similarly, Lennert and Hansmann[52] reported two cases of NLPHD followed by generalized lymphadenopathy with PTGC in which there was a humoral immunodeficiency (IgA or IgM deficiency). Immunologic studies on peripheral blood cells of patients with NLPHD have not shown excessive suppressor activity. However, in one patient with NLPHD and hypogammaglobulinemia the peripheral blood B lymphocytes showed insufficient maturation to plasma cells upon in vitro stimulation with pokeweed mitogen. These findings may be related to the absence of plasma cells in the lesions of NLPHD, to the scarcity of germinal center blasts in PTGC and NLPHD nodules, as well as to the expression of IgD on the L&H type RS cells in some of our cases. It is plausible that PTGCs and NLPHD are manifestations of an abnormal follicular center reaction based on B- or T-cell defects.

LARGE CELL LYMPHOMA

In the initial histologic study of NLPHD we described two cases with a transition to immunoblastic lymphoma and suggested that this might be the result of a further transformation of nodules with a predominance of L&H type RS cells.[6] Sarcomatous change of paragranuloma was earlier described by Robb-Smith[56] in 1964. He stated that the interval was usually 10 to 15 years. An increased risk for the development of subsequent non-Hodgkin's lymphomas in patients with NLPHD was subsequently documented by Miettinen et al.[57] They described 51 cases of NLPHD with a follow-up of 4 to 21 years. In five cases a diffuse large cell non-Hodgkin's lymphoma was diagnosed between 4 and 11 years after the primary diagnosis. They stated that it was unlikely that these were therapy induced, since only one of the patients had previously been irradiated. In addition, a number of case reports described "composite lymphomas" consisting of NLPHD and large cell lymphoma present in the same tumor mass.[58,59]

It is a relatively frequent finding to see nodules with an almost pure population of L&H type cells in otherwise classical cases of NLPHD.[6] Nevertheless, the general debate is whether the large cell lymphomas represent a separate, second malignancy or whether they are in fact a transition toward a lymphocyte depleted type of

Hodgkin's disease, or, finally, whether NLPHD just represents a precursor lesion of large cell lymphoma with further transformation of a subclone of B cells. This question has been addressed in a study of seven cases compiled from the NIH case consultation files that had NLPHD with large confluent sheets of L&H like cells, resembling large cell lymphoma.[60] All these patients had localized disease, and six of seven achieved long-term disease-free survival following radiation therapy or chemotherapy for Hodgkin's disease. None of these patients developed disseminated large cell lymphoma. Gene analysis studies performed in one of these cases demonstrated rearranged heavy and light chain immunoglobulin genes in this large cell population, demonstrating the presence of a clonal B-cell population. In another study, Hansmann and Lennert[61] found 14 cases (3 percent) of large cell lymphomas among a series of 441 cases of NLPHD. Six cases were classified as centroblastic (multilobated subtype), four as centroblastic (pleomorphic), three as immunoblastic, and one as Hodgkin's sarcoma. By immunohistochemistry a monoclonal staining for immunoglobulin light chains could be shown in five cases, an additional four cases were reactive with Ki-B3 (CD45Ra, B-cell restricted), and three cases were CD15+.

In conclusion, in some relatively large series of cases of NLPHD between 3 and 10 percent of the cases developed a large cell lymphoma, suggesting that there is indeed an underlying abnormal clone of B cells, most likely the L&H type RS cells that can further transform to a B-cell lymphoma. Although one would suspect a role for *bcl*-2, only one out of five cases of NLPHD tested by a PCR for *bcl*-2 was positive.[62] Also, no Epstein-Barr virus genome or virus related antigens have been demonstrated in NLPHD or in NLPHD related large cell lymphomas.[63,64]

DIFFUSE VARIANTS OF NLPHD (DIFFUSE PARAGRANULOMA)

There is some controversy as to whether a diffuse variant of nodular LPHD exists. Based on the finding that some cases of nodular LPHD have diffuse areas and other cases transform to a diffuse morphology, it appears likely that there are also primary diffuse variants. Such cases have the following histologic and immunohistologic features. They contain numerous L&H type RS cells that react with pan-B-cell reagents. In contrast to the nodular variant, they contain only a few small B lymphocytes. The predominant cells are small T lymphocytes that are CD4+ with a considerable proportion of CD57+ T cells participating in the T-cell rosettes around the L&H cells. In agreement with the absence of a nodular pattern, dendritic reticulum cells cannot be demonstrated with CD21 antibodies. The main differential diagnosis is with a T-cell-rich B-cell lymphoma. The distinguishing features are the presence of distinctive L&H type RS cells and the absence of other typical B cells, such as cleaved cells. The presence of CD57+ cell is also helpful. Immunoglobulin gene analysis studies show no clonal rearrangement in diffuse NLPHD, whereas cases of T-cell-rich B-cell lymphoma may show such rearrangement. In one of our cases an enlarged lymph node removed 2 years after the primary diagnosis showed only follicular hyperplasia with progressively transformed germinal centers.

CLINICAL FEATURES

NLPHD occurs in all age groups, with a peak incidence in the fourth decade in contrast to the third decade peak incidence of the nodular sclerosis subtype.[8] There is a male preponderance of 2.4:1, again different from the about equal numbers of patients with nodular sclerosis.[46] General symptoms, such as fever, night sweats, and weight loss, are found in only 10 percent of the patients.[65]

There is frequent involvement of cervical and axillary nodes, with less frequent inguinal or femoral nodal involvement. Mediastinal NLPHD is an extremely unusual finding.[8,65] Approximately 30 percent of the patients have advanced disease at the time of presentation.

The prognosis of NLPHD is favorable. The

life expectancy of stage I is about the same as that of the general population. Patients with splenic involvement (stage IIIS) or with stage IV have a poorer prognosis.[65] Recurrences develop in a relatively high percentage, regardless of original clinical stage, and multiple recurrences are not uncommon.[65,66] In 65 percent the recurrence occurred locally or regionally, but in 23 percent the recurrence was in a different region or the disease was generalized (12 percent).

Regula et al.[66] compared the clinical course of nodular and diffuse lymphocyte predominance cases in a series of 73 patients with NLPHD. The diffuse cases had a course similar to other types of Hodgkin's disease, with relapse and only two deaths due to Hodgkin's disease. Those with nodular type showed significantly more relapses, which were independent of stage or treatment and evenly distributed temporally up to 10 years after initial therapy. Despite these frequent relapses the patients with NLPHD followed an indolent course.

In other studies[67,68,69] no differences in relapse rate between nodular and diffuse cases were found, although unusually long intervals to relapse were observed in two patients with nodular histology.[68]

CONCLUSIONS

NLPHD has emerged as a distinct entity, different from other subtypes of Hodgkin's disease as well as from the follicular non-Hodgkin's lymphomas. The process can be identified as a polyclonal population of follicular B lymphocytes, CD4+ CD7+ germinal center T lymphocytes, and L&H type RS cells expressing B-cell markers and generally lacking CD15 and CD30. There appears to be a precursor lesion in the form of follicular hyperplasia with PTGC. Also, NLPHD transforms relatively frequently to a large cell lymphoma; nodules with increased numbers of L&H type RS cells may represent a transitional phase. Most of these large cell lymphomas are of B-cell immunophenotype, and in some cases monoclonality has been demonstrated by immunoglobulin gene analysis or chromosomal analysis. The preferred terminology for these tumors is *Hodgkin's disease, nodular lymphocyte predominance type, with coexistent large cell lymphoma.* In a few cases a proliferation of atypical T cells in combination with NLPHD has been found, but clonal T-cell receptor gene rearrangement was not detectable. It is possible that such cases represent further transformation of the CD4+ CD57+ T-cell population.

Clinically, NLPHD has a good prognosis, despite the fact that there may be relapses, including those in distant sites. The question whether NLPHD is a malignancy has not been resolved and needs further study. However, karyotyping of some cases has shown clonal chromosomal abnormalities, suggesting malignancy. Some cases progress to involve spleen and bone marrow. There is no reason to change the terminology for this disease, since it has a key characteristic in common with other subtypes of Hodgkin's disease, namely, the interaction of a majority of reactive lymphocytes with a minority of transformed lymphoid cells. Several questions remain unanswered. What is the functional significance of the increased numbers of CD4+ CD57+ T cells? What determines the transition of PTGC to NLPHD? What is the frequency and relevance of monoclonal versus oligoclonal versus polyclonal L&H cell populations? What are the mechanisms in the transformation to large cell lymphoma? Is it necessary to treat NLPHD with radiotherapy and/or chemotherapy, or is surgical excision sufficient? Long-term studies will be required to answer these questions.

REFERENCES

1. Jackson H, Parker F: Hodgkin's Disease and Allied Disorders. New York, Oxford University Press, 1947
2. Rappaport H, Winter WJ, Hicks EB: Follicular lymphoma. Cancer 9:792, 1956
3. Lukes RJ, Butler JJ: The pathology and nomenclature of Hodgkin's disease. Cancer Res 26: 1063, 1966
4. Lukes RJ, Craver LF, Hall TC et al: Report of the nomenclature committee. Cancer Res 26:1311, 1966

5. Lennert K, Mohri N: Histologische Klassifizierung und Vorkommen des Morbus Hodgkin. Internist 15:57, 1974
6. Poppema S, Kaiserling E, Lennert K: Hodgkin's disease with lymphocytic predominance, nodular type (nodular paragranuloma) and progressively transformed germinal centers—A cytohistological study. Histopathology 3:295, 1979
7. Poppema S, Kaiserling E, Lennert K: Nodular paragranuloma and progressively transformed germinal centers. Ultrastructural and immunohistologic findings. Virchows Arch [Cell Pathol] 31: 211, 1979
8. Poppema S, Kaiserling E, Lennert K: Epidemiology of nodular paragranuloma (Hodgkin's disease with lymphocytic predominance, nodular). Cancer Res Clin Oncol 95:57, 1979
9. Harris NL, Jaffe ES, Stein H et al: A revised European-American classification of lymphoid neoplasms: a proposal from the International Lymphoma Study Group. Blood 84:1361, 1994
10. Poppema S: The diversity of the immunohistological staining pattern of Sternberg-Reed cells. J Histochem Cytochem 28:788, 1980
11. Stein H, Hansmann ML, Lennert K et al: Reed-Sternberg and Hodgkin cells in lymphocyte-predominant Hodgkin's disease of nodular subtype contain J chain. Am J Clin Pathol. 86:292, 1986
12. Timens W, Visser L, Poppema S: Nodular lymphocyte predominance type of Hodgkin's disease is a germinal center lymphoma. Lab Invest 54: 457, 1986
13. Pinkus GS, Said JW: Hodgkin's disease, lymphocyte predominance type, nodular—a distinct entity? Am J Pathol 118:1, 1985
14. Coles FB, Cartun RW, Pastuszak WT: Hodgkin's disease, lymphocyte-predominant type: immunoreactivity with B cell antibodies. Mod Pathol 1: 274, 1988
15. Hansmann ML, Wacker HH, Radzun HJ: Paragranuloma is a variant of Hodgkin's disease with predominance of B-cells. Virchows Arch [Pathol Anat] 409:171, 1986
16. Poppema S: The nature of the lymphocytes surrounding Reed-Sternberg cells in nodular lymphocyte predominance and in other types of Hodgkin's disease. Am J Pathol 135:351, 1989
17. Doreen MS, Habeshaw JA, Stansfeld AG et al: Characteristics of Sternberg-Reed cells and related cells in Hodgkin's disease. Br J Cancer 49: 465, 1984
18. Poppema S, De Jong B, Atmosoerodjo J et al: Morphologic, immunologic, enzymehistochemical and chromosomal analysis of a cell line derived from Hodgkin's disease. Cancer 55:683, 1985
19. Poppema S, Visser L, de Jong B et al: Hodgkin's disease derived cell line–ZO–has typical Reed-Sternberg phenotype and Ig gene rearrangements indicating a B cell origin. Recent Res Cancer Res 117:67, 1989
20. Sherrod AE, Felder B, Levy N et al: Immunohistologic identification of phenotypic antigens associated with Hodgkin and Reed-Sternberg cells. Cancer 57:2135, 1986
21. Delsol G, Gatter KC, Stein H et al: Human lymphoid cells express epithelial membrane antigen. Implications for the diagnosis of human neoplasms. Lancet II:1124, 1984
22. Stein H, Mason DY, Gerdes J et al: The expression of Hodgkin's disease-associated antigen Ki-1 in reactive and neoplastic lymphoid tissue: evidence that Reed-Sternberg cells in histiocytic malignancies are derived from activated lymphoid cells. Blood 66:848, 1985
23. Chittal SM, Caveriviere P, Schwarting R et al: Monoclonal antibodies in the diagnosis of Hodgkin's disease. Am J Surg Pathol 12:9, 1988
24. Pinkus GS, Thomas P, Said JW et al: LeuM1—a marker for Reed-Sternberg cells in Hodgkin's disease: an immunoperoxidase study of paraffin embedded tissues. Am J Pathol 119:244, 1985
25. Dorfman RE, Gatter KC, Pulford KAF et al: An evaluation of the utility of anti-granulocyte and anti-leucocyte monoclonal antibodies in the diagnosis of Hodgkin's disease. Am J Pathol 123:508, 1986
26. Schmidt C, Sargent C, Isaacson PG: L and H cells of nodular lymphocyte predominant Hodgkin's disease show immunoglobulin light-chain restriction. Am J Pathol 139:1281, 1991
27. Momose H, Chen YY, Ben-Ezra J, Weiss LM: Nodular lymphocyte-predominant Hodgkin's disease study of immunoglobulin light chain protein and mRNA expression. Hum Pathol 23:1115, 1992
28. Hell K, Pringle JH, Hansmann ML et al: Demonstration of light chain mRNA in Hodgkin's disease. J Pathol 171:137, 1993
29. Stoler MH, Nichols GE, Symbula M, Weiss LM: Lymphocyte predominance Hodgkin's disease. Evidence for a κ light chain-restricted monotypic B-cell neoplasm. Am J Pathol 146:812, 1995
30. Weiss LM: Gene analysis and Epstein-Barr viral

genome studies of Hodgkin's disease. Int Rev Exp Pathol 33:165, 1992

31. Tamaru J, Hummel M, Zemlin M et al: Hodgkin's disease with a B-cell phenotype often shows a VDJ rearrangement and somatic mutations in the Vh genes. Blood 84:708, 1994
32. Kuppers R, Rajewski K, Zhao M et al: Hodgkin disease: Hodgkin and Reed-Sternberg cells picked from histological sections show clonal immunoglobulin gene rearrangements and appear to be derived from B cells at various stages of development. Proc Natl Acad Sci USA 91:10962, 1994
33. Delabie J, Tierens A, Wu G et al: Lymphocyte predominance Hodgkin's disease: lineage and clonality determination using a single-cell assay. Blood 84:3291, 1994
34. Poppema S, Elema JD, Halie MR: The localization of Hodgkin's disease in lymph nodes. A study with immunohistological, enzymehistochemical and rosetting techniques on frozen sections. Int J Cancer 24:532, 1979
35. Abdulaziz Z, Mason DY, Stein H et al: An immunohistological study of the cellular constituents of Hodgkin's disease using a monoclonal antibody panel. Histopathology 8:1, 1984
36. Poppema S, Timens W, Visser L: Nodular lymphocyte predominance type of Hodgkin's disease is a B cell lymphoma. Adv Exp Med Biol 186: 963, 1985
37. Lai R, Visser L, Poppema S: Tissue distribution of restricted leukocyte common antigens. A comprehensive study with protein and carbohydrate specific CD45R antibodies. Lab Invest 64:844, 1991
38. Pallesen G: The distribution of CD23 in normal human tissues and in malignant lymphomas p. 383. In McMichael AJ, Beverley PCL, Cobbold S et al (eds): Leucocyte Typing III. New York, Oxford University Press, 1987
39. Delespesse G, Sarfati M, Wu CY et al: The low affinity receptor for IgE. Immunol Rev 125:77, 1992
40. Pene J, Rousset F, Briere F et al: IgE production by normal human lymphocytes is induced by interleukin 4 and suppressed by interferons gamma and alpha and prostaglandin E2. Proc Natl Acad Sci USA 85:6880, 1988
41. Hansmann ML, Fellbaum C, Hui PK et al: Correlation of content of B cells and Leu7-positive cells with subtype and stage in lymphocyte predominance type Hodgkin's disease. J Cancer Res Clin Oncol 114:405, 1988
42. Timens W, Visser L, Poppema S: Nodular lymphocyte predominance type of Hodgkin's disease is a germinal center lymphoma. Lab Invest 4:457, 1986
43. Poppema S, Visser L, de Leij L: Reactivity of presumed natural killer cell antibody Leu7 with intrafollicular T lymphocytes. Clin Exper Immunol 54:834, 1983
44. Velardi A, Mingari MC, Moretta L et al: Functional analysis of cloned germinal center CD4+ cells with natural killer cell-related features. Divergence from typical T helper cells. J Immunol 137:2808, 1986
45. Bowen MB, Butch AW, Parvin CA et al: Germinal center T cells are distinct helper-inducer T cells. Hum Immunol 31:67, 1991
46. Butch AW, Chung G-H, Hoffmann J, Nahm MH: Cytokine expression by germinal center cells. J Immunol 150:39, 1993
47. Lederman S, Yellin MJ, Inghirami G et al: Molecular interactions mediating T–B lymphocyte collaboration in human lymphoid follicles: roles of T-cell–B-cell-activating molecule (5c8 antigen) and CD40 in contact dependent help. J Immunol 149:3817, 1992
48. Koopman G, Parmentier HK, Schuurman HJ et al: Adhesion of human B cells to follicular dendritic cells involves both the lymphocyte function associated antigen 1/intercellular adhesion molecule-1 and very late antigen 4/vascular adhesion molecule-1 pathways. J Exp Med 173:1297, 1991
49. Müller-Hermelink HK, Lennert K: The cytologic, histologic and functional basis for a modern classification of lymphomas. P. 1. In Uehlinger E (ed): Malignant Lymphomas Other Than Hodgkin's Disease: Histology, Cytology, Ultrastructure, Immunology. Handbuchder speziellen Pathologischen Anatomie und Histologie. Berlin, Springer, 1987
50. Burns BF, Colby TV, Dorfman RF: Differential diagnostic features of nodular L&H Hodgkin's disease, including progressive transformation of germinal centers. Am J Surg Pathol 8:253, 1984
51. Crossley B, Heryet A, Gatter KC: Does nodular lymphocyte predominant Hodgkin's disease arise from progressively transformed germinal centers? A case report with an unusually prolonged history. Histopathology 11:621, 1987
52. Lennert K, Hansmann ML: Progressive transformation of germinal centers: clinical significance and lymphocyte predominance Hodgkin's dis-

ease—the Kiel experience. Am J Surg Pathol 11: 149, 1987

53. Dorfman RF: Progressive transformation of germinal centers and lymphocyte predominant Hodgkin's disease—the Stanford experience. Am J Surg Pathol 11:150, 1987
54. Osborne BM, Butler JJ: Clinical implications of progressive transformation of germinal centers. Am J Surg Pathol 8:725, 1984
55. Poppema S: Current problems in Hodgkin's disease. p. 67. In Levy E (ed): Advances in Pathology. Oxford, Pergamon Press
56. Robb-Smith AHT: Treatment of Cancer and Allied Diseases. Vol 9, Lymphomas and Related Diseases. New York, Hoeber, 1964
57. Miettinen M, Franssila KO, Saxen E: Hodgkin's disease, lymphocyte predominance, nodular. Increased risk for subsequent non Hodgkin's lymphomas. Cancer 54:2293, 1983
58. Toner GC, Sinclair RA, Sutherland RC et al: Composite lymphoma. Am J Clin Pathol 86:375, 1986
59. Salter DM, Sheehan T, Krajewski AS et al: Immunohistological diagnosis of a case of composite lymphoma. Br J Haematol 66:479, 1987
60. Sundeen JT, Cossman J, Jaffe ES: Lymphocyte predominant Hodgkin's disease nodular subtype with coexistent ''large cell lymphoma:'' histological progression or composite malignancy? Am J Surg Pathol 12:599, 1988
61. Hansmann ML, Lennert K: Grosszellige maligne Lymphome bei nodulärem Paragranulom (lymphozytenreicher M. Hodgkin) Verh Dtsch Ges Pathol 70:597, 1986
62. Stetler-Stevenson M, Crush-Stanton S, Cossman J: Involvement of the *bcl*-2 gene in Hodgkin's disease. J Natl Cancer Inst 82:855, 1990
63. Said JW, Sassoon AF, Shintaku IP et al: Absence of *bcl*-2 major breakpoint region and JH gene rearrangement in lymphocyte predominance Hodgkin's disease. Am J Pathol 138:261, 1991
64. Algara P, Martinez P, Sanchez L et al: Lymphocyte predominance Hodgkin's disease (nodular paragranuloma)—a *bcl*-2 negative germinal centre lymphoma. Histopathology 19:69, 1991
65. Hansmann ML, Zwingers T, Boske A et al: Clinical features of nodular paragranuloma (Hodgkin's disease, lymphocyte predominance type, nodular). J Cancer Res Clin Oncol 108:321, 1984
66. Regula DP, Hoppe RT, Weiss LM: Nodular and diffuse types of lymphocyte predominance Hodgkin's disease. N Engl J Med 318:214, 1988
67. Borg-Grech A, Radord JA, Crowther D et al: A comparative study of the nodular and diffuse variants of lymphocyte-predominant Hodgkin's disease. J Clin Oncol 7:1303, 1989
68. Tefferi A, Zellers RA, Banks PM et al: Clinical correlates of distinct immunophenotypic and histologic subcategories of lymphocyte-predominance Hodgkin's disease. J Clin Oncol 8:1959, 1990
69. Crennan E, D'Costa I, Liew KH et al: Lymphocyte predominant Hodgkin's disease: a clinicopathologic comparative study of histologic and immunophenotypic subtypes. Int J Radiat Oncol Biol Phys 31:333, 1995

5

Classification of Non-Hodgkin's Lymphoma

Lawrence M. Weiss

Lymphoma classification has been the subject of numerous scholarly and sometimes less than scholarly debates. Much of the controversy has centered more on the differing philosophies of the individuals involved rather than on true disagreements about the specific types of lymphomas and their behavior. Some classifications have stressed the practical and clinical aspects of lymphomas, emphasizing morphologic approaches and clinical behavior. However, these classifications may overlook or minimize biologic findings. Others have stressed more biologic issues, often including schemes based on reputed cell of origin and cellular differentiation pathways, emphasizing immunologic and molecular biologic studies. However, these classifications may not be as clinically relevant, and our understanding of the human immune system is still incomplete, leaving gaps in the classification where there are gaps in our knowledge. Some classifications have been all-encompassing, including the lymphoid leukemias and Hodgkin's disease, while others have been more limited in scope. Some classifications strive to incorporate all lymphoma entities, while others limit their categories to the most common ones. This chapter will review some of the more important lymphoma classifications, with emphasis on the more recently proposed and widely used ones.

RAPPAPORT CLASSIFICATION

Henry Rappaport and colleagues proposed the first modern classification of non-Hodgkin's lymphoma in 1956 (Table 5-1). They emphasized that a classification should be "clinically useful, scientifically accurate, reproducible, and easily taught and readily learned."[2] They devised a relatively simple scheme based entirely on morphologic features that recognized the clinical differences between lymphomas with a nodular and a diffuse architecture and distinguished lymphomas with different cytologic characteristics. The Rappaport classification underwent several revisions. In 1966, the cytologic category of undifferentiated was added, and the incorrect term *reticulum cell* was replaced by *histiocytic* (which later also proved to be incorrect).[3] Later, the newly described entity of lymphoblastic lymphoma was incorporated, and it was recognized that some lymphomas such as undifferentiated and lymphoblastic lymphoma may not have nodular counterparts.[4] The utility of the classification was validated in many clinical studies,[5] and, although it was devised at a time when our knowledge of the immune system was very rudimentary, it was the primary lymphoma classification used by pathologists and clinicians for at least two decades.

Several other classifications were proposed in the mid-1970s that represented modifications of the Rappaport classification, including the British National Lymphoma Investigation (BNLI) classification,[6] the Dorfman classification,[7] and the World Health Organization (WHO) classification.[8] In part, these morphologic classifications provided more accurate terminology than the Rappaport classification (e.g., replacing *histiocytic* with *large lymphoid* in the schema of Dorfman) and in general included a wider spectrum of lymphoid neoplasia (e.g., the inclusion

Table 5-1. Original Rappaport Classification of 1956

Malignant Lymphoma	
Diffuse	Nodular ("Follicular")
1. Lymphocytic type, well differentiated	
2. Lymphocytic type, poorly differentiated	
3. Mixed type (lymphocytic and reticulum cell)	
4. Reticulum-cell type	
5. Hodgkin's type	

(From Rappaport et al.,[1] with permission.)

of plasma cell neoplasia in the BNLI and WHO classifications and mycosis fungoides in the Dorfman and WHO classifications). However, some of the new classifications may have unduly confused the unwary, introducing new terms for terms already used. For example, the WHO classification introduced the term *prolymphocytic* to include several cell types including *poorly differentiated lymphocyte* as used in the Rappaport classification. In addition, old terms were reintroduced with new meanings. For example, the term *poorly differentiated lymphocytic* was used in the BNLI classification as a synonym for *lymphoblastic,* while the new term *predominantly small follicle cell* replaced *poorly differentiated lymphocytic* in the Rappaport classification.

LUKES AND COLLINS CLASSIFICATION

In 1974, Lukes and Collins[9] introduced the first lymphoma classification based on cell of origin and alterations in lymphocyte transformation. Incorporating modern concepts of immunology, the classification emphasized a functional approach that integrated morphologic, cytochemical, and immunologic studies. Lukes and Collins recognized that the majority of the malignant lymphomas were B-lineage neoplasms, usually related to the germinal center. In the resulting classification, the initial separation of lymphomas was made on the basis of cell lineage, while the subsequent divisions were made by cytologic assessment (Table 5-2). Lymphoid leukemias were included in the classification.

New cytologic terms were introduced, including *small* and *large cleaved cells* and *small* and *large noncleaved cells,* cells all related to normal germinal center cells. In addition, the term *immunoblastic sarcoma* was first used. *Immunoblastic sarcoma of B cells* was used for a lymphoma closely related to the large noncleaved cell type, but derived from a cell residing outside the germinal center with somewhat farther differentiation toward the plasma cell. Thus, B immunoblasts tended to be large, with more cytoplasm, more pyroninophilia, and sometimes showed more plasmacytoid features than large noncleaved cells. *Immunoblastic sarcoma of T cells* was initially a theoretical concept only, but definitively identified with the report of Waldron and colleagues.[10]

Because the Lukes and Collins classification was primarily based on cellular immunology, recognition of the cell lineage of a given lymphoma was of critical importance. Lukes and Collins believed that an experienced hematopathologist could reliably assess B versus T lineage by morphology. This subsequently became a controversial point in the literature.[11] Furthermore, whether or not an experienced hematopa-

Table 5-2. Original Lukes and Collins Classification of 1974

I. U cell (undefined cell) type
II. T-cell types
    Mycosis fungoides and Sezary syndrome
    Convoluted lymphocyte
    ? Immunoblastic sarcoma (of T cells)
    ? Hodgkin's disease
III. B-cell types
    Small lymphocyte (CLL)
    Plasmacytoid lymphocyte
    Follicular center cell (FCC) types (follicular, diffuse, follicular and diffuse, and sclerotic)
        Small cleaved
        Large cleaved
        Small noncleaved
        Large noncleaved
    Immunoblastic sarcoma (of B cells)
IV. Histiocytic type
V. Unclassifiable

(From Lukes and Collins,[9] with permission.)

thologist could determine B versus T lineage was one matter, but what about the general surgical pathologist—does this mean that he or she could no longer classify non-Hodgkin's lymphomas? In addition, although the Lukes and Collins system had obvious biologic relevance, it did not immediately follow that the new classification would have clinical relevance. Lukes and Collins referred to preliminary survival studies, but the clinical validation was not provided until the Working Formulation study of 1982. The different categories within the Lukes and Collins system do not depend on architecture, which is an important feature in the Rappaport system. However, all cases with a follicular pattern were shown to be related to the follicular center cell types of Lukes and Collins. Nonetheless, it became another matter of controversy as to whether the favorable prognosis of follicular lymphoma was a manifestation of its architecture or of the generally favorable cell types comprising the follicles in most cases.

KIEL CLASSIFICATION

Also in 1974, the Kiel classification was introduced (Table 5-3).[12] This classification was largely based on the concepts of Lennert and Lukes, but introduced one major innovation. For the first time, there was a formal attempt to divide lymphomas into those of low grade and high grade. These distinctions were not based on clinical studies but rather on the cytologic characteristics of the cells. In general, neoplasms of low grade were those composed of cells with more mature cytologic characteristics, as indicated by the frequency of the suffixes "-cytic" or "-cytoid," while the high grade lymphomas were composed of cells with more immature cytologic characteristics, as indicated by the frequency of the suffix "-blast."

Table 5-3. Original Kiel Classification of 1974

Low-grade malignancy
Malignant lymphoma—lymphocytic (CLL and others)
Malignant lymphoma—lymphoplasmacytoid (immunocytic)
Malignant lymphoma—centrocytic
Malignant lymphoma—centroblastic-centrocytic—follicular, follicular and diffuse, diffuse; with and without sclerosis
High-grade malignancy
Malignant lymphoma—centroblastic
Malignant lymphoma—lymphoblastic
Burkitt type
Convoluted-cell type
Others
Malignant lymphoma—immunoblastic

(From Gerard-Marchant et al.,[12] with permission.)

There were many similarities between the original Kiel classification and that of Lukes and Collins. A comparison performed by Lennert, Collins, and Lukes revealed equivalence between 11 of the 13 major types of the Lukes and Collins classification and the Kiel classification.[13] Lymphoid leukemias were included in both schema. All lymphomas were considered to have a leukemic phase, but the incidence of involvement varied considerably from one type of lymphoma to another. Both classifications agreed that most lymphomas were of B-lineage origin and that many were of follicular center origin. Both systems also regarded the cytologic type to take precedence over architecture. However, the Kiel classification introduced yet another terminology, with *centrocytes* equivalent to Lukes and Collins' *cleaved cells* and *centroblasts* equivalent to *noncleaved cells.* All follicular lymphomas were considered to be composed of both cell types, with the recommendation that the pathologist state the approximate proportion of blast cells present in each case.

COMPARISON STUDY OF CLASSIFICATION

The numerous classifications, as well as the controversies among their authors, led to confusion among pathologists and clinicians. Much of the difficulty stemmed from the lack of objective data to assess the clinical relevance and reproducibility of the various classifications. Consensus meetings were convened, but failed largely because they could not provide adequate, meaningful data. Thus, a unique multi-institution, multiclassification, and multi-investigator study was planned, sponsored, and executed under the aegis of the National Cancer Institute of the National Institutes of Health. This study involved comparison of six major classification systems (the Rappaport, Dorfman, BNLI, WHO, Lukes and Collins, and Kiel schema) by 12 pathologists (one representing each classification system) and 6 experts at large using the diagnostic slides for 1,175 cases of malignant lymphoma with adequate follow-up collected and organized at four major institutions (Instituto Nazionale Tumori, Milan, Italy; University of Minnesota Hospitals, Minneapolis; Tufts–New England Medical Center, Boston; and Stanford University, Stanford, CA).[14] Immunologic methods were not employed in the study design.

In this landmark study, the major conclusion reached was that all six classifications were valuable and comparable in reproducibility and clinical correlations.[14] As a side issue, it was found that follicular architecture signaled clinical significance, independent of cell type. The study described a "working formulation" to separate the non-Hodgkin's lymphomas into 10 major types, with a larger number of subtypes (Table 5-4). Although the participants of the conference stated that this formulation was not proposed as a new classification but as a means of translation among the various systems and to facilitate clinical comparisons of case reports and therapeutic trials, the organization of the lymphoma types within three histologic grades suggests that the authors hoped that it might be used as a classification system in its own right.

Table 5-4. Working Formulation of Non-Hodgkin's Lymphomas for Clinical Usage

Low grade
- A. Small lymphocytic
  - Consistent with CLL; plasmacytoid
- B. Follicular predominantly small cleaved cell
  - Diffuse areas, sclerosis
- C. Follicular mixed small cleaved and large cell
  - Diffuse areas, sclerosis

Intermediate grade
- D. Follicular predominatly large cell
  - Diffuse areas, sclerosis
- E. Diffuse small cleaved cell
  - Sclerosis
- F. Diffuse mixed, small and large cell
  - Sclerosis; epithelioid cell component
- G. Diffuse large cell
  - Cleaved cell, noncleaved cell, sclerosis

High grade
- H. Large cell, immunoblastic
  - Plasmacytoid, clear cell, polymorphous, epithelioid cell component
- I. Lymphoblastic
  - Convoluted, nonconvoluted
- J. Small noncleaved cell
  - Burkitt's, follicular areas

Miscellaneous
- Composite, mycosis fungoides, histiocytic, extramedullary plasmacytoma, unclassifiable, other

(From Ref. 14, with permission.)

THE WORKING FORMUATION

The Working Formulation of Non-Hodgkin's Lymphomas for Clinical Usage, or *Working Formulation* as the new classification has become known, is essentially a modified Rappaport classification utilizing updated, expanded categories with altered terminology. The term *follicular* replaced *nodular,* the term *small cleaved* replaced *poorly differentiated lymphocytic,* and the term *large cell* replaced the term *histiocytic.* One major change in the Rappaport system was the subdivision of the Rappaport category of diffuse histiocytic lymphoma into intermediate grade; diffuse large cell; and high grade, large cell, immunoblastic categories, based on statistically significant survival differences between cases diagnosed as the large cell lymphomas of follicular cell type and large cell lymphomas of immunoblastic type (either T or B cell). It was noted, however, that consensus in the subcategorization of the large cell lymphomas was only achieved in a minority of cases.

Criticisms of the Working Formulation were offered by Lennert and Lukes in commentaries appended to the Working Formulation study.[14] Both pointed out that entitites that are biologically unrelated are grouped together. For example, the entities of *diffuse mixed* and *diffuse large cell* types must be heterogeneous. Conversely, entities that are biologically closely related are separated. Both investigators expressed the hope that the Working Formulation would not impede future lymphoma research by giving the impression that an ultimate lymphoma classification had been reached. Lukes, in particular, stressed his opinion that an immunologic classification recognizing immunologic types would ultimately be necessary. Nonetheless, the Working Formulation was widely embraced in the United States by both pathologists and clinicians as a practical classification system. One more recent criticism of the Working Formulation has been the lack of a capability to be updated. The term *Working* implied that the classification was temporary and could be modified as necessary; however, this has not occurred, perhaps because the Working Formulation was established by a study group no longer in existence. Therefore, more recently delineated clinicopathologic entities such as mantle cell (intermediately differentiated lymphocytic) lymphoma cannot be easily incorporated into the system.

REVISED KIEL CLASSIFICATION

The Working Formulation received less acceptance in Europe, where the Kiel system remained the primary lymphoma classification. In 1988, the Kiel classification was extensively updated (Table 5-5).[15] This revision contained several major changes from its original 1974 version. First, the primary separation was now done according to cell lineage, clearly distinguishing between B- and T-cell neoplasms. Within the categories of B- and T-cell neoplasms, separations based on low versus high grade were given, as in the first Kiel classification. A second major change was the introduction of an extensive subcategorization of the T-cell lymphomas, with 10 major types. Furthermore, the high grade B-cell category was expanded, with the additions of immunoblastic and large cell anaplastic. The authors suggested that the identification of more specific groups may eventually be shown to have greater clinical significance than a broad division into low, intermediate, and high grade lymphoma. Finally, the authors added a specific category of "rare types" to acknowledge the fact that the list of categories in their classification did not exhaust the total number of apparently distinct entities that had been described, only that it is not practical to include them all in a lymphoma classification.

Criticisms of the Kiel classification have highlighted its complexity. Mason and Gatter[16] state that "lymphoma pathologists [using the Kiel classification] sometimes appear to their clinical colleagues to insist on an arcane nomenclature with little relevance to patient management." They are particularly critical of the expansion of the large cell lymphomas of B-cell

Table 5-5. Updated Kiel Classification of Non-Hodgkin's Lymphomas

B cell	T cell
Low Grade	
Lymphocytic—chronic lymphocytic and prolymphocytic leukemia; hairy cell leukemia	Lynphocytic-chronic lymphocytic and prolymphocytic leukemia
Lymphoplasmacytic/cytoid	Lymphoepithelioid
Plasmacytic	Angioimmunoblastic
Centroblastic/centrocytic	T zone
Centrocytic	Pleomorphic, small cell
High grade	
Centroblastic	Pleomorphic, medium and large cell
Immunoblastic	Immunoblastic
Large cell anaplastic	Large cell anaplastic
Burkitt lymphoma	
Lymphoblastic	Lymphoblastic
Rare types	Rare types

(From Stansfeld et al.,[15] with permission.)

type into several types with several more subtypes, when pathologists generally cannot make these distinctions reproducibly. Similarly, Mason and Gatter state that the category of T-cell lymphomas has been overly subclassified. One study has demonstrated a very low reproducibility among the various subcategories of T-cell lymphoma within the Kiel system,[17] although some studies suggest that the separation of T-cell lymphoma into low and high grade categories may have clinical validity.[18]

REAL CLASSIFICATION

With this background, a group of 19 hematopathologists (representing 1 Asian, 6 American, and 10 European institutions) who call themselves the *International Lymphoma Study Group* proposed in 1994 a "Revised European-American Classification of Lymphoid Neoplasms" (the REAL classification, the acronym given by its originators) (Table 5-6).[9–21] They sought to enumerate the major distinct lymphoma types that could be recognized with the currently available morphologic, immunologic, and genetic techniques. Thus, it is a list of about 23 types of non-Hodgkin's lymphomas and four types of Hodgkin's disease, with four provisional entities, one subtype, four provisional subtypes, three provisional cytologic grades, and four provisional cytologic categories.

Broad in scope, it also includes plasmacytoma/plasma cell myeloma, at least eight types of lymphoid leukemia, as well as Hodgkin's disease. It also recognizes specific extranodal entities for the first time, including extranodal marginal zone B-cell lymphoma (mucosal-associated lymphoid tissue lymphoma [MALToma]). The list is organized by B and T/natural killer lineages and subdivided by precursor and peripheral neoplasms. In addition to morphologic assessment, the classification depends on a variety of techniques, including frozen and paraffin section immunohistochemistry and sometimes molecular studies.

Although there is no separation by grade, the specific entities recognized by the REAL classification are most similar to the 1988 Updated Kiel classification. However, there is no attempt to subdivide the B-cell diffuse large cell lymphomas other than recognizing a primary mediastinal subtype. In addition, there is much less subdivision of the peripheral T-cell lymphomas than in the updated Kiel classification. However, the REAL classification includes subcategories of intestinal T-cell lymphoma and angiocentric lymphoma, entities not included in the Kiel classification. In addition, there is a greater tendency to separate lymphoma categories by nodal versus extranodal pattern of involvement in the REAL classification.

Criticism of the REAL classification has come quickly, starting with an editorial accompanying the original publication of the system. In the editorial, Rosenberg[22] expresses the opinion that the classification is inadequate from a clinician's viewpoint. He states that it lacks essential clinical data such as frequency, age, sites of involvement, clinical course, prognosis, and curability. Rosenberg also notes that the REAL classification lacks data on reproducibility by other pathologists and ability to predict clinical behavior. Furthermore, he feels it is too encompassing by including entities such as multiple myeloma, which clinicians do not generally group with the non-Hodgkin's lymphomas, and Hodgkin's disease, which is too clearly distinct from the non-Hodgkin's lymphoma to be classified together. In addition, it includes information that is of limited use to the clinician (e.g., cell lineage), while excluding clinically useful information (such as a broad indication of grade).

The authors of the REAL classification have responded by pointing out that clinical data concerning the specific categories recognized in the classification largely already exist within the established literature.[16,23] Furthermore, they feel that their new classification is receiving greater scrutiny than any other newly proposed classification. This response may be true, but perhaps the Working Formulation study provided a new standard for rigor in validating lymphoma classifications to which all subsequent proposed classifications must be held. Additional studies, including some underway, may provide the

Table 5-6. Lymphoid Neoplasms Recognized by the International Lymphoma Study Group

B-cell neoplasms
- I. Precursor B-cell neoplasm: B-precursor lymphoblastic leukemia/lymphoma
- II. Peripheral B-cell neoplasms
  1. B-cell chronic lymphocytic leukemia/prolymphocytic leukemia/small lymphocytic lymphoma
  2. Lymphoplasmacytoid lymphoma/immunocytoma
  3. Mantle cell lymphoma
  4. Follicle center lymphoma, follicular
     Provisional cytologic grades: I (small cell), II (mixed small and large cell), III (large cell)
     Provisional subtype: diffuse, predominantly small cell type
  5. Marginal zone B-cell lymphoma
     Extranodal (Malt type ± monocytoid B cells)
     Provisional subtype: nodal (± monocytoid B cells)
  6. Provisional entity: splenic marginal zone lymphoma (± villous lymphocytes)
  7. Hairy cell leukemia
  8. Plasmacytoma/plasma cell myeloma
  9. Diffuse large B-cell lymphoma
     Subtype: primary mediastinal (thymic) B-cell lymphoma
  10. Burkitt lymphoma
  11. Provisional entity: high-grade B-cell lymphoma, Burkitt-like

T-cell and putative NK-cell neoplasms
- I. Precursor T-cell neoplasm: T-precursor lymphoblastic lymphoma/leukemia
- II. Peripheral T-cell and NK-cell neoplasms
  1. T-cell chronic lymphocytic leukemia/prolymphocytic leukemia
  2. Large granular lymphocyte leukemia (LGL), T- and NK-cell types
  3. Mycosis fungoides/Sezary syndrome
  4. Peripheral T-cell lymphoma, unspecified
     Provisional cytologic categories: medium-sized cell, mixed medium and large cell, large cell, lymphoepithelioid cell
     Provisional subtype: hepatosplenic $\gamma\delta$ T-cell lymphoma
     Provisional subtype: subcutaneous panniculitic T-cell lymphoma
  5. Angioimmunoblastic T-cell lymphoma (AILD)
  6. Angiocentric lymphoma
  7. Intestinal T-cell lymphoma (± enteropathy associated)
  8. Adult T-cell lymphoma/leukemia (ATL/L)
  9. Anaplastic large cell lymphoma (ALCL), CD30+, T- and null-cell types
  10. Provisional entity: anaplastic large cell lymphoma, Hodgkin's like

Hodgkin's disease
- I. Lymphocyte predominance
- II. Nodular sclerosis
- III. Mixed cellularity
- IV. Lymphocyte depletion
- V. Provisional entity: lymphocyte-rich classical Hodgkin's disease

(From Harris et al.[19] with permission.)

necessary data. The authors of the REAL classification counter the argument that omission of grade is a serious shortcoming by pointing out that many of the entities included in the REAL classification exhibit a spectrum of behavior ranging from indolent to aggressive. Thus, it is inappropriate to assign a specific grade to a specific category. This, however, may not help clinicians in selecting treatment for an individual patient unless there is close communication between the pathologist and clinician.

Pathologists raise the criticism that lymph node biopsies are received in formalin in most medical centers, and even if they were to be received fresh pathologists do not have sufficient access or financial resources (especially in this age of cost containment) to obtain the special studies necessary to diagnose cases in circumstances in which these studies are necessary for precise classification. Dehner[24] speaks for the general surgical pathologist, who remains the individual responsible for the diagnosis of the majority of diagnostic lymph node biopsies in the United States, when he states that "for a pathologic classification to have practical application in the everyday life of a pathologist, it must be something that can be used with the tools at hand, which for most of us is the light microscope." In addition, it is not clear how lymphomas of null or uncertain lineage fit into the REAL classification (other than CD30+ anaplastic large cell lymphoma of null lineage). Time will tell whether the REAL classification will gain acceptance for both pathologists and clinicians—and acceptance by both will be critical to its ultimate success.

FUTURE CONSIDERATIONS

As this book goes to press, the WHO is sponsoring a new lymphoma classification. About fifty pathologists from Europe and North America have been organized into 10 committees headed by Elaine Jaffe, Costan Berard, Karl Lennert, and Jacques Diebold. This effort may lead to a system of lymphoma classification that may address the concerns about the REAL classification.

REFERENCES

1. Rappaport H, Winter W, Hicks E: Follicular lymphoma. A reevaluation of its position in the scheme of malignant lymphoma, based on a survey of 253 cases. Cancer 9:792, 1956
2. Berard CW, Jaffe E, Rappaport H et al: Discussion II: roundtable discussion of histopathologic classification. Cancer Treat Rep 61:1037, 1977
3. Rappaport H: Tumors of the hematopoietic system. Series I, Section III, Armed Forces Institute of Pathology, Washington, DC, 1966
4. Nathwani B, Kim H, Rappaport H: Malignant lymphoma, lymphoblastic. Cancer 38:964, 1976
5. Jones S, Fuks Z, Bull M et al: Non-Hodgkin's lymphomas. IV. Clinicopathologic correlation in 405 cases. Cancer 31:806, 1973
6. Bennett MH, Farrer-Brown G, Henry K, Jelliffe AM: Classification of non-Hodgkin's lymphoma. Lancet ii:405, 1974
7. Dorfman RF: Classification of non-Hodgkin's lymphoma. Lancet i:1295, 1974
8. Mathe G, Rappaport H: Histological and cytological typing of neoplastic diseases of heamatopoietic and lymphoid tissues. 14, World Health Organization, Geneva, 1976
9. Lukes R, Collins R: Immunologic characterization of human malignant lymphomas. Cancer 34: 1488, 1974
10. Waldron JA, Leech JH, Glick AD et al: Malignant lymphoma of peripheral T-cell origin. Immunologic, pathologic, and clinical features in six patients. Cancer 40:1604, 1977
11. Jaffe ES: Predictability of immunologic phenotype by morphologic criteria in diffuse aggresive non-Hodgkin's lymphomas. Am J Clin Pathol 77: 46, 1982
12. Gerard-Marchant R, Hamlin I, Lennert K et al: Classification of non-Hodgkin's lymphomas. Lancet ii:406, 1974
13. Lennert K, Collins R, Lukes R: Concordance of the Kiel and Lukes-Collins classification of non-Hodgkin's lymphomas. Histopathology 7:549, 1983
14. Non-Hodgkin's lymphoma pathologic classification project. National Cancer Institute sponsored study of classifications of non-Hodgkin's lymphomas: summary and description of a Working Formulation for clinical usage. Cancer 49:2112, 1982
15. Stansfeld A, Diebold J, Kapanci Y et al: Updated Kiel classification for lymphomas. Lancet i:292, 1988
16. Mason DY, Gatter KC: Annotation. Not another lymphoma classification. Br J Haematol 90:493, 1995
17. Hastrup N, Hamilton-Dutoit S, Ralfkiaer E, Pallesen G: Peripheral T-cell lymphomas: an evaluation of reproducibility of the updated Kiel classification. Histopathology 18:99, 1991
18. Brittinger G, Bartels H, Common H et al: Clinical and prognostic relevance of the Kiel classification of non-Hodgkin lymphomas: results of a prospective multicenter study by the Kiel lymphoma study group. Hematol Oncol 2:269, 1984
19. Harris NL, Jaffe ES, Stein H et al: A revised European-American classification of lymphoid neoplasms. A proposal from the International Lymphoma Study Group. Blood 84: 1361, 1994
20. Chan JKC, Banks PM, Cleary ML et al: A revised

European-American classification of lympoid neoplasms: a proposal from the International Lymphoma Study Group. A summary version. Am J Clin Pathol 103:543, 1995
21. Chan JKC, Banks PM, Cleary ML et al: A proposal for classification of lymphoid neoplasms (by the International Lymphoma Study Group). Histopathology 25:517, 1994
22. Rosenberg SA: Classification of lymphoid neoplasms. Blood 84:1359, 1994
23. Harris NL, Jaffe ES, Stein H et al: Lymphoma classification proposal: clarification. Blood 85: 857, 1995
24. Dehner LP: Here we go again: a new classification of malignant lymphomas. A viewpoint from the trenches. Am J Clin Pathol 103:539, 1995

6

Low Grade B-Cell Neoplasms

Nancy Lee Harris

Since the mid-1980s, several new types of B-cell neoplasms composed predominantly of small cells, commonly referred to as *low grade B-cell lymphomas,* have been defined. The term *grade* is used differently in the two major lymphoma classifications, the Working Formulation (WF)[1] and the Kiel classification,[3] resulting in some confusion. In the WF, tumors are divided into three *prognostic groups* based on the survival of the patients in the original study; these prognostic groups are commonly referred to as *grades.* The Kiel classification, in contrast, defines grade as *histologic grade;* that is, all tumors composed of predominantly small cells with or without a minor component of large, transformed, or blast cells are called *low grade.* The WF defines only two major categories of low grade lymphoma: small lymphocytic and follicular lymphoma of predominantly small cleaved cell and mixed small cleaved and large cell types. However, as evidence that the prognostic groups defined by the WF do not really reflect the behavior of the tumors, many clinical trials of "low grade" lymphoma include diffuse small cleaved cell lymphoma, although this is technically *intermediate grade* in the WF. The original Kiel classification, in contrast, defined five types of low grade B-cell lymphoma, and the updated version[4] defines six types (excluding hairy cell leukemia and plasmacytoma), much more closely approximating reality as it is now seen by pathologists. Unfortunately, neither classification deals adequately with the important extranodal tumor described as *low grade B-cell lymphoma of mucosa-associated lymphoid tissue* (MALT); it is found in several categories of the WF and is officially excluded from the Kiel classification, which is restricted to node-based lymphomas.[4]

For these and other reasons, the International Lymphoma Study Group recently proposed a revised classification of lymphoid neoplasms,[1] which defines five accepted types (and one provisional one) of histologically low grade B-cell neoplasms, in addition to hairy cell leukemia and plasmacytoma/myeloma (Tables 6-1, 6-2). These definitions are based on a combination of morphologic, immunologic, genetic, and clinical features, all of which are important in defining a disease entity. Each of these neoplasms has a characteristic morphology, which may be sufficient in a given case to permit diagnosis and classification on morphologic grounds alone if well-prepared sections are available (Table 6-3). However, particularly in the low grade B-cell neoplasms, morphology alone may be insufficient to permit a confident diagnosis of lymphoma and to enable the pathologist to provide clinically useful subclassification. Immunophe-

Table 6-1. Low Grade B-Lymphoid Neoplasms Recognized By the International Lymphoma Study Group

1. B-cell chronic lymphocytic leukemia/small lymphocytic lymphoma
2. B-cell prolymphocytic leukemia
3. Lymphoplasmacytic lymphoma/immunocytoma
4. Mantle cell lymphoma
5. Follicle center lymphoma, follicular
6. Marginal zone B-cell lymphoma
   Extranodal (MALT type ± monocytoid B cells)
   Nodal (± monocytoid B cells)
7. Splenic marginal zone lymphoma (± villous lymphocytes)

Table 6-2. Comparison of the REAL Classification with the Kiel Classification and Working Formulation for Low-Grade B-Cell Lymphomas

Kiel	REAL	Working Formulation
B-Lymphocytic, CLL B-Lymphocytic, prolymphocytic leukemia Lymphoplasmacytoid immunocytoma	B-cell chronic lymphocytic leukemia/prolymphocytic leukemia/small lymphocytic lymphoma	Small lymphocytic, consistent with CLL Small lymphocytic, plasmacytoid
Lymphoplasmacytic immunocytoma	Lymphoplasmacytoid lymphoma	Small lymphocytic, plasmacytoid Diffuse, mixed small and large cell
Centrocytic Centroblastic, centrocytoid subtype	Mantle cell lymphoma	Small lymphocytic Diffuse, small cleaved cell Follicular, small cleaved cell Diffuse, mixed small and large cell Diffuse, large cleaved cell
Centroblastic/centrocytic, follicular	Follicular center lymphoma, follicular Grade I	Follicular, predominantly small cleaved cell
	Grade II	Follicular, mixed small and large cell
Centroblastic, follicular	Grade III	Follicular, predominantly large cell
Centroblastic/centrocytic, diffuse	Follicular center lymphoma, diffuse, small cell (provisional)	Diffuse, small cleaved cell Diffuse, mixed small and large cell
—	Extranodal marginal zone B-cell lymphoma of MALT type)	Small lymphocytic Diffuse, small cleaved cell Diffuse, mixed small and large cell
Monocytoid, including marginal zone Immunocytoma	Nodal marginal zone B-cell lymphoma (provisional)	Small lymphocytic Diffuse small cleaved cell Diffuse, mixed small and large cell Unclassifiable
—	Splenic marginal zone B-cell lymphoma (provisional)	Small lymphocytic Diffuse small cleaved cell

Abbreviations: REAL, Revised European-American Lymphoma Classification; CLL, chronic lymphocytic leukemia.

Table 6-3. Low Grade B-Cell Lymphomas: Morphologic Features

Neoplasm	Pattern	Small Cells	Transformed Cells
B-CLL/SLL	Diffuse with pseudofollicles	Round (occasionally cleaved)	Prolymphocytes Paraimmunoblasts
Lymphoplasmacytoid lymphoma	Diffuse; no pseudofollicles	Round (may be cleaved) Plasma cells	Centroblasts Immunoblasts
Mantle cell lymphoma	Diffuse, vaguely nodular, mantle zone, rarely follicular	Cleaved (rarely round or oval)	None
Follicle center lymphoma	Follicular ± diffuse areas, rarely diffuse	Cleaved	Centroblasts
Marginal zone B-cell lymphoma	Diffuse, interfollicular, marginal zone, follicular colonization	Heterogeneous: round (small lymphocytes), cleaved (marginal zone/monocytoid B cells), plasma cells	Centroblast-like Immunoblast-like

Table 6-4. Low Grade B-Cell Lymphomas: Immunohistologic and Genetic Features

Neoplasm	SIg; CIg (F/P)	CD5 (F)	CD10 (F)	CD23 (F/P)	CD43[a] (F/P)	Cyclin D1 (P)	Genetic Abnormality	Ig V Region Gene
B-CLL/SLL	+; −/+	+	−	+	+	−/+	Trisomy 12 (30%)	Unmutated
Lymphoplasmacytoid lymphoma	+; +	−	−	−	−/+	−	NA	Mutated
Mantle cell lymphoma	+; −	+	−	−	+	+	t(11;14); *bcl*-1R	Unmutated
Follicle center lymphoma	+;−	−	+/−	−/+	−	−	t(14;18); *bcl*-2R	Mutated, ongoing
Extranodal and nodal marginal zone lymphoma	+; +/−	−	−	−/+	−/+	−	Trisomy 3 (extranodal)	Mutated
Splenic marginal zone lymphoma	+; −/+	−	−	−	−	−/+	t(11;14) *bcl*-1R (15%)	Mutated

Abbreviations: SIg, surface immunoglobulin; CIg, cytoplasmic immunoglobulin; F, frozen sections; P, paraffin sections; B-CLL, B-cell chronic lymphocytic leukemia; SLL, small lymphocytic leukemia; R, rearrangement; +, >90% positive; +/−, >50% positive; −/+ <50% positive; −, <10% positive.

[a] Positivity may vary depending on antibody used.

noytping and, less often, genetic studies are therefore a useful adjunct to morphology in the diagnosis and subclassification of low grade B-cell neoplasms (Table 6-4).

In the Revised European-American classification of lymphoid neoplasms (abbreviated for convenience as The Revised European-American Lymphoma [REAL] classification), lymphomas and lymphoid leukemias are considered together since neoplasms that usually present as solid tumors of lymph nodes or extranodal sites can have bone marrow and peripheral blood involvement, and neoplasms that usually present with marrow and blood involvement can present with or develop involvement of solid tissues. To give the tumor a different name and treat it differently depending on how the patient presents can be confusing and may result in suboptimal management. Thus, B-cell chronic lymphocytic leukemia is discussed together with B-cell small lymphocytic lymphoma as different manifestations of the same neoplasm, and peripheral blood involvement by mantle cell or follicular lymphoma is considered here to be a leukemic phase of the disease rather than a different diagnosis. In this chapter, hairy cell leukemia and plasma cell myeloma/plasmacytoma are not discussed, since, although these are both neoplasms of cells of the lymphoid system, their diagnosis is usually straightforward and they are not often confused with the other diseases considered here.

B-CELL CHRONIC LYMPHOCYTIC LEUKEMIA/ SMALL LYMPHOCYTIC LYMPHOMA

Definition and Terminology

Most patients with B-cell chronic lymphocytic leukemia (B-CLL) have some degree of lymph node infiltration, which has a characteristic histologic pattern. Likewise, most patients whose lymph nodes contain the characteristic infiltrate associated with B-CLL will prove to have bone marrow and peripheral blood involvement at the time of the diagnosis or shortly thereafter; [3,5] however, some are nonleukemic at presentation, and it is possible that some may not develop leukemia. A term is needed for these cases, by analogy to granulocytic sarcoma or lymphoblastic lymphoma. The term *small lymphocytic lymphoma* (SLL) has in the past been used to encompass not only the nodal counterpart of B-cell CLL but also many MALT type lymphomas and probably also some T-cell neoplasms.[2,6] In the REAL classification, the term *small lymphocytic lymphoma* is restricted to tumors with the characteristic morphology and immunophenotype of B-CLL.

Morphology

Lymph Nodes

The lymph node infiltrate (Fig. 6-1) is composed predominantly of small lymphocytes, often slightly larger than normal lymphocytes, with condensed chromatin, round nuclei, and occasionally a small nucleolus. Larger lymphoid cells (prolymphocytes and paraimmunoblasts) with more prominent nucleoli and dispersed chromatin are always present, usually clustered in pseudofollicles (proliferation centers), imparting a vaguely nodular pattern at low magnification. Less often, these cells are distributed evenly throughout the node.[3,7,8] The term *prolymphocyte* refers to a cell that is larger than a lymphocyte, with more abundant, slightly basophilic cytoplasm, and a prominent central nucleolus. There is a spectrum of size from the small lymphocyte to the prolymphocyte to a larger cell, similar in size to an immunoblast, with a prominent central nucleolus, but with cytoplasm that is less strikingly basophilic than a typical immunoblast (paraimmunoblast). Pseudofollicles contain predominantly prolymphocytes, with rare paraimmunoblasts; the overall picture is reminiscent of an erythroid island in the bone marrow, with a gradual progression from the centrally located large, basophilic cells in the center to the smaller round lymphocytes at the periphery. This is in distinct contrast to the appearance of a true follicle of a follicular lymphoma or reactive lymph node, which contains two strikingly different cell types, the large, basophilic centroblast and the small, pale centrocyte, without intervening transitional forms.

The lymph node sinuses are usually not evident on routine stains, and the infiltrate often extends outside the lymph node capsule, particularly at areas of trabecular indentations. Destruction of the capsule, however, is usually not seen, and fibrosis is uncommon. Blood vessels are not increased in number, and those vessels that are present are usually small, with flat endothelium, although high endothelial venules may be present. Most cases have a low mitotic count; cases with more than 30 mitoses per 20 high power fields have been shown to have a worse prognosis.[9]

Bone Marrow

The infiltrate of B-CLL in the bone marrow may be nodular, interstitial, or diffuse. When nodular, it is usually randomly distributed and not specifically paratrabecular. The pattern of infiltration correlates with both clinical stage and prognosis, but is not an independent prognostic factor. Proliferation centers are usually not seen in the bone marrow, and the majority of the cells appear small and round. Prolymphocytes and paraimmunoblasts are inconspicuous or absent. Smears of the bone marrow or peripheral blood show a predominance of small lymphocytes with inconspicuous nucleoli and usually only a small number of prolymphocytes (larger cells with prominent central nucleoli). Cases with more than 10 percent prolymphocytes (CLL-PL) have been reported to have a worse prognosis. If the majority of the cells are prolymphocytes, a diagnosis of prolymphocytic leukemia is made (see below).[10]

Variants

Cleaved Cells. In some cases, the small and sometimes the larger cells show moderate nuclear irregularity, which can lead to a differential diagnosis of mantle cell lymphoma (see below). These cases have occasionally been diagnosed as "intermediate lymphocytic lymphoma"; however, studies have shown that cases diagnosed as intermediate lymphocytic lymphoma with pseudofollicles had a prognosis identical to that of B-CLL.[11] Therefore, if pseudofollicles and/or prolymphocytes and paraimmunoblasts

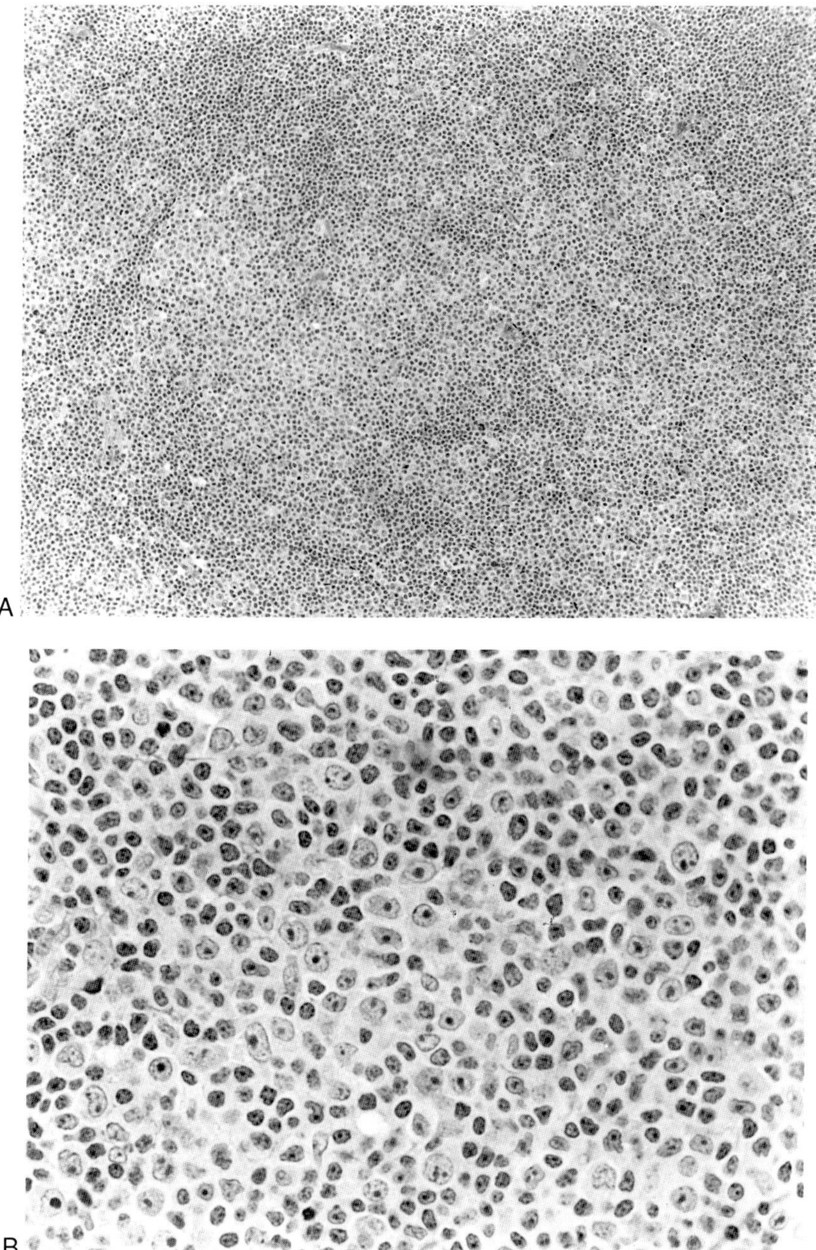

Fig. 6-1. B-cell chronic lymphocytic leukemia/small lymphocytic lymphoma. **(A)** Low magnification of lymph node, showing vague nodularity (pseudofollicles). **(B)** Higher magnification of center of pseudofollicle, showing prolymphocytes and paraimmunoblasts.

are present, a diagnosis of B-CLL should be made.[12]

Large Cells. Increased numbers or aggregates of prolymphocytes and paraimmunoblasts are seen in some cases, and some reports indicate that this finding may be associated with a more aggressive course.[3,5,13] The literature does not give clear guidelines for distinguishing cases that are likely to behave aggressively from the usual cases based on the number of large cells. In general, if the pseudofollicles contain a predominance of immunoblast-sized cells or are very large or destructive in their growth pattern, this should be mentioned in the report, with a suggestion that it may indicate a more aggressive lesion.[14]

Plasmacytoid Differentiation. Some cases with the characteristic morphology and immunophenotype of B-CLL can have plasmacytoid differentiation, with cytoplasmic immunoglobulin and often a small M component.[5,15] These cases correspond to the "lymphoplasmacyt*oid*" immunocytoma of the Kiel classification.[4] Since these tumors are morphologically and immunophenotypically virtually identical to typical B-CLL, the REAL classification regards these cases as a variant of B-CLL. However, in at least one study, cases of lymphoplasmacy*toid* immunocytoma (B-CLL with plasmacytoid features) had a worse prognosis than typical B-CLL.[14] This is an area that warrants further study, and therefore plasmacytoid features in B-CLL should be commented upon, if present.

Histologic Progression/Transformation

A gradual increase in prolymphocytes (prolymphocytoid transformation) may occur in B-CLL, with accompanying acceleration of the pace of the disease; however, this has been infrequently documented in the literature.[16,17] Abrupt development of a high grade lymphoma is a rare (5 percent of the cases) but well-documented phenomenon, called *Richter syndrome*.[18] In most cases these are diffuse large B-cell lymphomas, with the same immunoglobulin light chain and immunoglobulin gene rearrangement. In some cases, different light chains and/or different rearrangements have been found, suggesting a second B-cell neoplasm.[17,19]

Recently, cases of B-CLL associated with or transforming into a lesion resembling Hodgkin's disease have also been reported.[20–24] In some of these cases, Reed-Sternberg cells are admixed with the background infiltrate of B-CLL, while in others a distinct lesion with features of Hodgkin's disease develops in a patient with a history of B-CLL. In most cases, the Hodgkin's disease is of nodular sclerosis or mixed cellularity type and has the classic immunophenotype of Hodgkin's disease (CD15+ CD30+); however, a recent report describes two cases of simultaneous CLL and Hodgkin's disease of nodular lymphocyte predominance type. In most cases, the disease subsequently behaves like typical Hodgkin's disease with or without persistent CLL. In all cases studied, Epstein-Barr virus (EBV) genomes and antigens have been detected in the Hodgkin's disease like areas, suggesting involvement of this virus in the pathogenesis of the Hodgkin's disease. Interestingly, many of the recent patients have been treated with fludarabine, a purine analog that targets lymphoid cells, which can produce a defect in cellular immunity. It is possible that an altered immune state in these patients provides a setting for development of EBV-induced HD.[25,26]

Immunophenotype

The tumor cells of B-CLL have faint surface IgM with or without IgD. Rare cases with heavy chain class switch to IgG or IgA have been reported, but these are often CD5− and likely represent distinct diseases from typical B-CLL. The antigen specificity of the surface immunoglobulin in many cases has been shown to be against self-antigens, and these antibodies often have broad specificity, so-called cross-reactive idiotypes.[27,28] Cytoplasmic immunoglobulin is detectable in about 5 percent of the cases. B-cell-associated antigens (CD19, 20, 79a) are positive, but particularly CD20 may be very weak; tumor cells characteristically express both CD5 and

CD23. They are usually CD43+ and CD10−.[6,29,30] Myeloid antigens such as CD11c and CD13 may be expressed.[17] CD23 is particularly useful in distinguishing B-CLL/SLL from mantle cell lymphoma and should be evaluated in every case if possible.[6,31]

Genetic Features

Immunoglobulin Genes

Immunoglobulin heavy and light chain genes are rearranged. Analysis of the immunoglobulin gene sequences has shown that most cases (75 percent) do not show somatic mutation of their V regions, suggesting that they correspond to a cell that has not yet undergone antigen selection in the germinal center.[28,32,33] While several studies showed preferential utilization of a relatively small number of V region genes that were similar to those found in fetal B cells,[34–36] other studies have shown utilization of additional V region genes more commonly found in adult B cells.[28]

Genetic Abnormalities

No specific chromosomal or oncogene abnormality has been described in B-CLL. Trisomy 12 is reported in one-third of the cases,[37] and abnormalities of 13q are seen in up to 25 percent. t(11;14) and *bcl*-1 rearrangement have been reported;[38–40] some of these reported cases may be examples of leukemic mantle cell lymphoma. However, at least two clearcut cases of B-CLL have been reported with *bcl*-1 rearrangement or cyclin D1 overexpression; in both it was associated with an unusually aggressive clinical course.[41,42]

Postulated Normal Counterpart

Based on the combination of morphologic, immunophenotypic, and genetic features, most cases of B-CLL are thought to correspond to the recirculating CD5+ CD23+ naive or virgin B cells,[43] which are found in the peripheral blood, primary follicle, and follicle mantle zone.[28,44,45]

Clinical Features

B-CLL comprises 90 percent of chronic lymphoid leukemias in the United States and Europe. Most patients are older adults with bone marrow and peripheral blood involvement at diagnosis; generalized lymphadenopathy, hepatosplenomegaly, and extranodal infiltrates may occur.[2] The extent of the disease at the time of the diagnosis is the best predictor of survival[46]; however, chromosomal abnormalities and immunophenotype may also have prognostic importance.[17] Patients often have both hypogammaglobulinemia, which is associated with infectious complications, and autoimmune phenomena such as hemolytic anemia or thrombocytopenia.[17] Paradoxically, the antibodies mediating the autoimmune phenomena are usually IgG antibodies not related to the tumor immunoglobulin.[28] A small M component may be found

Table 6-5. Low Grade B-Cell Lymphomas: Clinical Features

Type	Age/Sex	Stage I	Extranodal	Outcome
CLL/SLL	60/M > F	None	Rare	Indolent, incurable
LP	60/M > F	None	Rare	Indolent, incurable
Mantle cell	60/M ≫ F	Rare	Many	Aggressive, incurable
Follicle center	50/M = F	Rare	Rare	Indolent, rare cure
MZ/MALT	50/M < F	Often	Usually	Indolent, curable

Abbreviations: CLL, chronic lymphocytic leukemia; SLL, small lymphocytic lymphoma; MZ, marginal zone; MALT, mucosa-associated lymphoid tissue.

in some patients[15]; thé paraproteins may have rheumatoid factor (anti-Ig) or other autoantigen specificity.[27] Occasional patients present with aleukemic nodal involvement, but most will ultimately be found to have or develop marrow and blood infiltration. Like most indolent hematologic malignancies, this disease is not usually considered curable with curently available therapy, and treatment with a single alkylating agent and prednisone have been the treatment of choice. Recently, purine analogs, particularly fludarabine, have been found to be remarkably effective in producing long-term remissions in patients with B-CLL.[17] A recent study found that loss of the *p53* gene on chromosome 17p was associated with shorter survival and decreased response to purine analogs.[47] Clinical features of B-cell lymphomas are presented in Table 6-5.

B-CELL PROLYMPHOCYTIC LEUKEMIA

Definition and Terminology

B-cell prolymphocytic leukemia B-PLL is characterized by a predominance (more than 55 percent) of prolymphocytes;[10,48,49] these cells are best evaluated on smears of peripheral blood or bone marrow. Although the French-American-British group definition of B-PLL makes it sound like a continuum with B-CLL (B-CLL = less than 10 percent prolymphocytes; CLL/PL = 10 to 55 percent prolymphocytes; PLL = more than 55 percent prolymphocytes), in fact most cases of CLL-PL have at most 20 to 30 percent prolymphocytes, and the vast majority of cases of B-PLL have 75 percent or more prolymphocytes.[10,49]

Morphologic Features

Prolymphocytes are most reliably recognized on smears of bone marrow or blood, and the disease is defined by these parameters. They are medium sized lymphoid cells (twice the size of an erythrocyte) with clumped chromatin but with a large, prominent central nucleolus and more abundant cytoplasm than typical CLL cells. Few descriptions of the morphologic features of B-PLL in tissue sections have been published;[4,50,51] these describe a diffuse infiltrate of medium sized cells with prominent nucleoli, involving both bone marrow and the splenic red and white pulp. Lymph node involvement is described as pseudonodular. Despite the immature appearance of the cells, mitotic activity is low.[50]

Immunophenotype

B-PLL may be CD5− or +, usually has strong surface Ig, and strongly express B-cell antigens. CD22 and FMC-7, which can be absent or faint in CLL by flow cytometry, are usually easily detected in B-PLL.[10]

Genetic Features

Immunoglobulin Genes

Analysis of the immunoglobulin gene shows that, like B-CLL, the cells of B-PLL show no somatic mutation in the V region genes.[52]

Genetic Abnormalities

No specific abnormality is reported; trisomy 12 is not seen. Up to 25 percent have been reported to have t(11;14).[53] The high frequency of this translocation raises the question of whether some reported cases of B-PLL are examples of mantle cell lymphoma.

Clinical Features

B-PLL is a very rare disorder, comprising only 1 to 2 percent of peripheral B-cell leukemias. Patients are slightly older than those with typical B-CLL and present with a very high white blood cell count and massive splenomegaly without lymphadenopathy. The disease tends to be refractory to treatment and has a more aggressive clinical course than typical B-CLL.[10,48,49]

LYMPHOPLASMACYTIC LYMPHOMA/IMMUNOCYTOMA

Definition and Terminology

The terms *lymphoplasmacytoid* or *lymphoplasmactyic lymphoma, plasmacytoid lymphocytic lymphoma,* and *immunocytoma* have been used to refer to heterogeneous lymphomas with plasmacytoid cells and plasma cells. Similarly, the term *Waldenstrom's macroglobulinemia* encompasses heterogeneous disorders that may produce a monoclonal IgM paraprotein. Many B-cell neoplasms may show maturation to plasmacytoid or plasma cells containing cytoplasmic immunoglobulin (CIg), including B-CLL, mantle cell, follicle center, and marginal zone cell lymphomas of extranodal, nodal, and splenic types. The Kiel classification restricts the term *immunocytoma* to B-cell neoplasms that lack features of follicle center, mantle cell, or monocytoid B-cell lymphoma. Two types are defined: one that resembles B-CLL and one that lacks features of B-CLL;[4,15] the former is called lymphoplasma*cytoid* and the latter lymphoplasma*cytic*. According to Lennert, the lymphoplasmacytoid type is mophologically, immunophenotypically, and clinically identical to B-CLL, differing only in the presence of cytoplasmic immunoglobulin in some cells and the presence of an M-component in some cases. The lymphoplasmacytic type lacks CD5, lacks proliferation centers, and is usually not leukemic; it is usually associated with Waldenstrom's macroglobulinemia.[4,15]

The International Lymphoma Study Group found this definition of immunocytoma to be confusing, splitting one disease (B-CLL) into two entities based on plasmacytoid features and lumping two distinct diseases (B-CLL and lymphoplasmacytic immunocytoma) into one category simply because of plasmacytoid features. It seems more logical to define immunocytoma as a tumor of small lymphoid cells that show maturation to plasmacytoid or plasma cells, without features of B-CLL or other lymphoma types.[6,29,30] Thus, the International Lymphoma Study Group proposed restricting the term *immunocytoma* to the lymphoplasma*cytic* type of the Kiel classification.[4,15] Since not all cases classified as lymphoplasma*cytic* in the Kiel classification have typical plasma cells, we felt that the term lymphoplasma*cytic* was too restrictive and proposed using the terms lymphoplasmacy*toid* lymphoma and immunocytoma interchangeably. However, the latter proposal has been criticized, since it results in confusion for those accustomed to the Kiel classification, and the term, lymphoplasma*cytic* seems preferable.

Morphology

Lymph Nodes and Spleen

The tumor consists of a diffuse proliferation of small lymphocytes, plasmacytoid lymphocytes (cells with abundant basophilic cytoplasm, but lymphocyte-like nuclei), and plasma cells with or without Dutcher bodies or Russell bodies. By definition, features of B-CLL, mantle cell, follicle center cell, or marginal zone lymphomas should not be seen. Specifically, pseudofollicles or marginal zone type cells should be absent. Immunoblast-like and centroblast-like large cells may be interspersed. There is considerable variation in the extent of plasmacytoid differentiation: some cases show predominantly lymphocytes with only scattered plasma cells or plasmactyoid cells, while others show numerous plasma cells and others have massive Dutcher or Russell body accumulation. The presence of plasma cells alone is not diagnostic of immunocytoma, and demonstration that they are part of the tumor (monotypic) by immunohistochemical stains is often necessary. The growth pattern is often interfollicular with sparing of the sinuses (Fig. 6-2). The sinuses may be widely dilated and contain eosinophilic, periodic acid-Schiff-

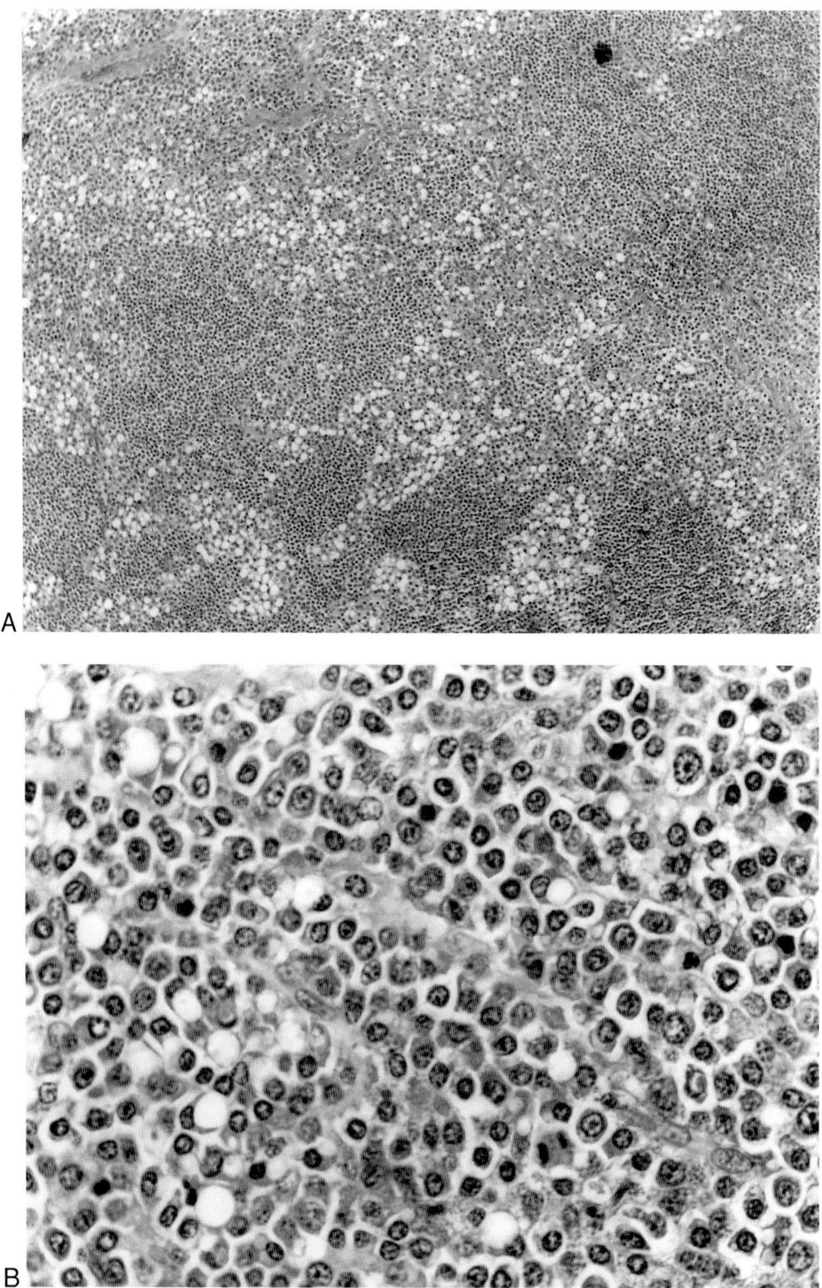

Fig. 6-2. Lymphoplasmacytoid lymphoma. **(A)** Low magnification of lymph node, showing diffuse pattern with open sinuses. **(B)** High magnification, showing small lymphoid cells, plasmacytoid cells, and plasma cells, many with intracytoplasmic vacuoles.

positive material. Mast cells are often numerous. A moderate amount of vascular proliferation may be seen, and both epithelioid histiocytes and reactive T cells may be numerous.[54]

These features may give rise to a differential diagnosis of either peripheral T-cell lymphoma (angioimmunoblastic or lymphoepithelioid cell type) or Hodgkin's disease of lymphocyte predominance or mixed cellularity type.[55] The presence of transitional forms between small lymphocytes and plasma cells should raise the possibility of immunocytoma. Immunoperoxidase stains for CIg should be done on any case of suspected peripheral T-cell lymphoma to exclude the possibility of immunocytoma.

In the spleen, both red and white pulp may be infiltrated. The major differential diagnosis in the spleen is with splenic marginal zone lymphoma/splenic lymphoma with villous lymphocytes (see below). There may be some overlap between these disorders, and precise criteria for distinguishing them have not been developed.

Bone Marrow

The bone marrow infiltrate may be either diffuse or nodular and is often interstitial and rather subtle. It is usually less massive than that of B-CLL. Plasma cells and plasmacytoid cells may be very inconspicuous in the marrow.

Variant: Immunoblast-Rich Immunocytoma

The original Kiel classification contained a subtype, polymorphous immunocytoma, that contained an admixture of centrocytes, centroblasts, and immunoblasts and that had a worse prognosis than typical immunocytoma.[3,56] In the updated version, this subtype was omitted since the authors thought it likely represented a wastebasket containing tumors of other types with plasmacytoid differentiation.[4] Nonetheless, some observers continue to distinguish a "large-cell-rich" variant of immunocytoma, with 20 to 50 percent immunoblasts or centroblasts, that has been shown to have a more aggressive clinical course.[57] Because of the possible prognostic importance of large cells, it is advisable to report cases containing more than 20 percent centroblast or immunoblast-like cells with a comment suggesting that they may have a more aggressive clinical course. Further clinicopathologic studies are required to elucidate the prognostic importance of large cells in this disorder and to determine whether histologic grading should be done.

Histologic Progression

As in B-CLL, transformation to a high grade B-cell lymphoma can occur in patients with lymphoplasmacytic immunocytoma

Immunophenotype

The cells have surface and (for some cells) cytoplasmic immonoglobulin, usually of IgM type, usually lack IgD, and strongly express B-cell-associated antigens (CD19, 20, 22, 79a). The cells are CD5−, CD10−, CD23−, CD43+/−; CD25 or CD11c may be faintly positive in some cases.[6,15,29,30] Lack of CD5 and CD23, strong surface immunoglobulin and CD20, and the presence of CIg are useful in distinction from B-CLL. As noted above, the presence of plasma cells is not in and of itself diagnostic of immunocytoma, since benign plasma cells can be present in many lymphomas. Immunoperoxidase stains on paraffin sections are the best method for demonstrating CIg and should be done in cases in which immunocytoma is suspected.

Genetic Features

Immunoglobulin Genes

Immunoglobulin heavy and light chain genes are rearranged. Recent studies show that immunoglobuin V region genes show somatic mutations in most cases of immunocytoma, suggesting that, in contrast to B-CLL, these cells arise from a population of B cells that has undergone some degree of antigen selection.[33]

Genetic Abnormalities

No specific chromosome translocation or oncogene abnormality is known.

Postulated Normal Counterpart

Lymphoplasmacytic lymphoma corresponds to a peripheral B lymphocyte stimulated to differentiate to a plasma cell, possibly corresponding to the primary immune response to antigen, or to a postgerminal center cell that has undergone somatic mutation but not heavy chain class switch.

Clinical Features

With the restrictive definition now used, lymphoplasmacytic lymphoma is a relatively rare disease. It occurs in the same general age group as B-CLL. Sites involved include bone marrow, lymph nodes, and spleen; less frequently peripheral blood or extranodal sites are involved. The majority of patients have a monoclonal serum paraprotein of IgM type (Waldenstrom's macroglobulinemia); hyperviscosity symptoms may occur.[4,6,15,29,30,58] As with B-CLL, the paraprotein may have autoantibody or cryoglobulin activity.[58] Recently, most cases of mixed cryoglobulinemia have been shown to be related to hepatitis C infection, even in patients who have demonstrable B-cell lymphoma in the bone marrow.[59] This observation raises the question of whether some cases of lymphoplasmacytic lymphoma may be antigen driven, similarly to MALT-type lymphoma (see below). The course is indolent, but has been reported to be more aggressive than typical B-CLL[56] like B-CLL, it has not generally been considered to be curable with conventional chemotherapy, but promising responses to purine analogs are being reported.

MANTLE CELL LYMPHOMA

Definition and Terminology

The Kiel classification in 1974 recognized an entity called *centrocytic lymphoma,*[60] which was composed exclusively of small, irregular lymphoid cells resembling normal germinal center centrocytes; it differed from another lymphoma composed of both centrocytes and centroblasts in having a predominantly diffuse growth pattern and a more aggressive clinical course.[56,61] Centrocytic lymphoma was not recognized in the United States. Instead, several groups reported cases of lymphoma that appeared to be ''intermediate'' in morphology between the ''well differentiated'' and ''poorly differentiated'' lymphocytic lymphomas of the Rappaport classification; these were variously called *intermediate lymphocytic lymphoma* (ILL) or *lymphocytic lymphoma of intermediate differentiation* (IDL).[62,63] Although centrocytic lymphoma was known to have a propensity for a partial or complete mantle zone pattern, the recognition that ILL could have such a pattern led to the recommendation that a distinct name, *mantle zone lymphoma,* be given to these cases.[64] Much confusion was generated by these papers, since the diagnostic criteria varied and distinction from CLL and ''PDL'' was not clearly defined. Finally, during the 1990s, identification of common immunophenotypic and genetic features between centrocytic lymphoma and a subset of ILL/IDL suggested that there was a distinct biologic entity that should be recognized.[11,38,65–76] Careful analysis of the literature and of individual cases clearly showed that the Kiel classification criteria identify a specific disease entity, which corresponds to many (but not all) cases classified by various authors as ILL/IDL.

Both terms, *centrocytic* and *ILL,* have significant drawbacks. The term *ILL* has been used inconsistently and may also cause confusion with the "intermediate grade" of the Working Formulation, while the term *centrocytic* implies a follicular center cell origin, which is now questioned. In addition, the term *mantle zone lymphoma*, which had been proposed for this entity, had previously been used for the nodular variant only. For this reason, the International Lymphoma Stody Group recently recommended that a new term be adopted. Because of the postulated origin of the neoplastic cell from the follicle mantle, the Study Group proposed the term *mantle cell lymphoma* to replace *centrocytic lymphoma*, *ILL*, *IDL*, and *mantle zone lymphoma*.[12]

In the original Working Formulation study, centrocytic lymphoma was included within the category of diffuse small cleaved cell lymphoma and comprised the majority of the cases of this subtype. Some cases with larger cells may fall within the diffuse mixed or large cleaved cell categories of the Working Formulation[2]; however, the tumor cells do not have basophilic cytoplasm and are distinct from the other lymphomas in these heterogeneous Working Formulation categories.

Morphology

The tumor is defined according to the Kiel classification criteria for centrocytic lymphoma.[3,4,12,61] In most cases it is composed exclusively of small to medium sized lymphoid cells, usually slightly larger than normal lymphocytes, with more dispersed chromatin, scant pale cytoplasm, and inconspicuous nucleoli (Fig. 6-3). In most cases, the nuclei are irregular or "cleaved"; however, in some cases the cells are nearly round and in others they may be very small and resemble small lymphocytes.[77] Transformed cells with basophilic cytoplasm (centroblast- or immunoblast-like cells) are by definition extremely rare or absent. The pattern is usually diffuse or vaguely nodular; well-defined follicles as in follicular lymphomas are occasionally seen. In many cases the tumor involves the mantle zones of at least some reactive follicles; less commonly, a pure mantle zone pattern occurs. Many cases contain individually scattered epithelioid histiocytes, creating a "starry-sky" appearance at low magnification, although these cells differ from usual starry-sky macrophages in that they do not usually contain apoptotic debris.

Morphologic Variants

Lymphoblastoid. A small proportion of the cases have larger nuclei with more dispersed chromatin and a high proliferation fraction.[6,69] Because some of these resemble lymphoblastic lymphoma, the term *blastic variant* has been applied. The terms *lymphoblastoid* and *blastoid* are preferable to emphasize the cytologic resemblance to lymphoblasts rather than to large transformed blasts (centroblasts or immunoblasts).

Centroblastoid. The updated Kiel classification defines a variant of *centroblastic* lymphoma, called *centrocytoid centroblastic*, in which the neoplastic cells are smaller than typical centroblasts and have round to oval nuclei, dispersed chromatin, and faintly basophilic cytoplasm. Although this was thought to be a variant of centroblastic lymphoma, recent studies have shown that the immunophenotype is typical of mantle cell (centrocytic) lymphoma and that these cases have *bcl*-1 rearrangement.[78] This suggests that the so-called centrocytoid centroblastic lymphoma is actually a *centroblastoid* variant of *centrocytic* (*mantle cell*) lymphoma.

Pleomorphic. The original Kiel classification recognized a variant of centrocytic lymphoma with larger nuclei, which was called *anaplastic* or *large cell* centrocytic lymphoma. Some cases of mantle cell lymphoma have larger cells than usual, with prominent nuclear clefts, often hyperchromatic nuclei, and a high mitotic rate with apoptosis. This appearance is often focal in an otherwise typical case and may also be seen in lymph nodes at relapse.[79]

Histologic Progression/Transformation

Transformation to a large cell lymphoma composed of centroblast or immunoblast-like cells does not appear to occur, although a grad-

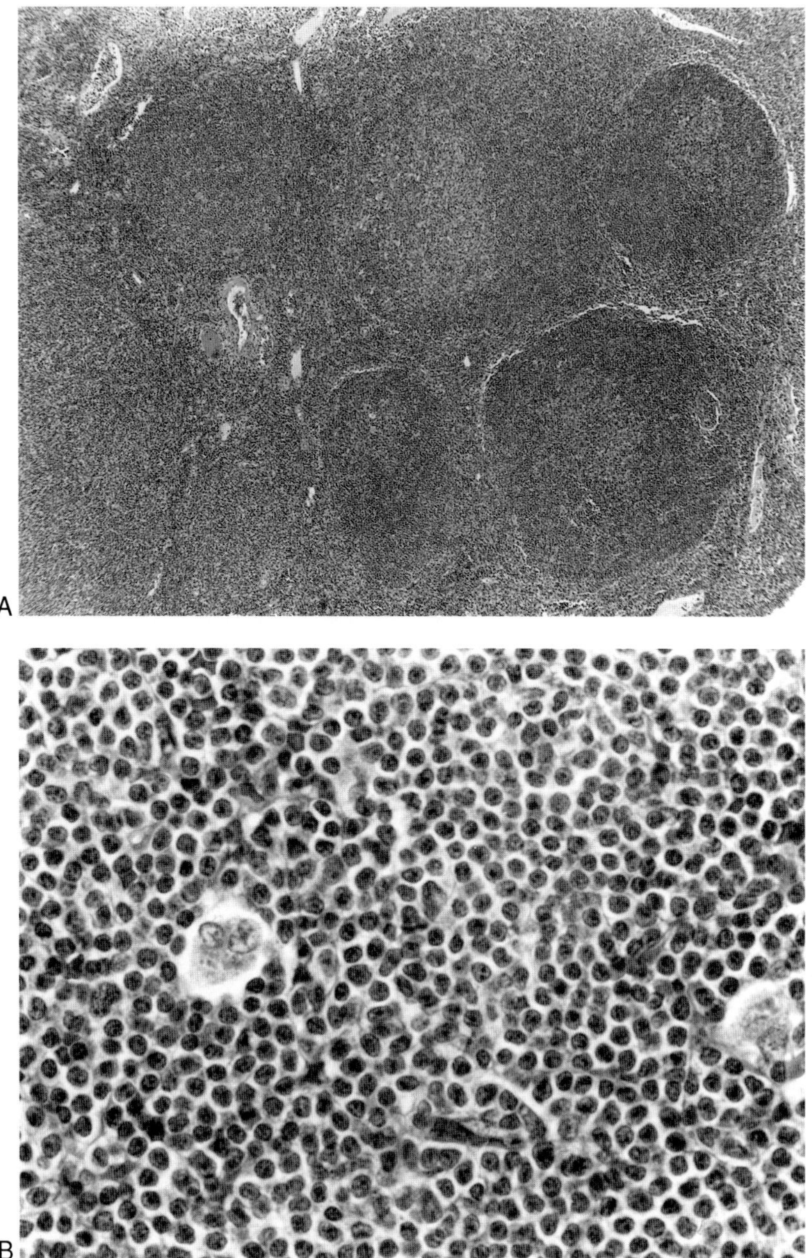

Fig. 6-3. Mantle cell lymphoma. **(A)** Low magnification of lymph node, showing mantle zone pattern, with reactive germinal centers. **(B)** High magnification, showing monotonous small, irregular lymphoid cells, with scattered single histiocytes. **(C)** ''Blastoid'' variant, showing larger cells with more nuclear irregularity and a high mitotic rate. **(D)** Immunoperoxidase stain for cyclin D1, showing dark staining neoplastic cells in mantle zones of reactive follicles. **(E)** Higher magnification, showing nuclear staining for cyclin D1. (*Figure continues.*)

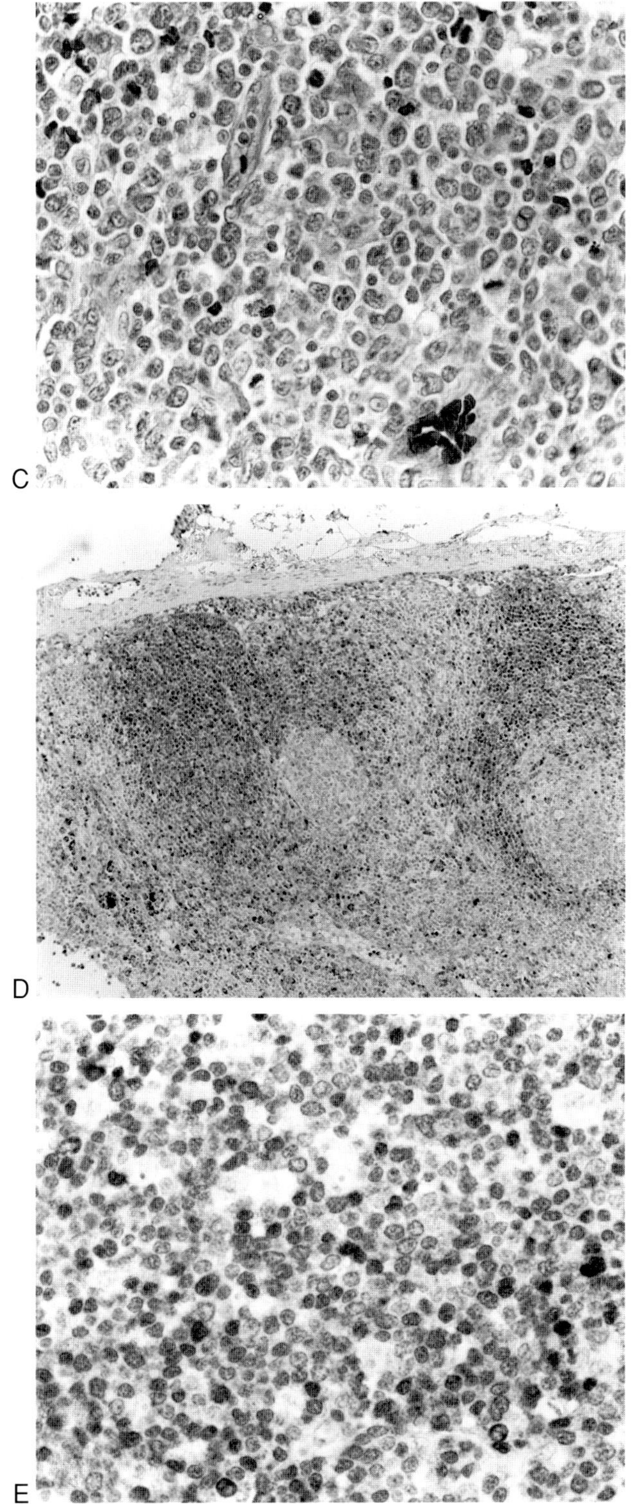

Fig. 6-3. (*continued*)

ual increase in the size of the tumor cells accompanied by an increase in proliferation fraction often occurs at relapse.[57,79]

Immunophenotype

The tumor cells are surface IgM+, usually IgD+, $\lambda > \kappa$, B-cell-associated antigen positive, CD5+, CD10−/+, CD23−, CD43+, and CD11c−. A prominent, disorganized meshwork of follicular dendritic cells is present. Absence of CD23 is useful in distinguishing mantle cell lymphoma from B-CLL; CD5 is useful in distinction from follicle center and marginal zone lymphomas.[6,29,31,61,80,81] The product of the cyclin D1 gene can be detected in the nuclei of neoplastic mantle cells in paraffin-embedded tissue sections with the immunoperoxidase technique; this may be a useful marker in distinguishing mantle cell lymphoma from other low grade B-cell lymphomas.[41,82]

Genetic Features

Immunoglobuin Genes

Immunoglobulin heavy and light chain genes are rearranged. Studies of the immunoglobulin V region genes indicate a relative lack of somatic mutations, consistent with a pregerminal center stage of differentiation, similar to the cells of B-CLL.[83]

Genetic Abnormalities

A chromosomal translocation t(11;14) involves the immunoglobulin heavy chain locus and the *bcl*-1 locus on the long arm of chromosome 11 in the majority of cases. This translocation results in overexpression of a gene known as *PRAD1* or *cyclin D1*, which encodes a cell cycle associated protein that is not normally expressed in lymphoid cells.[38,41,70,71,73–76,78]

Postulated Normal Counterpart

Stein and coworkers[29] postulated that the cell of centrocytic lymphoma might be a germinal center centrocyte of an early type that appeared before the centroblast and was distinct from the later centrocyte of follicular lymphomas. CD5+ B cells have been demonstrated in both germinal centers and follicle mantle zones.[45,84] CD5+ B cells make up less than 10 percent of peripheral blood B cells; expression of CD23 on these cells is variable, but at least some appear to be CD23−. Thus, it is possible that there are two types of CD5+ B cells, one that corresponds to B-CLL and one to mantle cell lymphoma.

Clinical Features

The tumor occurs in older adults, with a high male to female ratio; it is usually widespread at diagnosis. Sites involved include lymph nodes, spleen, Waldeyer's ring, bone marrow, blood, and extranodal sites, especially the gastrointestinal tract (lymphomatous polyposis).[85,86] The course is moderately aggressive, and it appears to be incurable with available treatment.[57,87–90] The median survival ranges from 3 to 5 years; the blastoid variant is reported in some studies to be more aggressive (median survival 3 years).[69,91]

FOLLICLE CENTER LYMPHOMA, FOLLICULAR (FOLLICULAR LYMPHOMA)

Definition and Terminology

This lymphoma is defined as a tumor composed of follicle center cells, usually a mixture of centrocytes (cleaved follicle center cells) and centroblasts (large noncleaved follicle center cells). The pattern is at least partially follicular, but diffuse areas may be present.[3] Centrocytes typically predominate; centroblasts are usually in the minority, but by definition are always present. Rare lymphomas with a follicular growth pattern consist almost entirely of centroblasts; since the follicular pattern implies a germinal center origin, these are included in the category of follicle center lymphoma.

The tumor defined in this manner comprises most cases found in the categories of nodular or follicular lymphomas in the Rappaport classification and WF; however, since the criteria in these classifications are based on pattern only, some cases of mantle cell lymphoma with a follicular pattern are also found in the category of follicular small cleaved cell or nodular poorly differentiated lymphocytic lymphoma. In addition, some cases of marginal zone B-cell lymphoma with follicular colonization could be called *follicular lymphoma* in the WF.

This tumor would be included in the categories of follicular center cell lymphoma of small or large cleaved cell type or large noncleaved cell type with a follicular pattern in the Lukes and Collins classification, but the Lukes and Collins classification does not distinguish between cases with a follicular or diffuse pattern or between cases that are composed entirely of one cell type and those that have a mixture of follicle center cells. In addition, Burkitt's lymphoma and some cases of diffuse large B-cell lymphoma are considered to be follicular center cell lymphomas in the Lukes and Collins classification.

Follicle center lymphoma corresponds most closely to centroblastic/centrocytic lymphoma in the Kiel classification. However, the category of centroblastic/centrocytic lymphoma excludes cases that have a follicular pattern but are composed entirely of large cells (centroblasts). Since data from some centers in the United States suggest that follicular large cell lymphomas do not behave identically to diffuse large cell lymphomas, it seems desirable to continue to separate them for diagnostic purposes.

For all these reasons, the term *follicle center lymphoma, follicular,* was proposed by the International Lymphoma Study Group to encompass most tumors classified as follicular lymphomas in the WF, most tumors with a follicular pattern classified as follicular center cell lymphoma in the Lukes and Collins classification, all cases in the Kiel classification category of centroblastic/centrocytic lymphoma with any follicular pattern, and centroblastic lymphoma with a purely follicular pattern. Although this term was selected as the most precise one, it is somewhat cumbersome. In practice, it seems reasonable simply to redefine the term *follicular lymphoma* with new precision, to refer only to a lymphoma of follicle center type with a follicular pattern and not to other lymphomas with a nodular or follicular growth pattern. The existence and clinical significance of a purely diffuse lymphoma composed of both centroblasts and centrocytes is controversial, and for this reason *follicle center lymphoma, diffuse,* is considered to be a provisional entity (see below).

Morphology

The cells of follicular lymphoma are virtually identical to those of the normal germinal center (Fig. 6-4). The centrocytes, while usually less than twice the size of small lymphocytes, have a spectrum of size and may be almost as large as centroblasts. The nuclei appear irregular or angulated in tissue sections; although the term *cleaved* is used, in fact a distinct nuclear cleft is seldom seen. The chromatin is paler than that of small lymphocytes and is evenly dispersed, giving the nucleus a grey-blue appearance. Single or multiple small nucleoli may be present. The cytoplasm is scant and pale and is not usually visible on H&E or Giemsa stained sections. Centroblasts are usually three to four times the size of small lymphocytes; the nuclei are round or oval, but may be irregular, indented, or even have a cleft. The nucleus is vesicular, with a clear center and some peripheral condensation of chromatin; there are one to three basophilic nucleoli, usually apposed to the nuclear membrane. There is a narrow rim of cytoplasm, which is intensely basophilic on Giemsa staining.

Grading

Cytology. Both the proportion of centroblasts and the size of the centrocytes vary among cases. Follicular lymphoma cannot be

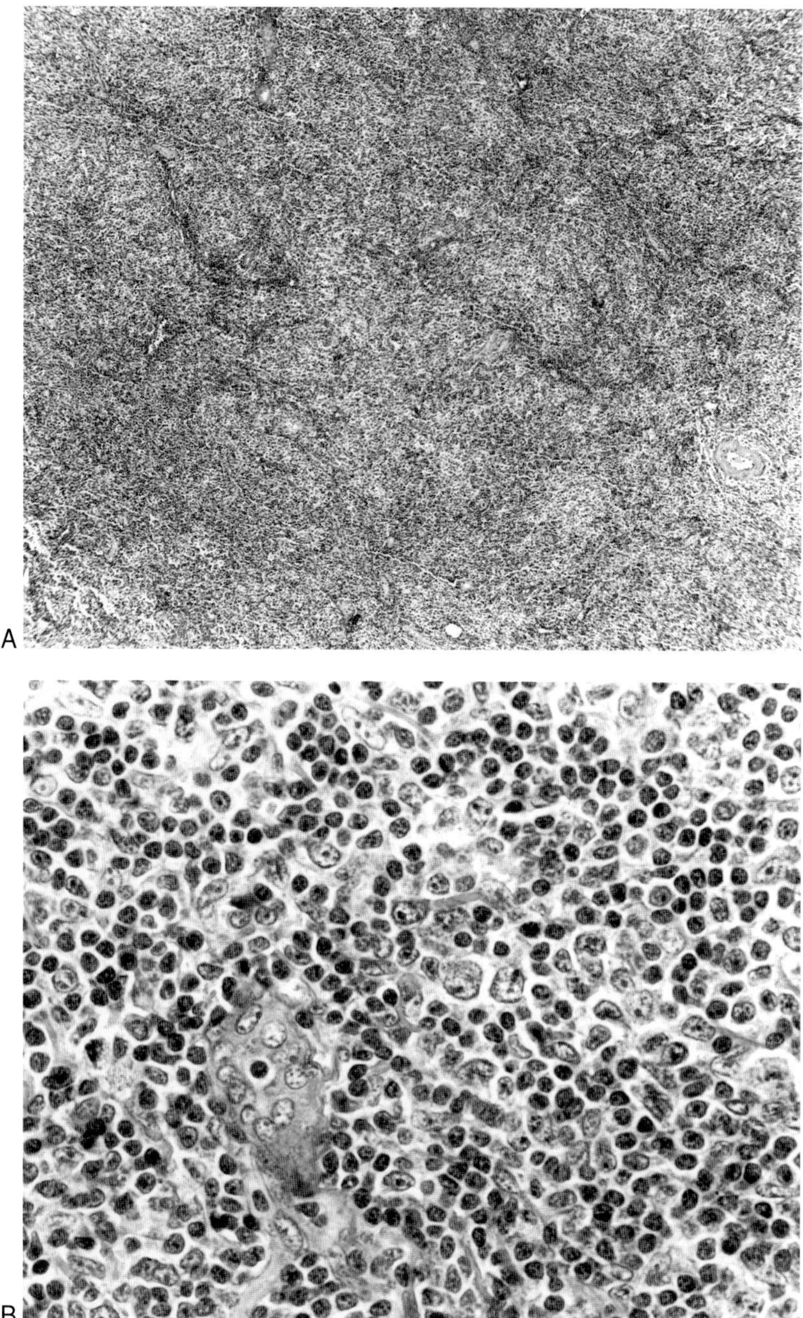

Fig. 6-4. Follicle center lymphoma, diffuse. **(A)** Low magnification, showing vague nodularity. **(B)** High magnification, showing mixture of centroblasts and centrocytes.

sharply divided into distinct subtypes, but rather shows a continuous gradation in the number of large cells.[92] Although this has been called *subclassification* in the past, it should be recognized as grading. It has been repeatedly shown that an individual pathologist can effectively predict outcome in follicular lymphoma by grading according to proportion of large cells, but studies have shown that this is difficult to reproduce among groups of pathologists.[93,94] By convention in the United States, cases of follicular lymphoma are separated into predominantly small, mixed small and large, and large cell categories. This terminology is not optimal for two reasons: first, it ignores the fact that all three categories are in fact "mixed," containing both centroblasts and centrocytes, and, second, it implies that there are three distinct tumor types rather than a continuum. For this reason, the International Lymphoma Study Group suggested the terms *follicular lymphoma, grade I, grade II,* and *grade III,* which are more analogous to terms used for other tumor types.

Unfortunately, there is no consensus among pathologists on the optimal method for grading follicular lymphomas. Several studies suggest that the "cell counting" method of Mann and Berard[92] is more reproducible and better at predicting prognosis than other methods.[93,94] In this method, the number of centroblasts (large nucleolated cells) per high power microscopic field are counted (10 to 20 high power fields in different follicles). A case with fewer than 5 per high power field is called *predominantly small cell;* 6 to 15 large cells is *mixed,* and more than 15 large cells is *large cell.*[92] In some studies, the number of centroblasts has been shown to correlate with prognosis.[95]

This method has a serious technical drawback, namely, it counts large cells *per high power microscopic field* rather than as a percent of all cells, and variation in ocular strength from one microscope to another can significantly affect the field size and potentially the grade of the tumor. Standardization of the field size using an ocular micrometer could resolve this problem. A more serious problem is the difficulty in an individual case of deciding which large cells are centroblasts: particularly on H&E sections, nuclei of histiocytes and dendritic cells, as well as those of large centrocytes, may be confused with centroblasts. A final problem is that, using the numerical cutoffs of Mann and Berard,[92] the spectrum of follicular large cell lymphoma may be very broad, ranging from cases with 16 large cells per high power field to cases in which the majority of the cells in the follicle are centroblasts.[96] Some authors have suggested modifying the Mann and Berard method so that cases are not called *large cell* unless at least 50 percent of the cells are centroblasts or large centrocytes (reviewed by Martin et al.[97]). One would hope that more objective methods such as counting Ki-67 + cells using an automated image analyzer would provide more unformity; however, a recent study[97] suggested that this method was less useful in predicting outcome than the Mann and Berard[92] counting method.

The criteria for diagnosis and grading of follicular lymphoma are very different in the Kiel classification, although since the vast majority of the cases have both a follicular pattern and a predominance of centrocytes, the differences in criteria result in only a few cases that would be classified differently. In the Kiel classification, cases are classified as centroblastic/centroyctic if they are composed of both centrocytes and centroblasts, regardless of pattern. They are further subclassified by pattern as follicular, follicular and diffuse, or diffuse. Cases that show a *solid growth of centroblasts,* even if only focally, are diagnosed as centroblastic lymphoma; these are further subclassified as follicular (about 10 percent of the cases), follicular and diffuse, or diffuse (the vast majority of the cases). If areas of typical centroblastic/centrocytic lymphoma are present in the same tissue, the case is diagnosed as "simultaneous" secondary centroblastic lymphoma; in the Kiel classification, these tumors have the same prognosis as cases that are purely diffuse.[4]

The International Lymphoma Study Group did not recommend specific criteria for grading follicular lymphoma, but suggested that, as with other tumors, each pathologist or institution should adopt a grading scheme and use it consistently until data from prospective clinical trials are available to suggest a uniform method. At our institution, we have for many years used a modification of the cell counting method, as summarized in Table 6-6.

Pattern. In addition to cellular composition, the proportions of follicular and diffuse areas vary from case to case. By convention in the United States, any follicular component, even if it is less than 10 percent of the tumor, means that the tumor is considered a follicular lymphoma.[2,96] In the Kiel classification, in contrast, the tumor is classified based on cell type (centroblastic/centrocytic) and further subclassified according to pattern (follicular, follicular and diffuse, or diffuse). Several studies suggest that the presence of diffuse areas may affect the prognosis, while others show no effect.[96,98–101] The impact of diffuse areas is much more important in cases classified as large cell (centroblastic): in these cases any diffuse area results in a worse outcome, suggesting that the presence of a diffuse component indicates histologic progression to diffuse large B-cell lymphoma.[96,98] These results tend to corroborate the practice of the Kiel classification, in which centroblastic lymphoma is considered a single entity, whether or not it has a follicular component. However, the study from Stanford,[96] showing that cases of *purely* follicular large cell lymphoma had a better prognosis than those with a diffuse component, suggests that centroblastic lymphoma with a *purely* follicular growth pattern should be distinguished from cases with a diffuse component.

Finally, some early studies of low grade follicular lymphoma may have included cases of mantle cell lymphoma in the small cleaved cell group; these lymphomas are more likely to have diffuse areas than are follicle center lymphomas and definitely have a worse prognosis. Additional studies using the current definition of follicular lymphoma might be useful in further assessing the impact of pattern on prognosis in follicular lymphoma of grades I and II.

Table 6-6. Grading of Follicular Lymphoma

Grade	Criteria
Grade 1:	0–5 centroblasts per hpf[a]
Grade 2:	6–15 centroblasts per hpf
Grade 3:	16 or more centroblasts per hpf *or* >50% centroblasts and large centrocytes

[a] With ×40 microscopic field; count 10 high power fields (hpf) in 10 different follicles.

(Adapted from Mann and Berard,[92] with permission.)

At present, treatment decisions for these patients do not depend on assessment of the proportion of follicular versus diffuse areas; however, patients with follicular grade III lymphoma are often treated as diffuse large cell lymphoma, particularly if they have diffuse areas. In our institution, we report the pattern as follicular (more than 75 percent follicular), follicular and diffuse (25 to 75 percent follicular), or focally follicular (less than 25 percent follicular). *For cases with a component of diffuse large B-cell lymphoma, we report them as diffuse large B-cell lymphoma and comment on the presence of a focal follicular pattern.*

Bone Marrow

Follicular lymphoma frequently involves the bone marrow, and this is the tumor that characteristically has a paratrabecular pattern in the marrow. Other low grade B-cell lymphomas produce nodular aggregates that are randomly distributed, and because they are numerous they can also be found in a paratrabecular location; however, they do not appear often to *selectively* involve paratrabecular regions, which seems to be the case with follicular lymphoma.

Variant: Follicle Center Lymphoma, Diffuse

Rare lymphomas composed of cells that resemble centrocytes, with a minor component of centroblasts, are entirely diffuse; if both the small and large cells have the phenotype of follicle center cells (see below), it may be assumed that they represent the diffuse counterpart of a follicle center lymphoma. This category corresponds to diffuse centroblastic/centrocytic lymphoma in the Kiel classification. Diffuse follicle center lymphomas typically have areas of sclerosis and numerous high endothelial venules and admixed T cells, similar to the interfollicular region of follicular lymphomas. Many of these cases can represent a sampling problem in some cases in which larger biopsies show follicular areas. Most have been called *diffuse small cleaved cell lymphoma* or *diffuse mixed small and large cell lymphoma* in the WF. This diagnosis should only be made if immunophenotyping studies show a B-cell phenotype of *both* the small and large cells and lack of CD5 and CD43; CD10 positivity and *bcl*-2 rearrangement are useful in confirming the diagnosis. If the number of centroblast-like cells is greater than about 25 percent, or if the small cells are T cells, the case should be classified as diffuse large B-cell lymphoma.

Histologic Transformation/Progression

Progression to diffuse large B-cell lymphoma occurs in 40 to 60 percent of the cases; the large cells may resemble centroblasts, immunoblasts, Burkitt's lymphoma cells, or even large anaplastic cells.[102] Transformation to large B-cell lymphoma may involve mutations in the *p53* gene; [103] rare cases of large cell, lymphoblastic, or Burkitt-like transformation involve c-*myc* translocation.[104–106]

Immunophenotype

The tumor cells of follicle center lymphoma are usually surface immunoglobulin positive; about 50 to 60 percent express IgM; about 40 percent express IgG; and rare cases express IgA. This frequency of IgG expression is greater than that seen in other low grade B-cell lymphomas and correlates with the fact that immunoglobulin heavy chain class switching occurs in the normal germinal center. The tumor cells express pan-B-cell associated antigens, about 60 percent are CD10+, and they are CD5−, CD23−/+, CD43−, and CD11c−. Tightly organized meshworks of follicular dendritic cells are present in follicular areas.[6,29,81,107,108] bcl-2 protein expression is useful in distinguishing reactive from neoplastic follicles, since it is absent from reactive follicles and present in most follicular lymphomas;[109,110] however, this is *not* useful in distinguishing follicle center from other types of low grade B-cell lymphoma, most of which also express bcl-2 protein. In addition, many grade III follicular lymphomas are bcl-2 negative. Lack of CD5 and CD43 is useful in distinguishing follicle center lymphoma from mantle cell lymphoma, and the presence of CD10 can be useful in distinguishing it from marginal zone B-cell lymphomas (see below).

Genetics

Immunoglobulin Genes

Immunoglobulin heavy and light chain genes are rearranged, and analysis of the immunoglobulin variable region genes shows that most cases have extensive somatic mutations, similar to normal germinal center cells. In addition, analysis of DNA from individual clones shows a high frequency of intraclonal diversity, indicating ongoing mutations—again, similar to findings in normal follicle center cells.[83,111–114]

Genetic Abnormalities

A translocation t(14;18), involving rearrangement of the *bcl*-2 gene, is present in 70 to 95 percent of the cases, resulting in expression of this "anti-apoptosis" gene, which is switched off at the translational level in normal germinal center cells; expression of the bcl-2 protein permits accumulation of long-lived centrocytes.[115–117] This translocation occurs at an early stage of B-cell development, during immunoglobulin gene rearrangement,[115] and occasional cells with rearranged *bcl*-2 genes can be detected in lymphoid tissues and peripheral blood lymphocytes in some normal individuals.[118] These observations suggest that when a resting B cell that carries the *bcl*-2 translocation undergoes blast transformation in response to antigen, failure to switch off the *bcl*-2 gene may contribute to development of a lymphoma.

Postulated Normal Counterpart

Germinal center B cells, both centrocytes (small cleaved follicular center cells) and centroblasts (large noncleaved follicular center cells), are postulated normal counterparts.[107,119,120]

Clinical Features

Follicular lymphoma is the most common adult lymphoma in the United States and Europe, comprising 35 to 40 percent of all non-Hodgkin's lymphoma, and 75 to 80 percent of low grade B-cell lymphomas. It affects predominantly older adults, with an equal male: female incidence.[2] Most patients have widespread disease at diagnosis, usually predominantly lymph nodes, but also spleen, bone marrow, and occasionally peripheral blood or extranodal sites. The clinical course is generally indolent, and it is not usually curable with available treatment. Both the number of centroblasts and the size of the centrocytes appear to correlate with prognosis.[3,92,94,121,122] Controversy exists over whether or not cases classified as follicular mixed cell type may be curable with aggressive therapy.[95,123] Follicular large cell (grade III) lymphomas are often treated similarly to diffuse large cell lymphomas, with aggressive chemotherapy regimens, and studies have shown that a proportion of these cases may be cured.[96,124,125] Like the proportion of centroblasts, the proportion of the tumor that has a follicular pattern is also related to prognosis.[96,98,100] The rare purely diffuse follicle center lymphomas appear to have a worse prognosis.[56] Histologic progression is generally regarded as an ominous event in follicular lymphoma, and these patients may be refractory to treatment; however, those who respond to aggressive therapy may be cured.[126]

MARGINAL ZONE B-CELL LYMPHOMA, EXTRANODAL (LOW GRADE B-CELL LYMPHOMA OF MUCOSA-ASSOCIATED LYMPHOID TISSUE) AND NODAL TYPES

Definition and Terminology

Extranodal infiltrates of small lymphoid cells, often associated with reactive germinal centers and plasma cells, were for many years considered to be benign, hyperplastic lesions called *pseudolymphomas*. The advent of immunologic marker studies in the 1970s and 1980s led to the recognition that the majority of these lesions expressed monotypic immunoglobulin and/or had clonal immunoglobulin gene rearrangement and were therefore low grade B-cell lymphomas. However, it rapidly became apparent that they were a clinically and immunophenotypically distinct type of low grade B-cell lymphoma, differing in many respects from the better known nodal types such as B-CLL/SLL, Waldenstrom's macroglobulinemia, mantle cell lymphoma, and follicular lymphoma. They differed from CLL and mantle cell lymphoma in lacking CD5, from follicular lymphoma in lacking CD10, and from all other low grade lymphomas in being frequently localized at the time of the diagnosis and potentially curable with local therapy.[127] In the mid-1980s, it was proposed that these tumors might arise from normal extranodal lymphoid tissue—the mucosa-associated lymphoid tissue (MALT).[128,129] It was noted that these tumors often contained an unusual type of cells, which were termed a *centrocyte-like* cell, since it had an irregular nucleus, similar to a germinal center centrocyte (cleaved cell), but had more abundant, pale cytoplasm. At about the same time, other observers described a lymphoma containing cells resembling nodal monocytoid B cells, which were called monocytoid B-cell lymphoma.[130,131] It soon became apparent that monocytoid B-cell lymphoma was common in extranodal sites, particularly the salivary gland (associated in many cases with Sjögren syndrome), and that patients with nodal disease often had a history of extranodal lymphoma or Sjögren syndrome.[132,133] In addition, although not identical, there were morphologic similarities between monocytoid B cells and centrocyte-like cells, leading Lennert to conclude that centrocyte-like cells were equivalent to a small monocytoid B cell.[134] All of these observations led many observers to conclude that monocytoid B-cell lymphoma and MALT lymphoma were essentially the same disease.[135,136]

Because of the confusion surrounding the nomenclature for these tumors[131–134] and the fact that they show morphologic evidence of differentiation at least in part into cells of marginal zone type,[137] which have the capacity to mature into both monocytoid B cells[138] and plasma cells, and display tissue-specific homing patterns,[139–147] the International Lymphoma Study Group proposed the term *marginal zone B-cell lymphoma* for this entity, with modifiers to indicate the clinical subtype: *extranodal* or *nodal*.

Morphology

Marginal zone B-cell lymphoma is characterized by cellular and architectural complexity. The neoplastic cell population is heterogeneous, in contrast to the relatively monomorphous character of the infiltrate in most other non-Hodgkin's lymphomas, and includes small lymphocytes, marginal zone (centrocyte-like) B cells, monocytoid B cells, and plasma cells (Fig. 6-5). Marginal zone B cells are small to medium sized cells resembling small cleaved follicular center cells or centrocytes, but with more abundant cytoplasm, similar to the cells found in the outer mantle zone of Peyer's patches, mesenteric lymph nodes, or splenic white pulp. Monocytoid B cells are larger cells, with more nuclear irregularity and more abundant, pale cytoplasm, identical to the monocytoid or parafollicular B cells found between the mantle zone and cortical or subcapsular sinuses of reactive lymph nodes. Occasional large basophilic blast cells (centroblast- or immunoblast-like) are present in most cases.

Reactive follicles are usually present, with the neoplastic marginal zone or monocytoid B cells occupying the marginal zone and/or the interfollicular region (Fig. 6-5); occasional follicles may contain an excess of marginal zone or monocytoid cells, giving them a neoplastic appearance (follicular colonization). Interfollicular monocytoid B cells may occupy the same locations in the lymphomas as they do in reactive nodes, causing difficulty in recognizing the process as neoplastic. In epithelial tissues, the marginal zone B cells typically infiltrate the epithelium, forming so-called *lymphoepithelial lesions*. In lymph nodes they may have a perisinusoidal, parafollicular, or marginal zone pattern of distribution (Fig. 6-5). Plasma cells are often distributed in distinct subepithelial or interfollicular zones and are neoplastic (monoclonal) in up to 40 percent of the cases.

Grading

There can be variability in the number of large cells (centroblast-like or immunoblast-like) in low grade MALT lymphomas; no specific criteria for determining when this represents a higher grade lymphoma have been developed. One group reported that large cells up to 25 percent of the total were not associated with a worse prognosis in gastric lymphomas.[148] The presence of solid sheets of blast cells, which would constitute evidence of high-grade lymphoma in another type of low grade lymphoma, should be considered evidence of high grade transformation. In such a case, we would generally make a diagnosis of diffuse large B-cell lymphoma, arising in marginal zone B-cell lymphoma.

Histologic Progression/Transformation

Like many other low grade lymphomas, there is a potential for marginal zone B-cell lymphoma to transform into a diffuse large B-cell lymphoma either in extranodal sites or in lymph nodes (Table 6-7). When large B-cell lymphomas of the stomach or lung are examined carefully, it is possible to find residual low grade

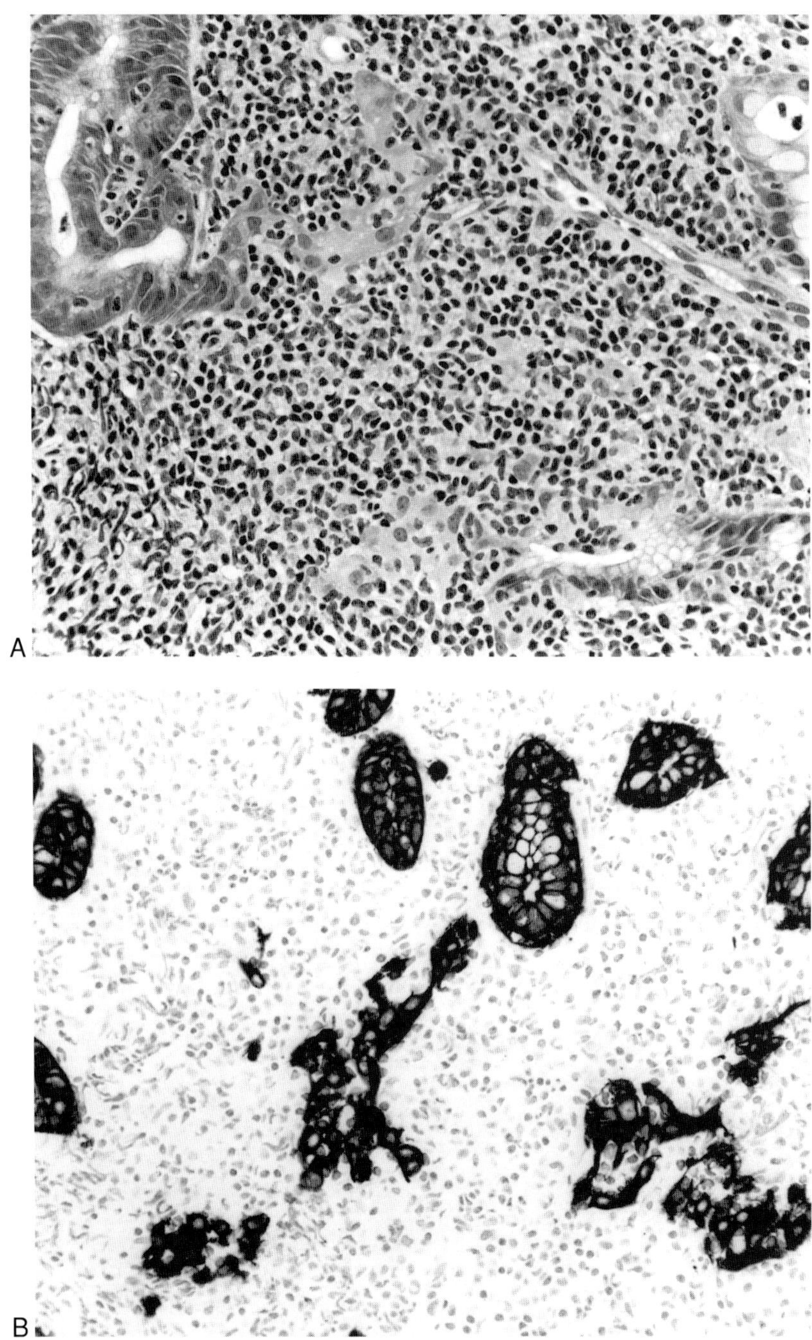

Fig. 6-5. Marginal zone B-cell lymphoma, extranodal, MALT type. **(A)** Gastric biopsy, showing a diffuse infiltrate of small lymphoid cells with focal infiltration of glands. **(B)** Immunoperoxidase stain for cytokeratin, showing disrupted epithelium. *(Figure continues.)*

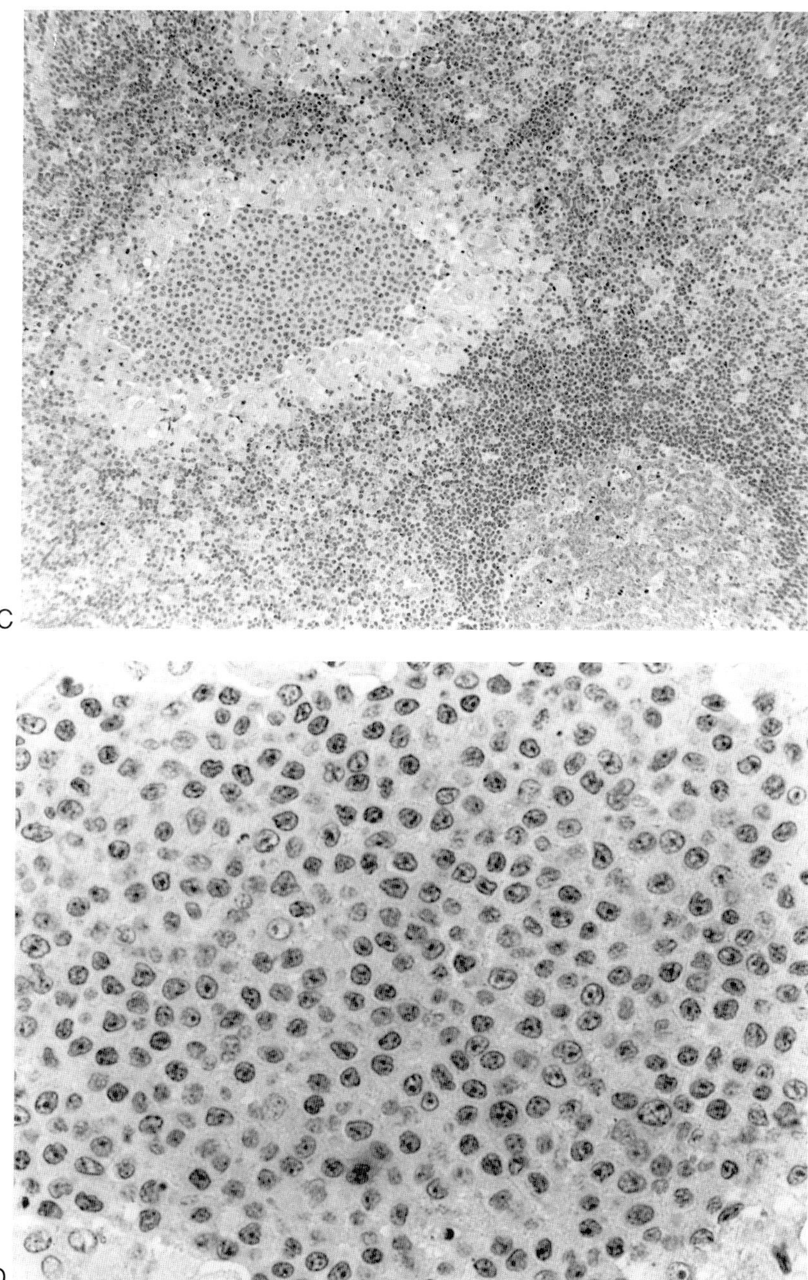

Fig. 6-5. *(Continued).* **(C)** Cervical lymph node biopsy from a patient with Sjögren syndrome, showing a cluster of monocytoid B cells surrounded by epithelioid histiocytes, in the interfollicular region. **(D)** Higher magnification, showing monocytoid B cells with irregular nuclei and pale cytoplasm. Both monocytoid cells and plasma cells expressed monotypic immunoglobulin. This lesion represents nodal involvement by an extranodal marginal zone (MALT lymphoma of the salivary gland).

Table 6-7. Histologic Diagnosis of Gastric MALT Lymphoma

Grade	Diagnosis	Histological Features
0	Normal	Scattered plasma cells; no follicles
1–2	Chronic active	Small clusters of lymphocytes with or without follicles
3	Suspicious, probably benign	Follicles surrounded by diffuse lymphocytic infiltrate, focally in epithelium
4	Suspicious, probably lymphoma	Follicles surrounded by diffuse infiltrate of MZ cells; rare LEL
5	MALToma	Diffuse infiltrate of MZ cells in lamina propria; prominent LEL

Abbreviations: MZ, marginal zone; LEL, lymphoepithelial lesions.
(Adapted from Wotherspoon et al.,[166] with permission.)

lymphoma at the periphery in 25 to 30 percent of the cases, suggesting that these tumors arose from pre-existing low grade MALT lymphomas.[149] These tumors have been referred to as high grade MALT lymphomas; it has been suggested but not proven that they may have a slightly more favorable prognosis than true primary large B-cell lymphomas of the same location.[148,150,151] (See Tables 6-7 for histologic diagnostic classification of gastric MALT lymphoma.)

Immunophenotype

The tumor cells of marginal zone lymphomas usually express surface immunoglobulin (M > G > A), lack IgD, and 40 to 60 percent have monoytpic CIg, indicating plasmacytoid differentiation. B-cell-associated antigens (CD19, 20, 22, 79a) are expressed, and the tumors are usually negative for CD5 and CD10, antigens that characterize SLL, mantle cell lymphoma, and follicular lymphoma, respectively. Expression of CD23, CD43, and CD11c is variable. Immunophenotyping studies are a useful adjunct to diagnosis in excluding B-CLL (CD5+), mantle cell (CD5+), and follicle center (CD10+ CD43−, CD11c−, usually CIg−) lymphomas.[6,152–154]

Genetic Features

Immunoglobulin Genes

Analysis of the immunoglobulin gene variable region indicates a high degree of somatic mutation, sometimes with intraclonal diversity, consistent with a postgerminal center stage of B-cell development.

Genetic Abnormalities

No rearrangement of *bcl*-2 or *bcl*- is seen.[155] Trisomy 3 and t(11;18) have been reported in both nodal and extranodal cases.[156]

Clinical Features

In Western countries, marginal zone B-cell lymphomas are usually tumors of adults, although patients may be in their 20s and 30s. A slight female predominance has been reported in some series.[6] Many patients have a history of autoimmune disease, such as Sjögren syndrome or Hashimoto's thyroiditis, or of *Helicobacter* gastritis. It has been suggested that "acquired MALT" secondary to autoimmune disease or infection in these sites may form the substrate for lymphoma development.[157] Proliferation of these cells at certain sites may depend on the presence of activated, antigen-driven T cells; in gastric tumors, it has been shown that the T cells are driven by *Helicobacter pylori* antigens.[158] The majority of patients present with localized stage I or II extranodal disease, involving glandular epithelial tissues of various sites, most frequently the stomach; however, skin and soft tissues may be the presenting site as well.[150,151,159–165] Dissemination or recurrence may occur, often in other extranodal sites, with long disease-free intervals.[165] Localized tumors may be cured with local treatment.[150,151,161] Recent studies suggest that therapy directed at the antigen (*H. pylori* in gastric lymphoma) may result in regression of early lesions.[166,167] The disease known as *Mediterraneal abdominal lymphoma, α heavy chain disease,* and *immunoproliferative small intestinal disease,* which occurs in young adults in Eastern Mediterranean countries, is also likely an example of a MALT-type lymphoma, which may respond to antibiotic therapy in its early stages.[157]

Tumors with morphologic features identical to those described for extranodal MALT-type or monocytoid B-cell lymphomas have occasionally been reported with isolated or disseminated nodal involvement in the absence of extranodal disease.[131–134,168] Other sites involved include bone marrow and, rarely, peripheral blood.[169] The clinical course is indolent and does not appear to be significantly different from other disseminated low grade B-cell lymphomas. A recent study[90] comparing disseminated (stage III and IV) nodal and extranodal marginal zone lymphomas found that the nodal cases had better survival than the extranodal cases. However, this study included cases of follicular lymphoma with monocytoid B cells in the category of monocytoid B-cell lymphoma; thus this result is difficult to interpret. When either extranodal or nodal marginal zone B-cell lymphomas are disseminated, patients are not usually curable with available therapy.

Postulated Normal Counterpart

Peripheral B cells with the capacity to differentiate into marginal zone, monocytoid, and plasma cells are the postulated normal counterpart.

SPLENIC MARGINAL ZONE LYMPHOMA, WITH OR WITHOUT VILLOUS LYMPHOCYTES

Definition and Terminology

This is a neoplasm of small B-lymphoid cells that involves the spleen (both red and white pulp, mantle and marginal zones), bone marrow, and usually the peripheral blood, with small lymphoid cells with abundant cytoplasm and small surface "villous" projections. A variety of terms have been used, including splenic immunocytoma, splenic marginal zone lymphoma, and splenic lymphoma with villous lymphocytes. This entity has been described relatively recently, and its precise definition is not clearly established.[153,154,170–172] However, it may comprise the majority of chronic B-cell leukemias that do not fit the defining criteria of B-CLL, mantle cell lymphoma, or hairy cell leukemia.

Morphology

The neoplastic cells occupy both the mantle and marginal zones of the splenic white pulp, usually with a central residual germinal center, which may be either atrophic or hyperplastic (Fig. 6-6).[53,154,173] Accentuation of the marginal zone (marginal zone pattern) is seen in some but not all cases. Red pulp involvement may be prominent and consists of both small nodular aggregates and diffuse infiltration. The neoplastic cells range from small lymphocytes in the mantle zone to larger cells with irregular nuclei and pale cytoplasm (marginal zone B cells) in the marginal zone.[173] The pattern of splenic involvement may resemble B-CLL, mantle cell, and follicular lymphomas; careful examination of sections stained for immunoglobulin, T- and B-cell antigens, and *bcl*-2 may be required to distinguish between them (see below). However, the pattern is completely different from that of hairy cell leukemia, which always involves the red pulp diffusely and spares the white pulp.

Immunophenotype

The tumor cells in the peripheral blood express strong surface immunoglobulin, usually IgM, B-cell-associated antigens including strong surface CD22, and variably CD10, CD23, CD11c, and CD25. A minority of the cases may express CD5 or CD103.[174] Thus, the immunophenotype may overlap with that of follicular

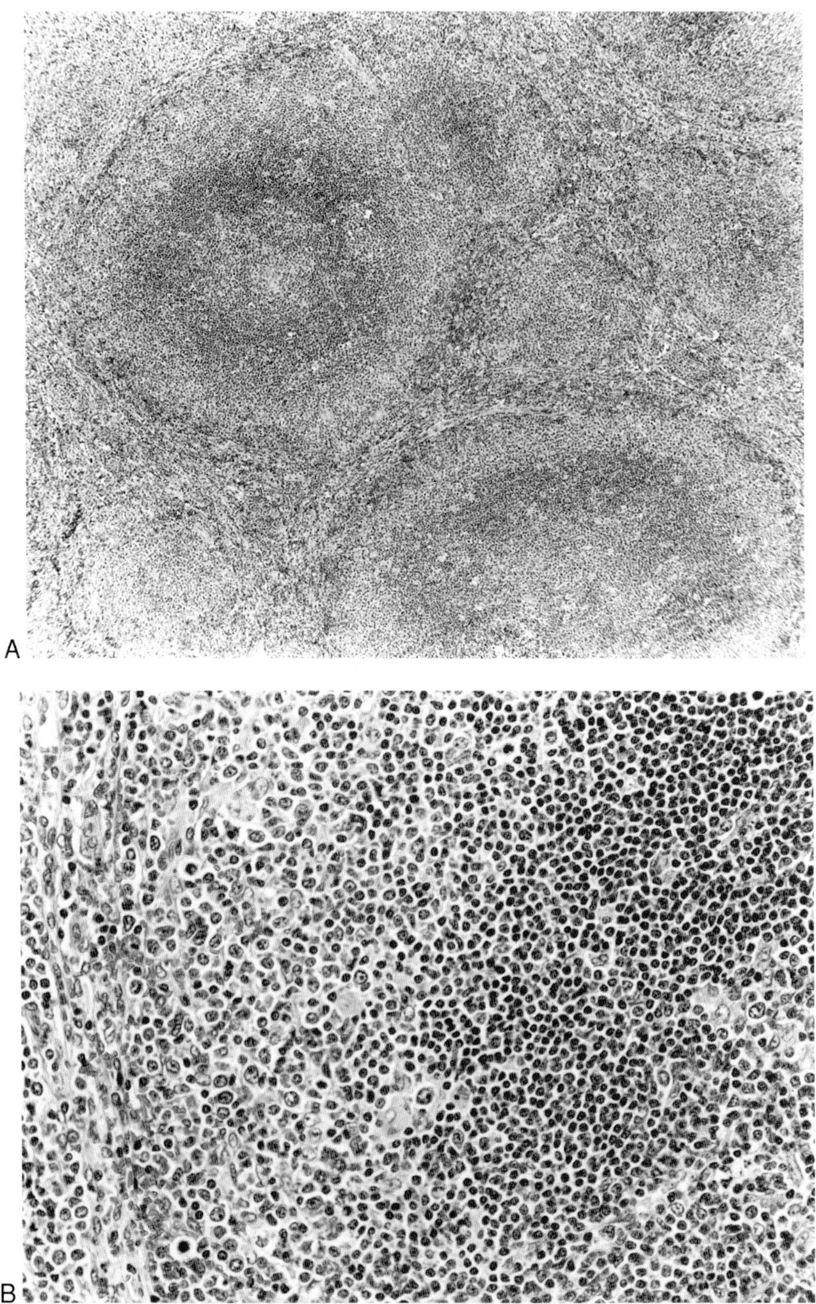

Fig. 6-6. Splenic marginal zone lymphoma. **(A)** At low magnification, there is expansion of both mantle and marginal zones, as well as red pulp involvement. **(B)** Neoplastic cells range from small round lymphocytes in the mantle zone (right) to larger, monocytoid-appearing cells in the marginal zone (left).

lymphoma, B-CLL, mantle cell lymphoma, and hairy cell leukemia. In the majority of the cases, strong surface immunoglobulin, strong CD22, and lack of CD5 will serve to distinguish this disorder from B-CLL, and lack of CD103 and CD25 are useful in distinguishing it from hairy cell leukemia.

In the spleen, immunoperoxidase stains on tissue sections reveal the complex architecture of the infiltrate, showing cells with monotypic immunoglobulin that are CD20+, *bcl*-2+, CD43− in the mantle and marginal zones, with small central *bcl*-2− follicles containing numerous T cells and a dense meshwork of CD21+ dendritic cells. In the differential diagnosis with mantle cell lymphoma and CLL, lack of CD43 may be useful on paraffin sections; recognition of the central benign follicle is useful in excluding follicular lymphoma.[173]

Genetic Features

Immunoglobulin Genes

Analysis of the immunoglobulin variable region indicates a high degree of somatic mutation but no intraclonal diversity, consistent with a postgerminal center stage B-cell development.[175]

Genetic Abnormalities

Most reported cases have an abnormal karyotype, but no consistent abnormality was found. The most common single chromosome abnormality in one series was t(11;14)(q13;132), similar to the abnormality found in mantle cell lymphoma, which was found in 15 percent.[176] Trisomy 3, found in nodal and extranodal marginal zone lymphoma, has not been detected.[156] As expected from the frequency of t(11;14), rearrangement of the *bcl*-1 locus and overexpression of the cyclin D1 gene was reported in 4 of 22 cases studied.[177] The possibility that the positive cases actually represent mantle cell lymphomas has not been excluded.

Clinical Features

Patients typically have bone marrow and peripheral blood involvement, usually without peripheral lymphadenopathy, and may have a small M component.[154] The course is extremely indolent, although the tumor may be surprisingly resistant to chemotherapy. Splenectomy may be followed by prolonged remission.

Postulated Normal Counterpart

Peripheral B cells with differentiation to splenic mantle and marginal zone cell are the postulated normal counterpart.

CONCLUSIONS

The recognition of new types of low grade B-cell lymphomas has been made possible largely because of advances in immunophenotyping and molecular genetics; thus, these techniques have paradoxically made lymphoma diagnosis both more complicated and yet more straightforward. Once the pathologist is familiar with the distinctive morphologic features of these neoplasms, most typical cases can be diagnosed without the need for immunophenotyping or genetic studies when an adequate amount of well-fixed tissue is available. However, in morphologically borderline or difficult cases, or when fixation or the amount of tissue is suboptimal, immunophenotyping studies can be very helpful in diagnosis. When neither good morphology nor tissue for immunophenotyping is available, it may be necessary simply to make a diagnosis of low grade B-cell lymphoma.

Although the various types of lymphoma described in this chapter do have significantly different natural histories, the treatments available are limited, and therefore many of them may be treated with similar regimens. Thus, if clinically important decisions do not require a precise subclassification, a diagnosis of low grade B-cell lymphoma may be sufficient to direct management. In other cases, such as a young patient with a differential diagnosis of B-CLL versus mantle cell lymphoma or mantle cell versus follicular lymphoma, re-biopsy may be indicated to obtain adequate tissue for subclassification. Although treatment options may be limited at present, the first step in developing better therapies is the recognition of distinct, specific disease entities by pathologists.

REFERENCES

1. Harris NL, Jaffe ES, Stein H et al: A revised European-American classification of lymphoid neoplasms: a proposal from the International Lymphoma Study Group. Blood 84:1361, 1994
2. Non-Hodgkin's lymphoma pathologic classification project. National Cancer Institute sponsored study of classifications of non-Hodgkin's lymphomas: summary and description of a Working Formulation for clinical usage. Cancer 49:2112, 1982
3. Lennert K: Malignant Lymphomas Other Than Hodgkin's Disease. Springer-Verlag, New York, 1978
4. Lennert K, Feller A: Histopathology of Non-Hodgkin's Lymphomas. 2nd Ed. Springer-Verlag, New York, 1992
5. Ben-Ezra J, Burke J, Swartz W et al: Small lymphocytic lymphoma: a clinicopathologic analysis of 268 cases. Blood 73:579, 1989
6. Zukerberg L, Medeiros L, Ferry J et al: Diffuse low-grade B-cell lymphomas: four clinically distinct subtypes defined by a combination of morphologic and immunophenotypic features. Am J Clin Pathol 100:373, 1993
7. Pangalis G, Nathwani B, Rappaport H: Malignant lymphoma, well differentiated lymphocytic: its relationship with chronic lymphocytic leukemia and macroglobulinemia of Waldenstrom. Cancer 39:999, 1977
8. Dick F, Maca R: The lymph node in chronic lymphocytic leukemia. Cancer 41:283, 1978
9. Evans H, Butler J, Youness E: Malignant lymphoma, small lymphocytic type: a clinicopathologic study of 84 cases with suggested criteria for intermediate lymphocytic lymphoma. Cancer 41:1440, 1978
10. Bennett J, Catovsky D, Daniel M-T et al: Proposals for the classification of chronic (mature) B and T lymphoid leukemias. J Clin Pathol 42: 567, 1989
11. Perry D, Bast M, Armitage J et al: Diffuse intermediate lymphocytic lymphoma: a clinicopathologic study and comparison with small lymphocytic lymphoma and diffuse small cleaved cell lymphoma. Cancer 66:1995, 1990
12. Banks P, Chan J, Cleary M et al: Mantle cell lymphoma: a proposal for unification of morphologic, immunologic, and molecular data. Am J Surg Pathol 16:637, 1992
13. Pugh W, Manning J, Butler J: Paraimmunoblastic variant of small lymphocytic lymphoma/leukemia. Am J Surg Pathol 12:907, 1988
14. Engelhard M, Brittinger G, Heinz R et al: Chronic lymphocytic leukemia (B-CLL) and immunocytoma (LP-IC): clinical and prognostic relevance of this distinction. Leuk Lymphoma (Suppl) 161, 1991
15. Lennert K, Tamm I, Wacker H-H: Histopathology and immunocytochemistry of lymph node biopsies in chronic lymphocytic leukemia and immunocytoma. Leuk Lymphoma (Suppl):157, 1991
16. Catovsky AED, O'Brien MO, Cerchi M et al: "Prolymphocytoid" transformation of chronic lymphocytic leukemia. Br J Haematol 41:9, 1979
17. O'Brien A, del Giglio A, Keating M: Advances in the biology and treatment of B-cell chronic lymphocytic leukemia. Blood 85:307, 1995
18. Richter M: Generalized reticular cell sarcoma of lymph nodes associated with lymphocytic leukemia. Am J Pathol 4:285, 1928
19. Matolcsy A, Inghirami G, Knowles DM: Molecular genetic demonstration of the diverse evolution of Richter's syndrome (chronic lymphocytic leukemia and subsequent large cell lymphoma). Blood 83:1363, 1994
20. Brecher M, Banks P: Hodgkin's disease variant of Richter's syndrome: report of eight cases. Am J Clin Pathol 93:333, 1990
21. Williams J, Schned A, Cotelingam JD et al: Chronic lymphocytic leukemia with coexistant Hodgkin's disease. Am J Surg Pathol 15:33, 1991
22. Momose H, Jaffe ES, Shin SS et al: Chronic lymphocytic leukemia/small lymphocytic lymphoma with Reed-Sternberg-like cells and possible transformation to Hodgkin's disease. Mediation by Epstein-Barr virus. Am J Surg Pathol 16:859, 1992
23. Rubin D, Hudnall AD, Aisenberg A et al: Richter's transformation of chronic lymphocytic leukemia with Hodgkin's like cells is associated

with Epstein-Barr virus infection. Mod Pathol 7:91, 1994

24. Weisenberg E, Anastasi J, Adeyanju M et al: Hodgkin's disease associated with chronic lymphocytic leukemia. Eight additional cases, including two of the nodular lymphocyte predominant type. Am J Clin Pathol 103:479, 1995
25. Harris N: The relationship between Hodgkin's disease and non-Hodgkin's lymphoma. Semin Diagn Pathol 9:304, 1992
26. Jaffe E, Zarate-Osorno A, Medeiros L: The interrelationship of Hodgkin's disease and non-Hodgkin's lymphomas—lessons learned from composite and sequential malignancies. Semin Diagn Pathol 9:297, 1992
27. Kipps TJ, Carson DA: Autoantibodies in chronic lymphocytic leukemia and related systemic autoimmune diseases. Blood 81:2475, 1993
28. Schroeder HW, Dighiero G: The pathogenesis of chronic lymphocytic leukemia: analysis of the antibody repertoire. Immunol Today 15:288, 1994
29. Stein H, Lennert K, Feller A et al: Immunohistological analysis of human lymphoma: correlation of histological and immunological categories. Adv Cancer Res 42:67, 1984
30. Harris N, Bhan A: B-cell neoplasms of the lymphocytic, lymphoplasmacytoid, and plasma cell types: immunohistologic analysis and clinical correlation. Hum Pathol 16:829, 1985
31. Dorfman DM, Pinkus GS: Distinction between small lymphocytic and mantle cell lymphoma by immunoreactivity for CD23. Mod Pathol 7: 326, 1994
32. Kuppers R, Ganse A, Rajewsky K: B cells of chronic lymphatic leukemia express V genes in unmutated form. Leuk Res 15:487, 1991
33. Aoki H, Takishita M, Kosaka M et al: Frequent somatic mutations in D and/or Jh segments of Ig gene in Waldenstrom's macroglobulinemia and chronic lymphocytic leukemia (CLL) with Richter's syndrome but not in common CLL. Blood 85:1913, 1995
34. Kipps TJ, Tomhavee E, Chen PP et al: Autoantibody-associated k light chain variable region gene expressed in chronic lymphocytic leukemia with little or no somatic mutation. J Exp Med 167:840, 1988
35. Kipps TJ, Fong S, Tomhave E et al: High-frequency expression of a conserved κ light-chain variable-region gene in chronic lymphocytic leukemia. Proc Natl Acad Sci USA 84:2916, 1987
36. Meeker TC, Grimaldi JC, O'Rourke R et al: Lack of detectable somatic hypermutation in the V region of the IgH chain gene of a human chronic B lymphocytic leukemia. J Immunol 141:3994, 1988
37. Knuutila S, Elonen E, Teerenhovi L et al: Trisomy 12 in B cells of patients with B-cell chronic lymphocytic leukemia. N Engl J Med 314:865, 1986
38. Athan E, Foitl D, Knowles D: *bcl*-1 rearrangement: frequency and clinical significance among B cell chronic lymphocytic leukemias and non-Hodgkin's lymphomas. Am J Pathol 138:591, 1991
39. Croce C, Tsujimoto Y, Erikson J et al: Chromosome translocations and B cell neoplasia. Lab Invest 51:258, 1984
40. Tsujimoto Y, Yunis J, Onorato-Showe L et al: Molecular cloning of the chromosomal breakpoint of B-cell lymphomas and leukemias with the t(11;14) chromosome translation. Science 224:14, 1984
41. Yang WI, Zukerberg LR, Mokotura I et al: BCL-1 (cyclin D1) protein expression in low grade B-cell lymphomas and reactive hyperplasia. Am J Pathol 145:86, 1994
42. Bosch F, Jares P, Campo E et al: PRAD-1/cyclin D1 gene overexpression in chronic lymphoproliferative disorders: a highly specific marker of mantle cell lymphoma. Blood 84:2726, 1994
43. Kipps T: The CD5 B cell. Adv Immunol 47: 117, 1989
44. MacLennan I, Liu Y, Oldfield S et al: The evolution of B-cell clones. Curr Top Microbiol Immunol 159:37, 1990
45. Inghirami G, Foitl D, Sabichi A et al: Autoantibody-associated cross-reactive idiotype-bearing human B lymphocytes: distribution and characterization, including Ig VH gene and CD5 antigen expression. Blood 78:1503, 1991
46. Rai KR, Sawitsky A, Cronkite EP et al: Clinical staging of chronic lymphocytic leukemia. Blood 46:219, 1975
47. Dohner H, Fischer K, Bentz M et al: *p53* gene deletion predicts for poor survival and non-response to therapy with purine analogs in chronic B-cell leukemias. Blood 85:1580, 1995
48. Galton D, Goldman J, Wiltshaw E et al: Prolymphocytic leukaemia. Br J Haematol 27:7, 1974
49. Melo J, Catovsky D, Galton D: The relationship

between chronic lymphocytic leukaemia and prolymphocytic leukaemia. I. Clinical and laboratory features of 300 patients and characterization of an intermediate group. Br J Haematol 63:377, 1985

50. Bearman RM, Pangalis GA, Rappaport H: Prolymphocytic leukemia. Clinical, histopathological and cytochemical observations. Cancer 42: 2360, 1978
51. Lampert I, Catovsky D, Marsh G et al: The histopathology of prolymphocytic leukaemia with particular reference to the spleen: a comparison with chronic lymphocytic leukemia. Histopathology 4:3, 1980
52. Wagner SD, Martinelli V, Luzzatto L: Similar patterns of Vk gene usage but different degrees of somatic mutation in hairy cell leukemia, prolymphocytic leukemia, Waldenstrom's macroglobulinemia, and myeloma. Blood 83:3647, 1994
53. Brito-Bapapulle V, Ellis J, Matutes E et al: Translocation t(11;14)(q13;q32) in chronic lymphoid disorders. Genes Chrom Cancer 5: 158, 1992
54. Ramsay A, Smith W, Isaacson P: T-cell-rich B-cell lymphoma. Am J Surg Pathol 12:433, 1988
55. Patsouris E, Noel H, Lennert K: Lymphoplasmacytic/lymphoplasmacytoid immunocytoma with a high content of epithelioid cells: histologic and immunohistochemical findings. Am J Surg Pathol 14:660, 1990
56. Brittinger G, Bartels H, Common H et al: Clinical and prognostic relevance of the Kiel classification of non-Hodgkin lymphomas: results of a prospective multicenter study by the Kiel lymphoma study group. Hematol Oncol 2:269, 1984
57. Berger F, Felman P, Sonet A et al: Nonfollicular small B-cell lymphomas: a heterogeneous group of patients with distinct clinical features and outcome. Blood 83:2829, 1994
58. Dimopoulos MA, Alexanian R: Waldenstrom's macroglobulinemia. Blood 83:1452, 1994
59. Pozzato G, Mazzaro C, Crovatto M et al: Low-grade malignant lymphoma, hepatitis C virus infection, and mixed cryoglobulinemia. Blood 84:3047, 1994
60. Gerard-Marchant R, Hamlin I, Lennert K et al: Classification of non-Hodgkin's lymphomas. Lancet ii:406, 1974
61. Tolksdorf G, Stein H, Lennert K: Morphological and immunological definition of a malignant lymphoma derived from germinal centre cells with cleaved nuclei (centrocytes). Br J Cancer 41:168, 1980
62. Nanba K, Jaffe E, Braylan R et al: Alkaline phosphatase-positive malignant lymphoma. A subtype of B-cell lymphomas. Am J Clin Pathol 68:535, 1977
63. Weisenburger D, Nathwani B, Diamond L: Malignant lymphoma, intermediate lymphocytic type: a clinicopathologic study of 42 cases. Cancer 48:1415, 1981
64. Weisenburger DD, Kim H, Rappaport H: Mantle-zone lymphoma: a follicular variant of intermediate lymphocytic lymphoma. Cancer 49: 1429, 1982
65. Weisenburger D, Linder J, Daley H et al: Intermediate lymphocytic lymphoma: an immunohistologic study with comparison to other lymphocytic lymphomas. Hum Pathol 18:781, 1987
66. Weisenburger DD, Sanger WG, Armitage JO et al: Intermediate lymphocytic lymphoma: immunophenotypic and cytogenetic findings. Blood 69:1617, 1987
67. Jaffe E, Bookman M, Longo D: Lymphocytic lymphoma of intermediate differentation—Mantle zone lymphoma. Hum Pathol 18: 877, 1987
68. Hollema H, Poppema S: Immunophenotypes of malignant lymphoma centroblastic-centrocytic and malignant lymphoma centrocytic: an immunohistologic study indicating a derivation from different stages of B cell differentiation. Hum Pathol 19:1053, 1988
69. Lardelli P, Bookman M, Sundeen I et al: Lymphocytic lymphoma of intermediate differentiation. Morphologic and immunophenotypic spectrum and clinical correlations. Am J Surg Pathol 14:752, 1990
70. Medeiros L, van Krieken J, Jaffe E et al: Association of *bcl*-1 rearrangements with lymphocytic lymphoma of intermediate differentiation. Blood 76:2086, 1990
71. Rimokh R, Berger F, Cornillet P et al: Break in the *BCL1* locus is closely associated with intermediate lymphocytic lymphoma subtype. Genes Chrom Cancer 2:223, 1990
72. Frizzera G, Sakurai M, Notohara K et al: t(11; 14)(q13;q32) in B-cell lymphomas (intermediately differentiated lymphocytic and follicular): a report of four cases. Am J Clin Pathol 95:684, 1991
73. Vandenberghe E, De Wolf-Peeters C, Van den Oord J et al: Translocation (11;14): a cytoge-

netic anomaly associated with B-cell lymphomas of non-follicle centre cell lineage. J Pathol 163:13, 1991

74. Rosenberg C, Wong E, Petty E et al: Overexpression of *PRAD1*, a candidate *BCL1* breakpoint region oncogene, in centrocytic lymphomas. Proc Natl Acad Sci USA 88:9638, 1991
75. Williams ME, Westermann CD, Swerdlow SH: Genotypic characterization of centrocytic lymphoma: frequent rearrangement of the chromosome 11 *bcl*-1 locus. Blood 76:1387, 1990
76. Williams M, Swerdlow S, Rosenberg C et al: Characterization of chromosome 11 translocation breakpoints at the *bcl*-1 and *PRAD1* loci in centrocytic lymphoma. Cancer Res (Suppl) 52: 5541, 1992
77. Zucca E, Stein H, Coiffier B: European lymphoma task force (ELTF): report of the workshop on mantle cell lymphoma (MCL). Ann Oncol 5:508, 1994
78. Ott M, Ott G, Kuse R et al: The anaplastic variant of centrocytic lymphoma is marked by frequent rearrangements of the *bcl*-1 gene and high proliferation indices. Histopathology 24:329, 1994
79. Norton AJ, Matthews J, Pappa V et al: Mantle cell lymphoma: natural history defined in a serially biopsied population over a 20 year period. Ann Oncol 6:249, 1995
80. Swerdlow S, Habeshaw J, Murray L et al: Centrocytic lymphoma: a distinct clinicopathologic and immunologic entity. Am J Pathol 113:181, 1983
81. Harris N, Nadler L, Bhan A: Immunohistologic characterization of two malignant lymphomas of germinal center type (centroblastic/centrocytic and centrocytic) with monoclonal antibodies: follicular and diffuse lymphomas of small cleaved cell types are related but distinct entities. Am J Pathol 117:262, 1984
82. Zukerberg LR, Yang W-I, Arnold A et al: Cyclin D1 expression in non-Hodgkin's lymphomas: detection by immunohistochemistry. Am J Clin Pathol 102:1995
83. Hummel M, Tamaru J, Kalvelage B et al: Mantle cell (previously centrocytic) lymphomas express Vh genes with no or very little somatic mutations like the physiologic cells of the follicle mantle. Blood 84:403, 1994
84. Caligeris-Cappio F, Gobbi M, Bofill M et al: Infrequent normal B lymphocytes express features of B chronic lymphocytic leukemia. J Exp Med 155:623, 1982
85. Isaacson P, MacLennan K, Subbuswamy S: Multiple lymphomatous polyposis of the gastrointestinal tract. Histopathology 8:641, 1984
86. O'Briain D, Kennedy M, Daly P et al: Multiple lymphomatous polyposis of the gastrointestinal tract: a clinicopathologically distinctive form of non-Hodgkin's lymphoma of centrocytic type. Am J Surg Pathol 13:691, 1989
87. Meusers P, Engelhard M, Bartels H et al: Multicentre randomized therapeutic trial for advanced centrocytic lymphoma: anthracycline does not improve the prognosis. Hematol Oncol 7:365, 1989
88. Bookman M, Lardelli P, Jaffe E et al: Lymphocytic lymphoma of intermediate differentiation: morphologic, immunophenotypic, and prognostic factors. J Natl Cancer Inst 82:742, 1990
89. Zukerberg L, Medeiros L, Ferry J et al: Diffuse low grade B-cell lymphomas: identification of four major immunophenotypic subtypes, abstracted. Lab Invest 62:87, 1991
90. Fisher RI, Dahlberg S, Nathwani BN et al: A clinical analysis of two indolent lymphoma entities: mantle cell lymphoma and marginal zone lymphoma (including the mucosa-asociated lymphoid tissue and monocytoid B-cell subcategories): a Southwest Oncology Group study. Blood 85:1075, 1995
91. Amrein P, Weissman DJ: Case record of the Massachusetts General Hospital: Case 43-1994. N Engl J Med 331:1576, 1994
92. Mann R, Berard C: Criteria for the cytologic subclassification of follicular lymphomas: a proposed alternative method. Hematol Oncol 1: 187, 1982
93. Metter G, Nathwani B, Burke J et al: Morphological subclassification of follicular lymphoma: variability of diagnosis among hematopathologists, a collaborative study between the Repository Center and Pathology Panel for Lymphoma Clinical Studies. J Clin Oncol 3:25, 1985
94. Nathwani B, Metter G, Miller T et al: What should be the morphologic criteria for the subdivision of follicular lymphomas? Blood 68:837, 1986
95. Anderson T, Bender R, Fisher R et al: Combination chemotherapy in non-Hodgkin's lymphoma: results of long-term follow-up. Cancer Treat Rep 61:1057, 1977
96. Bartlett NL, Rizeq M, Dorfman RF et al: Follicular large-cell lymphoma: intermediate or low grade? J Clin Oncol 12:1349, 1994

97. Martin AR, Weisenburger DD, Chan WC et al: Prognostic value of cellular proliferation and histologic grade in follicular lymphoma. Blood 85:3671, 1995
98. Warnke R, Kim H, Fuks Z et al: The co-existence of nodular and diffuse patterns in nodular non-Hodgkin's lymphomas. Cancer 40:1229, 1977
99. Hu E, Weiss L, Hoppe R et al: Follicular and diffuse mixed small cleaved and large cell lymphoma—a clinicopathologic study. J Clin Oncol 3:1183, 1985
100. Ezdinli E, Costello W, Kucuk O et al: Effect of the degree of nodularity on the survival of patients with nodular lymphomas. J Clin Oncol 5: 413, 1987
101. Paryani SB, Hoppe RT, Cox RS et al: Analysis of non-Hodgkin's lymphomas with nodular and favorable histologies, stages I and IL Cancer 52: 2300, 1983
102. Oviatt DL, Cousar JB, Collins RD et al: Malignant lymphomas of follicular center cell origin in humans. V. Incidence, clinical features, and prognostic implications of transformation of small cleaved cell nodular lymphoma. Cancer 53:1109, 1984
103. Sander CA, Yano T, Clark HM et al: *p53* mutation is associated with progression in follicular lymphomas. Blood 82:1994, 1993
104. Yano T, Jaffe ES, Longo DL et al: MYC rearrangements in histologically progressed follicular lymphomas. Blood 80:758, 1992
105. deJong D, Voetdujk B, Baverstock G et al: Activation of the c-*myc* oncogene in a precursor B-cell blast crisis of follicular lymphoma, presenting as composite lymphoma. N Engl J Med 318: 1373, 1988
106. Lee J, Innes D, Williams M: Sequential *bcl*-2 and c-*myc* oncogene rearrangements associated with the clinical transformation of non-Hodgkin's lymphoma. J Clin Invest 84:1454, 1989
107. Stein H, Gerdes J, Mason D: The normal and malignant germinal centre. Clin Haematol 11: 531, 1982
108. Stein H, Lennert K, Feller A et al: Immunological analysis of tissue sections in diagnosis of lymphoma. P. 127. In Hoffbrand A (ed): Recent Advances in Haematology, 11. Churchill Livingstone, New York, 1985
109. Ngan B, Chen-Levy Z, Weiss L et al: Expression in non-Hodgkin's lymphoma of the *bcl*-2 protein associated with the t(14;18) chromosomal translocation. N Engl J Med 318:1638, 1988
110. Pezzella F, Tse A, Cordell J et al: Expression of the *bcl*-2 oncogene protein is not specific for the 14-18 chromosomal translocation. Am J Pathol 137:225, 1990
111. Cleary M, Mecker T, Levy S et al: Clustering of extensive somatic mutations in the variable region of an immunoglobulin heavy chain gene from a human B cell lymphoma. Cell 44:97, 1986
112. Levy R, Levy S, Cleary M et al: Somatic mutation in human B-cell tumors. Immunol Rev 96: 43, 1987
113. Levy S, Mendel E, Kon S et al: Mutational hot spots in Ig V region genes of human follicular lymphomas. J Exp Med 168:475, 1988
114. Zelenetz AD, Chen TT, Levy R: Clonal expansion in follicular lymphomca occurs subsequent to antigenic selection. J Exp Med 176:1137, 1992
115. Tsujimoto T, Cossman J, Jaffe E et al: Involvement of the *bcl*-2 gene in human follicular lymphoma. Science 288:1440, 1985
116. Hockenbery D, Zutter M, Hickey W et al: BCL2 protein is topographically restricted in tissues characterized by apoptotic cell death. Proc Natl Acad Sci USA 88:6961, 1991
117. McDonnell T. Deane N, Platt F et al: *bcl*-2-immunoglobulin transgenic mice demonstrate extended B cell survival and follicular lymphoproliferation. Cell 57:79, 1989
118. Limpens J, de Jong D, van Krieken J et al: *bcl*-2 in benign lymphoid tissue with follicular hyperplasia. Oncogene 6:2271, 1991
119. Warnke R, Levy R: Follicular lymphoma: a model of B lymphocyte homing. N Engl J Med 298:481, 1974
120. Jaffe E, Shevach E, Frank M et al: Nodular lymphoma: evidence for origin from follicular B lymphocytes. N Engl J Med 290:813, 1974
121. Rappaport H: Tumors of the Hematopoietic System. Atlas of Tumor Pathology, Series I, Section III, Fascicle 8. Armed Forces Institute of Pathology, Washington, DC, 1966
122. Jones S, Fuks Z, Bull M et al: Non-Hodgkin's lymphomas IV. Clinicopathologic correlation in 405 cases. Cancer 31:806, 1973
123. Glick J, Barnes J, Ezdinli E et al: Nodular mixed lymphoma: results of a randomized trial failing to confirm prolonged disease-free survival with COPP chemotherapy. Blood 58:920, 1981
124. Glick J, McFadden E, Costello W et al: Nodular histiocytic lymphoma: factors influencing prog-

nosis and implications for aggressive chemotherapy. Cancer 49:840, 1982

125. Anderson JR, Vose JM, Bierman PJ et al: Clinical features and prognosis of follicular large-cell lymphoma: a report from the Nebraska Lymphoma Study Group. J Clin Oncol 11:218, 1993
126. Yuen AR, Kamel OW, Halpern J et al: Long-term survival after histologic transformation of low-grade follicular lymphoma. J Clin Oncol 13:1726, 1995
127. Harris N, Pilch B, Bhan A et al: Immunohistologic diagnosis of orbital lymphoid infiltrates. Am J Surg Pathol 8:83, 1984
128. Isaacson P, Wright D: Malignant lymphoma of mucosa associated lymphoid tissue. A distinctive B cell lymphoma. Cancer 52:1410, 1983
129. Isaacson P, Spencer J: Malignant lymphoma of mucosa-associated lymphoid tissue. Histopathology 11:445, 1987
130. Cousar J, McGinn D, Glick A et al: Report of an unusual lymphoma arising from parafollicular B lymphocytes or so-called "monocytoid" lymphocytes. Am J Clin Pathol 87:121, 1987
131. Sheibani K, Burke J, Swartz W et al: Monocytoid B cell lymphoma. Clinicopathologic study of 21 cases of a unique type of low grade lymphoma. Cancer 62:1531, 1988
132. Ngan B-Y, Warnke R, Wilson M et al: Monocytoid B-cell lymphoma: a study of 36 cases. Hum Pathol 22:409, 1991
133. Shin S, Sheibani K, Fishleder A et al: Monocytoid B-cell lymphoma in patients with Sjogren's syndrome: a clinicopathologic study of 13 patients. Hum Pathol 22:422, 1991
134. Nizze H, Cogliatti S, von Schilling C et al: Monocytoid B-cell lymphoma: morphological variants and relationship to low-grade B-cell lymphoma of the mucosa-associated lymphoid tissue. Histopathology 18:403, 1991
135. Isaacson P, Spencer J: Monocytoid B-cell lymphomas. Am J Surg Pathol 14:888, 1990
136. Harris NL: Lymphoma of mucosa-associated lymphoid tissue and monocytoid B-cell lymphoma: related entities that are distinct from other low-grade B-cell lymphomas. Arch Pathol 117:771, 1993
137. Liu Y-J, Oldfield S, MacLennan I: Memory B cells in T-cell dependent antibody responses colonise the splenic marginal zones. Eur J Immunol 18:355, 1988
138. Cardoso de Almeida P, Harris N, Bhan A: Characterization of immature sinus histiocytes (monocytoid cells) in reactive lymph nodes by use of monoclonal antibodies. Hum Pathol 15: 330, 1984
139. Gowans J, Knight E: The route of recirculation of lymphocytes in the rat. Proc R Soc Lond Biol 159:257, 1964
140. Gallatin W, Weissman I, Butcher E: A cell-surface molecule involved in organ-specific homing of lymphocytes. Nature 304:30, 1983
141. Van den Oord J, De Wolf-Peeters C, De Vos R et al: Immature sinus histiocytosis. Light- and electron-microscopic features, immunologic phenotype, and relationship with marginal zone lymphocytes. Am J Pathol 1985:266, 1985
142. Spencer J, Finn T, Pulford K et al: The human gut contains a novel population of B lymphocytes which resemble marginal zone cells. Clin Exp Immunol 62:607, 1985
143. Van den Oord J, De Wolf-Peeters C, Desmet V: The marginal zone in the human reactive lymph node. Am J Clin Pathol 86:475, 1986
144. Van den Oord J, De Wolf-Peeters C, Desmet V: Marginal zone lymphocytes in the lymph node. Hum Pathol 20:1225, 1989
145. Butcher E: Cellular and molecular mechanisms that direct leukocyte traffic. Am J Pathol 136: 3, 1990
146. Spencer J, Diss T, Isaacson P: A study of the properties of a low-grade mucosal B-cell lymphoma using a monoclonal antibody specific for the tumour immunoglobulin. J Pathol 160:231, 1990
147. Smith-Ravin J, Spencer J, Beverley P et al: Characterization of two monoclonal antibodies (UCL4D12 and UCL3D3) that discriminate between human mantle zone and marginal zone B cells. Clin Exp Immunol 82:181, 1990
148. Castrilli J, Montalban C, Obeso G et al: Gastric B-cell mucosa associated lymphoid tissue lymphoma: a clinicopathological study in 56 patients. Gut 33:1307, 1992
149. Chan J, Ng C, Isaacson P: Relationship between high-grade lymphoma and low-grade B-cell mucosa-associated lymphoid tissue lymphoma (MALToma) of the stomach. Am J Pathol 136: 1153, 1990
150. Li G, Hansmann M, Zwingers T et al: Primary lymphomas of the lung: morphological, immunohistochemical and clinical features. Histopathology 16:519, 1990
151. Cogliatti S, Schmid U, Schumacher U et al: Primary B-cell gastric lymphoma: a clinicopatho-

logical study of 145 patients. Gastroenterology 101:1159, 1991
152. Piris M, Rivas C, Morente M et al: Monocytoid B-cell lymphoma, a tumour related to the marginal zone. Histopathology 12:383, 1988
153. Schmid C, Kirkham N, Diss T et al: Splenic marginal zone cell lymphoma. Am J Surg Pathol 16:455, 1992
154. Melo J, Hegde U, Parreira A et al: Splenic B cell lymphoma with circulating villous lymphocytes: differential diagnosis of B cell leukaemias with large spleens. J Clin Pathol 40:642, 1987
155. Pan L, Diss T, Cunningham D et al: The *bcl*-2 gene in primary B-cell lymphomas of mucosa associated lymphoid tissue (MALT). Am J Pathol 135:7, 1989
156. Finn T, Isaacson P, Wotherspoon A: Numerical abnormality of chromosomes 3, 7, 12, and 18 in low grade lymphomas of MALT-type and splenic marginal zone lymphomas detected by interphase cytogenetics on paraffin embedded tissue. J Pathol 170:335, 1993
157. Isaacson PG: Gastrointestinal lymphoma. Hum Pathol 25:1020, 1994
158. Hussell T, Isaacson P, Crabtree J et al: The response of cells from low-grade B-cell gastric lymphomas of mucosa-associated lymphoid tissue to *Helicobacter pylori*. Lancet 342:571, 1993
159. Hyjek E, Isaacson P: Primary B cell lymphoma of the thyroid and its relationship to Hashimoto's thyroiditis. Hum Pathol 19:1315, 1988
160. Hyjek E, Smith W, Isaacson P: Primary B cell lymphoma of salivary gland and its relationship to myoepithelial sialadentiis (MESA). Hum Pathol 19:766, 1988
161. Medeiros L, Harmon D, Linggood R et al: Immunohistologic features predict clinical behavior of orbital and conjunctival lymphoid infiltrates. Blood 74:2121, 1989
162. Zukerberg L, Ferry J, Southern J et al: Lymphoid infiltrates of the stomach: evaluation of histologic criteria for the diagnosis of low-grade gastric lymphoma on endoscopic biopsy specimens. Am J Surg Pathol 14:1087, 1990
163. Pelstring R, Essell J, Kurtin P et al: Diversity of organ site involvement among malignant lymphomas of mucosa-associated tissues. Am J Clin Pathol 96:738, 1991
164. Sundeen J, Longo D, Jaffe E: CD5 expression in B-cell small lymphocytic malignancies: correlations with clinical presentation and sites of disease. Am J Surg Pathol 16:130, 1992
165. Mattia A, Ferry J, Harris N: Breast lymphoma: a B-cell spectrum including the low grade B-cell lymphoma of mucosa associated lymphoid tissue. Am J Surg Pathol 17:574, 1993
166. Wotherspoon A, Doglioni C, Diss T et al: Regression of primary low-grade B-cell gastric lymphoma of mucosa-associated lymphoid tissue type after eradication of *Helicobacter pylori*. Lancet 342:575, 1993
167. Pinotti G, Roggero E, Zucca E et al: Primary low-grade gastric MALT lymphoma, abstracted. Proc ASCO 14:393, 1995
168. Cogliatti S, Lennert K, Hansmann M et al: Monocytoid B cell lymphoma: clinical and prognostic features of 21 patients. J Clin Pathol 43:619, 1990
169. Carbone A, Gloghini A, Pinto A et al: Monocytoid B-cell lymphoma with bone marrow and peripheral blood involvement at presentation. Am J Clin Pathol 92:228, 1989
170. Neiman R, Sullivan A, Jaffe R: Malignant lymphoma simulating leukaemic reticuloendotheliosis: a clinicopathologic study of ten cases. Cancer 43:329, 1979
171. Audouin J, Diebold J, Schvartz H et al: Malignant lymphoplasmacytic lymphoma with prominent splenomegaly (primary lymphoma of the spleen). J Pathol 155:17, 1988
172. Hollema H, Visser L, Poppema S: Small lymphocytic lymphomas with predominant splenomegaly: a comparison of immunophenotypes with cases of predominant lymphadenopathy. Mod Pathol 4:712, 1991
173. Isaacson PG, Matutes E, Burke M et al: The histopathology of splenic lymphoma with villous lymphocytes. Blood 84:3828, 1995
174. Matutes E, Morilla R, Owusu-Ankomah K et al: The immunophenotype of splenic lymphoma with villous lymphocytes and its relevance to the differential diagnosis with other B-cell disorders. Blood 83:1558, 1994
175. Zhu D, Oscier DG, Stevenson FK: Splenic lymphoma with villous lymphocytes involves B cells with extensively mutated Ig heavy chain variable region genes. Blood 85:1603, 1995
176. Oscier DG, Matutes E, Gardiner A et al: Cytogenetic studies in splenic lymphoma with villous lymphocytes. Br J Haematol 85:487, 1993
177. Jadayel D, Matutes E, Dyer MJS et al: Splenic lymphoma with villous lymphocytes: analysis of *bcl*-1 rearrangements and expression of cyclin D1 gene. Blood 83:3664, 1994

7

Diffuse Aggressive Non-Hodgkin's Lymphomas

Lawrence M. Weiss and Bharat N. Nathwani

In this chapter, many of the diffuse aggressive lymphomas will be discussed, including lymphoblastic, small noncleaved cell, diffuse mixed, diffuse large cell, and large cell immunoblastic lymphomas. Peripheral T-cell lymphoma is discussed more comprehensively in Chapter 8 and anaplastic large cell lymphoma is discussed in Chapter 10. Additional details on the molecular biology of these neoplasms can be found in Chapter 1.

LYMPHOBLASTIC LYMPHOMA

Lymphoblastic lymphoma is a high grade lymphoma in the Working Formulation classification and included in both the B- and T/natural killer cell lymphoma categories as a precursor neoplasm in the Revised European-American Lymphoma (REAL) classification.[1,2] Similarly, in the updated Kiel classification, there is a category of lymphoblastic lymphoma including both a high grade B- and T-cell neoplasm.[3]

The aggressive nature of lymphoblastic lymphoma is readily apparent, at low magnification, by the presence of extensive infiltration of the pericapsular tissue, a single-file arrangement of the tumor cells, crush artifact, and invasion of vessel walls with tumor emboli.[4,5] Some of the medullary sinuses may be open and intertwined, and germinal centers may be preserved in some cases. Occasionally, a nodular appearance is imparted by the delineation of islands of tumor by fibrous septa, but a truly follicular pattern is never seen. Mitotic activity is usually quite high. In many cases, a "starry sky" appearance may be seen focally, but it is rarely seen throughout the tumor as is so common in small noncleaved lymphoma. At high magnification, the infiltrate almost always consists of a monomorphous population of neoplastic cells with few admixed small lymphocytes, although rare cases may have abundant plasma cells and eosinophils. The individual neoplastic cells have small to medium sized nuclei that average 15 μm in diameter, with a range of 10 to 20 μm (Figs. 7-1, 7-2). Regardless of the size, the neoplastic cells are extremely homogeneous with respect to the nuclear chromatin structure—very fine and delicate, with inconspicuous to absent nucleoli. The amount of cytoplasm is very sparse. The nuclear shape is quite variable in most patients (convoluted subtype); however, in a few cases the nuclei may be round (nonconvoluted subtype). The tumor cells are indistinguishable from the lymphoblasts of acute lymphoblastic leukemia.

Lymphoblastic lymphoma can generally be easily distinguished from other non-Hodgkin's lymphomas because, regardless of the size of the tumor cell nuclei, all of the tumor cells have a similar chromatin structure (very fine and delicate), and the larger cells do not contain large nucleoli. The latter feature is very common in all aggressive B-cell lymphomas and peripheral T-cell lymphomas. One recently described entity that must be distinguished from lymphoblastic lymphoma is the blastic variant of mantle cell lymphoma.[6] In this latter lymphoma, the mor-

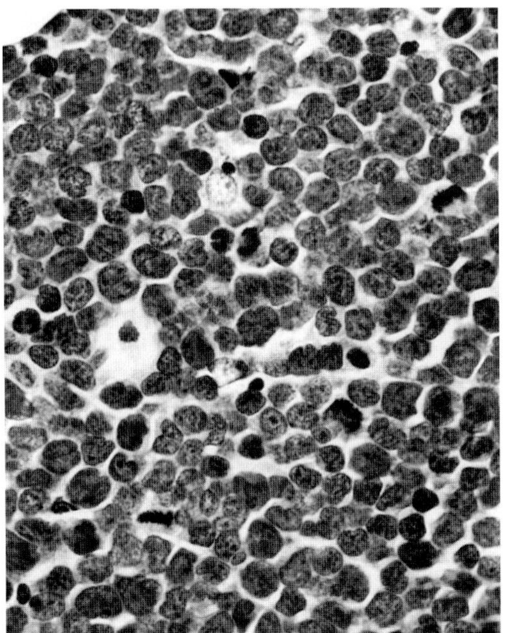

Fig. 7-1. Lymphoblastic lymphoma, convoluted variant. There is a monotonous proliferation of medium sized cells with a high mitotic rate. The nuclei have a fine chromatin pattern and generally lack discernible nucleoli.

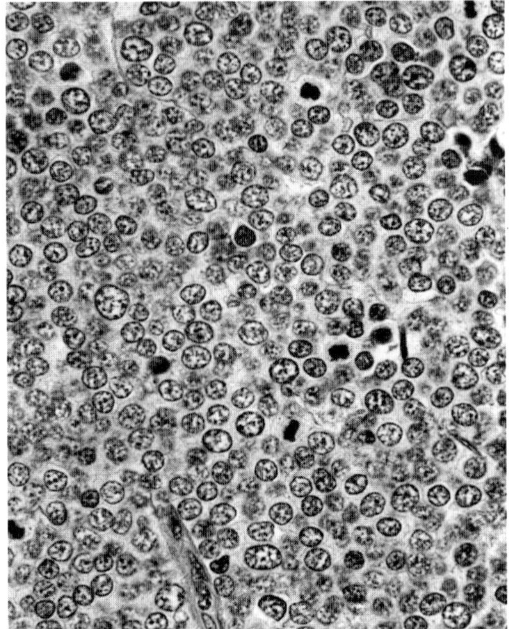

Fig. 7-2. Lymphoblastic lymphoma, nonconvoluted variant. Note the round nuclear outlines.

phology of the proliferating cells may be indistinguishable from those of lymphoblastic lymphoma. Often, there is a component of typical mantle cell lymphoma. In cases in which these latter cells are infrequent or absent, a history of prior mantle cell lymphoma may be a clue to the diagnosis. Immunophenotyping studies may be essential in difficult cases to establish a correct diagnosis.

The cells of virtually all cases of lymphoblastic lymphoma have been reported to be terminal deoxynucleotidyl transferase (Tdt) positive, a marker now reliable in formalin-fixed paraffin sections.[7–9] About 80 percent of cases are positive for CD45 (leukocyte common antigen).[10] About 90 percent of cases are of T lineage, and the majority show an immature thymocyte phenotype on comprehensive frozen section study (often with CD1 and coexpression of CD4 and CD8).[9,11] In paraffin sections, virtually all cases are CD43 positive, most cases are CD3 positive (although the positivity may be cytoplasmic only), but only about one-half of cases are CD45RO positive.[10,12] A minority of the T-lineage cases may also express markers of natural killer cell differentiation, including CD16 and CD57.[13]

About 10 percent of cases of lymphoblastic lymphoma are of B lineage, with the large majority of precursor B phenotype, similar to the common phenotypes of B-lineage acute lymphoblastic leukemia.[9,14] Many of these cases will express the B-lineage marker CD20. The most immature cases are often CD20 negative, but may be positive with the pan-B-cell marker CD79a.[15] A few cases have been reported to be surface immunoglobulin positive.[16] These cases may be Tdt negative and therefore difficult to distinguish from the blastic variant of mantle cell lymphoma, which is also Tdt negative. In this circumstance, evaluation of CD5 may be of use, as this is usually positive in mantle cell lymphoma but negative in B-lineage lymphoblastic lymphoma.

Clinically, most cases of T-lymphoblastic

lymphoma present as a mediastinal mass, often accompanied by pleural or pericardial effusions.[4,5] Although it may occur at any age, it is most common in childhood and adolescence; the male:female ratio is about 2:1. The tumor is high grade, and dissemination occurs in a high percentage. Peripheral blood, bone marrow, central nervous system, and gonadal involvement are very common. The involvement of peripheral blood and bone marrow raises consideration of acute lymphoblastic lymphoma, a disease that is closely related to lymphoblastic lymphoma. Generally, lymphoma is diagnosed when there is less than 10 percent circulating blasts in the peripheral blood and an absence of pancytopenia.[17] However, recognition that these two diseases probably represent a spectrum of the same biologic entity has led to adoption of successful multichemotherapy acute lymphoblastic leukemia regimens for the treatment of lymphoblastic lymphoma, with excellent results.[17] Although median survival was around 2 years in the early 1980s, the overall survival rate now is over 50 percent.

Lymphoblastic lymphoma expressing natural killer cell antigens may be more frequent in females and may be more aggressive.[18] B-lineage lymphoblastic lymphoma does not involve the mediastinum, but commonly presents as cutaneous nodules.[19]

SMALL NONCLEAVED CELL LYMPHOMA

Small noncleaved cell lymphoma is a high grade lymphoma in the Working Formulation and consists of Burkitt's and non-Burkitt's types.[1] In the REAL classification, Burkitt's lymphoma is in the category of peripheral B-cell neoplasms, while high grade lymphoma, Burkitt-like (non-Burkitt's) is only a provisional entity.[2] The latter includes cases of non-Burkitt's type and cases that do not fit in the categories of either Burkitt's or large cell lymphoma. In the Updated Kiel classification, only Burkitt's lymphoma is recognized as a specific entity.[3]

Small noncleaved lymphoma almost always shows diffuse effacement of architecture, although occasionally there is selective involvement of germinal centers. Generally, the mitotic rate is extremely high and a "starry-sky" appearance is conspicuous, with numerous tingible-body macrophages present (Figs. 7-3, 7-4). The sinuses are usually obliterated. Cytologically, the cells of Burkitt's lymphoma are extremely homogeneous, from case to case and within an individual case. The neoplastic cells measure between 15 and 20 μm. The nuclei are round, with a vesicular chromatin pattern, and have multiple, distinct nucleoli, some of which are located on the nuclear membrane. The cytoplasm is moderate in amount and highly pyrininophilic. The cytoplasms of adjacent cells tend to abut one another, giving an appearance of "squaring off." With the exception of tingible body macrophages, other reactive host cells are generally absent.

In the non-Burkitt's or Burkitt-like type, the low magnification appearance is similar to Bur-

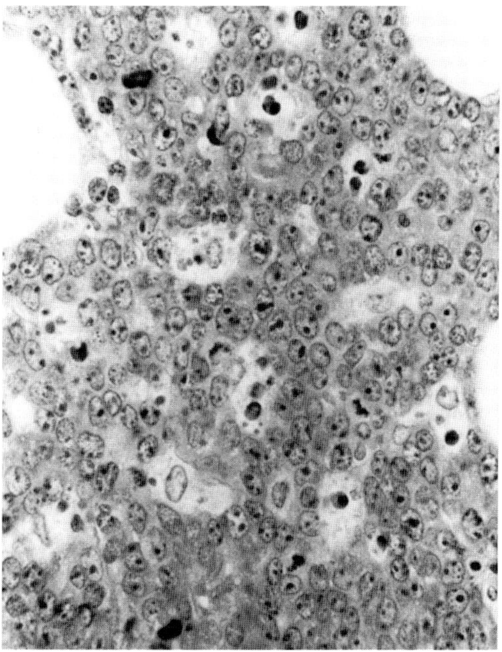

Fig. 7-3. Small noncleaved cell lymphoma, Burkitt's type. A starry-sky pattern is seen. The cells are monotonous, with medium sized nuclei with about three nucleoli per nucleus.

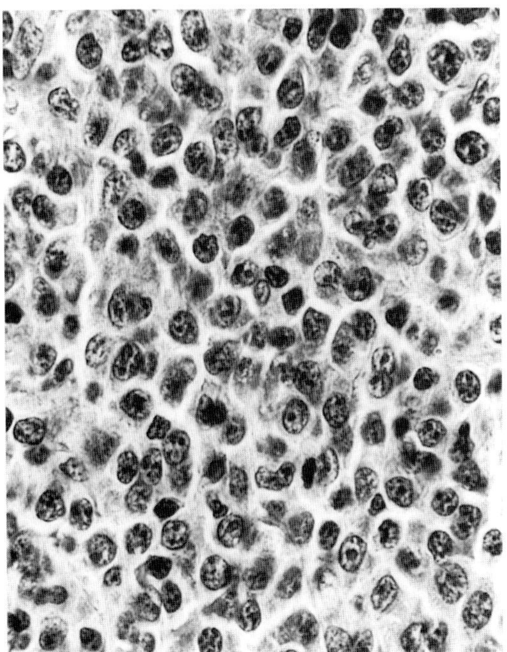

Fig. 7-4. Small noncleaved cell lymphoma, non-Burkitt's type. The cells are medium sized and very monotonous, but nuclear features classic for Burkitt's lymphoma are not present. Many nuclei have one moderately prominent nucleoli.

kitt's lymphoma, although a starry-sky pattern may sometimes not be seen. However, these lymphomas lack the cellular uniformity of Burkitt's lymphoma, and variation in the nuclear size is common. The nucleoli are prominent and sometimes solitary.

The histologic differential diagnosis of small noncleaved cell lymphoma includes other high grade lymphomas such as lymphoblastic lymphoma, large cell lymphoma, and immunoblastic lymphoma. In well-fixed sections, the presence of distinct nucleoli and a moderate rim of cytoplasm and the absence of fine chromatin should distinguish small noncleaved cell lymphoma from lymphoblastic lymphoma. Immunoblastic lymphoma may be difficult to distinguish from small noncleaved cell lymphoma, but the neoplastic cells in the former neoplasm are larger and more variable in size, with larger nuclei, more prominent nucleoli, and more abundant cytoplasm.

Small noncleaved cell lymphoma is a B-lineage lymphoma expressing monotypic immunoglobulins; it consistently expresses CD20 by paraffin section immunohistochemistry. In contrast to lymphoblastic lymphoma, cases of small noncleaved lymphoma never express Tdt. In frozen section studies, the cells of Burkitt's lymphoma express the phenotype of germinal center cells: CD5 negative, CD10 positive, CD21 negative, CD22 positive, and CD23 negative.[20] The cells of the non-Burkitt's subtype have a similar phenotype except that they may often be CD10 negative.

Clinically, Burkitt's lymphoma occurs in two forms: an endemic form, found in equatorial Africa and possibly also in South America, and a sporadic form, found in Western countries.[21] In the endemic form, children are mainly affected, with a male:female ratio of 2.5 : 1. The neoplasm tends to present in extranodal sites such as the jaw and gonads. In the sporadic form, there are peaks of incidence in childhood and in the elderly, and the male predominance is also seen.[1] In contrast to endemic Burkitt's lymphoma, abdominal presentations with bowel involvement are common in non-Burkitt's lymphoma. The clinical presentation is somewhat similar to the sporadic Burkitt's subtype, although lymph node presentations and bone marrow involvement are more common in the non-Burkitt's subtype.[22–24]

Small noncleaved lymphoma is an extremely aggressive neoplasm, with the highest doubling times of any human neoplasm. Although the median survival was less than 1 year only a decade ago, modern multichemotherapy regimens have led to cure rates of up to 90 percent.[25] In contrast to most lymphomas, surgical debulking may have a role in the treatment of small noncleaved lymphoma. The prognostic significance of the Burkitt's versus non-Burkitt's subtype is still not clear.[23,24]

Despite the close morphologic and clinical similarities between Burkitt's lymphoma and the non-Burkitt's subtype, it is not clear that they represent closely related entities from a biologic standpoint. As discussed in Chapter 1, Burkitt's lymphoma possesses characteristic chromosomal translocations involving the c-*myc* oncogene, while these translocations are less common in the non-Burkitt's subtype.[26] In contrast, some cases of the non-Burkitt's subtype possess the t(14;18), similar to diffuse large cell lymphoma. It is for this reason that the Revised European American Lymphoma (REAL) classification has separated out the Burkitt-like neoplasms from Burkitt's lymphoma as a provisional category of B-cell lymphoma.

DIFFUSE MIXED SMALL AND LARGE CELL LYMPHOMA

Diffuse mixed small and large cell lymphoma is an intermediate grade lymphoma in the Working Formulation[1] and has no equivalent in the REAL or the updated Kiel classifications. This omission is because this lymphoma subtype represents a morphologic category and not a true clinicopathologic or biologic entity; it includes several different biologic types of lymphoma, including diffuse varieties of follicular center cell lymphoma, T-cell-rich B-cell lymphoma, histiocyte rich B-cell lymphoma, lymphoplasmacytoid lymphoma with admixed large cells (polymorphous variant), marginal zone lymphoma with admixed large cells, and peripheral T-cell lymphoma.[27] It is still not clear whether T-cell-rich B-cell lymphoma represents a distinct biologic entity or a subtype of follicular center cell lymphoma. In addition, it is not certain whether histiocyte-rich B-cell lymphoma represents a unique entity or a variant of diffuse lymphocytic and histiocytic (L&H) lymphocyte predominance Hodgkin's disease. Diffuse mixed lymphoma of follicular center cell origin, T-cell-rich, and histiocyte-rich B-cell lymphoma are all probably classified as diffuse large cell B-cell lymphomas in the REAL classification, while most cases of diffuse mixed peripheral T-cell lymphoma are included in the category of peripheral T-cell lymphoma, not otherwise specified, unless a specific type of peripheral T-cell lymphoma can be recognized.

At low magnification, by definition, one sees diffuse effacement of the lymph node architecture. However, in some cases, a minor true follicular component may be found, and this morphologic feature serves as a marker to indicate that it is a follicular center cell lymphoma. Some studies have suggested that the diffuse component must account for greater than 75 percent of the tumor area for the neoplasm to have the prognostic significance of intermediate grade, diffuse mixed small and large cell lymphoma as opposed to low grade, follicular mixed small and large cell type.[28] The sinuses are usually completely obliterated, except in some cases of diffuse mixed peripheral T-cell lymphoma.

At high magnification, by definition, one can identify a mixture of small and large cells. However, different patterns may be seen in the various lymphoma types that comprise diffuse mixed lymphoma and may be clues to further classification of the lymphoma. In follicular center cell lymphomas showing a pattern of diffuse mixed lymphoma, both the small and large cells have features of cleaved and noncleaved cells (centrocytes and centroblasts) (Fig. 7-5). In ad-

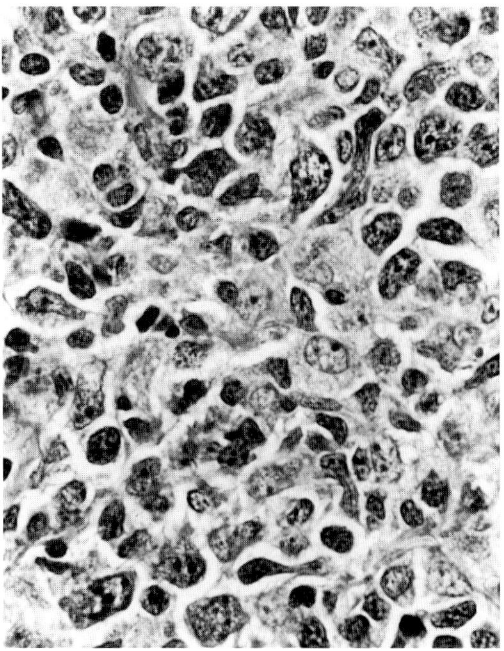

Fig. 7-5. Diffuse mixed small cleaved and large cell lymphoma of follicular center type. Both small and large cells show atypical nuclei. The large cells are a mixture of cleaved and noncleaved large cells.

dition, there are usually many small, round lymphocytes admixed, representing host reactive T cells. In T-cell-rich or histiocyte-rich B-cell lymphoma, the small cells, which often predominate in number, are all small with round, regular nuclei (representing host reactive T cells), while the large cells are usually noncleaved cell type, but may be multilobated (Fig. 7-6).[20–32] Nonepithelioid histiocytes are abundant in histiocyte-rich B-cell lymphoma.

In lymphoplasmacytoid lymphoma with admixed large cells, the small and large lymphoid cells both show plasmacytoid features, and admixed plasma cells may also be present. The small lymphocytes resemble the lymphoplasmacytic cells usually seen in lymphoplasmacytoid lymphoma, possessing mature lymphocytic or plasmacytic nuclei with small to moderate amounts of eccentrically placed basophilic cytoplasm, while the large cells usually have the morphologic appearance of immunoblasts with plasmacytoid features, possessing prominent, often centrally located nucleoli, and abundant basophilic cytoplasm. In marginal zone B-cell lymphoma with admixed large cells, the smaller lymphoid cells have the features of marginal zone B cells—cells with moderately abundant pale cytoplasm and nuclei with slightly irregular nuclear outlines and a bland chromatin pattern (monocytoid B cells). The large cells generally have the features of large noncleaved cells or plasmacytoid immunoblasts. Admixed plasma cells may also be present, and, when abundant, this lymphoma may be confused with lymphoplasmacytoid lymphoma.

In peripheral T-cell lymphomas resembling diffuse mixed lymphoma, a continuous spectrum of atypical lymphocytes is seen, with small, medium, and large lymphoid cells with irregular nuclear contours. Often, eosinophils, plasma cells, epithelioid histiocytes, and other host reactive cells are admixed and may mask the neoplastic process.

The results of phenotyping studies parallel those of the underlying lymphoma type. In dif-

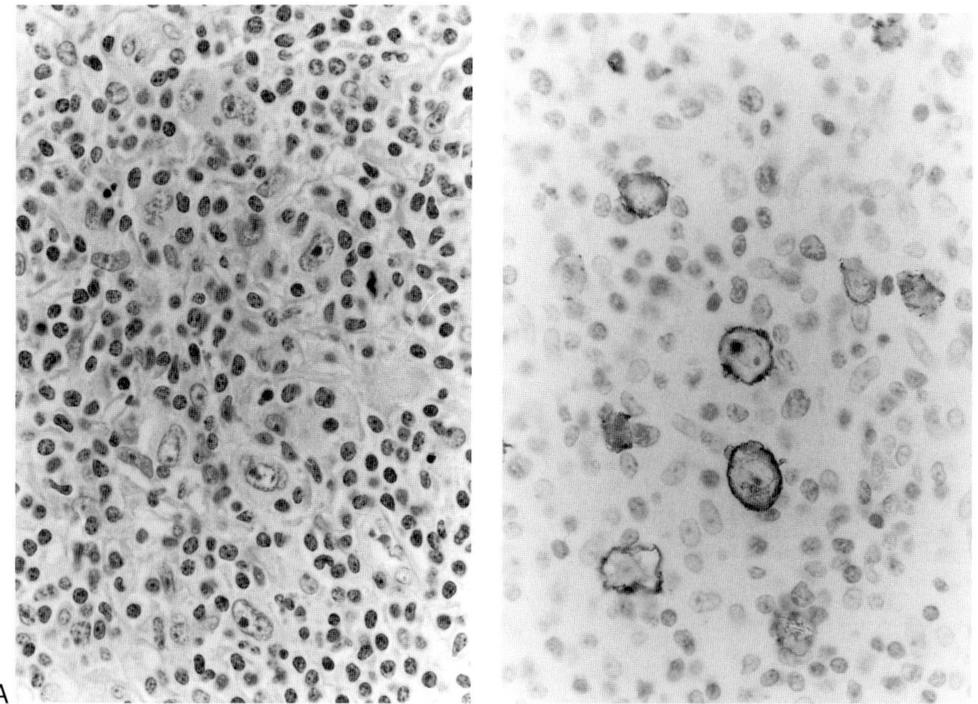

Fig. 7-6. T-cell-rich B-cell lymphoma. **(A)** Only scattered large cells are present. The small lymphocytes lack cytologic atypia and are marked as T lymphocytes. **(B)** Immunohistochemistry for CD20 identifies the large neoplastic B cells, leaving the small T cells unlabeled.

fuse mixed lymphoma of follicular origin, both the atypical small and large lymphoid cells are of B lineage, almost always expressing CD20. Although monotypic immunoglobulins generally cannot be demonstrated in paraffin sections, frozen section studies reveal immunoglobulin expression with light chain restriction in about 80 percent of cases. The neoplastic cells also express other antigens characteristic of germinal center cells, such as CD10, and almost always lack aberrant coexpression of CD5 or CD43. Scattered non-neoplastic T cells can always be found. In T-cell-rich and histiocyte-rich B-cell lymphoma, the malignant component of large cells are of B lineage and usually exhibit monotypic immunoglobulins in frozen sections and occasionally in paraffin sections.[29–32] Interestingly, epithelial membrane antigen (EMA) is occasionally positive, but CD30 is negative, similar to the phenotype observed in many cases of diffuse L&H lymphocyte predominance Hodgkin's disease. The characteristic feature of T-cell-rich B-cell lymphomas is that all the small lymphocytes represent phenotypically normal T cells and not B cells. Distinct from diffuse L&H lymphocyte predominance Hodgkin's disease, the T cells generally lack expression of CD57. In lymphoplasmacytic lymphoma, the neoplastic cells are monotypic B cells, often with aberrant coexpression of CD43, but usually not of CD5. Since plasmacytic differentiation is generally prominent, light chain restriction usually can be demonstrable in paraffin sections. Marginal zone B-cell lymphoma has a similar phenotype, but somewhat less commonly exhibits aberrant coexpression of CD43 and CD5. Light chain restriction may be demonstrable when plasmacytoid features are present. In peripheral T-cell lymphomas, a wide variety of aberrant T-cell phenotypes can be demonstrated, as discussed in greater detail in Chapter 8.

The most important differential diagnosis for diffuse mixed lymphoma is Hodgkin's disease, both mixed cellularity and L&H types. Mixed cellularity Hodgkin's disease lacks the small cell atypia seen in follicular and peripheral T-cell variants of diffuse mixed lymphoma. While a plasma cell component is commonly a feature in classical Hodgkin's disease, plasma cells are rarely abundant in number, and plasmacytoid lymphocytes are not seen. T-cell-rich B-cell lymphoma may closely resemble Hodgkin's disease, although eosinophils are not a prominent feature in the former.

Immunophenotyping studies may be very helpful in the differential diagnosis. The neoplastic cells in mixed cellularity Hodgkin's disease are always EMA negative, almost always CD45 negative, almost always CD30 positive, frequently CD15 positive, and occasionally CD20 positive (and usually only in a subset of cells), while the neoplastic cells in T-cell-rich B-cell lymphoma are sometimes EMA positive, almost always CD45 positive, usually CD30 negative and CD15 negative, and almost always CD20 positive. L&H lymphocyte predominance Hodgkin's disease may be extremely difficult to distinguish from T-cell-rich and histiocyte-rich B-cell lymphoma. A nodular appearance, even a vague one, would strongly favor L&H Hodgkin's disease, but diffuse variants of L&H Hodgkin's disease may occur. In L&H Hodgkin's disease, the background histiocytes are usually epithelioid, while they are nonepithelioid in histiocyte-rich Hodgkin's disease. Immunophenotyping studies may not always be discriminatory, since the large cells are almost always CD45 positive, CD15 negative, and CD20 positive in both neoplasms, and EMA and CD30 may also be positive in both. CD57 may be a valuable antibody, as increased numbers of CD57 positive T cells may be found in L&H Hodgkin's disease, particularly with ringing of the CD57 positive cells around the large cells.[33] As mentioned above, some hematopathologists believe that histiocyte-rich B-cell lymphoma may represent a variant of diffuse L&H lymphocyte predominance Hodgkin's disease.

The clinical features of diffuse mixed small and large cell lymphoma are very similar to those of diffuse large cell lymphoma, particularly the non-T-cell types. The median age of occurrence is the sixth decade with an equal incidence in males and females.[1] Extranodal presentations occur in 20 percent of cases. There appears to be no clinical distinctiveness to T-cell-rich large B-cell lymphoma.[34] Further clinical features, including therapy and prognostic factors, are discussed below.

DIFFUSE LARGE CELL LYMPHOMA

Diffuse large cell lymphoma is an intermediate grade lymphoma in the Working Formulation, with large cleaved and large noncleaved subtypes.[1] As a morphologic entity, it includes mostly B-cell, and much less commonly T-cell, neoplasms. Similar to diffuse mixed lymphoma, this neoplasm is highly heterogeneous and represents many different biologic types of lymphoma, some of which are awaiting better clarification. Diffuse large cell lymphoma may present de novo or may represent secondary transformation of another lymphoma. Both B-cell lymphomas (most commonly small lymphocytic lymphoma, follicular lymphoma, and marginal zone B-cell lymphoma) and peripheral T-cell lymphomas (such as mycosis fungoides and angioimmunoblastic lymphadenopathy-like T-cell lymphoma) may undergo such transformation. In the REAL classification, diffuse large cell lymphomas of B-cell lineage are included with the category of diffuse large cell B-cell lymphoma, along with diffuse mixed lymphoma and anaplastic large cell lymphoma of B lineage.[2] Most cases of diffuse large cell lymphoma of T-cell lineage are included within the category of peripheral T-cell lymphoma, not otherwise specified, unless a specific type of peripheral T-cell lymphoma can be recognized. In the updated Kiel classification, B-lineage varieties of diffuse large cell lymphoma include diffuse forms of centroblastic/centrocytic lymphoma (large cleaved cell in the Working Formulation) and centroblastic lymphoma, monomorphic, polymorphic, and multilobated types (large noncleaved cell and large cell not otherwise specified subtypes in the Working Formulation), while most T-lineage large cell lymphomas are probably found within the category of pleomorphic, medium, and large cell type.[3]

Diffuse large cell lymphoma usually involves tissues in a diffuse fashion. However, focal areas of follicularity may occasionally be present, which would indicate an origin in follicular lymphoma. In lymph nodes, involvement usually completely effaces the lymph node architecture with complete obliteration of the sinuses, but occasionally there is preferential paracortical involvement with sparing of the follicles or preferential sinusoidal involvement (sinusoidal large cell lymphoma). A coarse sclerosis delineating large aggregates of tumor may be present, a finding more commonly seen in diffuse large cell lymphomas of follicular center cell origin. A more fine, compartmentalizing sclerosis may also be found and is particularly common in mediastinal diffuse large cell B-cell lymphoma (see below) and occasionally in retroperitoneal and mesenteric lymphomas.

There are two major cytologic variants of diffuse large cell B-cell lymphoma.[1,35] In the large cleaved cell type (centroblastic/centrocytic), the predominant large cell type (greater than 75 percent) is a large lymphoid cell (13 to 30 μm) with twisted and contorted nuclear outlines and minimal cytoplasm (Fig. 7-7). Nucleoli are small

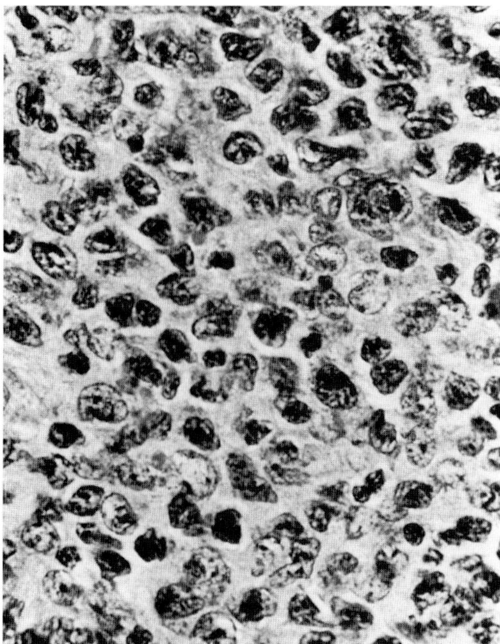

Fig. 7-7. Diffuse large cell lymphoma, cleaved cell type. Nucleoli are generally not prominent.

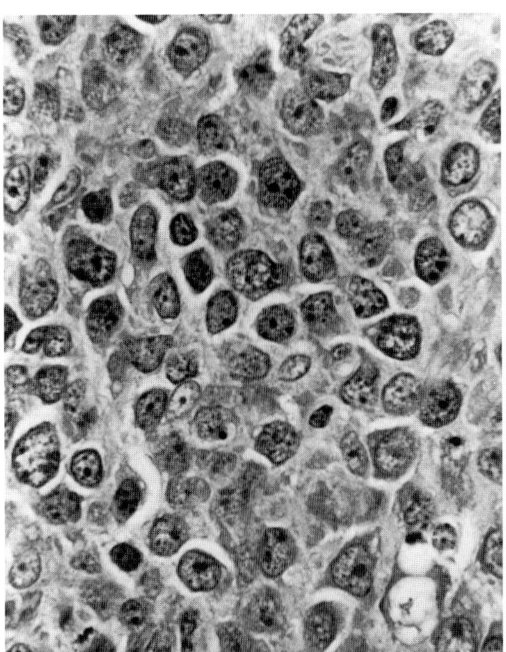

Fig. 7-8. Diffuse large cell lymphoma, noncleaved cell type. The chromatin is generally vesicular, and nucleoli are evident.

and inconspicuous. Virtually always, there are admixed small cleaved cells as well as small round lymphocytes (reactive host lymphocytes). In the large noncleaved cell type (centroblastic monomorphous), greater than 25 percent of the large cells represent large noncleaved cells (Fig. 7-8). These large lymphoid cells (20 to 40 μm) have a vesicular chromatin pattern, rounded or oval nuclear outlines that may vary in shape from one cell to another, and a slightly greater amount of cytoplasm than typically found in large cleaved cells. Nucleoli are one to several in number and are generally small but distinct; they are usually located on the nuclear membrane, but are occasionally solitary and centrally placed. Often, there are admixed small and large cleaved cells in varying numbers. In both variants, mitotic figures are usually readily identified. In a small number of cases, the large lymphoid cells may be multilobated (centroblastic multilobated).[36] This latter appearance may be found in both B- and T-cell lymphomas, particularly B-cell lymphomas primary in bone. Multilobated cells have greater than three lobes and usually have a chromatin pattern intermediate between large cleaved and noncleaved cells.

Large cell lymphomas of T lineage may be morphologically indistinguishable from B-cell large lymphomas, but typically they have a greater range of atypia and a greater spectrum of cell types. In addition, they usually have a more heterogeneous mixture of reactive cells, including eosinophils, histiocytes, epithelioid histiocytes, and plasma cells with vascular proliferation.

In cases of secondary diffuse large cell lymphoma of both B- and T-cell type, a residual component of the original lymphoma may be present. For example, large cell lymphoma complicating small lymphocytic lymphoma (Richter syndrome) may show a small lymphocytic component of neoplastic B cells, and large cell lymphoma complicating mycosis fungoides may show scattered foci of small cerebriform cells.

At least 80 percent of diffuse large cell lymphomas represent B-lineage neoplasms, expressing CD20 and other pan-B-cell markers.[37] A large subset of these cases is CD10 positive, presumably those of follicular center cell origin. Approximately two-thirds of the B-lineage cases express surface immunoglobulins, usually of IgM isotype. One-third of cases show aberrant loss of immunoglobulin, a finding that can be helpful in establishing a diagnosis of lymphoma. About 10 percent of cases show aberrant expression of the T-lineage marker CD5 or the T/myeloid marker CD43, findings that may also be exploited for diagnostic use.

In the Working Formulation, diffuse large cell lymphoma is of intermediate grade.[1] The median age of incidence is 57 years, and there is an equal incidence in males and females. About 60 percent present with nodal involvement. About 45 percent present in Ann Arbor stages I and II, while about 55 percent present in stages III and IV. Liver, spleen, and Waldeyer's ring involvement are common at presentation, but bone marrow involvement occurs at presentation in only about 10 percent of cases. Patients with diffuse large cell lymphoma are generally treated with multidrug chemotherapy regimens, with a remission rate of 80 percent and an overall survival rate of 60 percent.[38] The majority of those who show a complete response are cured.

Mediastinal (Thymic) B-Cell Lymphoma

In the REAL classification, primary mediastinal (thymic) B-cell large cell lymphoma is considered a clinicopathologic entity involving the mediastinum.[2] Synonyms for this lymphoma include primary mediastinal large cell lymphoma with sclerosis and mediastinal clear cell lymphoma, emphasizing some of the characteristic histologic features. This lymphoma is thought to derive from the normal thymic B cells.[39] This specific lymphoma type is not a part of any other major lymphoma classification, since none of the other systems of classification recognize site-specific neoplasms (with the exception of mycosis fungoides).

At low magnification, a diffuse pattern of infiltration is seen. Rather than primarily involving lymph node parenchyma, the neoplasm characteristically infiltrates fibrous tissue; in early cases, localization to the thymic medulla may be seen. Even in areas not recognizable as thymus, islands of thymic epithelium may be identified, suggesting that a hyperplasia of thymic epithelial cells is accompanying the lymphoma. A distinctive feature of this neoplasm is a hyaline sclerosis that is nearly always present (Fig. 7-9). This sclerosis is often finely trabecular, producing compartmentalization of the neoplasm, a feature that may mimic a poorly differentiated carcinoma or mediastinal seminoma.[40] Cytologically, the neoplastic cells may be cleaved, noncleaved, or multilobated. In addition, many neoplastic cells often have an abundant amount of cytoplasm that may be clear staining (formalin fixation) or pale staining (metal fixation).[41]

The immunophenotype of mediastinal (thymic) B-cell lymphoma tends to be similar to that of the normal thymic medulla B cell.[39] The cells are positive for pan-B-cell antigens, such as CD20, but are negative for CD10 and CD21 and do not show aberrant coexpression of CD5 and CD43. One major difference from the normal thymic medulla B cell is that the cells of mediastinal (thymic) B-cell lymphoma are often immunoglobulin negative.[42] It has been suggested that the neoplastic cells of mediastinal (thymic) B-cell lymphoma correspond to the terminal steps of B-cell differentiation.[43]

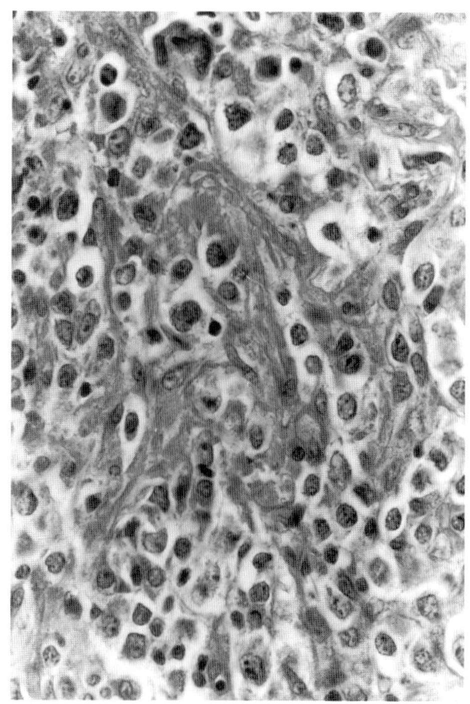

Fig. 7-9. Primary mediastinal large B-cell lymphoma. There is a hyaline sclerosis, showing a compartmentalizing effect. The nuclei are large, while the cytoplasm is moderate in amount and pale to clear in character.

The differential diagnosis of mediastinal (thymic) B-cell lymphoma is broad. The compartmentalizing fibrosis raises the differential of carcinoma and seminoma; immunohistochemical stains for keratin, placental alkaline phosphatase, CD45 (leukocyte common antigen), and CD20 should resolve that differential diagnosis in most cases (the latter two stains are positive in mediastinal B-cell lymphoma). In small biopsies, nodular sclerosing Hodgkin's disease may be extremely difficult to distinguish from mediastinal B-cell lymphoma, since both neoplasms show sclerosis and are composed of large cells with abundant clear to pale cytoplasm. Again, immunohistochemical stains are of great use as the lacunar cells of nodular sclerosing are usually CD45 −, CD15 +, CD30 +, and CD20 +/ −, while the cells of mediastinal B-cell lymphoma are CD45 +, CD15 −, CD30 −, and CD20 +.

Mediastinal (thymic) B-cell lymphoma subtype seems to have distinctive clinical features as well. It presents in a younger population than for other large cell lymphomas, with a median age of about 25 to 30 years.[39,40,42–45] Also in contrast to other large cell lymphomas, there is a female predominance, with a male:female ratio of 2:3. Most patients present with symptoms related to the mediastinum, with superior vena cava obstruction seen in about 60 percent of cases and pleural or pericardial effusions found in about 50 percent of cases. At the time of diagnosis, invasion of intrathoracic structures adjacent to the anterior mediastinum is found in 85 percent of cases. Although the early literature suggested that this lymphoma may be more aggressive than other large cell lymphomas,[46] recent studies employing combination multichemotherapy and radiotherapy have achieved a cure rate similar to that of other large cell lymphomas.[47]

Intravascular Large Cell Lymphoma

Although not recognized in any major classification, intravascular large cell lymphoma (intravascular lymphomatosis, angiotropic lymphoma, malignant angioendotheliomatosis) represents a distinct morphologic variant of diffuse large cell lymphoma that may also have characteristic clinicopathologic features.[48–50] This lymphoma is defined by its unique localization to the intravascular spaces.

Histologically, large cell lymphoma cells are found within the lumina of small to medium sized veins (Fig. 7-10). The tumor cells may lie free within the vascular space, they may appear to be attached to the wall, and occasionally they may be found in the subendothelial space. The involved blood vessels may show a reactive endothelial proliferation, which may complicate the diagnosis, and fibrin and platelets may be found admixed with the tumor cells within the lumen. Occasionally, tumor cells may be found in the media or the adventitia of the involved blood vessels or in the surrounding fibroadipose tissue. Rare cases have been associated with involvement of adjacent lymph nodes. Despite the presence of tumor cells apparently present in vascular spaces, the process is usually localized to specific organs, and only rarely can lymphoma cells be identified by examination of the peripheral smear. In addition, bone marrow involvement is uncommon.

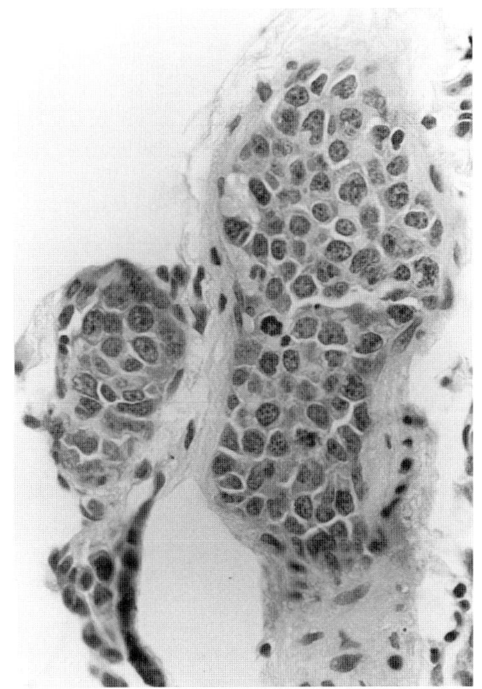

Fig. 7-10. Intravascular large cell lymphoma. The lymphoma cells are confined to medium sized veins, in this example from the lung.

Immunohistochemical studies have revealed that most cases are of B lineage, but T-lineage examples have also been reported.[49] The pathogenesis of this unique form of large cell lymphoma is not known, but a specific alteration in a homing/adhesion molecule that prevents or hinders migration through vessel walls is suspected.[51]

Clinically, the disease usually presents in older adults, with an equal sex ratio. There is a predilection for involvement of the central nervous system, skin, and adrenal gland, but essentially any organ can be affected.[50] Patients usually present with skin nodules or with neurologic deficits. When the neoplasm is not recognized, as is too often the case, there is rapid progression to death, usually from infarcts of vital organs. When prompt biopsy is performed, the correct diagnosis rendered, and appropriate treatment given (multichemotherapy), cures have been reported.

IMMUNOBLASTIC LYMPHOMA

The term *immunoblastic sarcoma* (lymphoma) was popularized by Lukes and Collins[35] in their classification in 1974 in reference to a neoplasm composed of the neoplastic equivalent of B immunoblasts. In the Working Formulation study, it was found that large cell lymphoma of presumed follicular center origin had a better prognosis than large cell lymphoma of presumed nonfollicular center origin.[1] Therefore, the high grade category of large cell immunoblastic was created to include not only the immunoblastic lymphoma as described by Lukes and Collins (plasmacytoid immunoblastic lymphoma) but also other morphologic variants that did not appear to be of follicular center cell origin (clear cell, polymorphous, and with an epithelioid cell component). It was presumed that many of the lymphomas comprising the latter three categories actually represented peripheral T-cell lymphomas; however, immunologic characterization was not a part of the Working Formulation study. In the REAL classification, there is no longer any immunoblastic subtype.[2] This is because many hematopathologists believe there are no distinct biologic differences between diffuse large cell B-cell lymphoma and immunoblastic B-cell lymphoma and because reproducibility studies have demonstrated little ability to distinguish reliably between these two morphologic variants. T-cell lymphomas with immunoblastic morphology are included in the classification under the most appropriate category of peripheral T-cell lymphoma, which would usually be the ''not otherwise specified'' group. In the updated Kiel classification, there is a category of immunoblastic lymphoma within both the high grade B- and T-cell lymphomas.[3]

At low magnification, immunoblastic lymphoma usually exhibits diffuse effacement of architecture. However, among the large cell lymphomas, immunoblastic lymphoma is the one that has the greatest propensity for partial lymph node involvement, preferentially involving either the paracortical region or the sinuses (sinusoidal large cell lymphoma).[52] If a sinusoidal pattern of involvement is present, one should strongly consider the possibility of CD30 positive anaplastic large cell lymphoma. The cells of immunoblastic lymphoma are uniformly large, greater than 20 μm in diameter (Fig. 7-11). The nuclei are large and usually round to oval, with a vesicular chromatin pattern. The nuclei either contain a solitary, centrally located nucleolus or

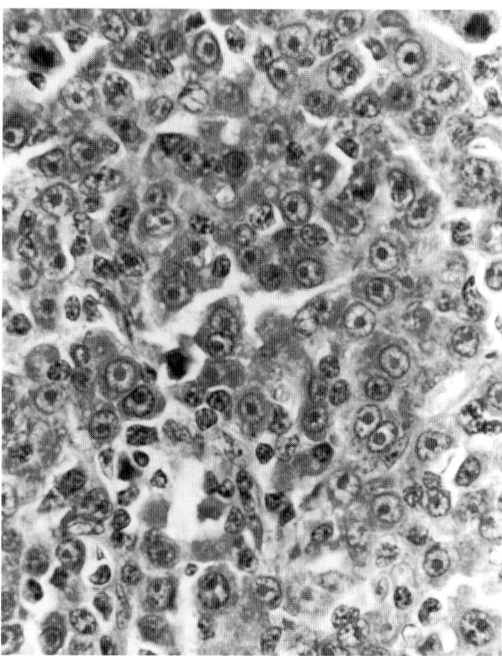

Fig. 7-11. Large cell immunoblastic lymphoma, plasmacytoid type. The nuclei are large, with a vesicular chromatin pattern and generally one prominent central nucleolus.

the nucleoli may be multiple, prominent, and centrally placed. Occasionally, however, the nucleoli are located peripherally. The mitotic rate is high.

In the plasmacytoid immunoblastic variant, the nuclei are usually eccentrically placed, and cytoplasm is moderate to abundant, deep staining, and strongly pyroninophilic.[1] The neoplasm may be monomorphic, or it may have admixed large noncleaved cells or transitional forms between large noncleaved cells and immunoblasts. Normal and abnormal plasma cells may also be evident. In the clear cell variant, the nucleus is centrally placed and the cytoplasm is abundant and pale to optically clear. According to Lukes and Collins[35] the nuclei of the clear cell variant have fine, evenly distributed chromatin and one or more small but distinct nucleoli. In the polymorphous variant, there is a mixture of atypical lymphoid cells with twisted nuclei lymphoid cells and large clear cell type immunoblasts. The clear cell and polymorphous variants were specifically included in the Working Formulation to encompass the wide spectrum of T-cell lymphomas. In the epithelioid variant, a prominent epithelioid histiocytic component is present in addition to the polymorphous neoplastic population; this subtype represents one form of Lennert lymphoma.

Immunoblastic lymphomas are usually of B-cell phenotype; the phenotype of T-cell lymphomas is discussed in Chapter 8. The B-cell lymphomas generally express CD45 (leukocyte common antigen) and pan-B antigens such as CD20 and CD79a, but those immunoblastic lymphomas that show well-developed plasmacytoid features may occasionally be negative for some of these markers. Correspondingly, as plasmacytoid features become more prominent, the neoplasms are more likely to express cytoplasmic immunoglobulin, usually of μ isotype.

As discussed above, the distinction between immunoblastic lymphoma and diffuse large cell lymphoma may be difficult and may not have great clinical significance. It is much more important not to mistake immunoblastic lymphoma for carcinoma or malignant melanoma; an immunohistochemical panel that includes keratin and S-100 may be important to exclude these possibilities. Immunoblastic lymphoma of plasmacytoid type may show histologic overlap with anaplastic plasmacytoma/multiple myeloma. The clinical setting is usually very helpful in making this distinction. Immunohistochemical studies may also be of use, as plasmacytoma/multiple myeloma is much more likely to be negative for CD45 and pan-B markers (except CD79a) and to express γ or α isotype immunoglobulins.

In the Working Formulation, large cell immunoblastic lymphoma was classified as high grade.[1] The median age was 51 years, somewhat younger than for the category of diffuse large cell lymphoma, and the male:female ratio was 1.5:1, higher than diffuse large cell lymphoma. Seventy percent of patients presented with nodal disease, with the gastrointestinal tract and spleen representing common extranodal sites of disease. About 50 percent present in Ann Arbor stages I and II; bone marrow involvement occurs in about 10 percent of patients at presentation. Immunoblastic lymphoma is generally treated similarly to diffuse large cell lymphoma, usually with multidrug chemotherapy. Recent studies have shown survival rates similar to those of other large cell lymphomas, additional evidence leading many hematopathologists to suggest that the histologic separation of these two groups may not be of great clinical importance.[53]

PROGNOSTIC FACTORS IN DIFFUSE MIXED, DIFFUSE LARGE CELL, AND LARGE CELL IMMUNOBLASTIC B-CELL LYMPHOMA

Since morphologic parameters have shown either a lack of prognostic significance or poor reproducibility, there has been great interest in determining if clinical and/or biologic factors can be used prospectively to identify subsets of patients with diffuse aggressive lymphomas with different long-term prognoses. The identification of low risk patients would enable clinicians to deliver a minimum of therapy in hopes of avoiding iatrogenic effects. The identification of high risk patients would enable clinicians to target these patients for the most aggressive regimens and would identify candidates for experimental protocols.

It has been known for many years that clinical parameters could be used to separate different prognostic groups among patients with diffuse aggressive lymphomas. The Ann Arbor staging system, originally applied to Hodgkin's disease, has been used for the staging of non-Hodgkin's lymphoma.[54] However, unlike Hodgkin's disease in which spread of disease occurs through involvement of contiguous sites, disease involvement in non-Hodgkin's lymphoma is more random, limiting the utility of the Ann Arbor system.[55] Nonetheless, it has been shown that patients with localized disease (Ann Arbor stages I and II) have a better prognosis than patients with advanced disease (Ann Arbor stages III and IV).[56–60] Similarly, other markers of tumor extent such as number of nodal and extranodal sites of disease, size of tumor, and lactate dehydrogenase concentrations have been shown to have prognostic significance.[56,58,60] Other clinical factors of prognostic significance include measures of host response and host competence. These include the Karnofsky performance index, presence of ''B'' symptoms, and patient age and sex.[56–60]

In a landmark paper published in 1993, a large group of investigators from multiple institutions pooled their data on over 2,000 patients to develop a model for predicting outcome in patients with aggressive non-Hodgkin's lymphoma on the basis of the patients' clinical characteristics before treatment.[61] This effort, the International Non-Hodgkin's Lymphoma Prognostic Factors Project, studied 12 variables and identified five pretreatment characteristics that remained independently significant in their analysis: age (more than 60 years), stage (III or IV), number of extranodal sites of disease (more than 1), performance status (at least 2), and serum lactate dehydrogenase level (greater than normal). In an index, called the *international index,* patients with 0 or 1 or the above risk factors are classified as low risk; 2, low intermediate risk; 3, high intermediate risk; or 4 or 5, high risk. These four groups had predicted 5 year survival rates of 73, 51, 43, and 26 percent, respectively. This system was found to be significantly more accutate than the Ann Arbor classification in predicting long-term survival. A second index, the age-adjusted international index, was developed for use in younger patients. It was found that tumor stage, performance status, and lactate dehydrogenase level remained independently significant prognostic factors in patients less than 60 years of age. In the age-adjusted international index, those patients with 0 risk factors are classified as low risk (83 percent 5 year survival); 1, low intermediate risk (69 percent 5 year survival); 2, high intermediate risk (46 percent 5 year survival); and 3, high risk (32 percent 5 year survival). These models may also be useful in predicting outcome in patients with other types of lymphoma as well.

Over the past several years, a number of biologic factors have been shown to be of prognostic significance in aggressive B-cell lymphomas, including proliferative rate, cytotoxic T-cell response, loss of molecules of immune recognition, loss of cell adhesion antigens, gain of drug resistance molecules, acquisition of aneuploidy, gain of specific oncogenes, and loss of specific tumor suppressor genes. An excellent review of many of these factors has been published.[62] Many of these parameters can be easily evaluated in paraffin or frozen section immunohistochemical studies, while some require molecular biologic studies. Some of the molecular studies are described in Chapter 1.

It is widely believed that the proliferative rate of a lymphoma may impact prognosis. Assessment of mitotic rates in lymphoma have led to conflicting results, perhaps due to the difficulty of their measurement. Measurement of radioactive tritiated thymidine incorporation and flow cytometric S-phase studies have shown a correlation between proliferative rates and lymphoma histologic grade,[63–65] but assessment of proliferation by Ki-67 antibody studies holds more promise as a practical test.[66] Ki-67 antibody labels a nuclear antigen found in cycling, but not resting, cells.[67,68] Although early studies utilizing Ki-67 were conflicting, in one well-controlled prospective study of a series of uniformly staged and treated intermediate and high grade patients, poor survival was found to correlate with Ki-67 values exceeding 80 percent of tumor cells, as determined by frozen section immunohistochemistry.[69] Cox regression analysis established Ki-67 staining as an independent prognostic variable with a relative risk of 17. A paraffin section antibody equivalent to Ki-67 (mib-1) is now available and may prove to be a more practical and as well as more effective measure of lymphoma proliferation, enabling better assessment of the Ki-67 positive and negative cells.[70]

The amount and character of the host response may also be important in determining the prognosis of lymphoma. The presence of T cells, particularly cytotoxic T cells, within tumor tissue may be an indication of the host response against the tumor. In one study of B-cell large cell lymphoma, the percentage of cytotoxic T cells in lymphoma tissues was correlated with patient outcome; when cytotoxic T cells fell below 6 percent, the patient invariably relapsed.[71] Loss of histocompatibility antigens may be one of the biologic explanations for a relative lack of host response. Class I and class II histocompatibility (HLA) antigens are critical to cell recognition and immunosurveillance. Class I antigens serve as self-recognition antigens for cytotoxic T cells, while class II antigens function similarly for helper T cells. In several studies, loss of class I or class II antigens on lymphoma cells has been found to result in a higher probability of relapse and shorter median patient survival.[72–74]

Loss of cell adhesion molecules may also predict poor prognosis in diffuse aggressive lymphomas. Cell adhesion molecules play important roles in cell-to-cell and cell-to-stroma interactions. For example, the leukocyte function-associated (LFA)-1 (CD11a-CD18) molecule and the intercellular adhesion molecule (ICAM)-1 (CD54) represent ligand/receptors for one other, and their interaction may be important in cell adhesion, particularly as a mediator of cytotoxic T-cell recognition and action. Loss of LFA-1 and/or ICAM-1 is common among diffuse aggressive lymphomas, and loss of both is characteristic of Burkitt's lymphoma, a high grade lymphoma that characteristically lacks a reactive host T-cell infiltrate.[75] In addition, loss of CD22, the B-cell homolog of neural cell adhesion molecule (NCAM) (CD56), has been correlated with poor survival in large cell lymphoma patients.[76] CD22 has ligands on both T cells (CD45RO) and B cells (CD75) and may be important in both B-cell cohesion and T-cell recognition and immunosurveillance.

Cell adhesion molecules also play an important role in lymphoid cell migration and homing, and alterations in these molecules may play a role in lymphoid neoplasia. One example may be CD44, a homing molecule that facilitates the migration of lymphocytes through adhesion to high endothelial venules. Several studies have found CD44 expression to be more frequent in high stage as opposed to low stage patients,[77,78] and several studies suggest that high level CD44 expression is an independent prognostic factor in malignant lymphoma.[77,79,80]

In addition to loss of critical antigens, gain of critical antigens may also lead to increased pathogenicity in diffuse aggressive lymphomas. One example of this may be the gain of the P-glycoprotein, the protein that acts as an efflux pump, removing a variety of cytotoxic agents from the cell. Detection of P-glycoprotein is uncommon in untreated patients, but found in about two-thirds of those with drugresistant disease.[81] It has proved difficult to detect P-glycoprotein reliably in standard immunohistochemical assays, but in some studies the presence of P-glycoprotein has been associated with poor response to therapy.[82,83] Drugs that competitively bind P-glycoprotein may benefit patients with P-glycoprotein positive lymphoma by reversing the clinical drug resistance.[81]

HUMAN IMMUNODEFICIENCY VIRUS ASSOCIATED MALIGNANT LYMPHOMAS

Malignant lymphomas are a major complication of human immunodeficiency virus (HIV) infection, and the occurrence of intermediate to high grade B-cell lymphomas in patients infected with HIV is part of the case definition of the acquired immune deficiency syndrome (AIDS).[84] Approximately 3 percent of AIDS patients develop non-Hodgkin's lymphoma, a greater than 60-fold incidence compared with the normal population,[85] and it is widely believed that this incidence will rise as patients with HIV infection live longer.[86] Currently, about 10 percent of all non-Hodgkin's lymphomas diagnosed in the United States are HIV related.[86] There may be as yet unknown cofactors in the development of non-Hodgkin's lymphomas, since a relatively high incidence is seen in hemophiliacs and a relatively low incidence is seen in patients born in the Carribean or Africa who obtained HIV by heterosexual contact. Factors associated with the development of lymphoma include a prior diagnosis of Kaposi sarcoma, cytomegalovirus disease, or oral hairy leukoplakia, all herpesvirus-associated diseases.[87]

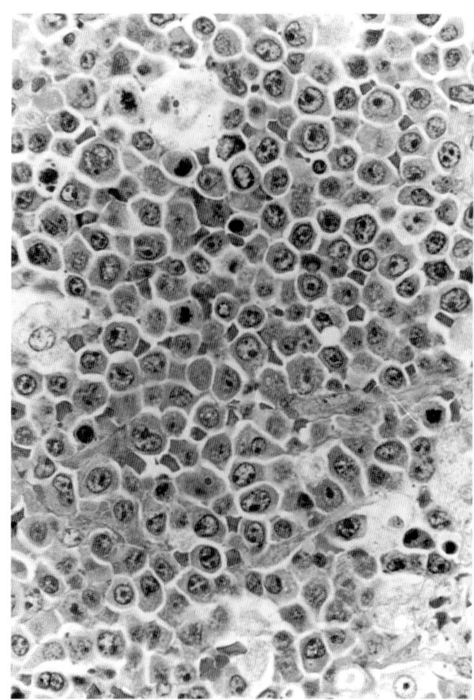

Fig. 7-13. HIV-associated non-Hodgkin's lymphoma. This case was a plasmacytoid immunoblastic lymphoma.

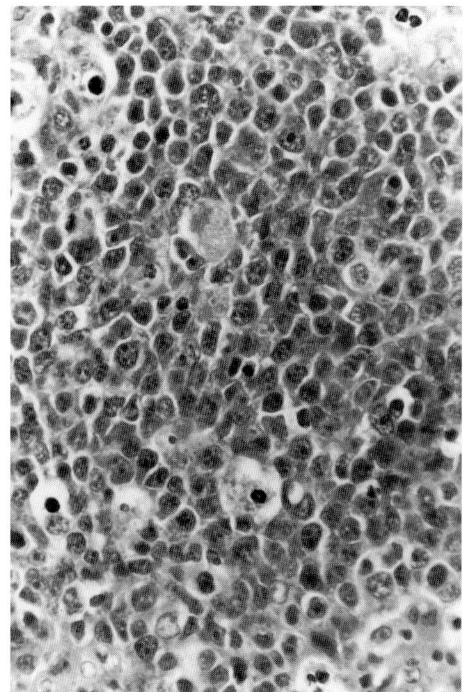

Fig. 7-12. HIV-associated non-Hodgkin's lymphoma. This case was classified as small noncleaved, non-Burkitt's type. Note, however, that the cells are somewhat plasmacytoid, and an occasional immunoblast is present.

About 90 percent of HIV-associated lymphomas represent intermediate to high grade B-cell lymphomas.[88–91] Two-thirds of cases present in stage IV.[92] One of the unusual features of HIV-associated lymphomas is that there is almost always involvement of extranodal sites at presentation. Although any site may be involved, the central nervous system, gastrointestinal tract, bone marrow, mucocutaneous sites, and the liver are most commonly involved.[88–90] There is a high incidence of "B" symptoms.[93]

About one-third of HIV-associated lymphomas represent small noncleaved lymphomas, about one-third are classified as large cell immunoblastic lymphomas, and one-third are other large cell lymphomas (Figs. 7-12 and 7-13).[88–91,94] However, they are frequently pleomorphic, and there are frequently cases that defy specific classification, seemingly representing transitions between these histologic types. Small noncleaved cell lymphomas are most likely to involve lymph nodes, the bone marrow, or soft tissues.[90] They usually occur at an early stage in the course of HIV infection[95] in patients without a history of AIDS-defining illnesses.[91] Histologically, about 40 percent have classical features of Burkitt's lymphoma.[90] About one-half of the non-Burkitt's variants have plasmablastic features, with medium sized malignant cells having a round, eccentric nucleus with one or more randomly located larger nucleoli and a well-defined paranuclear hof. The other cases show more pleomorphic features, with marked variation in cell size and shape and nuclear irregularity, with one to three iregularly sized nucleoli seen within nuclei with dispersed chromatin (Fig. 7-12). Some cells resembling immunoblasts are sometimes present.

HIV-associated immunoblastic lymphoma tends to involve extranodal sites, particularly the central nervous system, gastrointestinal tract, and oral cavity.[89,90] These cases are most likely to occur at a relatively late stage of HIV infection in patients with relatively low CD4 counts who have a previous history of AIDS-defining illness.[91,95] Histologically, the cases of immunoblastic lymphoma usually have well-developed plasmacytic features (Fig. 7-13).[90] HIV-associated large cell lymphoma, not otherwise specified, tends also to involve extranodal sites,[95] although lymph nodes may also be the presenting site of disease.[90] Similar to immunoblastic lymphoma, these cases are also most likely to occur in patients with relatively low CD4 counts.[95] Histologically, three variants have been observed: monomorphic, polymorphic, and multilobated.[90] Most cases are polymorphic, with a spectrum of cells from large noncleaved to immunoblastic.

Less than 5 percent of HIV-associated lymphoma cases represent highly anaplastic lymphomas, usually CD30 positive anaplastic large cell lymphomas.[96] Although most of these are of T or null lineage, a subset are of B-lineage origin. Many of these latter unusual cases have a marked predilection for involvment of the pleural or peritoneal cavities, giving rise to the appellation *body cavity based lymphoma* (Fig. 7-14).[97]

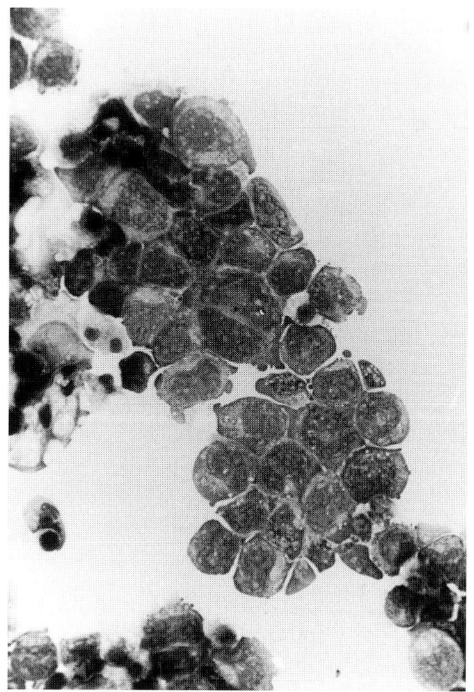

Fig. 7-14. HIV-associated non-Hodgkin's lymphoma, body cavity based type, in pleural fluid (case courtesy of Dr. Ethel Cesarman). This case had evidence of HHV-8.

Virtually all the B-lineage HIV-associated aggressive non-Hodgkin's lymphomas express B-lineage antigens, including CD19 and CD20.[89,94,98] The one exception is the body cavity based lymphoma, in which molecular studies are necessary to confirm the B-lineage derivation.[97] Almost all cases of small noncleaved cell lymphoma are immunoglobulin positive, but a significant subset of the large cell lymphomas, particular immunoblastic lymphoma, may be immunoglobulin negative.

Clonal rearrangements of the immunoglobulin heavy and light chain genes are found in most cases,[89,98,99] although some cases of allegedly polyclonal lymphoma have been reported by one group.[100] In a subset of cases more than two rearranged bands are identified, consistent with the presence of more than one clonal population, and study of different sites from the same patient have occasionally identified different clones, consistent with what has been observed in posttransplantation lymphoproliferative disorders.[89,99] Although *bcl*-1 and *bcl*-2 rearrangements have not been found in HIV-associated lymphomas, c-*myc* rearrangements are relatively common.[101,102] The c-*myc* oncogene activation occurs in almost all cases of small noncleaved lymphoma, but in less than half of the cases of large cell lymphoma. In addition, *p53* inactivation is found in about 60 percent of cases of small noncleaved cell lymphoma, but not in the large cell lymphoma categories.[102] In contrast, rearrangement of *bcl*-6 is found in about 20 percent of cases of large cell lymphoma, but not in small noncleaved cell lymphoma.[103] Mutations of *ras* genes occur in about 20 percent of cases, including both small noncleaved cell and immunoblastic lymphoma.[102] Abnormalities of the retinoblastoma gene have not been found.

Due to diminished immunocompetence, patients with HIV infection have abnormally high amounts of Epstein-Barr virus (EBV)-infected B cells in the peripheral blood and lymph nodes.[104–106] The identification of abnormally high amounts of EBV in benign lymph nodes has been correlated with metachronous or subsequent development of non-Hodgkin's lymphoma.[106] About 42 to 67 percent of cases of HIV-associated lymphomas are EBV positive,[91,102,107,108] including virtually all cases of central nervous system lymphoma. In contrast to post-transplantation lymphoma, both EBV types A and B have been identified.[94,107,109] In these positive cases, EBV has been localized to all or virtually all of the neoplastic cells by in situ hybridization.[94,107] EBV is most consistently identified in the immunoblastic lymphomas (about 75 to 100 percent of cases) and is least associated with small noncleaved cell lymphoma (15 to 50 percent).[94,102,107] The pattern of latency is unique among EBV-associated B-cell lymphomas, with most cases EBNA-1 positive, EBNA-2 negative, and LMP1 positive.[107]

The body cavity based lymphomas have been uniformly positive for EBV. However, they have also been found to be uniformly positive for the newly discovered Kaposi sarcoma-associated herpes virus (or human herpes virus [HHV]-8).[97] No other type of HIV-associated lymphoma has been found to be HHV-8 positive.

The above data suggest that HIV-associated lymphomas can be separated into two main types. The first, small noncleaved cell lymphoma, occurs relatively early in the course of HIV infection, is primarily nodal based, with alterations in c-*myc* and *p53* being important in the pathogenesis. On the other hand, the large cell lymphomas, particularly immunoblastic lymphoma, occurs as a late complication of HIV infection, occurs primarily in extranodal sites, is highly associated with EBV infection, with some cases associated with *bcl*-6 rearrangement. A rare and unique subset of cases may be caused by HHV-8, possibly working in concert with EBV.

HIV-associated lymphomas have been difficult to treat due to the intrinsic immunosuppression these patients have; however, some good results have been obtained with protocol employing good patient support such as hematopoietic growth factors.[110] Adverse prognostic factors in the setting include history of AIDS before lymphoma, Karnofsky performance status less than 70 percent, bone marrow involvement, CD4 counts less than 100/mm^3, and extranodal disease. The prognostic significance of histologic type is still not clear.[92,93]

REFERENCES

1. Non-Hodgkin's lymphoma pathologic classification project. National Cancer Institute sponsored study of classifications of non-Hodgkin's lymphomas: summary and description of a Working Formulation for clinical usage. Cancer 49:2112, 1982
2. Harris NL, Jaffe ES, Stein H et al: A revised European-American classification of lymphoid neoplasms. A proposal from the International Lymphoma Study Group. Blood 84:1361, 1994
3. Stansfeld A, Diebold J, Kapanci Y et al: Updated Kiel classification for lymphomas. Lancet i:292, 1988
4. Nathwani B, Kim H, Rappaport H: Malignant lymphoma, lymphoblastic. Cancer 38:964, 1976
5. Nathwani B, Diamond L, Winberg C et al:

Lymphoblastic lymphoma: a clinicopathologic study of 95 patients. Cancer 48:2347, 1981
6. Lardelli P, Bookman M, Sundeen J et al: Lymphocytic lymphoma of intermediate differentiation. Morphologic and immunophenotypic spectrum and clinical correlations. Am J Surg Pathol 14:752, 1990
7. Braziel RM, Keneklis T, Donlon JA et al: Terminal deoxynucleotidyl transferase in non-Hodgkin's lymphoma. Am J Clin Pathol 80:655, 1983
8. Orazi A, Caggoretti G, John K, Neimen RS: Terminal deoxynucleotidyl transferase staining of malignant lymphomas in paraffin sections. Mod Pathol 1994:582, 1994
9. Cossman J, Chused TM, Fisher RI et al: Diversity of immunological phenotypes of lymphoblastic lymphoma. Cancer Res 43:4486, 1983
10. Weiss LM, Arber DA, Chang KL: CD45: a review. Appl Immunohistochem 1:166, 1993
11. Weiss LM, Bindl JM, Picozzi VJ et al: Lymphoblastic lymphoma: an immunophenotype study of 26 cases with comparison to T cell acute lymphoblastic leukemia. Blood 67:474, 1986
12. Arber DA, Weiss LM: CD43: review. Appl Immunohistochem 1:88, 1993
13. Sheibani K, Winberg CD, Burke JS et al: Lymphoblastic lymphoma expressing natural killer cell-associated antigens: a clinicopathologic study of six cases. Leuk Res 11:371, 1987
14. Weiss LM, Bindl JM, Picozzi VJ et al: Lymphoblastic lymphoma: an immunophenotype study of 26 cases with comparison to T cell acute lymphoblastic leukemia. Blood 67:474, 1986
15. Mason DY, van Noesel CJ, Cordell JL et al: The B29 and mb-1 polypeptides are differentially expressed during human B cell differentiation. Eur J Immunol 22:2753, 1992
16. Stroup R, Sheibani K, Misset JL et al: Surface immunoglobulin-positive lymphoblastic lymphoma. A report of three cases. Cancer 65:2559, 1990
17. Coleman CN, Picozzi VJ, Cox RS et al: Treatment of lymphoblastic lymphoma in adults. J Clin Oncol 4:1628, 1986
18. Sheibani K, Nathwani BN, Winberg CD: Antigenically defined subgroups of lymphoblastic lymphoma: relationship to clinical presentation and biological behavior. Cancer 60:183, 1987
19. Link M, Roper M, Dorfman R et al: Cutaneous lymphoblastic lymphoma with pre-B markers. Blood 61:838, 1983
20. Garcia CF, Weiss LM, Warnke RA: Small noncleaved cell lymphoma: an immunophenotypic study of 18 cases and comparison with large cell lymphoma. Hum Pathol 17:454, 1986
21. Burkitt DP: A sarcoma involving the jaws in African children. Br J Surg 197:218, 1970
22. Aine R: Small non-cleaved follicular center cell lymphoma: clinicopathologic comparison of Burkitt and non-Burkitt variants in Finnish material. Eur J Cancer Clin Oncol 21:1179, 1985
23. Levine AM, Pavlova Z, Pockros AW et al: Small noncleaved follicular center cell (FCC) lymphoma: Burkitt and non-Burkitt variants in the United States. I. Clinical features. Cancer 52: 1073, 1983
24. Miliauskas JR, Berard CW, Young RC et al: Undifferentiated non-Hodgkin's lymphomas (Burkitt's and non-Burkitt's types). The relevance of making this histologic distinction. Cancer 50:2115, 1982
25. Bernstein JI, Coleman CN, Strickler JG et al: Combined modality therapy for adults with small non-cleaved cell lymphoma (Burkitt's and non-Burkitt's types). J Clin Oncol 4:847, 1986
26. Yano T, van Krieken J, Magrath I et al: Histogenetic correlations between subcategories of small noncleaved cell lymphomas. Blood 79: 1282, 1992
27. Nathwani B, Metter G, Gams R et al: Malignant lymphoma, mixed cell type, diffuse. Blood 62: 200, 1983
28. Hu E, Weiss L, Hoppe R, Horning S: Follicular and diffuse mixed small cleaved and large cell lymphoma—a clinicopathologic study. J Clin Oncol 3:1183, 1985
29. Macon WR, Williams ME, Greer JP et al: T-cell-rich B-cell lymphomas. A clinicopathologic study of 19 cases. Am J Surg Pathol 16:351, 1992
30. Chittal S, Brousset P, Voigt J, Delsol G: Large B-cell lymphoma rich in T-cells and simulating Hodgkin's disease. Histopathology 19:211, 1991
31. Ramsay A, Smith W, Isaacson P: T-cell-rich B-cell lymphoma. Am J Surg Pathol 12:433, 1988
32. Delabie J, Vandenberghe E, Kennes C et al: Histiocyte-rich B-cell lymphoma. A distinct clinicopathologic entity possibly related to lympho-

cyte predominant Hodgkin's disease, paragranuloma subtype. Am J Surg Pathol 16:37, 1992

33. Kamel OW, Gelb AB, Shibuya RB, Warnke RA: Leu7 (CD57) reactivity distinguishes nodular lymphocyte Hodgkin's disease, T cell rich B cell lymphoma and follicular lymphoma. Am J Pathol 142:541, 1993
34. Krishnan J, Wallberg K, Frizzera G: T-cell-rich large B-cell lymphoma. A study of 30 cases, supporting its histologic heterogeneity and lack of clinical distinctiveness. Am J Surg Pathol 18: 455, 1994
35. Lukes R, Collins R: Immunologic characterization of human malignant lymphomas. Cancer 34:1488, 1974
36. O'Hara C, Said J, Pinkus G: Non-Hodgkin's lymphoma, multilobated B cell type. Hum Pathol 17:593, 1986
37. Doggett R, Wood G, Horning S et al: The immunologic characterization of 95 nodal and extranodal diffuse large cell lymphomas in 89 patients. Am J Pathol 115:245, 1984
38. Urba WJ, Duffey PL, Longo DL: Treatment of patients with aggressive lymphomas: an overview. JNCI Monogr 10:29, 1990
39. Addis B, Isaacson P: Large cell lymphoma of the mediastinum: a B-cell tumor of probable thymic origin. Histopathology 10:379, 1986
40. Perrone T, Frizzera G, Rosai J: Mediastinal diffuse large-cell lymphoma with sclerosis: a clinicopathologic study of 60 cases. Am J Surg Pathol 10:176, 1986
41. Moller P, Lammler B, Erberlein-Gonska M: Primary mediastinal clear cell lymphoma of B-cell type. Virchows Arch 409:79, 1986
42. Yousem S, Weiss L, Warnke R: Primary mediastinal non-Hodgkin's lymphomas: a morphologic and immunologic study of 19 cases. Am J Clin Pathol 83:676, 1985
43. Moller P, Moldenhauer G, Momburg F et al: Mediastinal lymphoma of clear cell type is a tumor corresponding to terminal steps of B cell differentiation. Blood 69:1087, 1987
44. Davis RE, Dorfman RF, Warnke RA: Primary large cell lymphoma of the thymus: a diffuse B-cell neoplasm presenting as priamry mediastinal lymphoma. Hum Pathol 21:1262, 1990
45. Lamarre L, Jacobson J, Aisenberg A, Harris N: Primary large cell lymphoma of the mediastinum. Am J Surg Pathol 13:730, 1989
46. Trump DL, Mann RB: Diffuse large cell and undifferentiated lymphomas with prominent mediastinal involvement. A poor prognostic subset of patients with non-Hodgkin's lymphoma. Cancer 50:277, 1982
47. Jacobson J, Aisenberg A, Lamarre L et al: Mediastinal large cell lymphoma: an uncommon subset of adult lymphoma curable with combined modality therapy. Cancer 62:1893, 1988
48. Ferry JA, Harris NL, Picker LJ et al: Intravascular lymphomatosis (malignant angioendotheliomatosis). A B-cell neoplasm expressing surface homing receptors. Mod Pathol 1:444, 1988
49. Sheibani K, Battifora H, Winberg CD et al: Further evidence that ''malignant angioendotheliomatosis'' is an angiotropic large cell lymphoma. N Engl J Med 314:943, 1986
50. Stroup RM, Sheibani K, Moncada A et al: Angiotropic (intravascular) large cell lymphoma. A clinicopathologic study of seven cases with unique clinical presentations. Cancer 66:1781, 1990
51. Jalkanen S, Aho R, Kallajoki M et al: Lymphocyte homing receptors and adhesion molecules in intravascular malignant lymphomatosis. Int J Cancer 44:777, 1989
52. Osborne BM, Butler JJ, MacKay B: Sinusoidal large cell (histiocytic) lymphoma. Cancer 46: 2484, 1980
53. Kwak L, Wilson M, Weiss L et al: Clinical significance of morphologic subdivision in diffuse large cell lymphoma. Cancer 68:1988, 1991
54. Carbone PP, Kaplan HS, Musshoff K et al: Report of the committee on Hodgkin's disease staging classification. Cancer Res 31:1860, 1971
55. Rosenberg SA: Validity of the Ann Arbor Staging Classification for the non-Hodgkin's lymphomas. Cancer Treat Rep 61:1023, 1977
56. Velasquez WS, Jagannath S, Tucker SL et al: Risk classification as the basis for clinical staging of diffuse large-cell lymphoma derived from 10-year survival data. Blood 74:551, 1989
57. Shipp MA, Yeap BY, Harrington DP et al: The m-BACOD combination chemotherapy regimen in large-cell lymphoma: analysis of the completed trial and comparison with the M-BACOD regimen. J Clin Oncol 8:84, 1990
58. Hoskins PJ, Ng V, Spinelli JJ et al: Prognostic variables in patients with diffuse large-cell lym-

phoma treated with MACOP-B. J Clin Oncol 9: 220, 1991

59. Dixon DO, Neilan B, Jones SE et al: Effect of age on therapeutic outcome in advanced diffuse histiocytic lymphoma: the Southwest Oncology Group experience. J Clin Oncol 4:295, 1986
60. Coiffier B, Gisselbrecht C, Vose JM et al: Prognostic factors in aggressive malignant lymphomas: description and validation of a prognostic index that could identify patients requiring a more intensive therapy. J Clin Oncol 9:211, 1991
61. The International Non-Hodgkin's Lymphoma Prognostic Factors Project. A predictive model for aggressive non-Hodgkin's lymphoma. N Engl J Med 329:987, 1993
62. Grogan TM: Immunobiologic correlates of prognosis in lymphoma. Semin Oncol 5:58, 1993
63. Bauer KD, Merkel DE, Winter JN et al: Prognostic implication of ploidy and proliferative activity in diffuse large cell lymphomas. Cancer Res 46:3173, 1986
64. Braylan RC, Benson NA, Nourse VA: Cellular DNA of human neoplastic B-cells measured by flow cytometry. Cancer Res 44:5010, 1984
65. Bino GD, Silvestrini R, Costa A et al: Morphological and clinical significance of cell kinetics in non-Hodgkin's lymphomas. Eur J Basic Appl Histochem 30:197, 1986
66. Weiss L, Strickler J, Medeiros L et al: Proliferative rates of non-Hodgkin's lymphomas as assessed by Ki-67 antibody. Hum Pathol 18:1155, 1987
67. Gerdes J: Ki-67 and other proliferation markers useful for immunohistological diagnostic and prognostic evaluations in human malignancies. Semin Cancer Biol 1:199, 1990
68. Gerdes J, Lemke H, Baisch H et al: Cell cycle analysis of a cell-proliferation-associated human nuclear antigen defined by the monoclonal antibody Ki67. J Immunol 133:1710, 1984
69. Miller T, Grogan T, Dahlberg S et al: Prognostic significance of the Ki67 associated proliferation antigen in aggressive non-Hodkgin's lymphomas: a prospective Southwest Oncology Group Trial. Blood 83:1460, 1994
70. Cattoretti G, Becker MHG, Key G et al: Monoclonal antibodies against recombinant parts of the Ki-67 antigen (MIB1 and MIB3) detect proliferating cells in microwave-processed formalin-fixed paraffin sections. J Pathol 168:357, 1992
71. Lippman SM, Spier CM, Miller TP et al: Tumor-infiltrating T-lymphocytes in B-cell diffuse large cell lymphoma related to disease course. Mod Pathol 3:361, 1990
72. Miller TP, Lippman SM, Spier CM et al: HLA-DR (Ia) immune phenotype predicts outcome for patients wtih diffuse large cell lymphomas. J Clin Immunol 72:370, 1988
73. Mornburg F, Herrmann B, Moldenhauser G et al: B-cell lymphomas of high grade malginancy frequently lack HLA-DR, -DP and -DQ antigens and associated invariant chain. Int J Cancer 40: 598, 1987
74. Rybski JA, Spier CM, Miller TP et al: Prediction of outcome in diffuse large cell lymphoma by the major histocompatibility complex class I (HLA-A, B, C) and class II (HLA-DR, DP, DQ) phenotype. Leuk Lymphoma 6:31, 1991
75. Aiello A, Delia D, Fontanella E et al: Expression of differentiation and adhesion molecules in sporadic Burkitt's lymphoma. Hematol Oncol 8:229, 1990
76. Spier CM, Grogan TM, Lippman S et al: The aberrancy of immunophenotype and immunoglobulin status as indicators of prognosis in B cell diffuse large cell lymphoma. Am J Pathol 133:118, 1988
77. Jalkanen S, Joensuu H, Soderstrom KO et al: Lymphocyte homing and clinical behavior of non-Hodgkin's lymphoma. J Clin Invest 87: 1835, 1991
78. Pals ST, Host E, Ossekoppele GJ et al: Expression of lymphocyte homing receptor as a mechanism of dissemination in non-Hodgkin's lyphoma. Blood 73:885, 1989
79. Horst E, Meijer CJ, Radaszkiewicz T et al: Adhesion molecules in the prognosis of diffuse large-cell lymphoma: expression of a lymphocyte homing receptor (CD44), LFA-1 (CD11a/ 18), and ICAM-1 (CD54). Leukemia 4:595, 1990
80. Jalkanen S, Joensuu H, Klemi P: Prognostic value of lymphocyte homing receptor and S phase fraction in non-Hodgkin's lymphoma. Blood 75:1549, 1990
81. Miller TP, Grogan TM, Dalton WS et al: P-

glycoprotein expresion in malignant lymphoma and reversal of clinical drug resistance with chemotherapy plus high-dose verapamil. J Clin Oncol 9:17, 1991

82. Dan S, Esumi M, Sawada U et al: Expression of a multidrug resistance gene in human malignant lymphoma and related disorders. Leuk Res 15: 1139, 1991
83. Pileri SA, Sabattini E, Falini B et al: Immunohistochemical detection of the multidrug transport protein P170 in human normal tissues and malignant lymphomas. Histopathology 19:131, 1991
84. Centers for Disease Control and Prevention: Revision of the case definition of acquired immunodeficiency syndrome for national reported—United States. Ann Intern Med 103: 402, 1985
85. Beral V, Peterman T, Berkelman R, Jaffe H: AIDS-associated non-Hodgkin lymphoma. Lancet 337:805, 1991
86. Gail MH, Pluda JM, Rabkin CS et al: Projections of the incidence of non-Hodgkin's lymphoma related to acquired immunodeficiency syndrome. JNCL 83:695, 1991
87. Moore RD, Kessler H, Richman DD et al: Non-Hodgkin's lymphoma in patients with advanced HIV infection treated with zidovudine. JAMA 265:2208, 1991
88. Ziegler JL, Beckstead JA, Volberding PA et al: Non-Hodgkin's lymphoma in 90 homosexual men. Relation to generalized lymphadenopathy and the acquired immunodeficiency syndrome. N Engl J Med 311:565, 1984
89. Knowles DM, Chamulak GA, Subar M et al: Lymphoid neoplasia associated with the acquired immunodeficiency syndrome(AIDS): The New York University Medical Center experience with 105 patients (1981–1986). Ann Intern Med 108:744, 1988
90. Raphael M, Gentilhomme O, Tulliez M et al: Histopathologic features of high-grade non-Hodgkin's lymphomas in acquired immunodeficiency syndrome. Arch Pathol Lab Med 115:15, 1991
91. Pederson C, Gerstoft J, Lundgren JD et al: HIV-associated lymphoma: histopathology and association with Epstein-Barr virus genome related to clinical, immunological and prognostic features. Eur J Cancer 27:1416, 1991
92. Kaplan LD, Abrams DI, Feigal E et al: AIDS-associated non-Hodgkin lymphoma in San Francisco. JAMA 261:719, 1989
93. Levine AM, Sullivan-Halley J, Pike MC et al: Human immunodeficiency virus-related lymphoma. Prognostic factors predictive of survival. Cancer 68:2466, 1991
94. Hamilton-Dutoit S, Pallesen G, Franzmann M et al: AIDS-related lymphoma. Histopathology, immunophenotype, and association with Epstein-Barr virus as demonstrated by in situ nucleic acid hybridization. Am J Pathol 138:149, 1991
95. Roithman S, Tourani JM, Andrieu JM: AIDS associated non-Hodgkin's lymphoma. Lancet 338:884, 1991
96. Chadburn A, Cesarman E, Jagirdar J et al: CD30 (Ki-1) positive anaplastic large cell lymphomas in individuals infected with the human immunodeficiency virus. Cancer 72:3078, 1993
97. Cesarman E, Chang Y, Moore PS et al: Kaposi's sarcoma-associated herpesvirus-like DNA sequences in AIDS-related body-cavity-based lymphomas. N Engl J Med 332:1186, 1995
98. Raphael MM, Audouin J, Lamine M et al: Immunophenotypic and genotypic analysis of acquired immunodeficiency syndrome-related non-Hodgkin's lymphomas. Correlation with histologic features in 36 cases. Am J Clin Pathol 101:773, 1994
99. Pelicci PG, Knowles DM, Arlin Z et al: Multiple monoclonal B cell expansions and c-*myc* oncogene rearrangements in acquired immune deficiency syndrome-related lymphoproliferative disorders: implications for lymphomagenesis. J Exp Med 164:2049, 1986
100. Herndier BG, Shiramizu BT, McGrath MS: AIDS associated non-Hodgkin's lymphomas represent a broad spectrum of monoclonal and polyclonal lymphoproliferative processes. Curr Top Microbiol Immunol 182:385, 1992
101. Subar M, Neri A, Inghirami G et al: Frequent c-*myc* oncogene activation and infrequent presence of Epstein-Barr virus genome in AIDS-associated lymphoma. Blood 72:667, 1988
102. Ballerini P, Gaidano G, Gong JZ et al: Multiple genetic lesions in AIDS-related non-Hodgkin lymphoma. Blood 81:166, 1993
103. Gaidano G, LoCoco F, Ye BH et al: Rearrangements of the *bcl*-6 gene in acquired immunode-

ficiency syndrome-associated non-Hodgkin's lymphoma: association with diffuse large-cell subtype. Blood 84:397, 1994

104. Arber DA, Shibata D, Chen Y-Y, Weiss LM: Characterization of the topography of Epstein-Barr virus infection in human immunodeficiency virus-associated lymphoid tissues. Mod Pathol 5:559, 1992
105. Birx D, Redfield RR, Tosato G: Defective regulation of Epstein-Barr virus infection in patients with acquired immunodeficiency syndrome (AIDS) or AIDS related disorders. N Engl J Med 314:874, 1986
106. Shibata D, Weiss LM, Nathwani BN et al: Epstein-Barr virus in benign lymph node biopsies from individuals infected with the human immunodeficiency virus is associated with concurrent or subsequent development of non-Hodgkin's lymphoma. Blood 77:1527, 1991
107. Shibata D, Weiss LM, Hernandez AM et al: Epstein-Barr virus-associated non-Hodgkin's lymphoma in patients infected with the human immunodeficiency virus. Blood 81:2102, 1993
108. Hamilton-Dutoit SJ, Raphael M, Audouin J et al: In situ demonstration of Epstein-Barr virus small RNAs (EBER1) in acquired immunodeficiency syndrome-related lymphomas: correlation with tumor morphology and primary site. Blood 82:619, 1993
109. Re VD, Boiocchi M, Vita SD et al: Subtypes of Epstein-Barr virus in HIV-associated and HIV-unrelated Hodgkin's disease cases. Int J Cancer 54:895, 1993
110. Levine AM: Acquired immunodeficiency syndrome-related lymphoma. Blood 80:8, 1992

8

Peripheral T-Cell Lymphomas

Catherine P. Leith, William F. Kern, and Thomas M. Grogan

Peripheral T-cell lymphoma (PTL) is an immunologically defined category of non-Hodgkin's lymphomas that was not present in older morphologic classifications like the Working Formulation, but is emphasized in immunologically based classifications like the Kiel classification and the more recent Revised European-American Lymphoma (REAL) classification.[1] The emergence of PTL as a lymphoma category despite diverse morphology and outcome reflects several facts. First, its immunologic specificity is mature, activated T-cell status with "novel" aberrant pan T expression. Second, PTL as a broad category has spawned specific entities of etiologic definition (e.g., HTLV-I associated PTL), clinical distinctiveness (e.g., gluten-enteropathy associated PTL), organ specificity (e.g., hepatosplenic PTL), phenotypic specificity (e.g., CD56+ PTL), morphologic distinctiveness (e.g., Lennert's lymphoma), and cytogenetic definition (e.g., anaplastic large cell lymphoma with the t(2; 5) translocation).[1,2] In short, there has emerged under the rubric of PTL a number of distinct clinicopathologic entities not accounted for in the Working Formulation but now tabulated in the REAL scheme.[1] This chapter focuses on the newly listed PTL entities and adds some more recent provisional PTL entities of clinical import. In the end, this chapter seeks the middle ground by discussing many, but not all, published categories of PTL. The emphasis is placed on the morphologic, clinical, and biologic properties relevant to diagnosis, clinical characterization, and differential diagnostic features.

DEFINITION OF PTL

The term *peripheral T-cell lymphoma* is a broad immunologic category encompassing morphologically diverse lymphomas that are all characterized by a mature T-cell phenotype.[3–8] PTL represents 15 percent of all diffuse aggressive non-Hodgkin's lymphomas in the United States. The term signifies a post-thymic, peripheral lymphoid tissue origin in contrast with the central, thymic origin for immature T-cell lymphoblastic lymphomas.[3,8] PTL encompasses a broad spectrum of clinicopathologic entities, as listed in (Table 8-1).[9–27] Immunologically, PTL characteristically express an array of mature pan-T antigens without immature thymic cortex T-cell antigens (Figs. 8-1 and 8-2). Most PTL manifest aberrant pan T antigen expression with idiosyncratic loss of certain pan T antigens (Fig. 8-3). This frequent loss of pan T antigens is generally not found in T-cell inflammation and serves to herald true T-cell neoplasia.[6–8]

Morphologically, PTL are all diffuse and very heterogeneous with a broad spectrum of histologic types. The majority of PTL are classified in the Working Formulation as diffuse, mixed cell, or large cell type with a minority of diffuse small cell types of either cleaved or small cell type (Table 8-1).[1,5,7,9,10] These common morphologic PTL subtypes are illustrated in Figs. 8-4 through 8-6. Rare morphologic variants include, among others, Burkitt's-like PTL and signet cell PTL, which are illustrated because of their morphologic distinctiveness and their prospect for mistaken diagnosis (Figs. 8-7 and 8-8).[28–30] Histologically, PTL are characterized by

Table 8-1. Peripheral T-Cell Lymphoma Variants

Designation	Reference Nos.
Working Formulation category: all diffuse	1
Small cell (~15%)	
Mixed (~40%)	
Large cell (~45%)	1, 9, 10
Others (Burkitt's, signet cell; rare)	28–30
Additional morphologic categories	
Clear cell immunoblastic sarcoma (Lukes and Collins)	11
T-zone lymphoma (Lennert's)	12
Medium sized cell lymphomas (Japanese)	13
Plasmacytoid PTL	14
Anaplastic large cell	1, 86
Lymphokine-related categories	
Abundant epithelioid histiocytes (Lennert's lymphoma)	15 (16)
PTL with plasmacytosis and gammopathy	16
PTL with aberrant myelocytopoiesis and eosinophilia	17
Erythrophagocytic PTL simulating malignant histiocytosis	18, 19
PTL with hypercalcemia	20
Organ-associated categories	
CNS: CD56+ PTL	
Cutaneous: mycosis fungoides	
Subcutaneous: panniculitic PTL	
Gut: gluten sensitive, enteropathy associated	
Splenic: PTL simulating hairy cell leukemia	21
Blood: T-CLL, T-prolymphohistiocytic and large granular cell leukemia, Sezary syndrome	
Hepatosplenic: γ/δ T-cell lymphoma	
Vessel-associated categories	
Angioimmunoblastic lymphadenopathy-like (AILD-like)	22
Angiocentric, angiodestructive immunoproliferative lymphoma	23
Lymphomatoid granulomatosis (pulmonary)	
Midline malignant reticulosis (nasal)	24
Virus associated	
Adult T-cell lymphoma/leukemia of Japan and Carribbean (HTLV-I associated)	25–27
T-cell hairy cell leukemia (HTLV-II associated)	
HIV-associated PTL (HTLV-III associated)	
EBV associated	
Cytogenetic specific	
Anaplastic large cell [t(2;5)]	
Phenotype related	
NCAM positive PTL	
Ki-1 large cell lymphoma	
S100+ T-cell lymphoproliferative disease	

two words: pleomorphism and polymorphism. The pleomorphism may take the form of large polylobated Reed-Sternberg-like cells, which commonly obscures the diagnostic distinction of PTL from Hodgkin's disease. The polymorphism representing admixed eosinophils, plasma cells, fibroblasts, histiocytes, myelocytes, and vascular elements is largely due to the functional cytokines produced by PTL cells.[31] Commonly, in PTL these admixed reactive elements outnumber neoplastic elements, leading to great diagnostic difficulty. To the microscopist it presents a counterintuitive circumstance wherein a rare component (5 percent or less) of the pleomorphic cells heralds neoplasia, and the visually dominant inflammatory component (95 percent) is prominent but only secondary in pathogenesis. The extreme morphologic variability has led to a great variety of names and eponymic designations given to PTL. This diversity is reflected

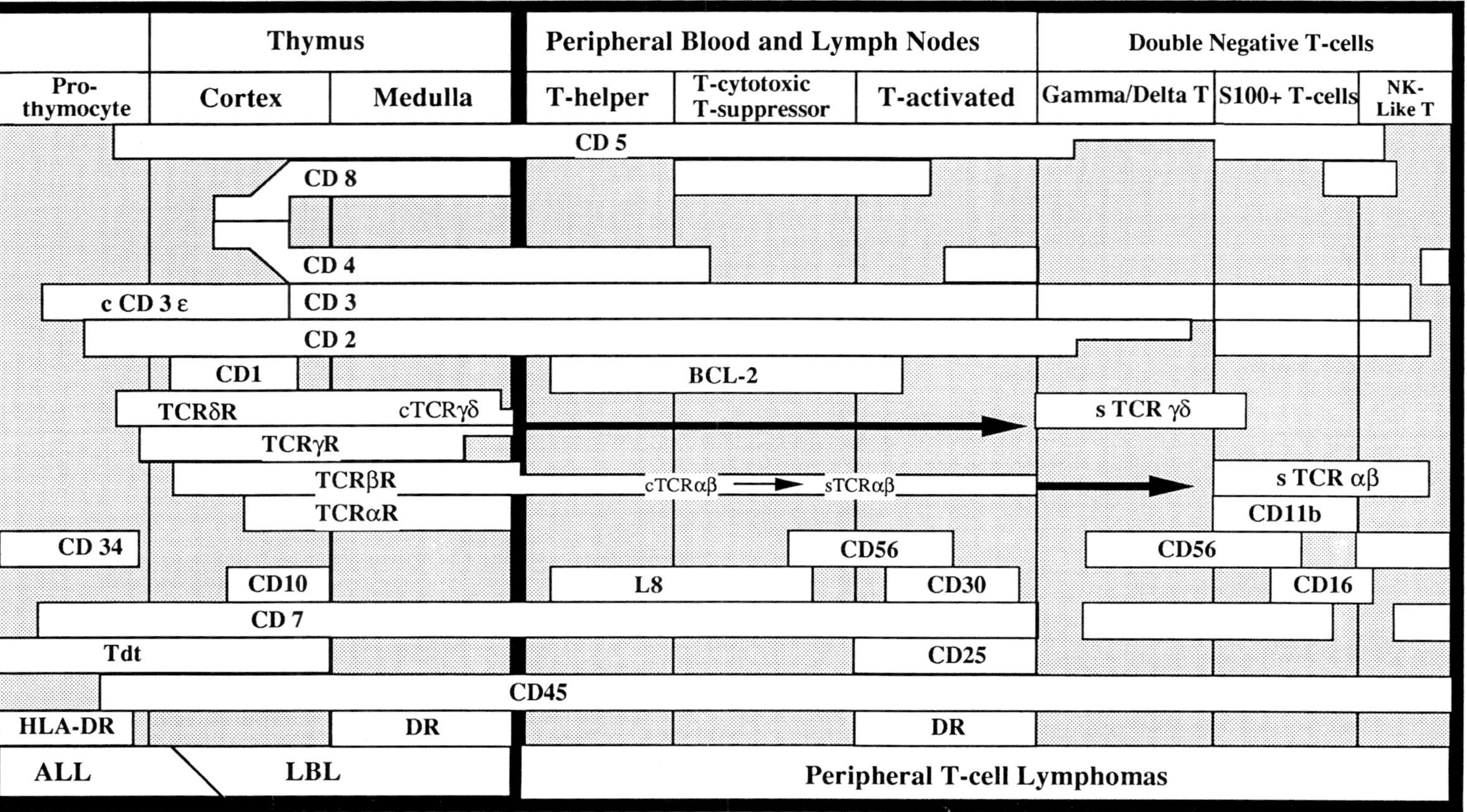

Fig. 8-1. T-cell neoplasia related to T-cell development.

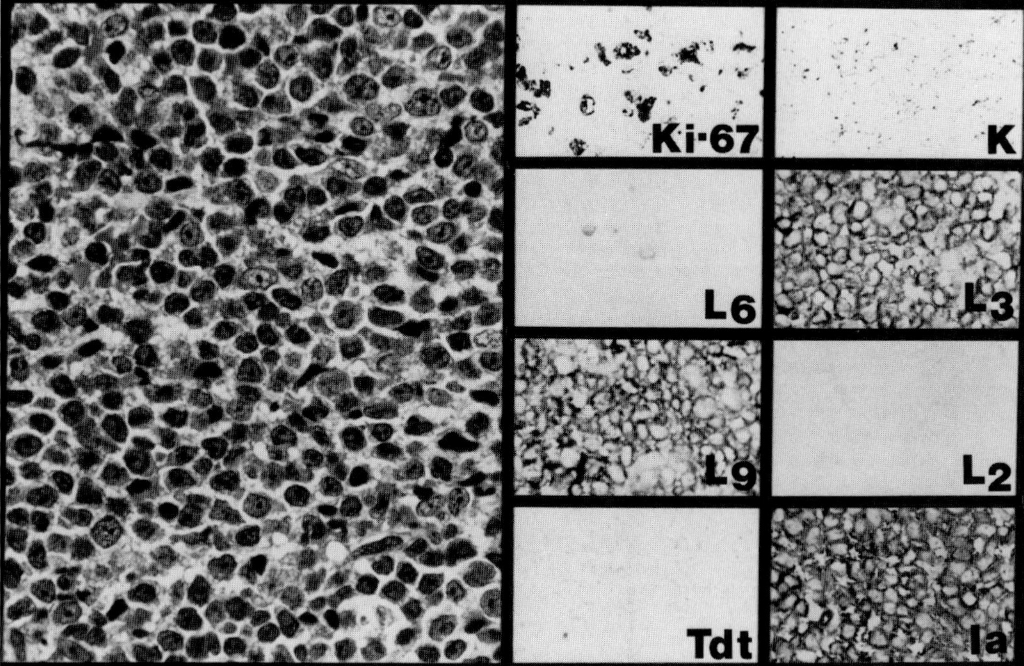

Fig. 8-2. Small lymphocytic PTL of mature T-helper phenotype with mature T-cell antigens and absent immature antigens. Tdt, terminal deoxynucleotidyl transferase.

in the length of Table 8-1, which supports the observation of Suchi et al.[32] that there are as many PTL categories as cases.

Clinically, most PTL patients are older (50 to 70 years of age, rarely under 20) with frequent generalized lymphadenopathy, a high frequency of extranodal stage IV disease, B symptoms, and a poor prognosis (median survival 9 to 22 months).[1,2,4,5] There is frequent involvement of the liver, lungs, marrow, blood (with mixed leukemia/lymphoma appearance), and skin. Cutaneous PTL involves the dermis and does not usually entail clustered epidermal invasion, in contrast with mycosis fungoides. Preceding autoimmune dysfunction (e.g., Sjögren syndrome) occurs in approximately 15 percent of PTL.[1,2,4,5]

Poor prognosis reflects that most PTL are intermediate to high grade neoplasms.[1] Among some single institution retrospective studies, PTL do not differ from B-cell non-Hodgkin's lymphoma of comparable histologic type.[1] Others have found more frequent relapse and shortened survival in PTL, signifying more aggressive disease requiring new therapeutic approaches.[33] A recent multi-institutional prospective trial in Europe by Group d'Etudes des Lymphoms Aggressives found that peripheral T-cell phenotype was associated with poor prognosis and that T-cell phenotype is independent of other adverse clinical prognostic factors.[34]

IMMUNOPHENOTYPIC FEATURES OF PTL

By definition, PTL are neoplasms of mature T cells that derive from peripheral lymphoid sites outside the thymus in contrast with the central thymic origin for immature T-cell lymphoblastic lymphomas.[1–4] As neoplastic cells derived from post-thymic T cells, these cells then expectedly express pan T cell antigens (e.g., CD2, 5, 7), lack immature antigens (e.g., CD1, 10, 34), and lack B-cell antigens, as shown in Figs. 8-1 and 8-2.

Physiologically, several distinct functional

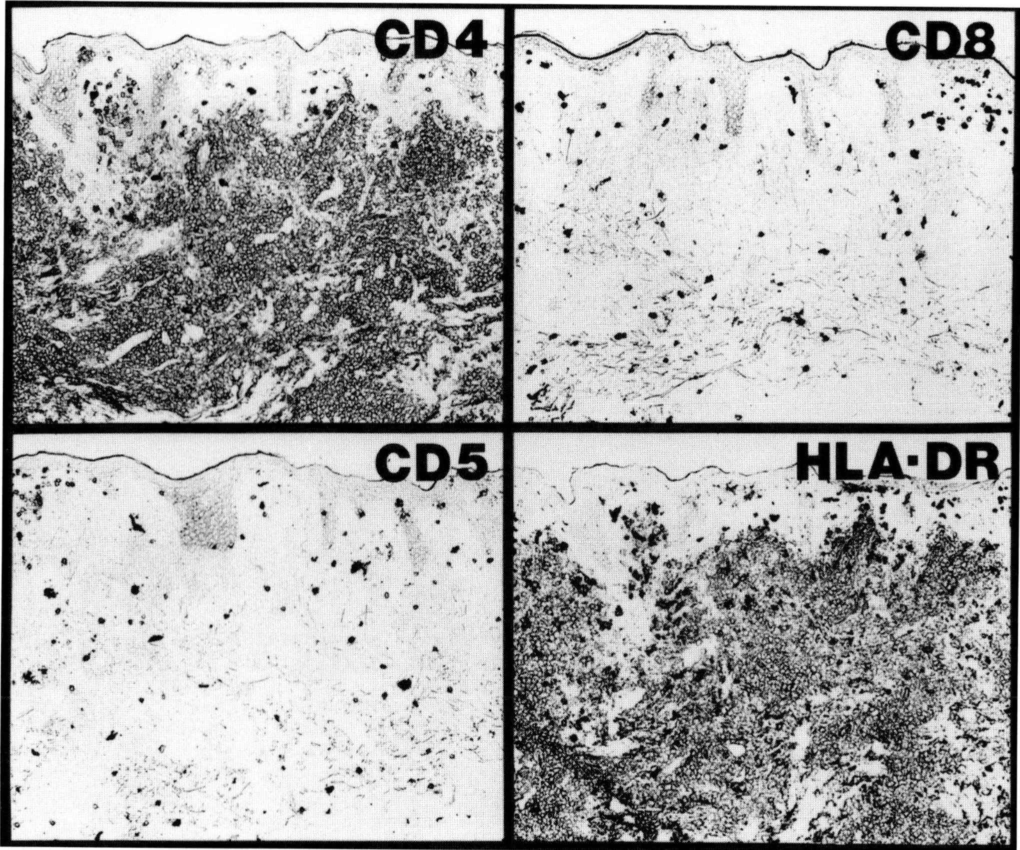

Fig. 8-3. Cutaneous PTL of T-helper phenotype (CD4+, CD8−) and aberrant loss of CD5 (see Fig. 8-1).

and genotypic subsets of mature T cells exist, and their neoplastic counterparts largely reflect the subset-restricted phenotype of the cell of origin, as shown in Fig. 8-1. Two major genotypic and phenotypic subpopulations of T cells have been described based on T-cell receptor (TCR) gene rearrangements and expressions. These include the "first" TCR receptor related to γ and δ gene rearrangements (TCR1) and the classical TCR receptor expression related to α and β genes (TCR2).[35] The TCR1 designation reflects the belief that progenitor thymocytes first undergo γ and δ gene rearrangement (as shown in Fig. 8-1), and, if no functional γ/δ receptor is produced, a further attempt is then made with α and β genes. The majority (more than 95 percent) of both thymocytes and circulating T cells express TCR α/β or TCR2, while a minority (less than 5 percent) express TCR1. TCR1 cells are frequently found in epithelium, including the skin and intestinal epithelium.[4] The majority of TCR2 cells function as either T-helper or T-cytotoxic/suppressor cells (CD4+8− or CD4−8+), while most TCR1+ cells are "double negatives" (CD4−8−), belonging to neither functional subgroup.[35] The TCR is critical for T-cell reactivity with nonself (foreign antigens). This reactivity with nonself antigen entails reactivity of the TCR two chain heterodimer (α and β TCR chains) with the major histocompatibility complex (MHC), as detailed below. Aside from nonself, T cells may also interact with self (e.g., B cells) mediated through a variety of molecules, including cell adhesion molecules, integrins (e.g., LFA-1), and their ligands.[2]

Functionally different subpopulations of T

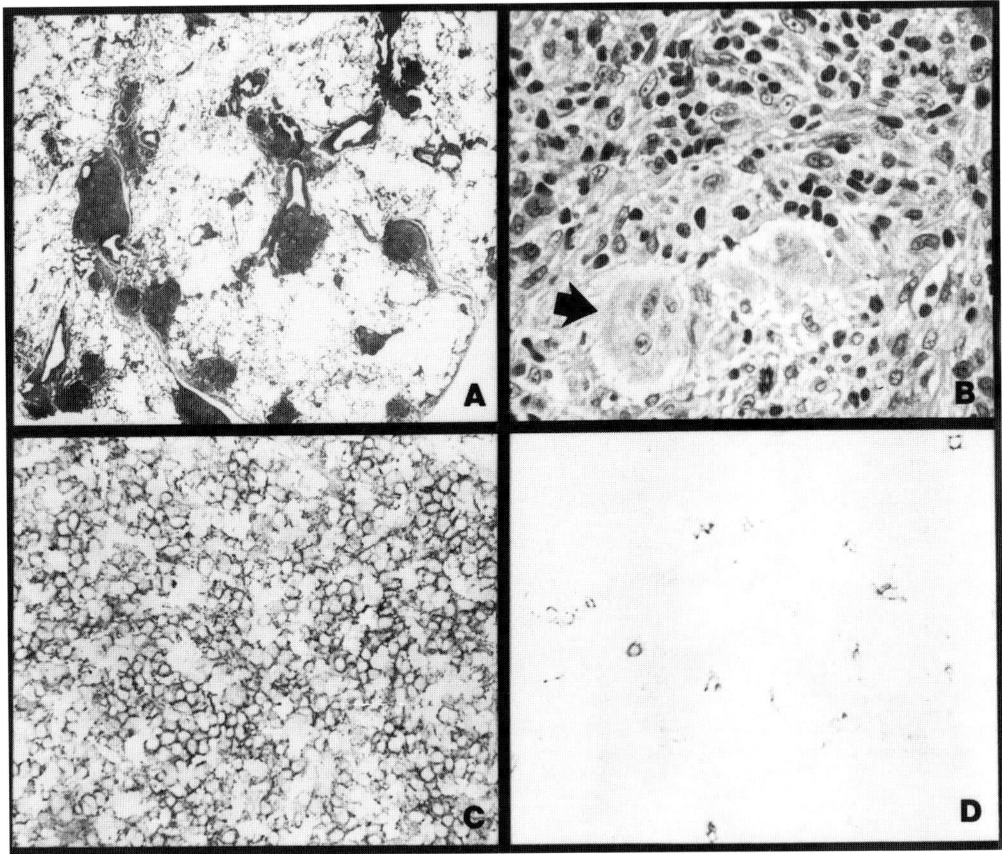

Fig. 8-4. **(A–D)** Pulmonary PTL of mixed cell type with admixed histiocytes forming granulomas (Lennert's lymphoma) with clonal expression of CD4, T-helper antigen **(C)** and absent CD8 **(D)**.

lymphocytes can be recognized by expression of either the CD4 or CD8 molecules, which occur respectively on helper/inducer T cells and cytotoxic/suppressor T cells.[2] CD8+ T cells via TCR2 recognize foreign antigen in association with MHC class I molecules and then function to eliminate foreign antigens and cells by direct cell contact (cell-mediated immunity). CD4+ T cells, also via TCR2, recognize foreign antigens associated with self MHC class II and thereby stimulate a B-cell humoral response.[2] Neoplasms derived from these functional subsets may sometimes dramatically retain these normal functional capacities as in the PTL with striking associated plasmacytosis due to functional T-helper activity.[16]

In the lymphoid tissues around the body, T cells generally outnumber B cells by 3:1 or 4:1 in an admixed polyclonal configuration.[2,36] Within specific lymphoid organs, T cells are found physiologically in the paracortex of lymph nodes, in the periarteriolar lymphoid sheath (PALS) of splenic white pulp, in the marrow paratrabeculum, and in the peripheral blood as the dominant lymphoid element (85 percent T cells).[36] Interestingly, while T-cells are predominant physiologically, T-cell lymphomas are a relative rarity compared with the far more common B-cell lymphomas. B-cell lymphomas predominate over PTL by a factor of 8 or 9 to 1.[4]

In the pathologic circumstance of T-cell neoplasia, the usual proportions of T-cell subsets are commonly altered, and the microanatomic context is also aberrant (Fig. 8-3 and 8-4). In

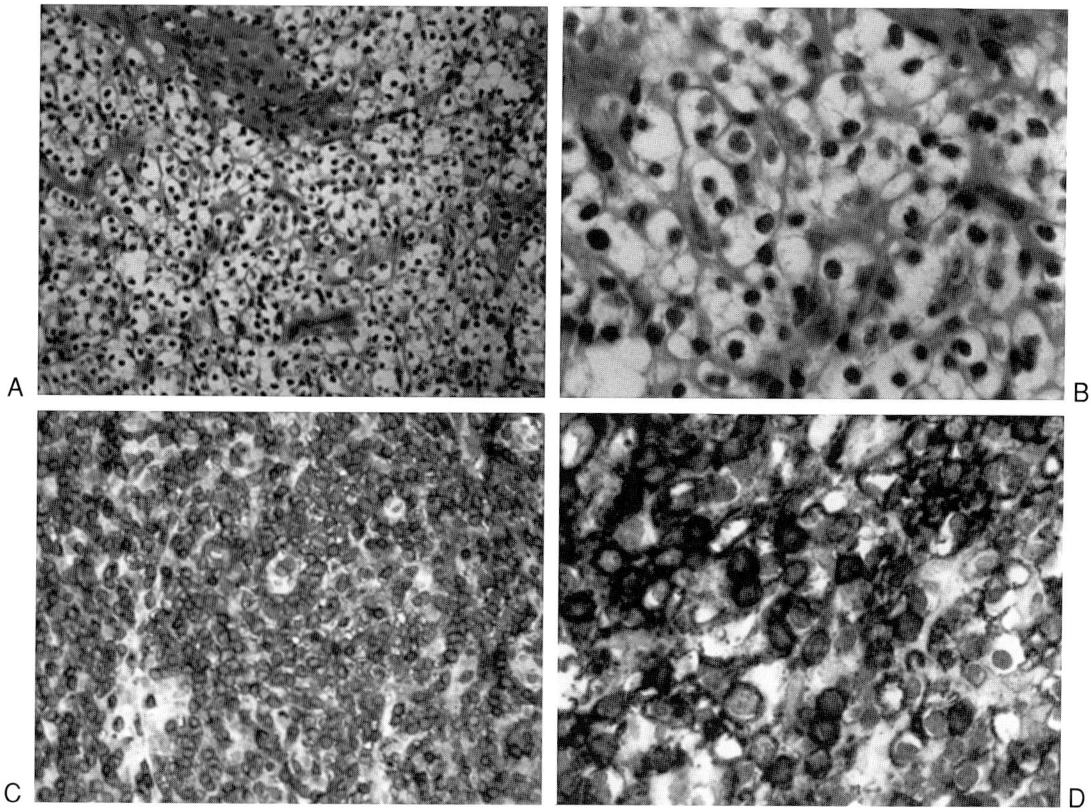

A B C D

Fig. 8-5. **(A–D)** Large cell PTL of clear cell type with coexpression of CD3 **(C)** and CD43 **(D)**.

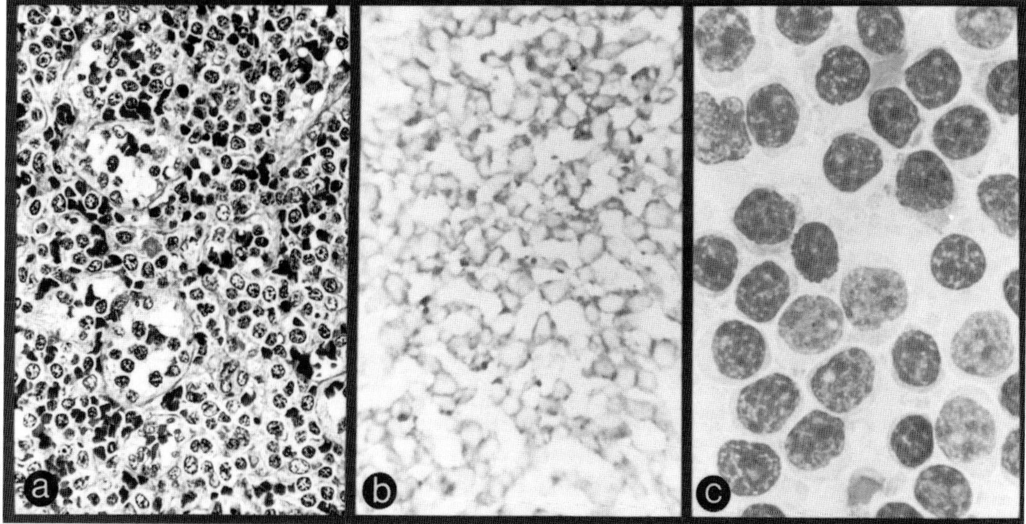

Fig. 8-6. **(A–C)** Small cell lymphocytic PTL simulating hairy cell leukemia in the spleen **(A)** with expression of CD3 **(B)** and cytologic mimicry of chronic lymphocytic leukemia cells.

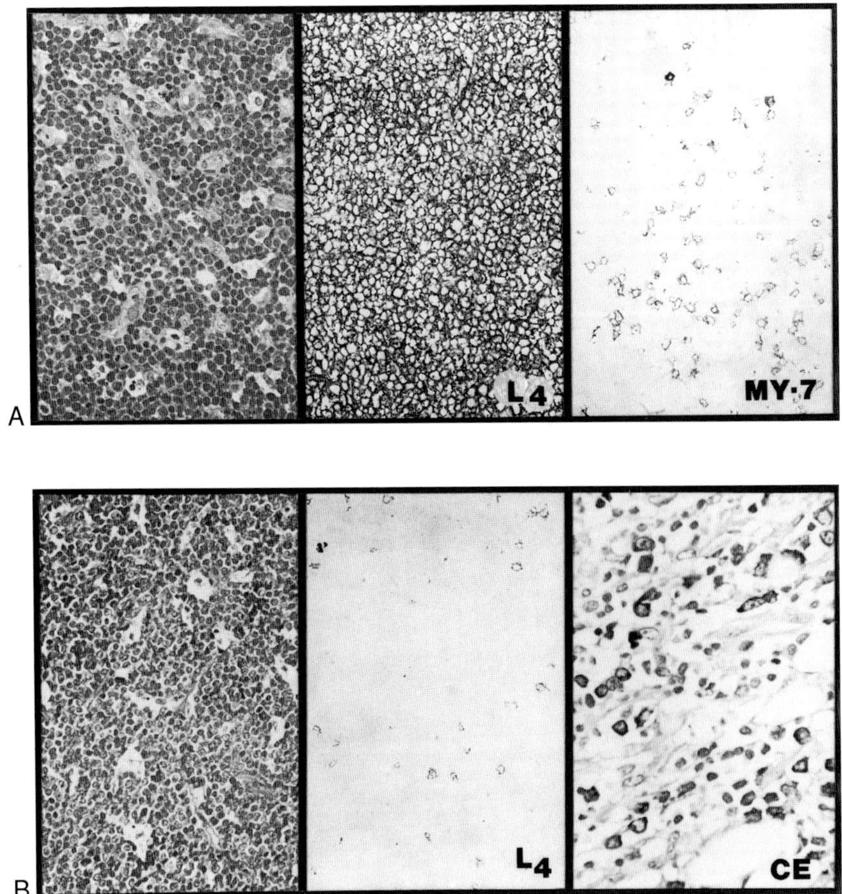

Fig. 8-7. **(A)** Burkitt's-like PTL with aberrant myelocytopoiesis with a predominance of L4, CD3+ T cells and admixed myelocytes (MY-7 CD33+ cells). This profile is contrasted with **(B)** a true granulocytic sarcoma with similar blastic morphology and with absent L4, CD3 and myeloid enzyme expression. CE, chloroacetate esterase.

particular, there may be expansion of the nodal paracortex, an expanded splenic PALS region, or increased marrow paratrabecular infiltration. The subset antigens may also be expressed in a mutually exclusive fashion (CD4+8− or CD4−8+), signifying a monoclonal T-helper/inducer or T-cytotoxic/suppressor cell malignancy, as shown in Figs. 8-3 and 8-4.[2] Most PTL (75 percent) are of T-helper subtype.[6–8] Since occasional non-neoplastic T-cell inflammatory proliferations may show very aberrant T-helper/suppressor ratios (e.g., 20:1 and vice versa),[37] the CD4/8 antigens are not reliable clonal markers as an isolated finding. In this circumstance, the judgement of T-cell monoclonality is greatly aided by immunoblot assessment of T antigen receptor genes to establish clonal rearrangements. However, even molecular assay of clonality may prove problematic unless both α/β and γ/δ assays are performed. Furthermore, phenotypically proven mature T-cell lymphomas without TCR rearrangements have been described.[38]

A more useful phenotypic finding of diagnostic import in PTL is the aberrant ''idiosyncratic'' loss of pan T antigens (CD2, 3, 5, 7) as illus-

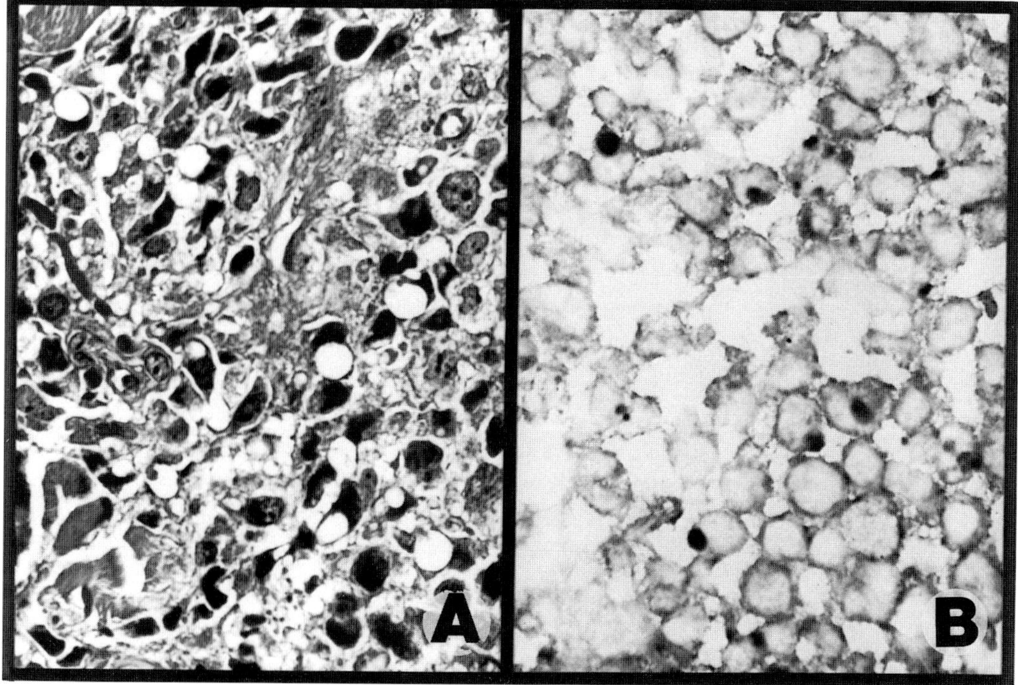

Fig. 8-8. **(A)** Cutaneous signet cell PTL with **(B)** expression of CD3. The signet cell formation led to an initial mistaken diagnosis of metastatic carcinoma. Marker studies showing sequestered pan T antigens established the correct tumor lineage.

trated in Figure 8-3.[7,8,39] In the majority of PTL (80 percent) there is loss of one or more pan T antigens. This phenotypic loss, which is inconsistent with the expected physiologic phenotype as shown in Fig. 8-3, is highly associated with clonal rearrangement of the T-cell antigen receptor genes in PTL and is decidedly not usual in benign inflammatory T-cell proliferations.[7,8,39] These abnormal PTL phenotypes have no corresponding counterpart in normal T ontogeny. This suggests that, unlike B-cell neoplasms, PTL are not as likely to slavishly recapitulate normal lymphoid development. This novel or idiosyncratic phenotype of PTL helps define PTL as a distinct aberrant immunologic entity, and the failure of PTL to mimic normalcy fully can serve a diagnostic purpose.[7,8,40] The use of pan T antigen loss to establish neoplasia has some caveats, notably that occasionally a pan T antigen (e.g., CD7 in cutaneous infiltrates) may be absent in inflammatory conditions.[4] Thus, the loss of more than one pan T (and in particular one in addition to CD7) is more reliable.

Besides loss of pan T antigens, another lineage-related phenomenon of PTL serves as a diagnostic aid: unusual cross-lineage coexpression. In particular, CD20 pan B antigen may be expressed rarely in some PTL.[41] In this instance the CD20+3+ PTL has a normal counterpart in the form of a rare (less than 1 percent) population of normal circulating T cells. However, in the neoplastic process the emergence of this rare clone to predominance is decidedly pathologic, and the unexpected cross-lineage pattern of markers is the key phenotypic clue.[41] The S100+ PTL is another example, as described below.

Besides the common T-helper PTL and less frequent T-cytotoxic PTL, other variants of PTL exist. These include rare cases of aberrant double expression of CD4 and CD8.[1,2,4] This CD4+8+ PTL mimics the thymic cortex phenotype except that terminal deoxynucleotidyl transferase is absent, and it is in fact a mature aberrant PTL phenotype. There are also PTL with absence of both CD4 and 8, known as "double negative" PTL.[1,2,4] These include PTL with γ/δ rearrangements without CD4 and CD8, as shown in Fig. 8-1, and S100+ PTL with some natural killer cell (NK)-like antigen coexpressions.[1] Finally, there are double negative PTL without S100 and with NK antigens (e.g., CD56), which represent NK-like PTL variants.[1]

Lastly, many PTL are mature T-cell neoplasms derived from activated T cells and therefore have abundant expression of activation antigens (e.g., HLA-DR), IL-2 receptors (CD25), T-cell activation antigen (TAC), and CD30 Ki-1 antigen, a nerve growth factor receptor.[1]

The polymorphous cellular composition of many PTL has led to several dilemmas, including difficulty in distinguishing the phenotype of reactive elements (tumor-infiltrating T-lymphocytes [T-TIE]) from neoplastic cells and difficulty in distinction from Hodgkin's disease. In some PTL the reactive T- and B-cell and histiocytic elements may greatly outnumber the neoplastic cells. Tissue section typing then produces a "hodge-podge" effect of both neoplastic and reactive cells. Several maneuvers may aid correct interpretation: (1) double labeling (pan T and Ki-67 nuclear proliferation antigen) may reveal that the large polylobated proliferating cells are of T-cell lineage and (2) phenotyping with paraffin sections (even though limited to fewer CD markers) may give clearer histology, allowing clearer interpretation. This contrasts with the often used snap frozen tissue section phenotyp-

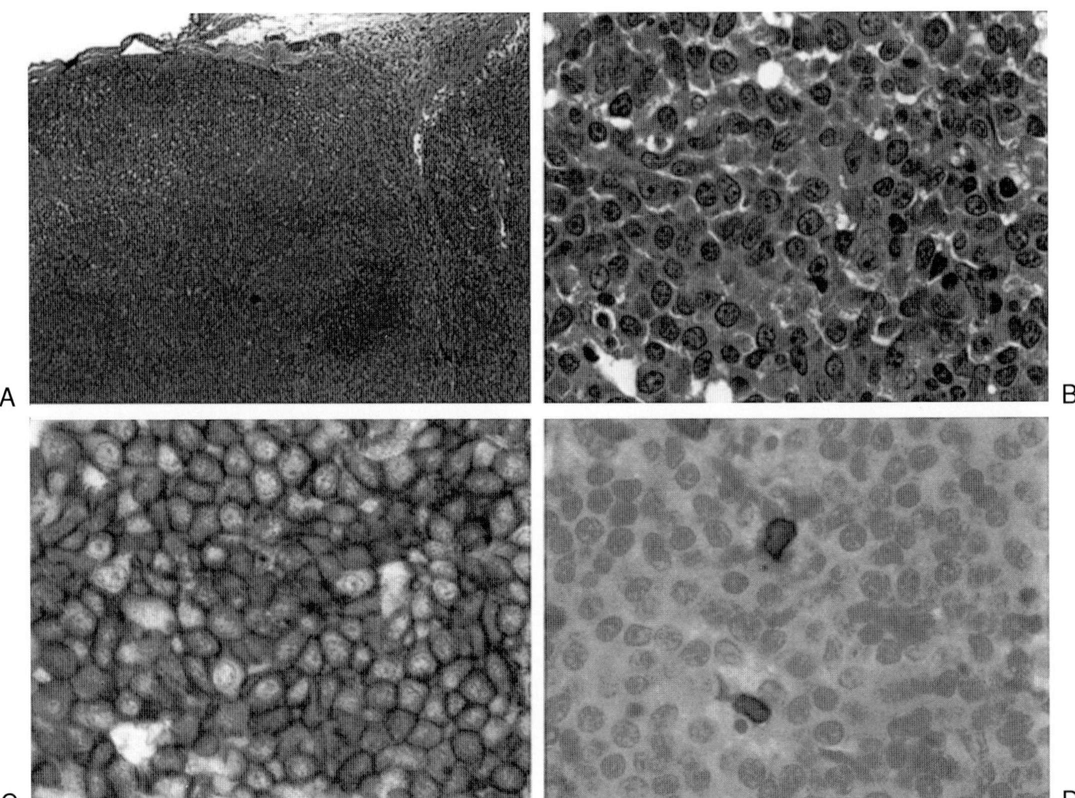

Fig. 8-9. (A–D) Extramedullary acute myelomonocytic leukemia mistakenly called PTL. This myeloid leukemia showed paracortical effacement **(A)** and CD43 expression **(C),** but absent CD3 **(D)** failed to confirm T-cell lineage. A subsequent marrow established an acute myeloid leukemia.

ing, which favors use of multiple pan T antibodies and thus provides greater assurance of delineation of pan T antigen loss particularly given the above caveat that delineation of more than one pan T antigen loss is a more reliable indicator of PTL neoplasia.

Regarding delineation from Hodgkin's disease, this differential may be difficult given the sometimes substantial morphologic similarity between large polylobated PTL Hodgkin's-like cells and true Reed-Sternberg cells. Nonetheless, phenotypic distinction is usually straightforward, as Hodgkin's disease typically (85 percent) expresses CD15 and 30 and lacks CD45 and pan T antigens. In contrast, PTL typically express pan T antigens and CD45, may express CD30, and only rarely express CD15. The *absence* of CD45 and pan T antigens on Reed-Sternberg cells frequently is the key determinant, since CD15 and CD30 coexpression is possible in both.

Diagnosis can be further confounded by the nonspecificity of certain markers (e.g., CD43, UCHL1, CD4). For example, CD43 utilized in isolation can mistakenly suggest a diagnosis of T-cell lymphoma, as illustrated in Fig. 8-9. In this instance, a confirmatory CD3 proved negative and a myeloperoxidase was positive, indicating that the paracortical lymph node infiltrate was due to an acute myelomonocytic leukemia and not PTL. Similarly, UCHL1 and CD30 may cross-react with plasmacytoma cells, and CD4 may be expressed on histiocytes in reactive histiocytic or Langerhans cell proliferations. It is also noteworthy that all of the so-called pan T antigens with the exception of TCR determinants and CD3 may be found on myeloid cells and their neoplasms.

USE OF GENOTYPING IN THE DIAGNOSIS OF T-CELL LYMPHOMA.

A vast variety of antigens are recognized by a population of mature T cells because of the diversity of antigen binding TCR, which are expressed through the mechanism of rearrangement of the TCR genes. The resultant rearranged TCR gene is unique to the individual T cell and its progeny and encodes a TCR protein with unique antigen recognition sequences.[42] Benign T-cell proliferations contain expansions of numerous T-cell clones, each with a uniquely rearranged TCR. In contrast, neoplasms of mature T cells are all derived from a single T cell and thus will show an identical rearrangement of the TCR.[42–44]

Analysis of TCR gene rearrangement either by Southern blotting or the polymerase chain reaction (PCR) is thus a useful method to assess clonality in T-cell populations. In Southern blotting, rearrangements of the TCR are detected in DNA digested with restriction enzymes using probes to portions of the TCR gene (normally α/β T, γ/δ T).[42] Clonal TCR rearrangements appear as discrete bands distinct from the germline bands of nonlymphoid tissue (Fig. 8-10).[42,43] Clonal TCR rearrangements can also be detected with PCR by using pairs of oligonucleotide

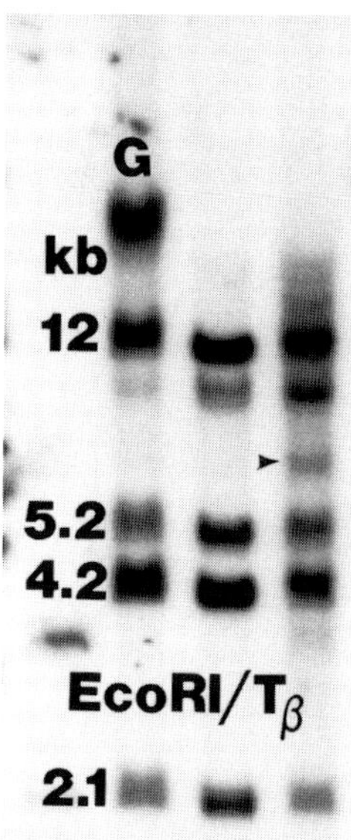

Fig. 8-10. Southern blot demonstration of TCRβ (Tβ) chain gene rearrangement (*arrowhead*) in *Eco*RI digests from a patient with peripheral T-cell lymphoma (right-hand column). G designates the germline bands seen in control placental DNA and DNA from a non-neoplastic control node (middle column). Molecular weights of germline bands in kb (kilobases).

primers complimentary to the V and J regions to amplify tissue DNA and then analyzing the PCR products, for example, by gel electrophoresis to look for PCR products of identical size.[42,45]

Both techniques may be very useful in confirming the presence of a clonal T-cell population and thus in the context of deranged nodal architecture are very helpful in confirming a suspected T-cell malignancy.[44,46] However, interpretation of the results is not always straightforward, as both technical and biologic variables may lead to unexpected results. Thus gene rearrangement studies should always be interpreted in the context of the clinical history and morphologic and immunophenotypic findings of the case.[42,47]

Detection of TCR gene rearrangement does not always equate with malignancy; as these molecular studies are applied to a greater variety of diseases, TCR gene rearrangements have been detected in lymphomatoid papulosis, PLEVA, granulomatous slack skin, and a variety of other T-cell proliferations that generally follow a benign clinical course.[42,46,47] Although T-cell lymphomas can develop in patients with these diseases, arguing that these ''benign'' lesions may be T-cell lymphoma precursors, the current evidence does not indicate that clonal gene rearrangements in these diseases predict disease evolution. Clonal TCR gene rearrangements have also been detected in T cells after Epstein-Barr virus (EBV) infection, further evidence that clonality does not equal malignancy. Thus detection of a clonal TCR rearrangement must be put

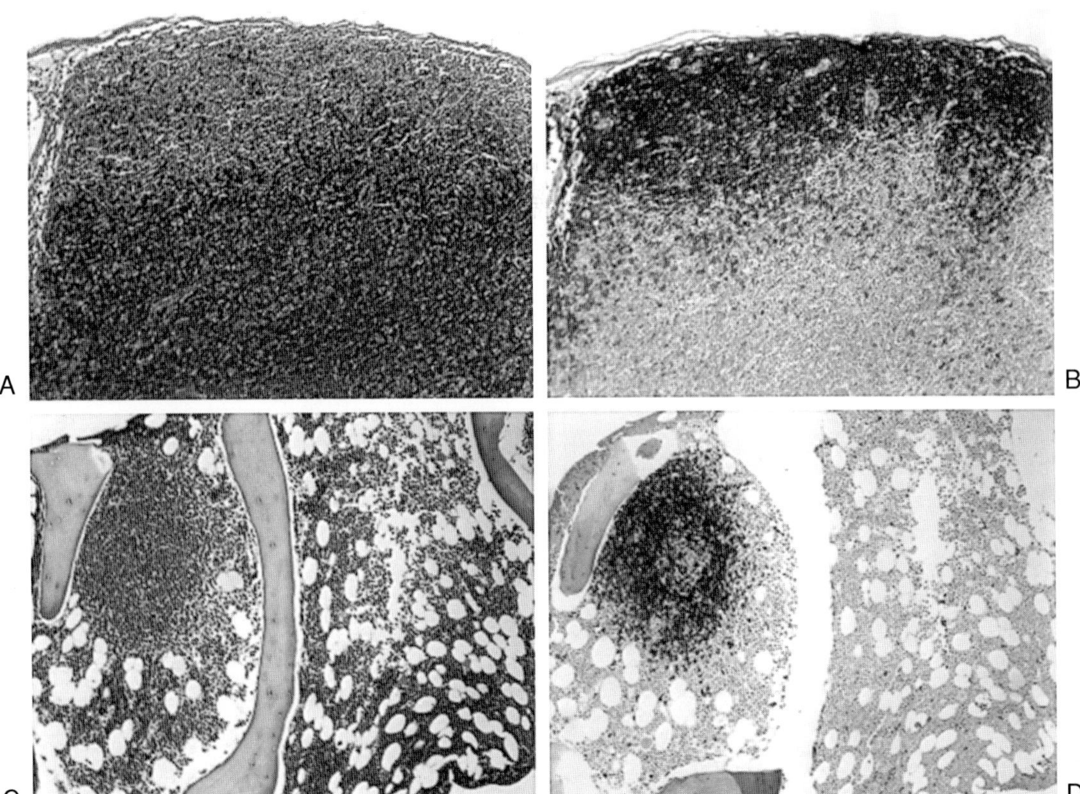

Fig. 8-11. (A–D) Diffuse mixed B-cell lymphoma mimicking a PTL. As shown in Figs. A and B, phenotyping initially mistakenly suggested a PTL due to a predominance of T cells (**A,** CD3) and a minority of B cells primarily located in the subcapsular sinus (**B,** CD20). Subsequent lymph node and bone marrow biopsies **(C & D)** showed emergence of a monoclonal B-cell lymphoma with CD20 expression **(D).**

in the context of the histologic findings before a diagnosis of malignancy is made.

Detection of a clonal TCR gene rearrangement in the context of "malignant" morphologic findings does not necessarily denote that the neoplasm is of T-cell lineage, as both B-cell and myeloid malignancies may also show TCR gene rearrangements.[42,47,48] To prevent assigning a neoplasm to the wrong lineage, genotypic studies should include analysis of both TCR and immunoglobulin gene rearrangements. Results of these assays should be correlated with morphologic and immunophenotypic data. This allows assessment of whether the band intensity of the rearranged genes is appropriate for the malignant infiltrate seen. A case in point is illustrated in Figures 8-11 and 8-12. This patient had adenopathy and B symptoms compatible with high grade lymphoma. The lymph node shown was largely effaced by a polymorphous T-cell infiltrate including immunoblasts, some irregular small cells, and histiocytes. Small foci of B cells were also present particularly in the subcapsular sinuses. Gene rearrangement studies showed a T-cell receptor and immunoglobulin gene rearrangement that appeared to involve about 10 percent of the cells. This appeared incompatible with the percentage of T cells in the lymph node by phenotype. Subsequent bone marrow biopsy and aspirate showed obvious paratrabecular aggregates of B cells that were monoclonal; in retrospect, the case was most likely a B-cell lymphoma with an exuberant associated clonal T-cell response in the node. Alternatively, the malignant B cells might have rearrangement of both immunoglobulin heavy chain and TCR genes.

Genotyping may also give false negative results: besides the technical factors detailed in Chapter 1, 10 to 15 percent of T-cell malignancies, particularly the angioimmunoproliferative disorders, lack TCR gene rearrangements, although they are morphologically and clinically malignant.[42,47,49] The precise reason for this phenomenon has not yet been clearly established. Thus the absence of a TCR rearrangement does not necessarily denote a benign disease.[49]

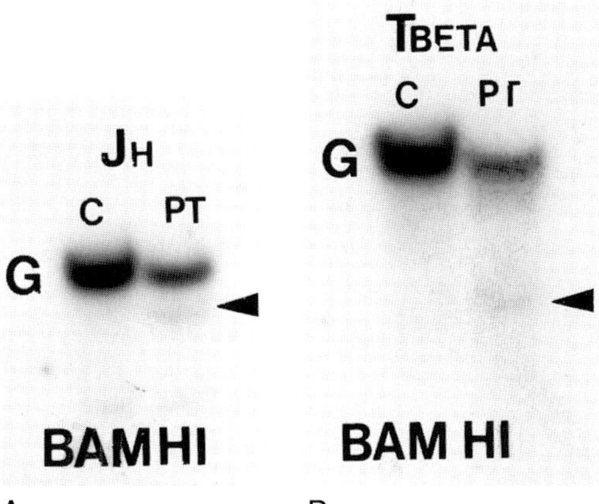

Fig. 8-12. (A–B) Southern blot demonstration of both **(A)** immunoglobulin (J_H, *BAM*HI) gene and **(B)** Tβ gene rearrangements (Tβ, *BAM*HI) gene in the initial lymph node biopsy illustrated in Figure 8-11. The faint Tβ rearrangement band appears inappropriate given the phenotypic prominance of T cells, while the faint J_H band appropriately reflects the minority malignant B-cell component.

PERIPHERAL T-CELL LYMPHOMA VARIANTS

While Table 8-1 lists a complex array of PTL entities, we have selected only a portion of these for further discussion, mainly choosing those with clear defining properties. These PTL variants have achieved diagnostic status through their distinct morphologic, immunologic, genotypic, epidemiologic, etiologic, or clinical properties. These entities belong to five basic groupings and will be discussed in order: (1) phenotype related, (2) cytokine related, (3) vessel related, (4) virus associated, and (5) organ based.

Phenotype Related

S100β-Positive T-Cell Lymphoproliferative Disease

Definition. This is a lymphoproliferative disorder derived from S100+ mature T cells, which is characterized by lymphocytosis and prominent splenomegaly. Despite the morphologic appearance of a relatively low grade disorder, the disease is rapidly progressive, with most patients dying, often from central nervous system disease, within 1 year of diagnosis.

Morphology. The major abnormalities are found in the blood and spleen; peripheral adenopathy is not generally a presenting feature of this disease, although small palpable nodes may develop with disease progression. Lymph nodes show effacement by a lymphoid infiltrate that expands the subcapsular and medullary sinuses and spills into the paracortex, compressing residual follicles.[50,51] The infiltrate is composed of small lymphocytes with irregular or indented nuclei, clumped chromatin, moderately conspicuous nucleoli, and quite abundant amphophilic cytoplasm. Some cells are plasmacytoid. The spleen is massively enlarged. There is prominent red pulp infiltration by small, irregular lymphocytes similar to those found in lymph nodes and other sites. The infiltrates found in the liver are sinusoidal (Fig. 8-13). Bone marrow involvement may be very inconspicuous[51] to diffusely replaced.[50] The blood shows a mild to marked lymphocytosis. The circulating lymphocytes have round to indented nuclei, with condensed chromatin and quite distinct nucleoli, and moderately abundant cytoplasm. Cytologically they may resemble prolymphocytes.

Phenotype. The neoplastic cells are derived from a CD2+ CD8+ CD11b+ S100+ T cell of the suppressor/cytotoxic subset present at very low levels in normal blood, thymus, and spleen.[52] When fresh cells are phenotyped, the malignant cells can show expression of pan T-

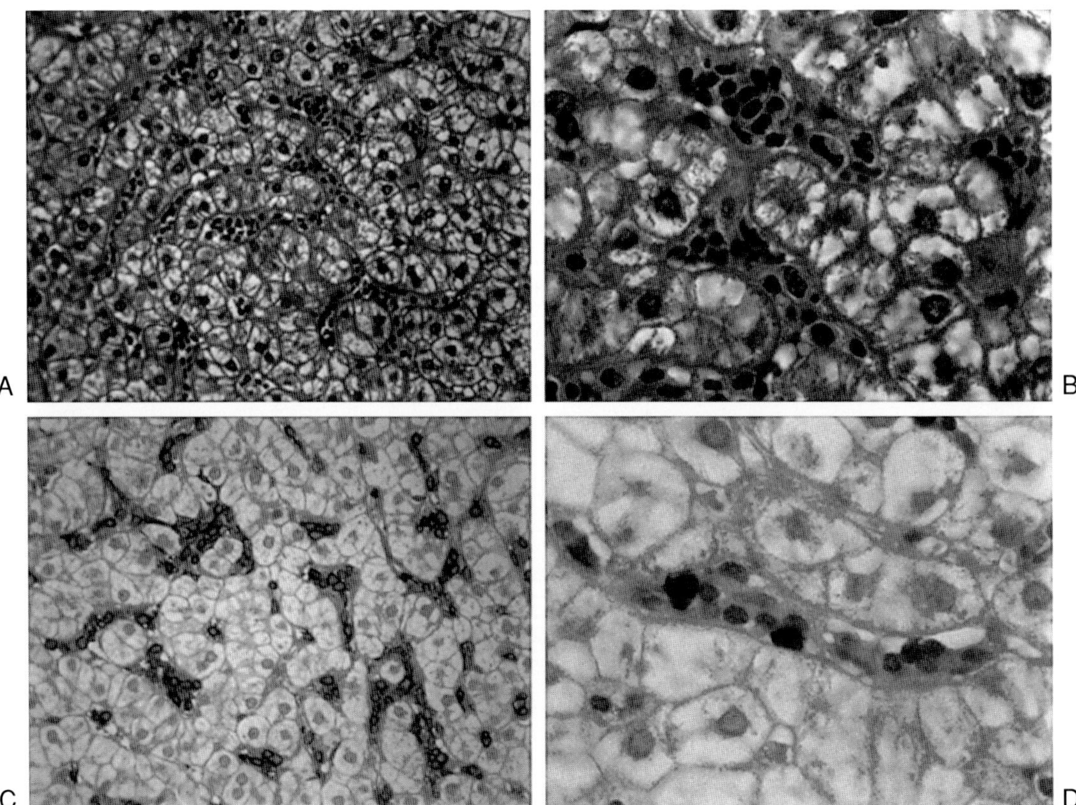

Fig. 8-13. S100-*βb*+ PTL involving the liver sinusoids (**A & B,** H&E). **(C)** CD3 expression and **(D)** S100 expression (nuclear) are present.

cell antigens including CD2, CD3, CD5, CD7.[53,54] However, like other post-thymic T-cell malignancies, aberrant loss of CD2, CD5, and CD7 has been described. Therefore, testing with multiple antibodies is recommended. In addition, expression of TCR1 may be low or absent in these cases even though TCR1 and TCR RNA is detectable by Northern analysis. Unlike their normal counterparts, these tumors usually are double negative for CD4 and CD8.[53,54] This is an unusual finding, as in normal T cells the CD3+ CD4− CD8− phenotype is usually found among T cells bearing the γ/δ TCR rather than the α/β receptor as described in these cases.[55]

These cases may also express NK-associated antigens, including CD11b, CD16, and CD56. Their NK antigen expression is incomplete, as CD57 is typically negative. Expression of CD56 may explain the propensity of these cases to involve the central nervous system (see below).

The defining immunophenotypic marker in these cases is expression of the S100 protein (Fig. 8-13). S100 expression can be readily detected in these cases on cytospin preparations of peripheral blood lymphocytes or on tissue sections of involved tissues (Fig. 8-13). S100 is a calcium binding protein formerly considered specific for the nervous system.[52] Subsequently it was recognized in a variety of tumor cells, including neurogenic tumors, melanomas, Langerhans cell histiocytosis, pleomorphic adenomas of the salivary gland, bronchioalveolar carcinoma of the lung, and cartilage tumors. In the normal peripheral blood it is specifically the β subunit of S100 that is found within a minor subset of T cells as described above.[52] These suppressor/cytotoxic T cells uniquely coexpress CD11b and are thought to function in tumor immunosurveillance, as S100+ CD11b+ T cells are decreased in association with tumor progression.[56]

Genotype. Genotyping shows clonal rearrangement of the TCRβ chain gene. Interestingly, in the two cases described by Hanson et al.[51] rearrangements were also found in the TCRγ and TCRδ chain genes (see Fig. 8-1).

Clinical Features. Importantly, while this entity appears histologically indolent, it is clinically highly aggressive, underscoring the importance of the S100 assays in recognition of this aggressive disease. Patients may present with constitutional symptoms or symptoms related to thrombocytopenia. At presentation, patients show massive splenomegaly, often with hepatomegaly.[57] Peripheral adenopathy may develop with disease progression.[53–55] The peripheral blood shows a lymphocytosis, which initially may be quite modest. There is thrombocytopenia without anemia or neutropenia. Liver function tests are abnormal. Patients frequently develop central nervous system involvement. The disease is generally characterized by rapid progression despite chemotherapy. Death is from multisystem failure frequently within 1 year.[53–55]

Differential Diagnosis. The differential diagnosis includes T-cell prolymphocytic leukemia (PLL), large granular lymphocytosis, and HTLV-I associated leukemia/lymphoma. Differentiation from T-cell PLL will rely on immunophenotypic analysis, as the morphologic appearance of these entities is quite similar in the blood. S100+ T-cell lymphoproliferative disorder, in contrast to the usual CD4+ T-cell PLL, will lack expression of CD4 and CD8, and will express NK-associated markers. In addition, S100+ T-cell lymphoproliferative disorder is S100+ by definition; this marker will presumably differentiate these cases from the more common T-cell PLL, although no systematic studies of the latter for S100 expression have been performed.

Large granular lymphocytosis is characterized by a very slowly progressive clinical course, neutropenia, and frequently autoimmune disease. By definition the lymphoid cells in this disease have intracytoplasmic azurophilic granules, unlike S100+ T-cell lymphoproliferative disorder, which typically lacks granules.

Differentiation from HTLV-I associated T-cell leukemia/lymphoma can be made based on (1) the distinctive multilobated nuclei seen in the latter, (2) presence of HTLV-I circulating antibodies, and (3) clinical features including hypercalcemia and bone lesions.

CD56 (NCAM) Positive Peripheral T-Cell Lymphomas

Definition. This PTL entity is defined by the expression of the neural cell adhesion molecule (NCAM, CD56) on the cell surface.[58–60] NCAM positive PTL are derived from NK-like T cells. These are MHC unrestricted cytotoxic T cells that coexpress CD3 and rearrange their TCR2 receptor and also coexpress NK antigens such as CD56, CD16, or CD57.[61] These aggressive PTL, usually of intermedlate/high grade morphology, have a striking predilection for unusual sites of involvement, including the central nervous system, the endocrine glands, skeletal muscle, and the gastrointestinal tract.[58–60] Interestingly, these anatomic sites are naturally high expressors of NCAM, and the like–like homophilic attraction of NCAM might account for the preferrential homing of NCAM positive lymphomas to these sites.[59,62]

Morphology. The majority of CD56+ NK-like T-cell PTL are extranodal.[2,3,6] The most common histologic classification is either diffuse large cell lymphoma or diffuse mixed; a minority (one-third) are of diffuse small cleaved cell type.[58] Azurophilic granules may be found in some cases.[59,60,63] Vascular invasion with associated coagulative necrosis is frequent.[60] No histologic feature, other than perhaps azurophilic granules, distinguishes NCAM positive PTL from NCAM negative PTL; the diagnosis must be made by phenotyping.[58] Occasionally, circulating blasts with azurophilic granules are found. Both large cell size and a blastic appearance distinguish these neoplastic cells from patients with T-cell large granular lymphocytic leukemia, which is more indolent.[64] Occasionally erythrophagocytosis by tumor cells and lymphoepithelial lesions in mucosal surfaces are identified.[58,63]

Phenotyping. By definition all these PTL cases express CD56 and coexpress surface CD3.[58–60,63] Variable expression of other T-cell antigens includes CD2, 4, 5, and 8 and NK antigens (CD16 and CD57 [rarely]). The tumor cells are typically CD45+ and lack S100 or TCR1 rearrangement or protein.[58–60,63] Western blotting of neoplastic NK-like T cells sometimes reveals an unusual type of glycosylation,[65] in particular a high content of α2,8 polysialic acid as found in embryogenesis.[66] The prominence of this embryonic NCAM suggests the presence of an oncodevelopmental antigen in some PTL.[58,65] Furthermore, it is known that α2,8 polysialic acid, an NCAM associated carbohydrate, is a neuroinvasive determinant in *Neisseria meningitides* and *Escherichia coli,* bacteria species that cause meningitis.[67] α2,8 polysialic acid specifically facilitates meningeal invasion by these bacteria in neonates. Recent findings suggest that NCAM positive lymphomas are similarly predisposed to central nervous system metastasis by the same neurodeterminant.[58,65]

Genotyping. NCAM positive NK-like PTL expectedly show TCRβ chain rearrangements and not rearrangement of TCRγ chain as found in γ/δ T-cell lymphomas.[63] Immunoglobulin genes are generally germline. TCR "silent" CD56+ cases without TCR1 or TCR2 rearrangements are typically true NK tumors (see below). As a point of information, some "TCR silent" PTL lack the framework determinant (BFI) of TCRβ rearrangements but nonetheless show actual TCRβ rearrangements, suggesting that BFI TCR gene products can be either a nonproductive rearrangement of TCR genes or a post-transcriptional defect due to neoplasia.[68] This loss of TCR framework determinants is similar to the loss of other T-cell markers in the aberrant T-cell phenotype of PTL and may serve as a diagnostic factor.[68] This feature also confounds ready interpretation of "TCR silent" status.

Clinical Features. NCAM positive NK-like T-cell PTL are generally aggressive extranodal lymphomas presenting predominantly in middle aged males with stage III and IV disease and B symptoms (fever, night sweats, weight loss).[58–63] Extranodal sites include central nervous system (brain, meninges, cerebrospinal fluid, and cranial nerves), endocrine organs (pituitary, parathyroids, adrenals), skeletal muscle, and gastrointestinal and hepatosplenic involvement.[58,59] The neuroendocrine propensity could reflect a like–like NCAM homophilic effect. The central nervous system involvement could reflect α2,8 polysialic acid expression, and hepatosplenic/gut involvement could reflect the known origin of extrathymic NK-like T cells in the hepatic sinusoids and gut submucosa.[65,69,70] Absolute lymphocytosis and leukemic phase occurs in some cases. Many NK-like PTL are found in chronically immunosuppressed patients, especially including those in the post-transplantation state.[63] The latter PTL in particular are apt to have evidence of EBV presence (e.g., EBER transcripts or EB-related latent membrane protein 1).[63]

Differential Diagnosis. CD56 expression is not specific for NK-like T-cell PTL.[71] It is found in a variety of mature T-cell leukemias and lymphoma. These entities may be placed in two broad categories: TCR rearranged/expressed and TCR nonrearranged (silent). The TCR rearranged entities include S100+ T-cell lymphoproliferative disorder, γ/δ T-cell lymphoma, and T-cell large granular lymphocyte leukemia.[71] The nonrearranged, silent TCR include the true NK lymphomas, both adult and fetal NK types and some TCR "silent" true T-cell as described above.[72,73] These entities are compared with NK-like PTL in order:

1. S100+ T-cell lymphoproliferative disorder is similar to NK-like PTL both phenotypically and clinically by virtue of coexpression of CD56, CD3, and an α/β TCR and frequent central nervous system involvement.[74,75] It differs largely in expres-

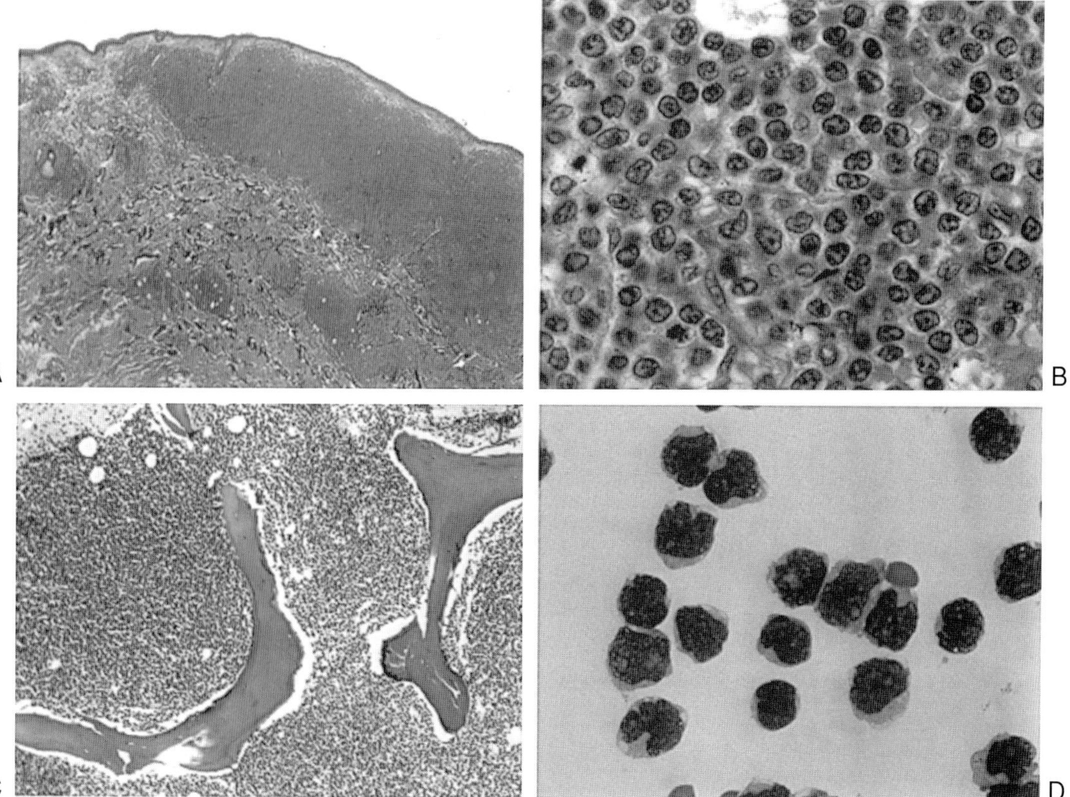

Fig. 8-14. **(A–D)** True NK cell tumor with cutaneous **(A)**, marrow **(C)**, and peripheral blood involvement **(D)**. The neoplastic cells are medium sized **(B)** and have irregular nuclear outlines and azurophilic granules **(D)**. Phenotyping is shown in Figure 8-15.

sion of S100 and CD8 and clinically by having frequent nodal involvement, leukemia, and marked splenomegaly. Morphologically the S100+ neoplastic cells are small or medium sized in contrast with the frequently large NK-like PTL cells.[74,75]

2. γ/δ T-cell lymphoma is frequently CD56+ but manifests a γ/δ not α/β rearrangement of TCR.[76,77] The cells are typically small to medium in size with decidedly sinusoidal infiltrates of spleen, liver, and lymph nodes. Phenotypically, the cells are typically double negatives (CD4−8−), although expression of CD8 is described.[76,77] Occasionally TCRβ chain rearrangement is seen in some cases with a concomitant TCRγ chain rearrangement.[77]
3. CD56+ large granular lymphocytic leukemia differs from NK-like PTL both phenotypically by more frequent expression of CD8, 16, and 57 and clinically by following a more indolent course with prominent neutropenia.[78] Morphologically, the leukemic cells of NK-like T-cell lymphoma often exhibit marked nuclear pleomorphism with blastic nuclear chromatin unlike the denser chromatin of chronic large granular lymphocyte leukemia.[63] A more aggressive form of large granular lymphocyte leukemia has been described.[79]
4. True NK lymphomas differ fundamentally by absence of TCR gene rearrangements. Reflecting true NK origin, they express CD16, CD56 or CD57 and some T-cell markers (CD2 and 7) but not CD3 or CD5 (Figs. 8-14 and 8-15).[72,73] Most cases are CD4−8−. There is reactivity with TIA-1 cytotoxic granules.[72,73] While NK lymphoma cells are expectedly lacking surface CD3 in concert with a lack of TCR2 rearrangement, they nonetheless express cytoplasmic CD3e as described in fetal NK cells and in activated adult NK cells.[80,81] Clinically, compared with NK-like PTL, the NK lymphomas have a younger age at presentation (44 years) with very frequent nasal involvement (75 percent).[72,73,81–83] Among non-nasal cases, the presentation frequently entails involvement of bone marrow, blood, liver, spleen, and skin (Figs. 8-14).[82,83] Morphologically the neoplastic cells range from pleomorphic me-

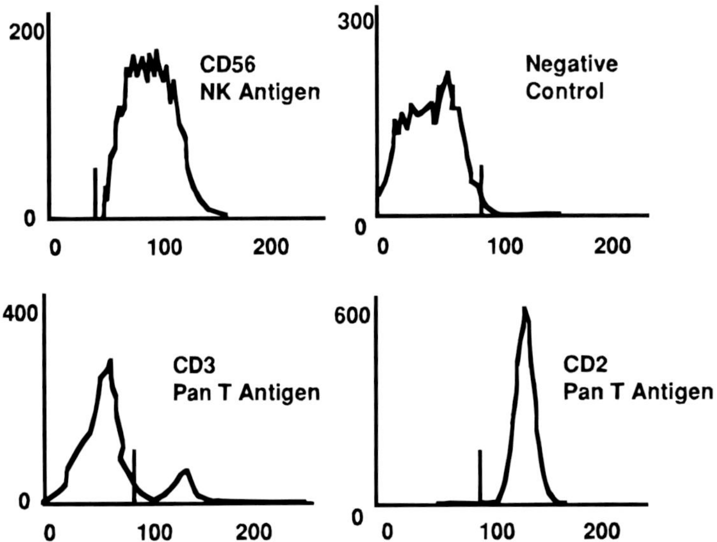

Fig. 8-15. (A–D) Flow cytometric assay of the peripheral blood tumor cells in Figure 8-14 reveals a coexpression of NK (CD56) and pan T antigens (CD2) without surface CD3, consistent with an NK cell phenotype.

dium to large cell size (Fig. 8-14). Azurophilic granules are present in some.[72,73]

CD30 Positive Ki-1 Anaplastic Large Cell Lymphoma

Definition. This is a neoplasm comprised of anaplastic, large blastic lymphoid cells that express the Ki-1 (CD30) antigen.[1]

Morphology. The characteristic features are the large blastic cells with elaborate polylobated "wreath-like" nuclei growing in a sinusoidal, cohesive pattern (Figs. 8-16). This sinusoidal pattern strongly raises suspicion of possible metastatic carcinoma, seminoma, or melanoma prior to immunotyping.[84–86] The tumor cells of anaplastic large cell lymphoma are typically much larger (two to three times) the usual large cell lymphoma cells. Lymphohistiocytic and small cell variants are described. There are two major histologic variants: (1) the classical variant, which occurs in a sinusoidal pattern as above; and (2) a Hodgkin's-like variant, which has morphologic similarity to Hodgkin's disease by virtue of nodular growth pattern, syncytial growth, large polylobated cells and surrounding bands of fibrous sclerosis (Fig. 8-17).[2]

Phenotyping. By definition the tumor cells are CD30+ (Fig. 8-16). Additionally, most (70 percent) are of mature T-cell lineage with variable expression of CD3 and 4.[84–86] There is typically strong CD25 expression. There are several antigens that are highly associated with anaplastic large cell lymphoma and may therefore be considered anaplastic large cell lymphoma associated antigens: BNH9,[87] EMA,[88] and CBF78[89]

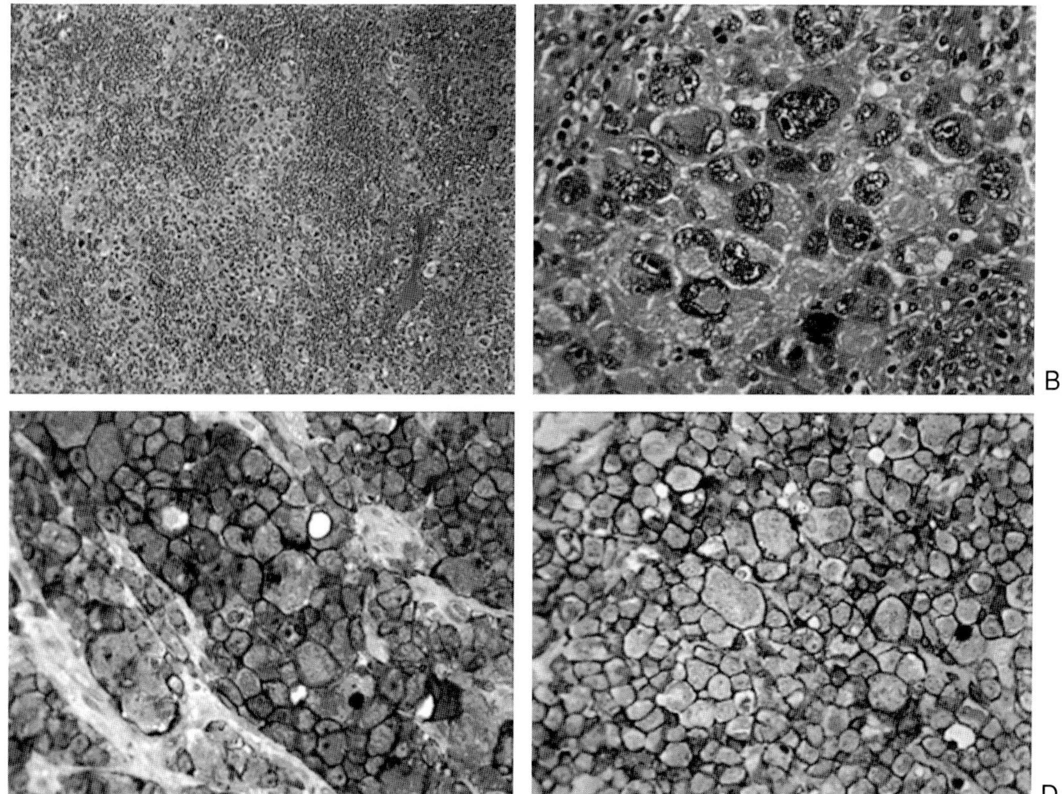

Fig. 8-16. **(A–D)** Anaplastic large cell PTL (classic variant) with cohesive groups **(A)** of large polylobated cells with "wreath-like" nuclei filling sinuses. Phenotype reveals coexpression of CD30 **(C)** and CD3 **(D)**.

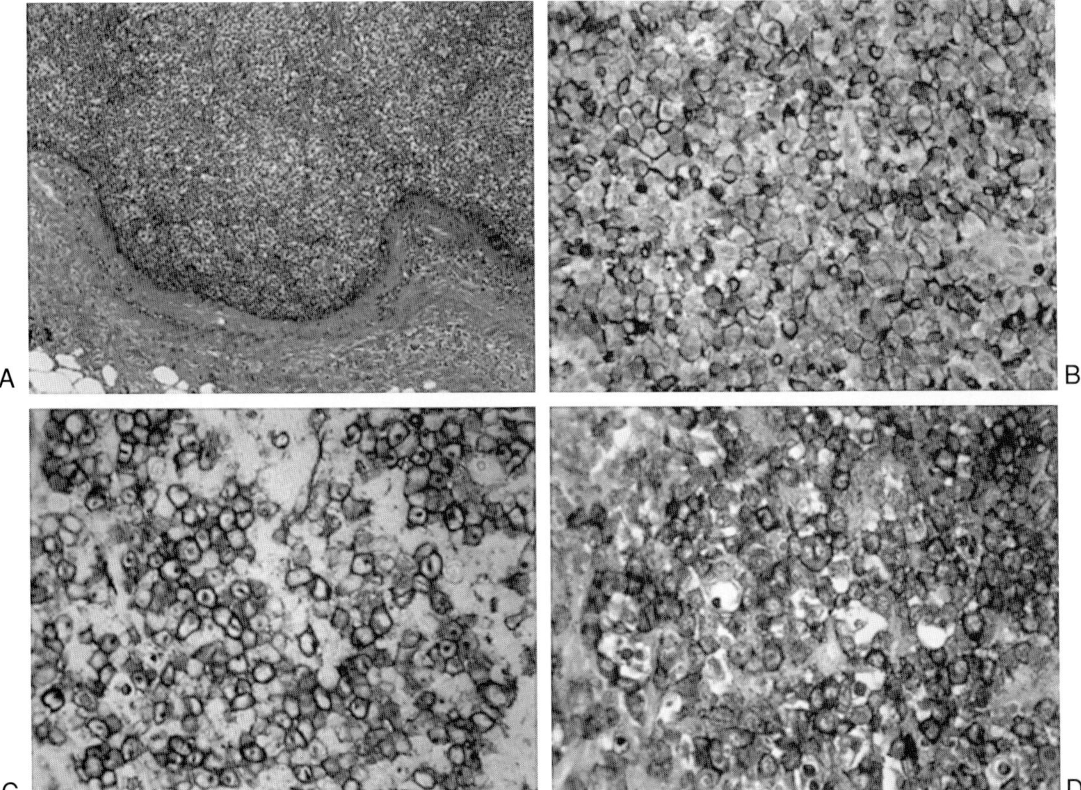

Fig. 8-17. Anaplastic large cell PTL (Hodgkin's-like variant) with syncytial growth of large polylobated cells with surrounding fibrous sclerosis **(A)** and anaplastic associated antigen co-expression including CB7F78 **(B)**, BNH9 **(C)**, and EMA **(D)**.

(Fig. 8-17). Occasionally CD30+ anaplastic large cell lymphomas are of null or B-cell lineage.

Genotype. TCR2 gene rearrangements occur in 60 percent of cases, with 40 percent being TCR2 silent.[85] Cytogenetic studies reveal that some cases (12 to 50 percent) have a unique translocation t(2;5)(p23;q35) that results in the fusion of the nucleophosmin gene on 5q35 with a novel anaplastic lymphoma kinase gene on chromosome 2p23.[90–93] A higher percentage of t(2;5) is observed in pediatric cases.[90–93]

Clinical Features. Clinically two major profiles relevant to outcome are described: systemic and cutaneous anaplastic large cell lymphoma.[94,95] The latter type typically presents in localized cutaneous form, and it may either regress spontaneously or follow an indolent but nonetheless incurable course. The systemic form is disseminated and has a more aggressive course, although complete cure is possible at the rate (35 to 40 percent) described in regular large cell lymphoma. Among the disseminated systemic forms of anaplastic large cell lymphoma the classical subset matches the clinical profile of a diffuse non-Hodgkin's large cell lymphoma.[94,95] In contrast, the Hodgkin's-like variant has shown a high propensity to involve the mediastinum in young females, once again mimicking Hodgkin's disease.[96] However, phenotypic distinction from Hodgkin's disease is unequivocal, as described below.

Differential Diagnosis. Since the large polylobated nuclei of Reed-Sternberg cells in Hodgkin's disease also express CD30, distinction of anaplastic large cell lymphoma from

Hodgkin's disease may be difficult both morphologically and immunologically. Anaplastic large cell lymphoma differs from Hodgkin's disease by its usual phenotypic profile (CD30+ CD15− CD45+ pan T+ or pan B+), which contrasts with the usual Hodgkin's phenotype (CD30+ CD15+ CD45− T− B−). There are also newly delineated anaplastic-associated antigens (CBF78, BNH9, and EMA) that are characteristically expressed in anaplastic large cell lymphoma and not Hodgkin's disease.[87–85] Finally the t(2;5) translocation is also highly associated with anaplastic large cell lymphoma and not Hodgkin's disease.

LYMPHOKINE RELATED

PTL Associated with Paraneoplastic Syndrome Abnormal Myelopoiesis

Definition. This is a PTL associated with paraneoplastic features, probably secondary to production of cytokines by the malignant cells.

Morphology and Clinical Features. The clinical features of PTL may be overshadowed by a paraneoplastic syndrome, which can prove to be a clinical conundrum.[97] The etiology of these paraneoplastic features is likely due to production of cytokines or other factors by the malignant cells. Paraneoplastic features may include constitutional symptoms, aberrant elevated myelopoiesis, eosinophilia, hypergammaglobulinemia, plasmacytosis, the hemophagocytic syndrome (described below), pancytopenia, coagulopathy, and hypercalcemia and lytic bone lesions (as described below).[16–20,97,98] Eosinophilic vasculitis has also rarely been associated with PTL. An illustrative example of the paraneoplastic effect is the PTL patient with hypergammaglobulinemia and striking plasmacytosis with circulating plasma cells causing confusion with plasma cell leukemia.[16] The neoplastic cells in this PTL are of T-helper phenotype, and the reacting proliferating plasma cells are polyclonal, representing recruitment of B cells by tumor related T-helper lymphokines.[16] PTL with compartmentalizing fibrosis also reflect recruitment of fibroblasts into PTL, producing a sclerosing effect. Another example of PTL-associated paraneoplastic syndrome is illustrated in Fig. 8-7. In this instance, a peripheral T-cell (PTL) phenotype is found in a tumor with Burkitt's-like morphology.[28] Surprisingly, this PTL Burkitt's-like lymphoma appears to have aberrant admixed myelocytes probably due to lymphokine stimulation of myelocytopoiesis. Clearly confusion with a granulocytic sarcoma, as shown, is possible unless extensive phenotyping is employed.[28]

In some cases, the paraneoplastic syndrome may be so complex as to suggest a diagnosis of collagen vascular disease, systemic infection, or severe liver disease, and the diagnosis of lymphoma may be obscured. In the three cases described by Diez-Martin et al.,[97] the patients not only had complex clinical presentations, with multiple paraneoplastic complications, but they lacked peripheral adenopathy as well. Thus the diagnosis of PTL in these patients was very difficult. Peripheral T-cell lymphomas should be a diagnostic consideration when evaluating a patient with unexplained complex constitutional symptoms.

PTL with Excess of Epithelioid Histiocytes (Lennert's Lymphoma)

Definition. This is an intermediate or high grade mature T-cell malignancy with a prominent multifocal epithelioid histiocytic reaction commonly misdiagnosed as inflammatory, granulomatous disease. Lennert's lymphoma characteristically presents in elderly men with widespread involvement of the reticuloendothelial system.[15,99–105]

Morphology. As illustrated (Figs. 8-4, 8-18), Lennert's PTL are highly heterogenous lymphomas typically of either diffuse mixed or large cell type with prominent associated granulomas.[15,99] There is commonly widespread visceral organ (lung, liver, spleen) involvement with minimal nodal involvement.[15] Frequently initial biopsies come from percutaneous liver or marrow biopsies (Fig. 8-18), and the numerous

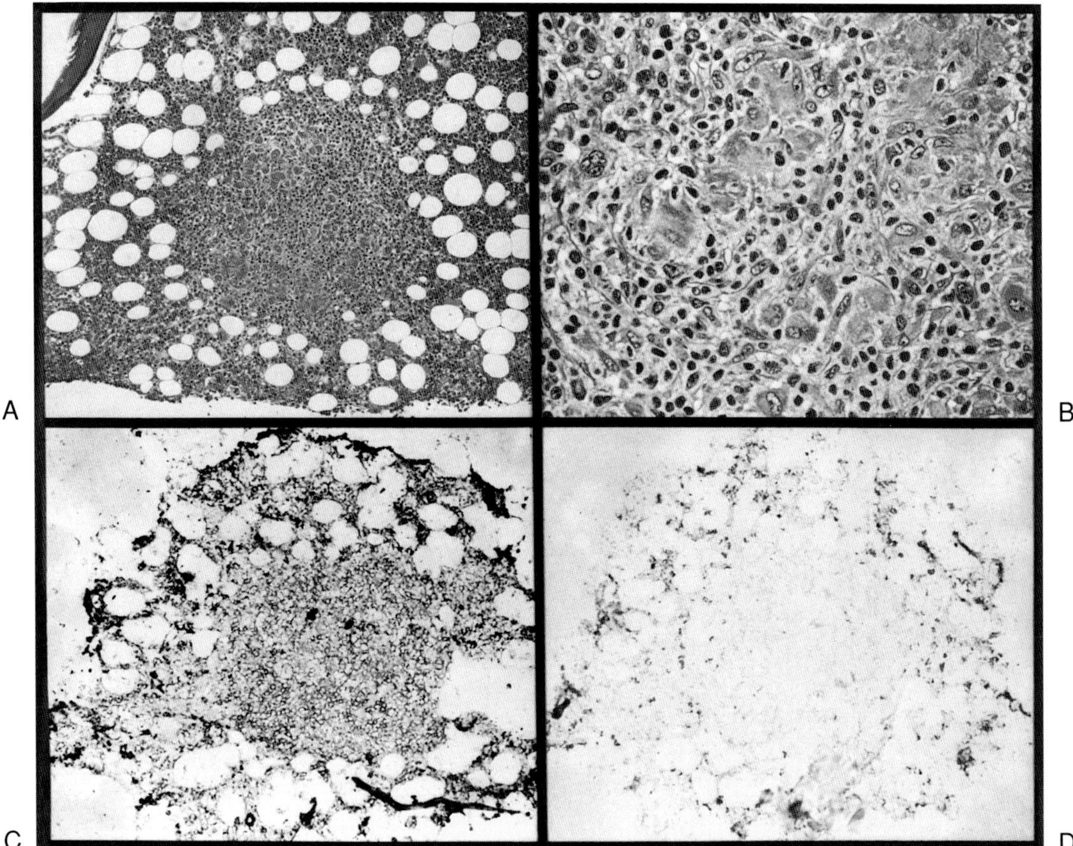

Fig. 8-18. Lennert's lymphoma involving the marrow (**A & B**) with expression of CD4 (**C**) and not CD8 (**D**).

small aggregates of benign appearing epithelioid histiocytes lead to a benign diagnosis.[105] It is specifically the atypicality of the admixed smaller or larger polylobated cells that is pivotal to correct diagnosis.

Phenotyping. Typically, it is a malignancy of mature T helper cells with "novel" idiosyncratic loss of some pan T-cell antigens (Figs. 8-4, 8-18).[103,104] Rare cases with coexpression of both T-helper and cytotoxic antigens (CD4+8+) are described. The excess histiocytes are thought to reflect an untoward cytokine effect derived from neoplastic, but still functional, T cells.

Clinical Features. Lennert's lymphoma characteristically occurs in elderly males with B symptoms and stage IV disease. In particular, there is prominent reticuloendothelial organ involvement of spleen, liver, and marrow and less prominent nodal involvement. The clinical course is typically aggressive with a median survial of less than 20 months.[15]

Differential Diagnosis. Occasionally intermediate/high grade lymphomas with excess histiocytes may be of B-cell lineage.[105] These B-cell Lennert's lymphomas are morphologically indistinguishable from T-cell Lennert's PTL. Like T cells, some B cells are known to stimulate lymphokine-driven histiocytes.[106] Since the B-cell variant has a more favorable prognosis, establishing lineage is clinically useful. Misdiagnosis of Lennert's lymphoma of either lineage is common. In one study,[105] the initial histiologic diagnosis was incorrect in 10 of 11 patients. The initial diagnoses were Hodgkin's disease, granulomatous disease, and other non-Hodgkin's lymphomas. In these cases the median delay in correct diagnosis was 10 months (1 to 45 months).[105]

Confusion with Hodgkin's disease is common given the occurrence of scattered pleomorphic, polylobated Reed-Sternberg-like cells in Lennert's lymphomas. The critical distinction lies in the atypicality of the small and medium sized cells found in abundance in Lennert's and not Hodgkin's disease. The phenotypic distinction is more obvious with pan T antigens and CD45RO expression and absent CD15 usual in Lennert's and absent pan T and CD45RO and presence of CD15 usual in Hodgkin's disease. Cell clonality of Lennert's may sometimes be obvious with phenotyping, as shown in Figure 8-4.[4,18]

Hemophagocytic Syndrome in Peripheral T-Cell Lymphoma

Definition. Hemophagocytic syndrome can occur in association with PTL. The hemophagocytic syndrome is a serious and frequently fatal complication of PTL in these patients. In these patients it is believed to be secondary to secretion of a cytokine by the malignant T cells.[18,19,107] EBV has been implicated in the pathogenesis of some of these PTLs.[108–111]

Morphology. Predominant sites of disease are generally the liver, spleen, and bone marrow; there is usually little or no peripheral adenopathy. When lymph nodes are involved, the architecture is at least partially effaced by an infiltrate of numerous benign phagocytozing histiocytes admixed with atypical lymphocytes. The atypical lymphocytes range in size from small to large; atypia is more easily seen in the larger lymphocytes, some of which may even resemble Reed-Sternberg cells.[110,112] The bone marrow and spleen are similarly effaced by an infiltrate of phagocytes and atypical lymphocytes. The marrow is hypercellular and shows bone marrow fibrosis, leading to a ''dry tap''; only patchy islands of residual recognizable marrow elements may be identified. The spleen shows red pulp infiltration, with white pulp involution; while in the liver, the infiltrate affects the portal areas.

Phenotype. The benign, phagocytizing histiocytes express macrophage-associated antigens such as CD11b, CD11c, CD14, CD68.[93] The atypical neoplastic cells show a peripheral T-cell phenotype (CD3 +, CD43 +, CD45RO + in paraffin sections). Frozen section immunohistochemistry reveals expression of pan T-cell antigens as well as CD4 and/or CD8.[107] In only exceptional cases are the activation antigens CD25 and CD30 expressed. In contrast, the T cells in EBV-associated hemophagocytic syndrome often express these activation antigens.

Genotype. Clonal rearrangement of the TCRβ chain gene can be detected in many cases.[108] However, some cases fail to show gene rearrangement of the TCR despite immunophenotypic data in support of a T-cell phenotype in the neoplastic cells.[109]

Clinical Features. Hemophagocytic syndrome may be the initial presentation of disease[10,110] or may develop months to years after diagnosis of PTL.[18,108] Patients are middle aged and more frequently male. The syndrome presents acutely with high fever, weight loss, and constitutional symptoms. Marked hepatosplenomegaly is always present; skin lesions and adenopathy are uncommon. Pancytopenia, generally severe, is invariably found. Liver enzymes are elevated.[98,107] The clinical course is rapid and frequently fatal, with most patients dying within weeks or months of diagnosis, even when the underlying PTL is recognized and the patient is treated with aggressive chemotherapy.[98,107] In some patients, an angiocentric PTL generally involving extranodal sites such as lung or nasopharynx precedes the syndrome by months to years;[15,108,113] in such cases hemophagocytic syndrome may develop at relapse of the lymphoma or even while the disease is in clinical remission. Florid, fatal hemophagocytic syndrome is also commonly associated with the subcutaneous nodules found in subcutaneous panniculitic PTL.

Differential Diagnosis. The differential diagnosis includes infection-related hemophagocytic syndrome, the hemophagocytic lymphohistiocytosis of children, and malignant histiocytosis (MH). The clinical picture of hemophagocytic syndrome can be very similar regardless of the underlying disease etiology. In some cases, infection-related hemophagocytic syndrome may be clinically distinguished from PTL-associated hemophagocytic syndrome if the disease occurs in an immunocompromised patient or following a recent viral illness. However, in general distinction of PTL-associated hemophagocytic syndrome and cases of reactive etiology relies largely on careful histologic and immunophenotypic examination of involved disease sites. In both cases, there is a predominant infiltration of involved disease sites with benign appearing phagocytic histiocytes. The involved marrow in PTL is uniformly hypercellular, in contrast to infection-associated hemophagocytic syndrome, where cellularity is variable.[114] The key to the diagnosis of PTL-associated hemophagocytic syndrome is the demonstration of pleomorphic, neoplastic-appearing cells with a T-cell phenotype admixed with the histiocytic infiltration. These atypical lymphocytes are generally CD25− CD30− in distinction to the reactive lymphoid cells found in infection-associated disease. MH is historically a second differential consideration in these cases; however, since the advent of immunophenotyping and genotyping, it has become apparent that many of the cases originally classified as MH really represent PTL-associated hemophagocytic syndrome.[115] The diagnosis of MH is now reserved for those cases where the histio-

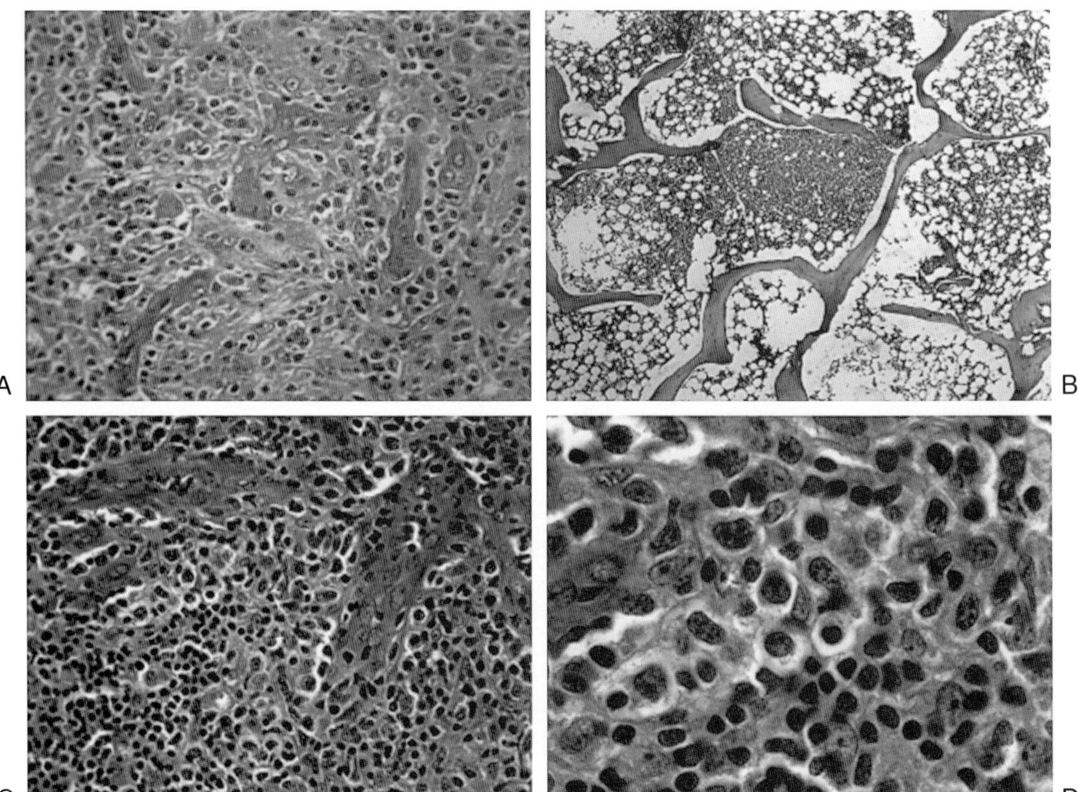

Fig. 8-19. Angioimmunoblastic lymphadenopathy (AILD) in the lymph node (**A**) and bone marrow (**B**) are hypocellular and show a vascular prominence. In contrast, AILD-like lymphoma (**C & D**) shows greater cellularity and clusters of large clear cells (**D**).

cytic derivation of the neoplastic cells is proven by immunophenotyping. A single report has associated hemophagocytic syndrome with B-cell lymphoma; immunophenotyping should distinguish such rare cases from PTL.[116]

Vessel Associated

Angioimmunoblastic Lymphadenopathy/ Angioimmunoblastic Lymphadenopathy with Associated T-Cell Lymphoma

Definition. Angioimmunoblastic lymphadenopathy with dysproteinemia (AILD) is a rare acute systemic disease characterized by lymphadenopathy, hepatosplenomegaly, a Coombs positive hemolytic anemia, skin rashes, weight loss, fever, and hypergammaglobulinemia.[112–124] While occasional remissions are described, transition to T-cell lymphoma (AILD-like PTL) (rarely B-cell lymphomas) commonly occurs.[122,123] There are now morphologic critieria that establish the diagnosis of AILD PTL.[123,125] However, the correlation between morphologic and genotypic evidence of malignancy is poor. This difficulty in correlating the presence of a clonal lymphoid population with morphologic evidence of neoplasia, as well as the inexorable downhill course of some patients whose disease is not clonal (and therefore "benign"), has challenged our thinking in terms of the boundary between neoplasia and benignancy.[126–131]

In the early 1970s, similar lymphoma-like syndromes with the same constellation of clinical findings (generalized lymphadenopathy, hepatosplenomegaly, hemolytic anemia, rashes, and hypergammopathy) were independently described and separately termed *lymphogranulomatosis* X (LGX) by Lennert,[124] immunoblastic lymphadenopathy by Lukes and Tindle,[119] and angioimmunoblastic lymphadenopathy (AILD) by Frizzera et al.[117] While these early studies noted progression to immunoblastic lymphoma in a proportion of patients, LGX, immunoblastic lymphadenopathy, and AILD were nonetheless considered benign abnormal immune responses or benign lymphoproliferative disorders. However, in subsequent reports strong similarities were shown between AILD and T-cell lymphomas described by Watanabe et al.[130] as adult T-cell lymphoma with hypergammoglobulinemia. This suggested a spectrum of disorders in which the diagnostic distinction between benignancy and neoplasia is problematic.

Morphology. The histologic features of immunoblastic lymphadenopathy and AILD include a characteristic nodal effacement by arborizing venules and an associated stromal prominence due to both lymphoid cell depletion and the accumulation of amorphous eosinophilic deposits (Fig. 8-19).[117–124] The lymphocyte loss and stromal prominence give the AILD node a decidedly "pink" cast on hematoxylin and eosin stain. The anastomosing network of small vessels has plump hyperplastic endothelial cells (Fig. 8-19). These proliferating venules may be surrounded by hyperplastic dendritic cells.[129]

In AILD, normal follicles are generally absent. However, abnormal follicle remnants (naked germinal centers, burned out follicles or follicles with Castleman-like changes) may be seen in a minority of cases. Residual or burned out germinal centers are present in AILD, not in immunoblastic lymphadenopathy, while amorphous eosinophilic sludge is essential to the diagnosis of immunoblastic lymphadenopathy, not AILD.[117–124] These represent minor descriptive differences in two highly related if not identical conditions. The burned out germinal centers in AILD are largely comprised of the proliferating reticulum cells that surround arborizing venules.

The lymphoid infiltrate characteristic of AILD is a polymorphous mixture of small morphologically unremarkable lymphocytes, plasma cells, immunoblasts, a scattering of individual large cells with clear cytoplasm, and a sprinkling of eosinophils (Fig. 8-19).[116–119] However, in distinction to AILD-like T-cell lymphoma, neither clear cell nor immunoblast clusters are seen. Furthermore, in distinction to the cellular nodal effacement seen in non-Hodgkin's lymphoma, AILD lymph nodes typically appear hypocellular at low power. Additionally, unlike non-Hodgkin's lymphoma, the sinuses are frequently patent with preservation in particular of the peripheral sinus.[116–119]

The polymorphous, vascular, stromal prominent "tumors" of AILD may also be seen outside the lymph nodes at sites including the bone marrow, liver, spleen, and skin (Fig. 8-19). These "tumors" further challenge the true benignancy of AILD. Nonetheless, the AILD designation is judged appropriate as long as the AILD extranodal nodules remain polymorphous and not pleomorphic or do not contain clusters of large clear cells or immunoblasts.[122]

Three salient features herald the transition to AILD-like lymphoma: (1) greater cellularity, (2) greater pleomorphism, and (3) the emergence of clusters of transformed large cells (Fig. 8-19).[121–125] AILD-like T-cell lymphoma, like AILD, shows nodal effacement by a polymorphous lymphoid infiltrate, with associated arborizing vascular proliferation, and the presence of rare burned out germinal centers. In contrast to hypocellular AILD, the overall cellularity of the node tends to be normal or increased. The pathognomonic feature distinguishing AILD-like T-cell lymphoma from AILD is the presence of large transformed lymphoid cells occurring in clusters or sheets.[121–125] In particular, clusters of large transformed cells with clear or amphophilic cytoplasm are essential for diagnosis.[121–125] An additional feature of AILD lymphoma is an increased pleomorphism with greater lymphoid cell atypicality, more blastic appearance, and greater nuclear polylobation (Fig. 8-19).

Immunophenotype. The lymphoid infiltrate in AILD is generally composed predominantly of T cells, usually with a predominance of helper T cells and without loss of normal T-cell differentiation antigens. Loss of pan T-cell antigens is more typically found in AILD-like T-cell lymphoma.[126] Unfortunately, loss of pan T-cell antigens has also been reported in AILD and thus may not be a reliable way to differentiate the two diseases.[122] Characteristically expanded follicular dendritic cell clusters may be found surrounding proliferating venules.[124] Hyperplasia of these cells beyond the follicles is said to be a characteristic immunophenotypic feature of AILD.[129] This feature persists in AILD-like lymphoma and does not serve as a differential feature.[129]

Genotype. Just as the morphologic features of AILD and AILD-like PTL show some overlap, genotyping of these lesions is not straightforward.[126–129] Clonal rearrangement of the TCRβ chain locus can be found in most cases (75 percent) of AILD-like PTL. Similar gene rearrangements are also detected in cases of AILD that lack morphologic evidence of malignant lymphoma.[126] It is said by Weiss et al.[126] that "AILD that contain clonal T-cell populations probably represent peripheral T-cell lymhomas." In contrast, clonal gene rearrangements may be lacking in cases that morphologically fit AILD-like lymphoma. Despite the lack of clonal disease in such patients, the disease may be highly aggressive, leading to early death.[126,127] Thus, in keeping with the difficulty in morphologic distinction between the entities, a similar grey zone is present when gene rearrangement studies are performed.[126–129] Further complicating interpretation, the IgH gene may be present as a co-existing rearrangement with TCRβ in 10 percent of AILD-like PTL.[1]

Interphase cytogenetic studies have revealed a further level of complexity in this disease; AILD-like PTL with multiple unrelated aberrant clones have been detailed, indicating that multiple clones may be present in patients with a "clonal" disease.[128] Patients with a morphologic diagnosis of AILD have also been shown to have clonal cytogenetic abnormalities. It has been suggested that patients with clonal disease should probably be treated as malignant lymphomas even when morphologic evidence of AILD-like PTL is lacking, since multiagent chemotherapy may be beneficial in AILD-like PTL.[131]

In a recent review, Frizzera et al.[123] proposed that three different AILD related disorders (AILD, AILD-like dysplasia, AILD-like PTL) could be recognized by a combination of immunophenotyping and molecular genetic and cytogenetic parameters. In this pragmatic approach true AILD lacks clonal rearrangement or karyotypic change and is polyclonal by immunophenotyping. At the other extreme true AILD lymphoma is clonal by both genotyping and phenotyping and has karyotypic aberrancy. AILD-like dysplasia is an intermediate group with some but not all the defects associated with AILD PTL.[123]

Clinical Features. The disease affects the elderly and is manifested by generalized lymphadenopathy, fever, hepatosplenomegaly, hemolytic anemia, a skin rash, and polyclonal hypergammaglobulinemia.[121,122] Although transient steroid responsiveness and occasional spontaneous remissions are described, the disease frequently runs a rapid and fatal course; overall over 60 percent of patients die.[131] A worse prognosis is found among patients who have morphologic evidence of AILD-associated PTL rather than AILD;[129] among patients who fail to respond to the initial chemotherapy; among patients whose lymph nodes show clonal TCR gene rearrangements;[129] and among patients with a high proliferative index as measured by the monoclonal antibody Ki-67 (Ki-67 more than 25 percent).[132]

Differential Diagnosis. PTL unrelated to AILD may be similar to AILD-like PTL; however, the combination of prominent arborizing vascular proliferation, polymorphous less cellular background proliferation, expanded follicular dendritic cell clusters, and the characteristic clinical symptoms distinguish AILD-like PTL. In some AILD-like PTL, the presence of Reed-Sternberg-like cells in an effaced node with an accompanying polymorphous lymphoid infiltrate including eosinophils and plasma cells may lead to a consideration of Hodgkin's disease. However, the overall milieu including the presence of immunoblasts, clusters of clear cells, and arborizing blood vessels is not correct for Hodgkin's disease. In general, it is the constellation of polymorphous lymphocyte depletion with a vascular proliferation in a characteristic clinical setting that characterizes AILD-related PTL.

Angiocentric T-Cell Lymphoma

Definition. An angiocentric, angioinvasive pattern of infiltration can be seen in both nodal and extranodal T-cell lymphomas, typically resulting in necrosis of both tumor and normal tissue.[24,133–136] Among nodal lymphomas, this angiocentric pattern does not define a specific subtype of peripheral T-cell lymphoma. In contrast, angiocentricity was a key feature in the initial descriptions of the extranodal angioimmunoproliferative lesions involving lung (lymphomatoid granulomatosis), upper aerodigestive tract (midline malignant reticulosis and polymorphic reticular nasal T-cell lymphoma), central nervous system, and skin (lymphomatoid vasculitis).[4] However, recent insights into the biology of extranodal lymphomas have resulted in the recommendation to rename these angioimmunoproliferative lesion-type angiocentric lymphomas.[133] In particular, nasal angiocentric T-cell lymphomas are now recognized as most commonly true NK cell neoplasms without TCR1 or TCR2 rearrangements.[73] In contrast, lymphomatoid granulomatosis, formally an angiocentric T-cell lymphoma, is now recognized commonly to represent a B-cell proliferation with EBV localized to the large B cells, with the prominent admixed T cells representing a reactive component.[137] It currently appears that angiocentricity is of less importance as a defining property of PTL than is either phenotype or the site of disease.[137]

Morphology. *Angiocentricity* had been defined as "preferential concentration of tumor cells around and within blood vessels, with destruction of the blood vessel wall"; a perivascular infiltrate of lymphoid cells is insufficient to term a lymphoma angiocentric.[4] This pattern of infiltration can be seen in both nodal and extranodal lymphomas. There is often associated tissue necrosis due to vascular destruction. Erythrophagocytosis by benign histiocytes may be seen.

Phenotype. True nasal T/NK-cell lymphomas have a T-cell, NK-like T-cell, or true NK-cell phenotype (CD2+, CD3−, CD56+), with the latter phenotype predominating (Fig.

8-20).[133–136] In contrast, angiocentric nodal T-cell lymphomas generally have a T-cell phenotype (CD3+).

Genotype. Angiocentric T-cell lymphomas involving lymph node show a similar frequency of TCR gene rearrangement as T-cell lymphomas lacking this pattern of infiltration. In contrast, most nasal T/NK lymphomas lack rearrangement of their TCR gene, including both TCR1 and TCR2, although they typically show clonal integration of EBV.[4,35,135]

Clinical Features. Nodal T-cell lymphomas with an angiocentric component probably have a clinical behavior similar to other node-based peripheral T-cell lymphomas. Clinical correlates among nasal T/NK lymphomas are more difficult because of the confusion in the histologic and phenotypic classification of these extranodal diseases. However, it appears that patients with relatively low grade histology may have a better prognosis than those with higher grade lesions.[136] Furthermore, among patients with nasal T/NK lymphomas localized stage I disease is generally radiosensitive. Dissemination is typically extranodal, involving the stomach, gastrointestinal tract, skin, and subcutaneous tissues. Spread to distant sites is associated with a poor prognosis. Nasal T/NK lymphoma patients also show an increased risk of an associated hemophagocytic syndrome.

Differential Diagnosis. An angiocentric pattern of lymph node infiltration is not confined to T-cell lymphomas, but is also seen in B-cell lymphomas, including the unusual angiotropic B-cell lymphomas. Thus lineage of the neoplastic cells should always be confirmed, for example, by immunohistochemistry, before making the diagnosis of peripheral T-cell lymphoma with an angiocentric component. Differential of the disseminated nasal T/NK lymphomas includes lymphomatoid granulomatosis, NK-cell leukemia/lymphoma, and AML. Lymphomatoid granulomatosis has features very similar to the low grade nasal lymphomas, but may be distinguished in expert hands by detection of EBV sequences in the (putatively malignant) CD20+ B cells within the lesions. Distinction of an extranodal T-cell lymphoma from monocytic sarcoma/granulocytic sarcoma depends on demonstration of staining with two or more T-cell markers and lack of staining with myeloid markers (e.g., specific esterase).

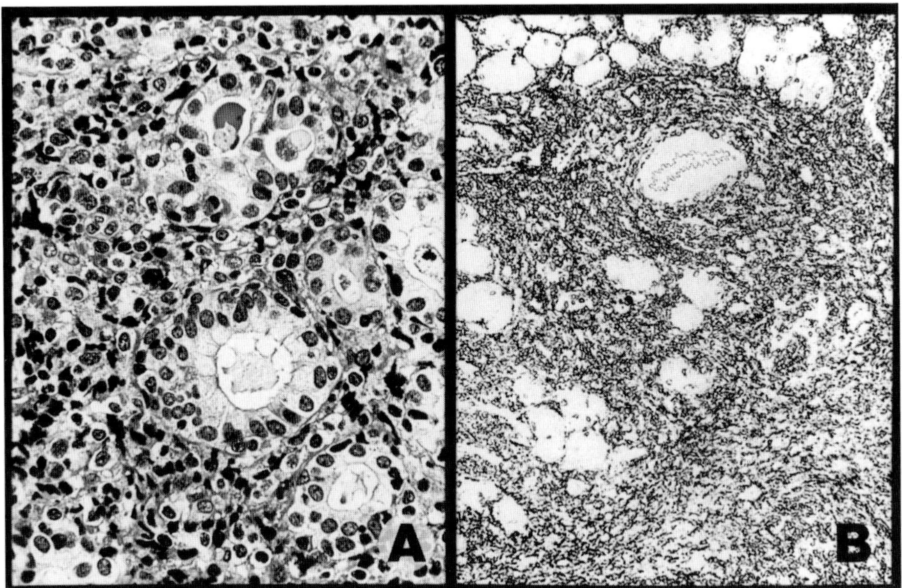

Fig. 8-20. Nasal NK-like T-cell PTL with submucosal, pleomorphic lymphoid infiltrate (**A**) and co-expression of CD3 (**B**) and CD56 (not shown).

Virus Associated

HTLV-I Associated Japanese T-Cell Lymphoma Leukemia

Definition. This is a mature T-cell lymphoma/leukemia caused by the human retrovirus known as human T-cell leukemia virus III (HTLV-III) that is endemic in Southwestern Japan, the Caribbean, and Southeastern United States.[138–147]

Morphology. Pronounced nuclear pleomorphism with hyperlobated nuclei (flower cells or clover leaf cells) (Fig. 8-21) are found in the peripheral blood.[142] The nodes are involved with a heterogeneous mix of small and large lymphoid cells with some multinucleate cells similar to Reed-Sternberg cells.[144] Common sites of involvement include lymph nodes, skin, liver, spleen, central nervous system, bone marrow, and peripheral blood, with widespread stage IV presentation most frequent.[138–142]

Phenotyping. Typical HTLV-I associated neoplastic cells have a natural T-helper cell phenotype with coexpression of CD2, 3, 4, and 5 with absent CD7 (Fig. 8-21). The IL-2 receptor (CD25) is commonly highly expressed. The occasional admixed large Reed-Sternberg cells may be CD30+ or CD15+, adding to diagnostic difficulty.[141,142,144]

Genotype. TCR2 genes are typically clonally rearranged. Demonstration of monoclonal or oligoclonal integration of HTLV-I provirus by Southern blotting provides definitive proof of etiology. More recently PCR methodologies have demonstrated proviral sequences in DNA extracted from tissues fixed in formalin and embedded in paraffin.[145,148]

Clinical Features. This entity occurs in adults in the endemic areas of Kyushu, Japan, the Caribbean, and the southern United States.

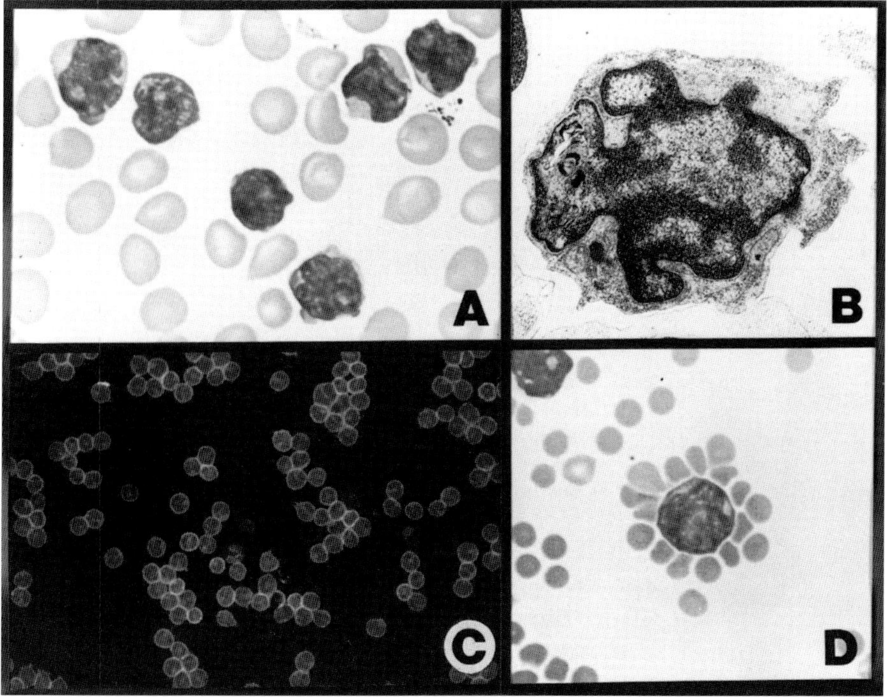

Fig. 8-21. Japanese T-cell lymphoma/leukemia, HTLV-I associated. There are circulating flower or clover leaf cells **(A & B).** Phenotyping shows T-helper (CD3) surface antigen by immunofluorescence **(C)** and pan T markers CD2 by E rosetting **(D).**

The latter patients are largely but not exclusively blacks.[143,144] The acute form presents with a high peripheral blood white cell count, hepatosplenomegaly, hypercalcemia, and lytic bone lesions with an aggressive course (survival less than 1 year).[142] Rarely it may occur as chronic or smoldering subtypes, frequently with a predominance of cutaneous involvement.

Hypercalcemia and lytic bone lesions are commonly found. Biopsies of lytic bone lesions typically show increased osteoclastic activity with bony resorption and evidence of local bony involvement by lymphoma/leukemia. The focal osteoclastic activity appears to be an untoward effect of the ''tax'' gene product of HTLV-I, which induces a parathyroid-like hormone resulting in osteoclast activity and hypercalcemia.[149]

Differential Diagnosis. Cutaneous involvement may be confused with mycosis fungoides/Sézary syndrome. In particular, epidermal clustered lymphoid invasion may occur in the form of Pautrier's microabscesses, greatly mimicking mycosis fungoides.[138–142] HTLV-I associated disease resembles the d'emblee variant of mycosis fungoides without a chronic premycotic phase. As a differentiating point, the typical acute fulminant course of HTLV-I associated T-cell lymphoma/leukemia contrasts with the indolent disease course of mycosis fungoides. Ultimately Southern blot or PCR evidence of HTLV-I virus allows definitive distinction.[145,148]

HTLV-II Associated T-Cell Lymphoproliferative Disorders

HTLV-II infection has been associated with both T-cell hairy cell leukemia[150–152] and large granular lymphocyte leukemia of T-cell type or variants.[150–152] However, the role of HTLV-II infection in these lymphoproliferative disorders is unclear. Studies on New Mexican Native American and Hispanic populations in whom there is a high endemic incidence of HTLV-II infection have not shown an excess incidence of hairy cell leukemia, chronic lymphocytic leukemia, or mycosis fungoides. Thus the role of HTLV-II infection in these disorders must await larger studies, preferably on groups with a high endemic HTLV-II incidence.

EBV-Related Peripheral T-Cell Lymphoma

Definition. This peripheral T-cell lymphoma demonstates the presence of EBV within malignant lymphoid cells.[153–161] The role of EBV in some of these neoplasms is unclear in part because the percentage of malignant cells that are EBV positive varies considerably.[161]

Morphology. EBV may be detected in 10 percent or more of PTL.[157,158] EBV infection is particularly common in nasopharyngeal T-cell lymphomas (T/NK nasal lymphomas), where over 80 percent of cases may be EBER (EBV-encoded RNA) positive,[156] and is also found in over 60 percent of extranodal PTL with the CD56+ phenotype from other sites.[153] Among nodal lymphomas, EBV-related PTL are generally intermediate or high grade (diffuse mixed, large cell, or immunoblastic in the Working Formulation). EBV is detected particularly commonly in AILD-type T-cell lymphoma.[159] Interestingly, in AILD Epstein-Barr transcripts (EBER) may be found in immunoblasts of B- or T-cell phenotype. Despite the association of EBV with particular entities, no specific morphologic features distinguish nodal PTL associated with EBV. Demonstration of EBV infection of malignant cells depends on phenotypic or genotypic studies.

Immunophenotype. EBV-encoded latent membrane protein (LMP-1) can be detected by immunohistochemistry. LMP-1 protein expression does not always correlate with detection of EBERs, as the LMP does not always appear to be transcribed in EBV infected cells.[160,161] In particular, LMP-1 expression is detected in approximately 50 percent of EBER positive cases.

Genotype. EBV DNA can be detected by PCR. However, this does not distinguish EBV infection of malignant cells and physiologic bystander cells. Alternatively, viral RNA transcripts can be detected by reverse transcriptase PCR (RT PCR). In situ hybridization techniques allow detection of EBERs in malignant cells; double labeling techniques can confirm the phenotype of the EBER+ cells identified by costaining with monoclonal antibodies directed against B or T cells. Detection of EBERs does not always correlate with LMP expression, with the EBER+/LMP− phenotype being found particularly in EBV infected bystander cells.[161] The percentage of EBER+ malignant cells can vary considerably, making definitive statements about the role of EBV in PTL difficult.

Clinical Features. Some studies have found that patients with EBV associated PTL have a worse prognosis than those with EBV− PTL and that EBV-associated PTL may be associated with a terminal hemophagocytic syndrome.[155,158] Further studies on larger numbers of uniformly treated patients are needed to determine if EBV+ PTL, other than those associated with T/NK nasal lymphoma, represent a clinically distinct entity.

PTL Associated with Immunodeficiency States Including HIV-1 (HTLV-III) Associated

Definition. Immunosuppressed patients are at greatly increased risk of developing non-Hodgkin's lymphomas, usually of B-cell phenotype. However, T-cell lymphomas may also arise in immunosuppressed patients, including organ transplant recipients, AIDS (HTLV-III+) patients, and some patients with inherited immunodeficiencies.[167–171] Unlike immunosuppression-associated B-cell lymphomas, which are almost always EBV related, EBV is only sometimes associated with these T-cell lymphomas.[170] Other cases have been associated with HIV infection.[168]

Morphology. T-cell lymphomas arising in the context of immunosuppression usually have a large cell component, being classified as diffuse mixed, large cell, or immunoblastic.[162,163,165,168,170] However, lymphoblastic lymphoma and large granular lymphocytic leukemia have also been reported.[166,167]

Phenotype. These lymphomas have a T-cell phenotype, expressing pan T antigens such as CD2, CD3, CD7. Tumors may lack both CD4 and CD8.[162,170] A T-cell phenotype can also be demonstrated by paraffin section immunohistochemistry with antibodies such as CD45RO and CD43. However, discrepant results have been reported with paraffin section immunohistochemistry, emphasizing the need for care in the interpretation of these results.[170]

Genotype. Like most peripheral T-cell lymphomas, PTL in immunosuppressed patients show rearrangement of the TCR2 locus.

Clinical Features. In the post-transplant setting, these lymphomas can occur months to years after transplantation. The interval appears to depend in part on the immunosuppressive regimen used, with more aggressive immunosuppression being associated with a shorter interval to development of lymphoma.[164] Most patients have systemic disease at the time of diagnosis and frequently die of disease. Improved survival is found among patients with localized disease.[164]

Organ Associated

Subcutaneous Panniculitic PTL

Definition. Panniculitic peripheral T-cell lymphomas are lymphomas that involve primarily the subcutaneous tissues, morphologically resembling panniculitis, hence their name.[172–175] The classical case is associated with a hemophagocytic syndrome.

Morphology. These lymphomas primarily involve the subcutaneous tissues, with some infiltration of the deep dermis (Fig. 8-22). Superficial dermal and epidermal involvement are not characteristic, but have been described in occasional cases.[172] Lymphoid cells infiltrate between fat cells, creating a ''lace-like'' pattern that is morphologically similarity to panniculitis (Fig. 8-22). Focal aggregates and small sheets of lymphoid cells are also seen. The lymphoid

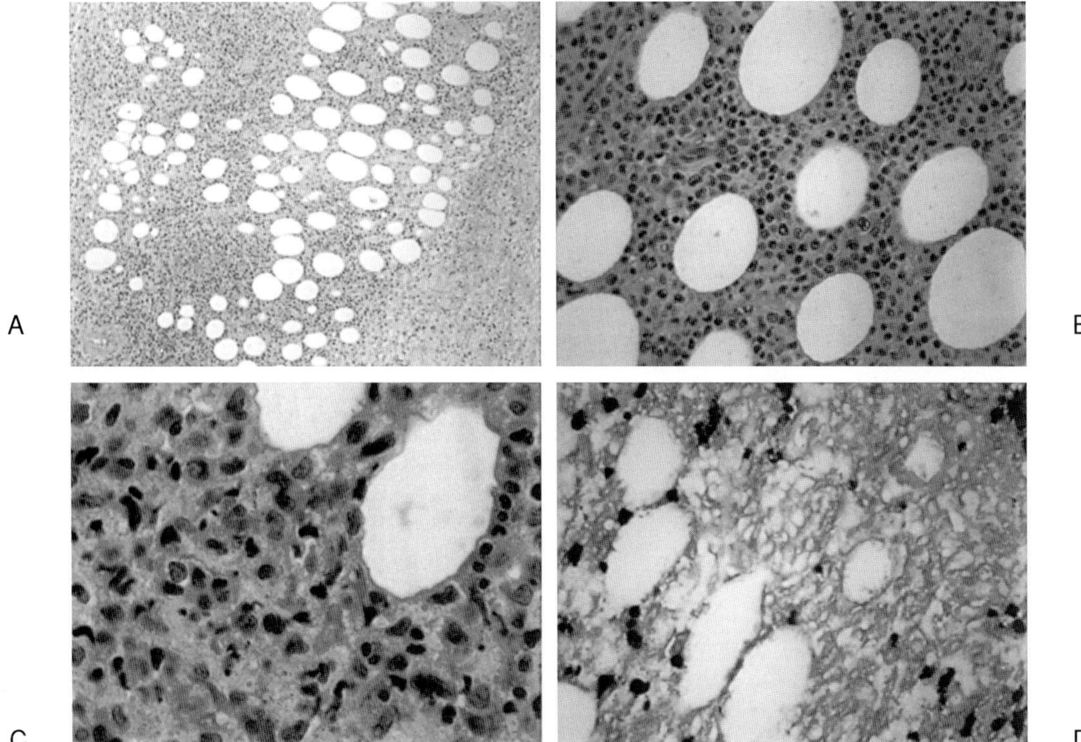

Fig. 8-22. Subcutaneous panniculitic PTL with subcutaneous lymphoid infiltrate between fat cells **(A & B)**. The lymphoid infiltrate is mixed with both small and large cells with associated mitoses and karyorrhexis **(C)**. Phenotyping revealed CD4 reactivity on frozen section **(D)**.

infiltrate may be quite bland in early lesions, making differentiation from benign panniculitis difficult. More advanced lesions show a mixed infiltrate of small and large cells with irregular nuclear outlines and coarsely clumped chromatin (Fig. 8-22). Most of these infiltrates would be classified as diffuse mixed small cleaved and large cell, or diffuse large cell, immunoblastic, under the Working Formulation or as mixed medium and large cell, or large cell by the REAL classification scheme.[172–175]

Karyorrhexis and frequent mitotic figures are characteristic (Fig. 8-22). Larger lesions show necrosis of connective tissue and fat. Scattered single benign histiocytes, granulomas, and foreign body giant cells may be seen within these areas of necrosis. In cases associated with the hemophagocytic syndrome, erythrophagocytosis by histiocytes is present. Unlike the angiocentric T-cell lymphomas, angiocentricity and angioinvasion are not characteristic.[172–175]

The lymph nodes from patients with panniculitic PTL are not involved by lymphoma but may show sinus histiocytosis and erythrophagocytosis.

Phenotype. With paraffin section immunohistochemistry, panniculitic PTL stains with the T-cell associated antigen CD45RO and may also stain with other T-cell markers such as CD43. Detailed immunophenotypic data are limited in this disease; four of five patient samples tested by Gonzalez et al.[172] were CD4+; the remaining case was CD8+. Antigenic aberrancy may be observed.[4,172]

Genotype. Rearrangement of the TCRβ chain gene is characteristic of the disease in the

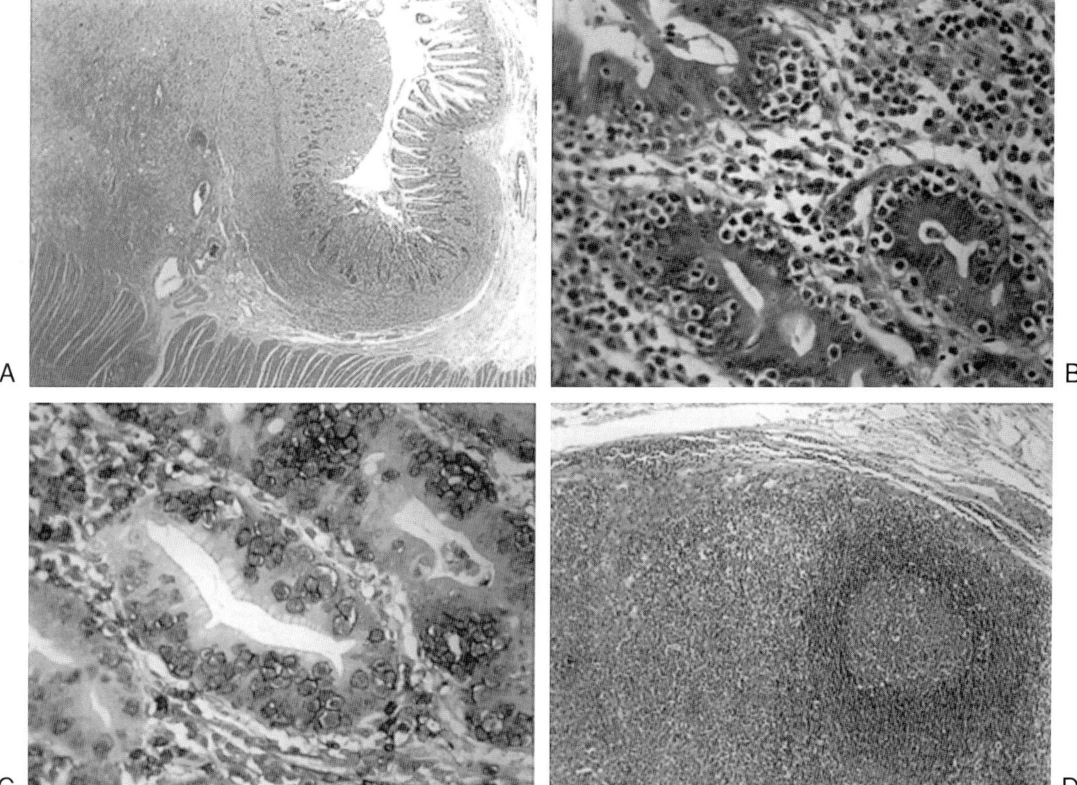

Fig. 8-23. Intestinal T-cell lymphoma involving the jejunum (**A**) with intraepithelial clustered invasion (**B**) by CD3+ T cells (**C**) and spread to paracortex of adjacent mesenteric nodes (**D**).

few cases tested, but may not be identified in every case.[172,173]

Clinical Features. Patients are adults (reported age range 19 to 54 years) who present with subcutaneous nodules 1 to 13 cm in size, classically of the extremities. Most patients develop an associated hemophagocytic syndrome, either at the time of diagnosis of panniculitic PTL or subsequently in the disease course. The hemophagocytic syndrome has been attributed to cytokine production by the malignant T cells.[175] The hemophagocytic syndrome is generally florid and is often fatal. Interestingly, several reports describe patients who initially presented with skin lesions that clinically and morphologically resembled benign panniculitis several years before developing a morphologically recognizable panniculitic PTL in tandem with a hemophagocytic syndrome.[173–175] Whether these represent precursor lesions of PTL is as yet unknown.

Differential Diagnosis. The differential of the skin lesions lies between panniculitic PTL and the different subtypes of benign panniculitis (erythema nodosum, erythema induratum, Weber-Christian disease), as well as the different types of cutaneous PTL. Differentiation from benign panniculitis may be made in cases that show atypia of the lymphoid infiltrate; a clinical history of hemophagocytosis may also support the diagnosis. However, in bland lesions, molecular genetic studies may be the only reliable method to determine if a clonal process is present. Panniculitic PTL can be differentiated from angiocentric immunoproliferative lesions, as this disease does not have the predilection for angioinvasion and destruction seen in the latter.

The differential of panniculitic hemophagocytic syndrome includes viral associated hemophagocytic syndrome. Patients with the latter disease may have a skin exanthem from a viral illness but do not show the subcutaneous infiltrate seen in panniculitic PTL. Furthermore, they lack the pleomorphism found in panniculitic PTL.

Enteropathy Associated T-Cell Lymphoma (Intestinal T-Cell Lymphoma)

Definition. This is a peripheral T-cell lymphoma derived from the intraepithelial mucosal T cells of the small bowel, frequently associated with celiac disease.[176–183]

Morphology. Enteropathy associated T-cell lymphoma usually involves the small bowel, in particular the jejunum, where over 70 percent of the neoplasms are found, and is frequently multifocal.[176,177] The tumor infiltrates the lamina propria and overlying epithelium and may invade through the muscularis propria, leading to thickening of the bowel wall (Fig. 8-23). Malignant cells invade the epithelium singly and in groups, giving rise to tumor cell collections resembling Pautrier's microabscesses in mycosis fungoides and also resembling the lymphoepithelial lesions of clustered mucosal invasion found in mucosa-associated B-cell lymphomas (MALTomas) (Fig. 8-23).[179] More extensive epithelial involvement leads to extensive mucosal ulceration and associated inflammation. The tumor cells are usually large or immunoblastic, although in a minority of cases, a predominant small cell component is found. Scattered Reed-Sternberg-like cells are frequently found. Admixed plasma cells and eosinophils may be found. In areas grossly uninvolved by neoplasm, there may be a background of celiac disease changes with villous atrophy and increased numbers of normal appearing intraepithelial T cells. Microscopic foci of intramucosal tumor may be found within this background of celiac disease distant from the main tumor mass.[176] Background celiac disease type changes, however, are not seen in a significant number of cases.

Involved lymph nodes show paracortical infiltration by malignant cells (Fig. 8-23). Generalized disease can involve not only lymph nodes, but other sites including spleen, liver, and lung.[176,177]

Phenotype. The neoplastic cells are T cells, with a characteristic CD3+, CD7+, CD4−, CD8− or CD8+ phenotype. CD5 and HLA-DR are generally absent.[176] The CD3+, CD7+, CD4, and CD8 "double negative" phenotype is also found in a proportion of intraepithelial T cells in normal small intestine. Interestingly, it is this same T-cell subset that is expanded in celiac disease.[181] The tumor cells also frequently express HML-1, an antigen expressed by, though not specific for, intestinal intraepithelial T cells.[181,183] By paraffin immunohistochemistry, the neoplastic cells stain with CD3 and CD45RO. CD30 is also frequently expressed[178] and may be a useful marker to detect malignant cells in areas where the neoplastic infiltrate is obscured by acute inflammation from mucosal ulceration. The tumor cells also express *p53* and generally show a very high proliferative index when stained with MIB1, a marker of proliferating cells.[178]

Genotype. Genotyping shows rearrangement of the TCRβ chain gene. Interestingly, this rearrangement is also frequently detected in areas of the small bowel unaffected by tumor, but involved by celiac disease[178,182] and has also been described in small bowel biopsies from a patient with adult onset celiac disease who lacked histologic evidence of malignant lymphoma, suggesting that the celiac disease lesions may in fact be precursor T-cell lymphoma lesions in some cases.[182]

Clinical. Enteropathy associated T-cell lymphoma is a disease of older patients, with a median age of about 60 years. Although controversial, it is generally believed that the disease is strongly associated with celiac disease. Many patients present with celiac disease type symptoms, with months to years of abdominal pain and weight loss. However, a significant number present as an acute abdominal emergency with perforation or obstruction[176] without antecedent celiac disease symptoms.

The disease is generally aggressive with frequent recurrences. The majority of patients die within 6 months of diagnosis. Survival is better in patients with localized (stage I) than advanced disease.[176]

Differential Diagnosis. These lymphomas may be mistaken for high grade MALT-type B-cell lymphomas because of the epitheliotropism (mucosal lymphoepithelial lesions) of the lymphoid cells. Immunohistochemistry will reliably distinguish these two entities.

Hepatosplenic γ/δ T-Cell Lymphoma

Definition. This is a neoplasm of γ/δ "double negative" T cells that is characteristically associated with hepatosplenomegaly, but minimal lymph node involvement.[184–186]

Morphology. In the spleen there is sinusoidal infiltration of the red pulp by fairly uniform, medium sized lymphoid cells that have oval or folded nuclei, somewhat condensed chromatin, and moderate amounts of pale cytoplasm.[184] Splenic involvement may lead to massive splenic enlargement. A similar lymphoid infiltrate is seen in the hepatic sinusoids. Lymph node involvement is likewise characterized by a sinusoidal and interfollicular neoplastic infiltrate leading to partial or complete nodal effacement.

Phenotype. The neoplastic cells phenotype as CD3+ TCRδ1+ α/β TCR−. Characteristically they lack both CD4 and CD8 expression and are double negative by typing (Fig. 8-1). Expression of the other pan T-cell antigens, CD2 and CD5, may be weak or absent.[185,186] Most of the cases described express the NCAM CD56.[184–186] In paraffin section immunohistochemistry, the neoplastic infiltrate phenotypes as a T-cell infiltrate (CD3+ CD45RO+ CD43+). When paraffin section immunohistochemistry is performed, it is important not to rely exclusively on CD43 staining, as myeloid leukemia likewise will be CD43+ and may show a similar sinusoidal infiltration pattern (Fig. 8-9).

Genotype. All cases show rearrangement of the γ/δ TCR and, additionally, may show α/β TCR rearrangement.[184–186]

Clinical Featores. The disease may be aggressive, requiring multiagent chemotherapy. Patients typically present with fever, myalgia, arthralgia, and weight loss. This may lead to a clinical evaluation for fever of unknown origin. Splenomegaly or hepatomegaly may be presenting signs or develop during the course of the illness. The peripheral blood shows a normal white blood cell count and anemia. There may be either thrombocytopenia or thrombocytosis. Although the white cell count is normal, examination of the peripheral smear reveals the presence of atypical lymphocytes, although these may account for only a small percentage of cells at initial presentation. The disease may sometimes not respond to multiagent chemotherapy.

Differential Diagnosis. Differential diagnosis of the splenic infiltrate lies between T-cell lymphoma, hairy cell leukemia, and myeloid leukemia. The differential diagnosis in the lymph nodes would lie between T-cell lymphoma and a leukemic infiltrate. Immunophenotyping either on fresh or paraffin fixed tissue is essential to ensure the correct diagnosis. Since helper and cytotoxic T-cell antigens are absent, demonstration of the γ/δ TCR1 framework determinants is essential. Furthermore, an absence of S100 is essential in excluding S100+ PTL, which may also have a sinusoidal hepatosplenic pattern of involvement.

Lymph Nodes in Mycosis Fungoides/ Sezary Syndrome

Definition. Mycosis fungoides (MF) is a neoplasm of mature helper (CD4+) T cells that have a propensity for dermal and epidermal localization (e.g., Pautrier's microabcesses) (Fig. 8-24). The skin disease generally progresses slowly over a period of years from erythroderma to plaque-type lesions and finally to frank skin tumors. Many patients develop an associated lymphadenopathy during the course of disease, while some in addition show circulating atypical

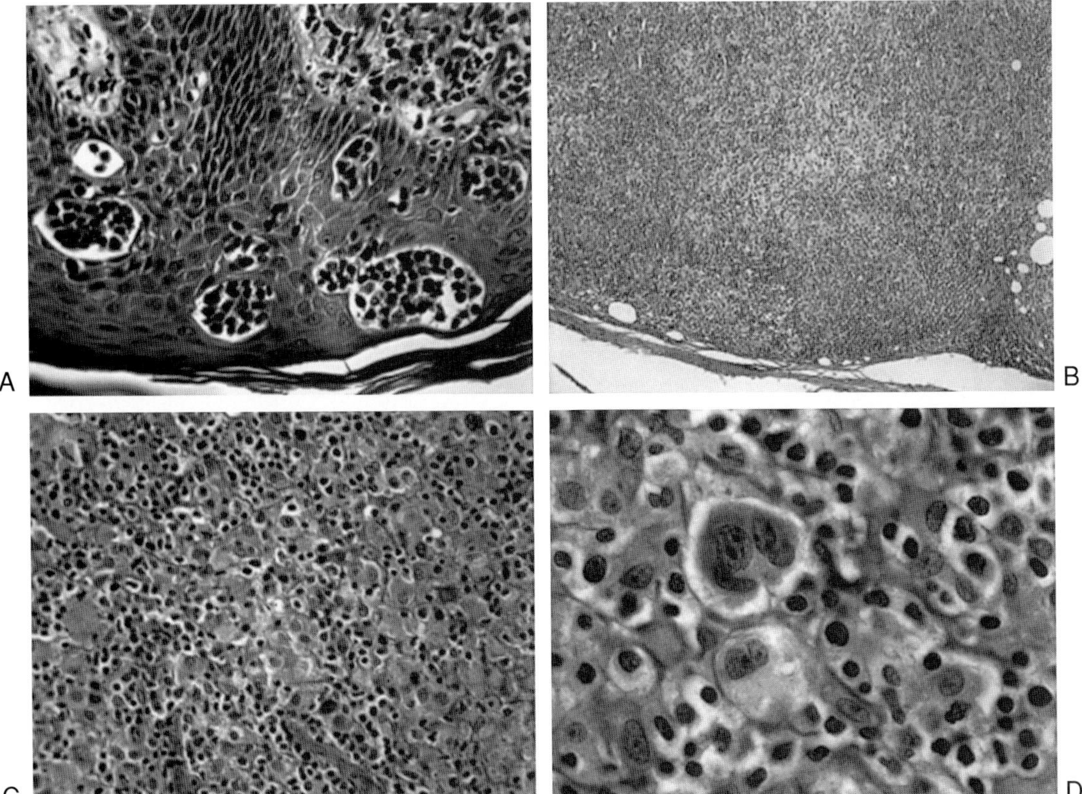

Fig. 8-24. (A–D) Mycosis fungoides involving the epidermis **(A),** in association with dermatopathic lymphadenopathy (LN1) **(B).** Fig. C is another example with more frequent atypical, cerebriform cells (LN2) that progressed to LN4 with Reed-Sternberg cells **(D).**

lymphocytes. This latter constellation of findings is termed Sezary syndrome. The discussion that follows is limited to the lymph node findings in MF/SS.[182–197]

Morphology. Patients with MF frequently develop lymphadenopathy in the course of their disease (Fig. 8-24). Histologic examination of excised lymph nodes shows one of three patterns in these patients: (1) lymph node hyperplasia (uncommon), (2) dermatopathic lymphadenopathy, or (3) frank lymphomatous effacement.

Dermatopathic lymphadenopathy is commonly found in lymph nodes draining areas of erythroderma in MF. Dermatopathic lymphadenopathy is characterized by a paracortical proliferation of histiocytes, Langerhans cells, and interdigitating reticulum cells, which impart a characteristic pale, mottled appearance to the paracortex at low power. Some of the histiocytes contain melanin. Intermixed within the T-cell zone are small lymphocytes and scattered plasma cells. Residual follicles may be compressed, but are preserved. Careful examination will also frequently reveal atypical lymphocytes either singly or in clusters admixed with the histiocytic infiltrate.[192] These atypical lymphocytes range from small lymphocytes with condensed chromatin and convoluted nuclei to immunoblasts and multinucleated/multilobated cells resembling Reed-Sternberg cells (Fig. 8-24).[189] The presence of these atypical cells suggests these dermatopathic nodes are partially involved by lymphoma and has led to efforts to quantify the extent of nodal involvement by enumerating the number of atypical cells present. The resulting grading systems developed, however, have not been of clear predictive value for clinical course in mulitvariate analysis.[187–194] Moreover, identification of atypical lymphoid cells in the context of dermatopathic lymphadenopathy is not limited to cases of MF/SS, but can also be seen in dermatopathic lymphadenopathy associated with a variety of benign skin disorders.[193]

Nodal Involvement by Frank Lymphoma in MF/SS

Nodal effacement by lymphoma can be seen both in MF and SS. In MF the neoplastic infiltrate is composed predominantly of large cells or immunoblasts with a varying number of admixed smaller atypical convoluted lymphocytes. Reed-Sternberg-like cells may also be present. The backgound may contain reactive plasma cells, eosinophils, and foci of fibrosis as well as residual dermatopathic changes. In contrast to the predominance of large cells seen in nodes effaced by MF, the lymph nodes in SS characteristically show a monotonous infiltrate of medium sized atypical lymphocytes with irregular or convoluted nuclei. Dermatopathic changes are generally not seen.[195]

Phenotype. The neoplastic cells in MF and SS phenotype as helper T cells (CD3 + CD4 +). The neoplastic cells show characteristic absence of CD7 expression. While a population of CD7 − T cells can be detected in morphologically benign cutaneous lymphoid infiltrates,[196] the presence of a significant population of such CD7 − T cells in lymph node is strongly supportive of T-cell neoplasia.[40] Like other T-cell neoplasms, the neoplastic infiltrate in MF or SS may show loss of other pan T-cell antigens such as CD5 or CD2.

Genotype. The neoplastic cells in MF/SS show clonal TCRβ gene rearrangement. Rearrangement of the TCRβ can be detected by Southern blotting in MF/SS nodes that are partially or totally effaced by lymphoma, as well as in some dermatopathic nodes that contain atypical T cells. Interestingly, patients whose dermatopathic nodes show clonal gene rearrangements have significantly poorer clinical outcome than those with similar lymph node histology but whose nodes lack a clonal T-cell population.[197]

Differential Diagnosis. In some cases of nodal involvement by MF, the presence of Reed-Sternberg-like malignant cells as well as a background of plasma cells, eosinophils, and fibrosis may raise the differential of Hodgkin's disease; however, the presence of atypical lymphocytes in the background milieu should exclude this possibility.

ACKNOWLEDGEMENT

This chapter was supported in part by SWOG Lymphoma Biology Repository grant CA32102

REFERENCES

1. Harris NL, Jaffe ES, Stein H et al: A revised European-American classification of lymphoid neoplasms: a proposal from the International Lymphoma Study Group. Blood 84:1361, 1994
2. Grogan TM, Spier CM, Richter LC et al: Immunologic approaches to the classification of non-Hodgkin's lymphomas. P. 3. In Bennett JM, Foonk A (eds): Immunologic Approaches to the Classification and Management of Lymphomas and Leukemias. Norwell, MA, Kluwer Academic Publishers, 1988
3. Waldron JA, Leech JH, Glick AD et al: Malignant lymphoma of peripheral T-lymphocyte origin. Cancer 40:1604, 1977
4. Jaffe E: Post-thymic lymphoid neoplasia. P. 344. in Jaffe E (ed): Surgical Pathology of the Lymph Nodes and Related Organs. Major Problems in Pathology, 16. 2nd Ed. Philadelphia, WB, Saunders, 1995
5. Weisenburger D, Linder J, Armitage J: Peripheral T-cell lymphoma. A clinicopathologic study of 42 cases. Hematol Oncol 5:175, 1987
6. Borowitz M, Reichert T, Brynes R, et al: The phenotypic diversity of peripheral T-cell lymphomas. The Southestern Cancer Study Group experience. Hum Pathol 17:567, 1986
7. Weiss LM, Crabtree GS, Rouse RV et al: Morphologic and immunologic characterization of

50 peripheral T-cell lymphomas. Am J Pathol 118:316, 1985

8. Grogan TM, Fielder K, Rangel C et al: Peripheral T-cell lymphoma—aggressive disease with heterogeneous immunotypes. Am J of Clin Pathol 83:279, 1985
9. Foucar K, Armitage J, Dick F: Malignant lymphomas, diffuse mixed small and large cell. A clinicopathologic study of 47 cases. Cancer 51: 2090, 1983
10. Medeiros L, Lardelli P, Stetler-Stevenson M et al: Genotypic analysis of diffuse, mixed cell lymphomas: comparison with morphologic and immunophenotypic findings. Am J Clin Pathol 95:547, 1991
11. Luke RJ, Collins RD: New approaches to the classification of the lymphomata. Br J Cancer 31:1, 1975
12. Lennert K: Malignant Lymphomas Other Than Hodgkin's Disease: Histology, Cytology, Ultrastructure, Immunology. New York, Spinger-Verlag 1978
13. Watanabe S, Nakajima T, Shimosato Y, et al: T-cell malignancies: subclassification and interrelationship. Jpn J Clin Oncol 9:423, 1979
14. Muller-Hermelink HK, Steinmann G, Stein H, Lennert K: Malignant lymphoma of plasmacytoid T cells. Morphologic and immunologic studies characterizing a special type of T cell. Am J Surg Pathol 7:849, 1983
15. Kim H, Jacobs C, Warnke RA, Dorfman RF: Malignant lymphoma with a high content of epithelioid histiocytes. A distinct clinicopathologic entity and a form of so-called "Lennert's lymhoma." Cancer 41:620, 1978
16. Tamaki T, Katagiri S, Kanayama Y et al: Helper T-cell lymphoma with marked plasmacytosis and polyclonal hypergammaglobulinemia. Cancer 53:1590, 1984
17. Prastohofer EF, Grizzie WE, Prchal JT, Grossi CE: Plasmacytoid T-cell lymphoma associated with chronic myeloproliferative disorder. Am J Clin Pathol 9:380, 1985
18. Kadin ME, Kamoun M, Lamberg J: Erythrophagocytic T gamma lymphoma: a clinicopathologic entity resembling malignant histiocytosis. N Engl J Med 304:648, 1981
19. Chott A, Augustin I, Wra F, Hanak H, et al: Peripheral T-cell lymphomas—a clinicopathologic study of 75 cases. Hum Pathol 21:1117, 1990
20. Greer JP, York JC, Cousar JB, et al: Peripheral T-cell lymphoma: a clincopathologic study of 42 cases. J Clin Oncol 2:788, 1984
21. Greenberg BR, Grogan TM, Takasug GJ, et al: A unique malignant T-cell lymphoproliferative disorder with neutropenia simulating hairy cell leukemia. Cancer 56:2823, 1985
22. Shimoyama M, Mirato K, Saito H, et al: Immunoblastic lymphadenopathy (IBL)-like T-cell lymphoma. Jpn J Clin Oncol 9:347, 1979
23. Jaffe ES: Pathologic and clinical spectrum of post-thymic T-cell malignancies. Cancer Invest 2:413, 1984
24. Lippman SM, Grogan TM, Spier CM et al: Lethal midline granuloma with a novel T-cell phenotype as found in peripheral T-cell lymphoma. Cancer 59:936, 1987
25. Jaffe ES, Blattner EA, Blaynew DW et al: The pathologic spectrum of adult T-cell leukemia/ lymphoma in the United States. Human T-cell leukemia/lymphoma virus-associated lymphoid malignancies. Am J Surg Pathol 8:263, 1984
26. Uchiyama T, Yodoi J, Sagawa K, et al: Adult T-cell leukemia: clincial and hematologic features of 16 cases. Blood 50:481, 1977
27. Blattner WA, Kalyanaraman VS, Robert-Guroff M et al: The human type-C retrovirus, HTLV, in blacks from the Caribbean region and relationship to adult T-cell leukemia/lymphoma. Int J Cancer 30:2457, 1982
28. Oliver JD, Grogan TM, Payne CM et al: Burkitt's-like lymphoma of T-cell type. Mod Pat 1: 15, 1988
29. Grogan TM, Payne CM, Richter LC, Rangel CS: Signet-ring cell lymphoma of T-cell origin. An immunocytochemical and ultrastructural study relating giant vacuole formation to cytoplasmic sequestration of surface membrane. Am J Surg Pathol 9:684, 1985
30. Weiss L, Wood G, Dorfman R: T-cell signet-ring cell lymphoma. Am J Surg Pathol 9:273, 1985
31. Wright DH: T-cell lymphomas. Histopathology 10:321, 1986
32. Suchi T, Lennert K, Tu L-Y: Histopathology and immunohistochemistry of peripheral T-cell lymphomas: a proposal for their classification. J Clin Pathol 40:995, 1987
33. Lippman SM, Miller TP, Spier CM et al: The prognostic significance of the T-cell phenotype in diffuse large cell lymphoma: a comparative study of the T-cell and B-cell phenotype. Blood 72:436, 1988

34. Coiffier B, Brousse N, Peuchmaur M et al: Peripheral T-cell lymphomas have a worse prognosis than B-cell lymphomas: a prospective study of 361 immunophenotyped patients treated with the LNH-84 regimen. Ann Oncol 1:45, 1990
35. Waldmann TA, Davis MM, Bongiovanni KF: Rearrangements of genes for the antigen receptor on T cells as markers of lineage and clonality in human lymphoid neoplasms. N Engl J Med 313:776, 1985
36. Stein H, Bonk A, Tolksdorf G: Immunohistologic analysis of the organization of normal lymphoid tissue and non-Hodgkin's lymphomas. J Histochem Cytochem 28:746, 1980
37. Collins RD, Waldron JA, Glick AD: Results of multiparameter studies of T-cell lymphoid neoplasms. Am J Clin Pathol 72:699, 1979
38. Weiss L, Picker L, Grogan T et al: Absence of clonal beta and gamma T-cell receptor gene rearrangements in a subset of peripheral T-cell lymphomas. Am J Pathol 130:436, 1988
39. Hastrup N, Ralfkiaer E, Pallesen G: Aberrant phenotypes in peripheral T-cell lymphomas. J Clin Pathol 42:398, 1989
40. Picker L, Weiss LM, Medeiros LJ et al: Immunophenotypic criteria for the diagnosis of non-Hodgkin's lymphoma. Am J Pathol 128:181, 1987
41. Quintanilla-Martinez L, Preffer F, Rubin D, et al: CD20+ T-cell lymphoma: neoplastic transformation of a normal T-cell subset. Am J Clin Pathol 102:483, 1994
42. Sklar J: Antigen receptor genes: structure, function, and techniques for analysis of their rearrangements. p. 211. In Knowles D. (ed): Neoplastic Hematopathology. Williams & Wilkins, Baltimore, 1992
43. Medeiros LJ, Bagg A, Cossman J: Application of molecular genetics to the diagnosis of hematopoietic neoplasms. p. 299. In Knowles D (ed): Neoplastic Hematopathology. Williams & Wilkins, Baltimore, 1992
44. Picker LJ, Brenner MB, Michie S, Warnke RA: Expression of T cell receptor delta chains in benign and malignant T lineage lymphoproliferations. Am J Pathol 132:401, 1988
45. Trainor KJ, Brisco MJ, Wan JH et al: Gene rearrangement in B- and T-lymphoproliferative disease detected by the polymerase chain reaction Blood 78:192, 1991
46. Davis RE, Warnke RA, Dorfman RF, Cleary ML: Utility of molecular genetic analysis for the diagnosis of neoplasia in morphologically and immunophenotypically equivocal hematolymphoid lesions. Cancer 67:2890, 1991
47. Medeiros LJ, Bagg A, Cossman J: Molecular genetics in the diagnosis and classification of lymphoid neoplasms. P. 58. In Jaffe E (ed): Surgical Pathology of the Lymph Nodes and Related Organs. WB Saunders, Philadelphia, 1985
48. Sheibani K, Wu A, Ben-Ezra J et al: Rearrangement of K-chain and T-cell receptor β-chain genes in malignant lymphomas of "T-cell" phenotype. Am J Pathol 129:201, 1987
49. Weiss LM, Picker LJ, Grogan TM et al: Absence of clonal beta and gamma T-cell receptor gene rearrangements in a subset of peripheral T-cell lymphomas. Am J Pathol 130:436, 1988
50. Zarate-Osorno A, Raffeld M, Berman EL et al: S100-positive T-cell lymphoproliferative disorder: a case report and review of the literature. Am J Clin Pathol 102:478, 1994
51. Hanson CA, Bockenstedt PL, Schnitzer B et al: S100-positive, T-cell chronic lymphoproliferative disease: an aggressive disorder of an uncommon T-cell subset. Blood 78:1803, 1991
52. Ferrari C, Sansoni P, Rowden G et al: One half of the CD11b+ human peripheral blood T lymphocytes coexpresses the S100 protein. Clin Exp Immunol 72:357, 1988
53. Suzushima H, Asou N, Hattori T, Takatsuki K: Adult T-cell leukemia derived from S100 positive double-negative (CD4− CD8−) T cells. Leuk Lymphoma 13:257, 1994
54. Ruco LP, Stoppacciaro A, Barsotti P et al: S100+ lymph node neoplasm: report of a case with histological and immunological features intermediate between T-cell lymphoma and malignant histiocytosis. Virchows Arch (A) 404: 351, 1984
55. Takahashi K, Ohtsuki Y, Sonobe H et al: S100 positive T-cell leukemia. Blood 71:1299, 1988
56. Takahashi K, Yoshino T, Hayashi K, et al: S100 beta positive T lymphocytes: their characteristics and behavior under normal and pathologic conditions. Blood 70:214, 1987
57. Chan JKC, Ng CS, Chu YC, Wong KF: S100 protein-positive sinusoidal large cell lymphoma. Hum Pathol 18:756, 1987
58. Kern WE, Spier CM, Miller TP, Grogan TM: NCAM (CD56)-positive malignant lymphoma. Leuk Lymphoma 12:1, 1993
59. Kern WF, Spier CM, Hanneman EH, et al: Neu-

ral cell adhesion moleule-positive peripheral T-cell lymphoma: a rare variant with a propensity for unusual sites of involvement. Blood 79: 2432, 1992

60. Wong KF, Chan JK, Ng CS et al: CD56 (NKH-1)-positive hematolymphoid malignancies: an aggressive neoplasm featuring frequent cutaneous/mucosal involvement, cytoplasmic azurophilic granules, and angiocentricity. Hum Pathol 23:798, 1992
61. Lanier LL, Le AM, Ding A et al: Expression of Leu-19 (NKH-1) antigen on IL 2-dependent cytotoxic and noncytotoxic T-cell lines. J Immunol 138:2019, 1987
62. Hoffman S, Edelman GM: Kinetics of homophilic binding by embryonic and adult forms of the neural cell adhesion molecule. Proc Natl Acad Sci USA 80:5762, 1983
63. Macon WR, Williams ME, Greer JP et al: Natural killer-like T-cell lymphomas: CD56+ peripheral T-cell lymphomas of large granular lymphocytes with aggressive clinical course. Blood 87:1474, 1996
64. Aisenberg A, Wilkes B, Harris N et al: Chronic T-cell lymphocytosis with neutropenia: report of a case studied with monoclonal antibody. Blood 58:818, 1981
65. Grogan TM, Guptill V, Mullen J et al: Polysialated NCAM as a neurodeterminant in malignant lymphoma (ML). Acad Pathol Abstr 1994
66. Edelman GM: Cell adhesion molecules in the regulation of animal form and tissue pattern. Annu Rev Cell Biol 2:81, 1986
67. Troy FA: Polysialylation: from bacteria to brains. Glycobiology 2:5, 1992
68. Henni T, Gaulard P, Divine M et al: Comparison of genetic probe with immunophenotype analysis in lymphoproliferative disorders: a study of 81 cases. Blood 72:1937, 1988
69. Van Tol EAF, Verspaget HW, Pena S, et al: The CD56 adhesion molecule is the major determinant for detecting non-major histocompatibility complex-restricted cytotoxic mononuclear cells from the intestinal lamina propria. Eur J Immunol 22:23, 1992
70. Abo T: Extrathymic pathways of T-cell differentiation: a primitive and fundamental immune system. Microbiol Immunol 37:247, 1993
71. Kingma DW, Raffeld M, Jaffe ES: Differential diagnosis of CD3+, CD56+ T-cell leukemias. Blood 85:1675, 1994
72. Emile J, Boulland M, Haioun C et al: CD5− CD56+ "TCR silent peripheral T-cell lymphomas" are natural killer cell lymphomas. Blood 87:1466, 1996
73. Suzumiya J, Takeshita M, Kimura N et al: Expression of adult and fetal natural killer cell markers in sinonasal lymphomas. Blood 83: 2255, 1994
74. Zarate-Osorno A, Raffeld M, Berman EL et al: S100 positive T-cell lymphoproliferative disorder: a case report and review of the literature. Am J Clin Pathol 102:478, 1994
75. Hanson CA, Bockenstedt PL, Schnitzer B, et al: S100-positive, T-cell chronic lymphoproliferative disease: an aggressive disorder of an uncommon T-cell subset. Blood 78:1803, 1991
76. Farcet J, Gaulard P, Marolleau J, et al: Hepatosplenic T-cell lymphoma: sinusal/sinusoidal localization of malignant cells expressing the T-cell receptor γ/δ. Blood 75:2213, 1990
77. Gaulard P, Bourquelot P, Kanavaros P et al: Expression of the alpha/beta and gamma/delta T-cell receptors in 57 cases of peripheral T-cell lymphomas: identification of a subset of γ/δ T-cell lymphomas. Am J Pathol 137:617, 1990
78. Loughran T: Clonal diseases of large granular lymphocytes. Blood 82:1, 1993
79. Gentile TC, Uner AH, Hutchinson RE et al: CD3+, CD56+ aggressive variant of large granular lymphocyte leukemia. Blood 84:2315, 1994
80. Phillips JH, Hori T, Nagler A, Bhat N, Lanier LL. Ontogeny of human natural killer (NK) cells: fetal NK cells mediate cytotoxic function and express cytoplasmic CD3ϵ, δprotein. J Exp Med 175:1055, 1992.
81. Lanier LL, Chang C, Spits H, Phillips JH. Expression of cytoplasmic CD3ϵ proteins in activated human adult natural killer (NK) cells and CD3 γ, δ, ϵ complexes in fetal NK cells. J Immunol 149:1876, 1992.
82. Imamura N, Kusunoki Y, Kawa-Ha K, Yumura K, Hara J, Oda K, Abe K, Dohy H, Inada T, Kajihara H, Kuramoto A. Aggressive natural killer cell leukaemia/lymphoma: report of four cases and review of literature. British J of Haematology 75:49-59, 1990.
83. Sun T, Brody J, Susin M, Marino J, Teichberg S, Koduru P, Hall W, Urmacher C, Hajdu S. Aggressive natural killer cell lymphoma/leukemia. Am J Surg Pathol 17:1289-1299, 1993.
84. Falini B, Pileri S, Stein H, Dienenmann D, Dallenbach F, Delsol G, Minelli O, Poggi S, Mar-

telli M, Pallesen G, Palestro G. Variable expressio of leucocyte-common (CD45) antigen in CD30 (Kil)-positive anaplastic large-cell lymphoma: Implications for the differential diagnosis between lymphoid and nonlymphoid malignancies. Hum Pathol 21:624, 1990.

85. Herbst H, Tippelmann G, Anagnostopoulos I et al: Immunoglobulin and T-cell receptor gene rearrangements in Hodgkin's disease and Ki-1-positive anaplastic large cell lymhoma: dissociation between phenotype and genotype. Leuk Res 13:103, 1989
86. Agnarsson B, Kadin ME: Ki-1 positive large cell lymphoma: a morphologic and immunologic study of 19 cases. Am J Surg Pathol 12: 264, 1988
87. Delsol G, Blancher A, Al Saati T, et al: Antibody BNH9 detects red blood cell-related antigens on anaplastic large cell (CD30+) lymphomas. Br J Cancer 64:321, 1991
88. Delsol G, Al Saati T, Gatter K, et al: Coexpression of epithelial membrane antigen (EMA), Ki-1, and interleukin-2 receptor by anaplastic large cell lymphomas: diagnostic value in so-called malignant histiocytosis. Am J Pathol 130:59, 1988
89. Saati TA, Tkaczuk J, Krissansen G, et al: A novel antigen detected by the CBF.78 antibody further distinguishes anaplastic large cell lymphoma from Hodgkin's disease. Blood 86:2741, 1995
90. Mason D, Bastard C, Rimokh R et al: CD30-positive large cell lymphomas (''Ki-1 lymphoma'') are associated with a chromosomal translocation involving 5q35. Br J Haematol 74: 161, 1990
91. Bitter MA, Franklin WA, Larson RA et al: Morphology in Ki-1 (CD30)-positive non-Hodgkin's lymphoma is correlated with clinical features and the presence of a unique chromosomal abnormality, t(2;5)(p23;q35). Am J Surg Pathof 14:305, 1990
92. Bullrich F, Morris SW, Hummel M et al: Nucleophosmin (NPM) gene rearrangements in Ki-1-positive lymphomas. Cancer Res 54:2873, 1994
93. Downing JR, Shurtleff SA, Zielenska M, et al: Molecular detection of the (2;5) translocation of non-Hodgkin's lymphoma by reverse transcriptase-polymerase chain reaction. Blood 85: 3416, 1995
94. de Bruin PC, Beljaards RC, Van Heerde P et al: Differences in clinical behaviour and immunophenotype between primary cutaneous and primary nodal anaplastic large cell lymphoma of T-cell or null cell phenotype. Histopathology 23:127, 1993
95. Kadin ME, Sako D, Berliner N et al: Childhood Ki-1 lymphoma presenting with skin lesions and peripheral lymphadenopathy. Blood 68:1042, 1986
96. Pileri S, Bocchia M, Baroni CD et al: Anaplastic large cell lymphoma (CD30+/Ki-1+): results of a prospective clinico-pathological study of 69 cases. Br J Haematol 86:513, 1994
97. Diez-Martin JL, Lust JA, Witzig TE, et al: Unusual presentation of extranodal peripheral T-cell lymphomas with multiple paraneoplastic features. Cancer 68:834, 1991
98. Falini B, Pileri S, De Solas I et al: Peripheral T-cell lymphoma associated with hemophagocytic syndrome. Blood 75:434, 1990
99. Lennert K, Mestdeagh J: Hodgkin's disease with constantly high content of epithelioid cells. Virchows Arch 344:1, 1968
100. Kim H, Nathwani BN, Rappaport H: So-called ''Lennert's lymphoma'': is it a clinicopathologic entity? Cancer 45:1379, 1980
101. Burke JS, Butler JJ: Malignant lymphoma with a high content of epithelioid histiocytes (Lennert's lymphoma). Am J Clin Pathol 66:1, 1976
102. Braylan RC, Long JC, Jaffe ES et al: Malignant lymphoma obscurred by concomitant extensive epithelioid granulomas. Cancer 39:1146, 1977
103. Palutke M, Varadachari C, Weise RW, et al: Lennert's lymphoma: a T-cell neoplasm. Am J Clin Pathol 69:643, 1978
104. Feller AC, Griesser GH, Mak TW, Lennert K: Lymphoepithelioid lymphoma (Lennert's lymphoma) is a monoclonal proliferation of helper/inducer T-cells. Blood 68:663, 1986
105. Spier C, Miller T, Lippman S, Grogan T: Lennert's lymphoma. Cancer 61:517–24, 1988
106. Grey HM, Colon SM, Chestnut RW: Requirements for the processing of antigen by antigen-presenting B-cells: II. Biochemical comparison of the fate of antigen in B-cell tumors and macrophages. J Immunol 129:2389, 1982
107. Simrell CR, Margolick JB, Crabtree GR et al: Lymphokine-induced phagocytosis in angiocentric immunoproliferative lesions (AIL) and malignant lymphoma arising in AIL. Blood 65: 1469, 1985
108. Yao M, Cheng A-L, Su I-J et al: Clinicopatho-

logical spectrum of haemophagocytic syndrome in Epstein-Barr virus-associated peripheral T-cell lymphoma. Br J Haematol 87:535, 1994

109. Su I-J, Hsu Y-H, Lin M-T et al: Epstein-Barr virus-containing T-cell lymphoma presents with hemophagocytic syndrome mimicking malignant histiocytosis. Cancer 72:2019, 1993
110. Craig FE, Clare CN, Sklar JL, Banks PM: T-cell lymphoma and the virus-associated hemophagocytic syndrome. Am J Clin Pathol 97:189, 1992
111. Gaffey MJ, Frierson HF, Medeiros LJ, Weiss LM: The relationship of Epstein-Barr virus infection-related (sporadic) and familial hemophagocytic syndrome and secondary (lymphoma-related) hemophagocytosis: an in situ hybridization study. Hum Pathol 24:657, 1993
112. Pileri S, Sabattini E, Falini B: Lymphohistiocytic T-cell lymphoma and peripheral T-cell lymphoma associated with haemophagocytic syndrome: two recently recognized entities which mimic malignant histiocytosis. Leuk Lymphoma 6:317, 1992
113. Chubachi A, Imai H, Nishimura S, et al: Nasal T-cell lymphoma associated with hemophagocytic syndrome. Immunohistochemical and genotypic studies. Arch pathol Lab Med 116:1209, 1992
114. Henter J-I, Elinder G, Öst A et al: Diagnostic guidelines for hemophagocytic lymphohistiocytosis. Semin Oncol 18:29, 1991
115. Wilson MS, Weiss LM, Gatter KC et al: Malignant histiocytosis: a reassessment of cases previously reported in 1975 based on paraffin section immunophenotyping studies. Cancer 66:530, 1990
116. Okada Y, Nakanishi I: Angiotropic B-cell lymphoma with hemophagocytic syndrome. Pathol Res Pract 190:718, 1994
117. Frizzera G, Moran EM, Rappaport H: Angioimmunoblastic lymphadenopathy with dysproteinaemia. Lancet 1:1070, 1974
118. Frizzera G, Moran EM, Rappaport H: Angioimmunoblastic lymphadenopathy: diagnosis and clinical course. Am J Med 59:803, 1975
119. Lukes RJ, Tindle BH: Immunoblastic Lymphadenopathy. Workshop on the Classification of Non-Hodgkin's Lymphoma. University of Chicago, Chicago, June 25–29, 1973
120. Lukes RJ, Tindle BH: Immunoblastic lymphadenopathy: a hyperimmune entity resembling Hodgkin's disease. N Engl J Med 292:1, 1975
121. Nathwani BN, Jaffe ES: Angioimmunoblastic lymphadenopathy (AILD) and AILD-like T-cell lymphomas. In Jaffe E (ed): P. 390. Surgical Pathology of the Lymph Nodes and Related Organs. 2nd Ed. WB Saunders, Philadelphia, 1995
122. Frizzera G: Atypical lymphoproliferative disorders. P. 459. In Knowles DM (ed): Neoplastic Hematopathology. Williams & Wilkins, Baltimore, 1992
123. Frizzera G, Kaneko Y, Sakurai M: Angioimmunoblastic lymphadenopathy and related disorders: a retrospective look in search of definitions. Leukemia 3:1, 1989
124. Lennert K: Pathologisch-histologische Klassifizierimg der malignen lymphome. P. 181. In Stacher A (ed): Leukaemien und Maligne lymphome. Urban & Schwarzenberg, Munich, 1973
125. Nathwani BN, Rappaport H, Moran EM et al: Malignant lymphoma arising in angioimmunoblastic lymphadenopathy. Cancer 41:578, 1978
126. Weiss LM, Stricler JG, Dorfman RF et al: Clonal T-cell populations in angioimmunoblastic lymphadenopathy and angioimmunoblastic lymphadenopathy-like lymphoma. Am J Pathol 122:392, 1986
127. Knecht H, Odermatt BF, Hayoz D et al: Polyclonal rearrangements of the T-cell receptor beta-chain in fatal angioimmunoblastic lymphadenopathy. Br J Haematol 73:491, 1989
128. Schelgelberger B, Zhang Y, Weber-Matthiesen K, Grote W: Detection of aberrant clones in nearly all cases of angioimmunoblastic lymphadenopathy with dysproteinemia-type T-cell lymphoma by combined interphase and metaphase cytogenetics. Blood 84:2640, 1994
129. Feller AC, Griesser H, Schilling CV et al: Clonal gene rearrangement patterns correlate with immunophenotype and clinical parameters in patients with angioimmunoblastic lymphadenopathy. Am J Pathol 133:549, 1988
130. Watanabe S, Shimosato Y, Shimayama M: Adult T-cell lymphoma with hypergammaglobulinemia. Cancer 46:2472, 1980
131. Siegert W, Agthe A, Griesser H, et al: Treatment of angioimmunoblastic lymphadenopathy (AILD)-type T-cell lymphoma using prednisone with or without the COPBLAM/IMVP-16 regimen. A multicenter study. Ann Intern Med 117: 364, 1992
132. Knecht H, Odermatt BF, Maurer R, Riittner JR: Diagnostic and prognostic value of monoclonal

antibodies in immunophenotyping of angioimmunoblastic lymphadenopathy/lymphogranulomatosis X. Br J Haematol 67:19, 1982

133. Jaffe ES, Chan JKC, Su I-H, et al: Report of the workshop on nasal and related extranodal angiocentric T/NK-cell lymphomas. Definitions, differential diagnosis, and epidemiology. Am J Surg Pathol 20:103, 1996
134. Pinkus GS, Said JW: Peripheral T-cell lymphomas. P. 837. In Knowles D (ed): Neoplastic Hematopathology. Williams & Wilkins, Baltimore, 1982.
135. Medeiros LJ, Peiper SC, Elwood L, et al: Angiocentric immunoproliferative lesions: a molecular analysis of eight cases. Hum Pathol 22:1150, 1991
136. Ho FCS, Choy D, Loke SL et al: Polymorphic reticulosis and conventional lymphomas of the nose and upper aerodigestive tract: a clinicopathologic study of 70 cases, and immunophenotypic studies of 16 cases. Hum Pathol 21: 1041, 1990
137. Guniee U, Jaffe E, Kingma D et al: Pulmonary lymphomatoid granulomatosis: evidence of Epstein-Barr virus infected B-lymphocytes with a predominant T-cell component and vasculitis. Am J Surg Pathol 18:753, 1994
138. Uchiyama T, Yodoi J, Sagawa K, et al: Adult T-cell leukemia: Clinical and hematologic features of 16 cases. Blood 50:481, 1977.
139. Poiesz B, Ruscetti F, Gazdar A: Detection and isolation of type C retrovirus particles from fresh and cultured lymphocytes of a patient with cutaneous T-cell lymphoma. Proc Natl Acad Sci USA 77:7415, 1980
140. Tokunaga M, Sato E: Non-Hodgkin's lymphomas in a southern prefecture in Japan: an analysis of 715 cases. Cancer 46:1231, 1980
141. Yamada Y: Phenotypic and functional analysis of leukemic cells from 16 patients with adult T cell leukemia/lymphoma. Blood 61:192, 1983
142. Jaffe E, Blattner W, Blayney D et al: The pathologic spectrum of adult T-cell leukemia/lymphoma in the United States. Am J Surg Pathol 8:263, 1984
143. Swerdlow S, Habeshaw J, Rohatiner A et al: Caribbean T-cell lymphoma/leukemia. Cancer 54:687, 1984
144. Duggan D, Ehrlich G, Davey F et al: HTLV-1 induced lymphoma mimicking Hodgkin's disease. Diagnosis by polymerase chain reaction amplification of specific HTLV-1 sequences in tumor DNA. Blood 71:1027, 1988
145. Chadburn A, Athan E, Wieczorek R, Knowles D: Detection and characterization of HTLV-I associated T neoplasms in an HTLV-I non-endemic region by polymerase chain reaction. Blood 70:1500, 1991
146. Kikuchi M, Mitsui T, Takeshita M et al: Virus associated adult T-cell leukemia (ATL) in Japan: clinical, histological and immunological studies. Hematol Oncol 4:67, 1987
147. Abrams M, Sidawy M, Novich M: Smoldering HTLV-associated T-cell leukemia. Arch Intern Med 145:2257, 1985
148. Kiyokawa T, Yamaguchi K, Takeya M et al: Hypercalcemia and osteoclast proliferation in adult T-cell leukemia. Cancer 59:1187, 1987
149. Shibata D, Tokumaga M, Sasaki N, Nanba K: Detection of human T-cell leukemia virus type I proviral sequences from fixed tissues of seropositive patients. Am J Clin Pathol 95:536, 1991
150. Hjelle B: Human T-cell leukemia/lymphoma viruses: life cycle, pathogenicity, epidemiology, and diagnosis. Arch Pathol Lab Med 115:440, 1991
151. Sohn CC, Blayney DW, Misset JL et al: Leukopenic chronic T cell leukemia mimicking hairy cell leukemia: association with human retroviruses. Blood 67:949, 1986
152. Kalyanaraman VS, Sarngadharan MG, Robert-Guroff M et al: A new subtype of human T-cell leukemia virus (HTLV II) associated with a T-cell variant of hairy cell leukemia. Science 218: 571, 1982
153. Tsang WYW, Chan JKC, Yip TTC, et al: In situ localization of Epstein-Barr virus encoded RNA in non-nasal/nasopharyngeal CD56-positive and CD56-negative T-cell lymphomas. Hum Pathol 25:758, 1994
154. Ott G, Ott M, Feller AC, et al: Prevalence of Epstein-Barr virus DNA in different T-cell lymphoma entities in a European population. Int J Cancer 51:562, 1992
155. Cheng A-L, Su I-J, Chen Y-C, et al: Characteristic clinicopathologic features of Epstein-Barr virus-associated peripheral T-cell lymphoma. Cancer 72:909, 1993
156. Chan JKC, Yip TTC, Tsang WYW, et al: Detection of Epstein-Barr viral RNA in malignant lymphomas of the upper aerodigestive tract. Am J Surg Pathol 18:938, 1994
157. Hamilton-Dutoit SJ, Pallesen G: A survey of

Epstein-Barr virus gene expression in sporadic non-Hodgkin's lymphomas. Detection of Epstein-Barr virus in a subset of peripheral T-cell lymphomas. Am J Pathol 140:1315, 1992

158. Su I-J, Hsieh H-C, Lin K-H et al: Aggressive peripheral T-cell lymphomas containing Epstein-Barr viral DNA: a clinicopathologic and molecular analysis. Blood 77:799, 1991
159. Anagnostopoulos I, Hummel M, Finn T et al: Heterogeneous Epstein-Barr virus infection patterns in peripheral T-cell lymphoma of angioimmunoblastic lymphadenopathy type. Blood 80: 1804, 1992
160. Suzushima H, Asou N, Fujimoto T et al: Lack of the expression of EBNA-2 and LMP-1 in T-cell neoplasms possessing Epstein-Barr virus. Blood 85:480, 1995
161. Korbjuhn P, Anagnostopoulos I, Hummer M et al: Frequent latent Epstein-Barr virus infection of neoplastic T cells and bystander B cells in human immunodeficiency virus-negative European peripheral pleomorphic T-cell lymphoma. Blood 82:217, 1993
162. Garvin AJ, Self S, Sahovic ES et al: The occurrence of a peripheral T-cell lymphoma in a chronically immunosuppressed renal transplant patient. Am J Surg Pathol 12:64, 1988
163. Griffith RC, Saha BK, Janney CM et al: Immunoblastic lymphoma of T-cell type in a chronically immunosuppressed renal transplant recipient. Am J Clin Pathol 93:280, 1990
164. van Gorp J, Doornewaard H, Verdonck LF et al: Posttransplant T-cell lymphoma. Cancer 73: 3064, 1994
165. Kaplan MA, Jacobson JO, Ferry JA, Harris NL: T-cell lymphoma of the vulva in a renal allograft recipient with associated hemophagocytosis. Am J Surg Pathol 17:842, 1993
166. Feher O, Barilla D, Locker J et al: T-cell large granular lymphocytic leukemia following orthotopic liver transplantation. Am J Hematol 49: 216, 1995
167. Lippman SM, Grogan TM, Carry P et al: Posttransplantation T cell lymphoblastic lymphoma. Am J Med 82:814, 1987
168. Herndier BG, Shiramizc BT, Jewett NE et al: Acquired immunodeficiency syndrome-associated T-cell lymphoma: evidence for human immunodeficiency virus type 1-associated T-cell transformation. Blood 79:1768, 1992
169. Thomas JA, Cotter F, Hanby AM et al: Epstein-Barr virus-related oral T-cell lymphoma associated with immunodeficiency virus immunosuppression. Blood 81:3350, 1993
170. Kumar S, Kumar D, Kingma DW, Jaffe ES: Epstein-Barr virus-associated T-cell lymphoma in a renal transplant patient. Am J Surg Pathol 17: 1046, 1993
171. Meropol NJ, Hicks D, Brooks JJ et al: Coincident Kaposi sarcoma and T-cell lymphoma in a patient with the Wiskott-Aldrich syndrome. Am J Hematol 40:126, 1992
172. Gonzalez CL, Medeiros LJ, Braziel RM, Jaffe ES: T-cell lymphoma involving subcutaneous tissue. A clinicopathologic entity commonly associated with hemophagocytic syndrome. Am J Surg Pathol 15:17, 1991
173. Perniciaro C, Zalla MJ, White JW, Menke DM: Subcutaneous T-cell lymphoma. Report of two additional cases and further observations. Arch Dermatol 129:1171, 1993
174. Aronson IK, West DP, Variakojis D et al: Panniculitis associated with cutaneous T-cell lymphoma and cytophagocytic histiocytosis. Br J Dermatol 112:87, 1985
175. Burg G, Dummer R, Wilhelm M, et al: A subcutaneous delta-positive T-cell lymphoma that produces interferon gamma. N Engl J Med 325: 1078–81, 1991
176. Chott A, Dragosics B, Radaszkiewicz T: Peripheral T-cell lymphomas of the intestine. Am J Pathol 141:1361, 1992
177. O'Farelly C, Feighery C, O'Brian DS et al: Humoral response to wheat protein in patients with coeliac disease and enteropathy-associated T-cell lymphoma. BMJ 293:908, 1986
178. Murray A, Cuevas EC, Jones DB, Wright DH: Study of the immunohistochemistry and T cell clonality of enteropathy-associated T cell lymphoma. Am J Pathol 146:509, 1995
179. Foucar K, Foucar E, Mitros F et al: Epitheliotropic lymphoma of the small bowel. Report of a fatal case with cytotoxic/suppressor T-cell immunotype. Cancer 54:54, 1984
180. Spencer J, MacDonald TT, Diss TC et al: Changes in intraepithelial lymphocyte subpopulations in coeliac disease and enteropathy associated T cell lymphoma (malignant histiocytosis of the intestine). Gut 30:339, 1989
181. Spencer J, Cerf-Bensussan N, Jarry A et al: Enteropathy-associated T cell lymphoma (malignant histiocytosis of the intestine) is recognized by a monoclonal antibody (HML-1) that defines

a membrane molecule on human mucosal lymphocytes. Am J Pathol 132:1, 1988

182. Wright DH, Jones DB, Clark H et al: Is adult-onset coeliac disease due to a low-grade lymphoma of intraepithelial T lymphocytes? Lancet 337:1373, 1991
183. Möller P, Mielke B, Moldenhauer G: Monoclonal antibody HML-1, a marker for intraepithelial T cells and lymphomas derived thereof, also recognizes hairy cell leukemia and some B-cell lymphomas. Am J Pathol 136:509, 1990
184. Wong KF, Chan JKC, Matutes E et al: Hepatosplenic $\gamma\delta$ T-cell lymphoma. A distinctive aggressive lymphoma type. Am J Surg Pathol 718, 1995
185. Mastovitch S, Ratech H, Ware RE et al: Hepatosplenic T-cell lymphoma: an unusual case of a $\gamma\delta$ T-cell lymphoma with a blast-like terminal transformation. Hum pathol 25:102, 1994
186. Gaulard P, Bourqueltot P, Kanavaros P et al: Expression of the alpha/beta and gamma delta T-cell receptors in 57 cases of peripheral T-cell lymphomas. Identification of a subset of $\gamma\delta$ T-cell lymphomas. Am J Surg Pathol 137:617, 1990
187. Matthews M, Gazdar A, quoted in Clendenning WE, Rappaport H: Report on the committee on pathology of cutaneous T cell lymphomas. Cancer Treat Rep 63:719, 1979
188. Scheffer E, Meijer CJLM, van Vlote WA: Dermatopathic lymphadenopathy and lymph node involvement in mycosis fungoides. Cancer 45: 137, 1980
189. Sausville EA, Worsham GF, Matthews MJ et al: Histologic assessment of lymph nodes in mycosis funcoides/Sézary syndrome (cutaneous T-cell lymphoma): clinical correlations and prognostic import of a new classification system. Hum Pathol 16:1098, 1985
190. Sausville EA, Eddy JL, Makuch RW et al: Histopathologic staging at initial diagnosis of mycosis fungoides and the Sézary syndrome: definition of three distinctive prognostic groups. Ann Intern Med 109:372, 1988
191. Colby TV, Burke JS, Hoppe RT: Lymph node biopsies in mycosis fungoides. Cancer 47:351, 1985
192. Wood GS, Matthew MJ: Diagnosis of T-cell malignant lymphoproliferative disorders in the skin. P. 413. In Jaffe ES (ed): Surgical Pathology of the Lymph Nodes and Related Organs. 2nd Ed. WB Saunders, Philadelphia, 1995
193. Burke JS, Colby TV: Dermatopathic lymphadenopathy. Comparison of cases associated and unassociated with mycosis fungoides. Am J Surg Pathol 5:343, 1981
194. Vonderheid EC, Diamohd LW, Lai S-M et al: Lymph node histopathologic findings in cutaneous T-cell lymphoma: a prognostic classification system based on morphologic assessment. Am J Clin Pathol 97:121, 1992
195. Scheffer E, Meijer CJLM, van Vloten WA, Willemze R: A histologic study of lymph nodes from patients with the Sézary syndrome. Cancer 57:2375, 1986
196. Knowles DM: Immunophenotypic and immunogenotypic approaches useful in distinguishing benign and malignant lymphoid proliferations. Semin Oncol 20:583, 1993
197. Bakels V, van Oostveen JW, Geerts M-L et al: Diagnostic and prognostic significance of clonal T-cell receptor beta gene rearrangements in lymph nodes of patients with mycosis fungoides. J Pathol 170:249, 1993

9

Posttransplant Lymphoproliferative Disorders

Michael A. Nalesnik and Glauco Frizzera

The ability to induce chronic iatrogenic immunosuppression has helped to ensure the success of clinical organ transplantation. Unfortunately, the indiscriminate nature of the immunosuppression produced by current regimens also predisposes to infection with an ever-expanding assortment of opportunistic microorganisms. One outstanding example of this problem is the development of virus-associated lymphoid hyperplasias and neoplasias that constitute the syndrome of posttransplantation lymphoproliferative disorders (PTLD).[1–7]

The original proposal of a single conceptual entity to encompass both hyperplastic and neoplastic lymphoid growths was buttressed by a common denominator of the intralesional presence of Epstein-Barr virus (EBV) in the index series of transplant patients.[1] Subsequent series have confirmed a strong association between EBV and PTLD. However, the association is not universal, and cases exist in which no evidence of this virus is detectable.[4,7–9]

Posttransplant lymphoproliferations can be recognized and categorized from a morphologic perspective regardless of the presence or absence of EBV. This chapter begins with a brief clinical overview of PTLD followed by a discussion of the evolution of classifications useful in subdividing this syndrome. The narrative incorporates currently extant classification systems and does not introduce any new form of organization. The histopathology of these lesions within lymphoid tissues is next presented, followed by a consideration of phenotype, clonal status, oncogene/tumor suppressor gene abnormalities, and cytogenetics. The singular role of EBV is emphasized by a discussion of methodologies useful for detecting this agent within tissue specimens. The groundwork for an appreciation of these techniques is laid by the interposition of a short account of the host–EBV interaction in the normal and immunosuppressed states. Next, the pathologic differential diagnosis of PTLD is discussed. Since many of these lesions can occur outside of lymphoid tissues, a description of PTLD at various extranodal sites is also presented.

CLINICAL ASPECTS

Frequency

The frequency of PTLD varies among recipients of different allograft types and with different therapeutic regimens.[10,11] Renal transplant patients have been reported to have a 1 percent and liver recipients a 2 percent PTLD frequency. Figures for heart recipients range from 1.8 to 9.8 percent, for heart/lung patients from 4.6 to 9.4 percent, and for bone marrow patients from 0.6 to 7.4 percent.[12] Higher figures cited in the literature usually reflect early experience at individual centers or the use of high dose drug regimens.[13,14]

Other risk factors for the development of PTLD that have thus far been identified include seronegative EBV status at the time of transplant[15,16] and possibly pediatric status (M. Green, personal communication). Frequency figures can only give a static estimate of disease risk in the pediatric population. One longitudinal study of a pediatric liver transplant population showed a 2.8 percent actuarial risk of developing PTLD per year.[17] The study was terminated after 7 years, at which time the cumulative PTLD risk had leveled off at approximately 20 percent.

Signs and Symptoms

PTLDs can present with a heterogeneous array of clinical signs and symptoms. Several authors have used related terminologies to group these clinical manifestations into prototypic subclasses. Hanto et al.[1] and Frizzera et al.[2,12] separated infectious mononucleosis-like diseases from solid tumor presentation. The former occurred at a mean of 9 months and the latter at a mean of 5.3 years posttransplant in this azathioprine-treated population. Nalesnik et al.[4] observed three types of clinical presentation. One group had disease primarily confined to the head and neck and often presented with mononucleosis-like symptoms. A second category had involvement of the gastrointestinal tract. This group constituted 26 percent of this series of 43 patients and presented with abdominal pain typically accompanied by impending or frank bowel perforation. A third category demonstrated signs and symptoms referable to solid organ involvement. Lymphadenopathy was variable among all patients, and the clinical categories were not mutually exclusive. Mean onset time of PTLD was 4.4 months in this cyclosporine-treated population. Malatack et al.[17] divided their patients into those with lymphadenopathic, systemic, or lymphomatous presentations.

In EBV-related mononucleosis-like syndromes, exudative tonsillitis may be seen, and this is usually accompanied by cervical adenopathy together with fever, fatigue, and pharyngitis. Variations that normally occur in infectious mononucleosis may likewise be seen when this syndrome occurs in the transplant population. Cheeseman[18] divided the clinical presentations of infectious mononucleosis in the nonimmunosuppressed host into the anginose type, with predominance of tonsillitis; the glandular type, in which lymphadenopathy overshadows other manifestations; and the febrile type, in which an extended prodrome of fever and malaise could precede the development of lymphadenopathy.

In contrast, the clinical onset of some PTLDs may be fulminant, with multisystem involvement. Symptoms as diverse as pancreatitis, meningoencephalitis, and pneumonitis have been observed in this subgroup.[17] These patients are often septic due to concomitant opportunistic infection.

Clinical presentation in the form of one or more tumors represents the most common clinical subtype of PTLD, occurring approximately twice as frequently as a mononucleosis-like syndrome in one series.[19]

Signs and symptoms are dependent on the location of the tumors. Tumorous PTLDs are notorious for their multicentricity and tendency to involve extranodal as well as nodal locations. No region is exempt from possible involvement,[20,21] although there is a tendency to involve specific sites. The allograft itself may be involved, in which case symptoms such as tenderness and swelling may mimic rejection.[22–25] In one series, allograft lung involvement occurred in 80 percent of cases (n = 5), whereas allograft heart involvement occurred in 0 percent.[26] PTLD involved allograft liver, kidney, or bone marrow in about one-third of cases occurring in patients who received those respective transplants.[26]

Gastrointestinal involvement was seen in 26 percent of PTLDs reported from two separate series.[4,6] Central nervous system involvement by PTLD was seen in 23 percent of cases in one autopsy series.[27]

PATHOLOGIC FEATURES

Posttransplant lymphoproliferative disorders is a term applied in a nonuniform fashion to encompass a restricted set of lymphoid lesions that arise in transplant patients and that have a close (but not invariant) association with EBV. The lesions are conveniently divided into three general categories: hyperplasias, polymorphic lymphoproliferations, and lymphoid neoplasias. Some authors use the term *PTLD* as an umbrella designation for all of these categories. Others use it to refer to lymphoid hyperplasias and polymorphic lymphoproliferations and apply the term *posttransplant lymphoma* for obvious lymphoid neoplasias. Still others may restrict use of *PTLD* to polymorphic lymphoproliferations alone. For these reasons it is important for the pathologist to realize that the term *PTLD* is not a specific diagnosis and that it must be further qualified according to specific histopathologic criteria. It is also inappropriate to refer to all posttransplant lymphoid growths as *posttransplant lymphomas* as is occasionally done in the clinical literature.

Gross Pathology

The gross appearance of PTLD in lymphoid tissue is most often that of a rounded fleshy tan pink mass with or without regional necrosis. The latter may present as gray flecks on the surface and/or interior of the lesion, or it may comprise the bulk of the specimen. Total and diffuse nodal involvement is almost always the case. Rarely, partial involvement may be seen.

Since PTLD represents a range of disorders, the gross appearance may vary accordingly. Lesions at the lower end of the spectrum may show only diffuse enlargement of a well-preserved node without evidence of nodules. More advanced lesions may infiltrate into adjacent tissues, distorting the capsular–soft tissue interface.

PTLD that occurs in extranodal sites may assume an infiltrative or tumorous appearance. Vascular infiltration or simply the rapid growth rate of the tumor may lead to secondary infarction or hemorrhage, imparting a mottled aspect to the exterior and cut surfaces. In the gut, ulcerating masses with overgrown borders may be seen.

Histology

It is to be emphasized that PTLD is a syndrome that encompasses both hyperplastic and neoplastic lymphoproliferations. Hyperplasias currently thought to be closely related to or actually representative of one end of the family of PTLD lesions include uncomplicated infectious mononucleosis[28] and plasma cell hyperplasia.[7]

Infectious mononucleosis is typically characterized by paracortical expansion with retention of follicles (Fig. 9-1).[29–31] Spillover of the mononuclear inflammation beyond the capsule is frequent, but destruction of underlying architecture is minimal and is evidenced by small foci of necrosis (Fig. 9-2). Intense activation of lymphoid cells imparts a heterogeneous appearance to paracortical regions. Plasma cells may be frequent. Occasional foci of large transformed cells may be observed, again with retention of underlying architecture. Reed-Sternberg-like cells may be observed in small numbers.[32–34] The germinal centers may be hyperplastic in tonsil specimens, but this is not a prominent finding at other sites and it may be necessary to employ the reticulin stain to highlight follicles.[32]

Plasma cell hyperplasia consists of a diffuse proliferation of benign-appearing plasma cells that may be admixed with smaller numbers of lymphoid cells (Fig. 9-3).[4,7] Germinal centers may be difficult or impossible to find. The sinusoids appear intact, and no evidence of architectural destruction is observed.

Polymorphic PTLDs are comprised of two histologic subtypes: polymorphic diffuse B-cell hyperplasia and polymorphic B cell lymphoma.[2,12] Polymorphic diffuse B-cell hyperplasia is characterized by a diffuse effacement of the lymph node due to a heterogeneous lymphoid infiltrate that contains variable numbers of small round or angulated and large centroblast-like cells together with immunoblasts and plasma cells (Fig. 9-4). The proportion of cells may vary from field to microscopic field, and it is this feature that underscores designation of the term *polymorphic* to these lesions. Overall, however, there is a tendency toward promi-

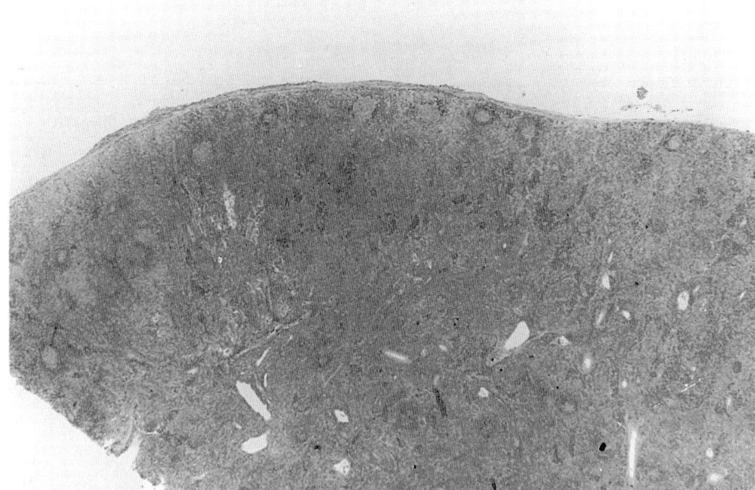

Fig. 9-1. Residual follicles are present in a setting of marked paracortical expansion in this lymph node from an organ transplant patient with infectious mononucleosis. Such pronounced changes are typical of EBV-associated lymphadenitis, but must be distinguished from other virus-associated lymphadenitides. Demonstration of EBV proteins or nucleic acid within more than an occasional cell in the lesion strongly implicates this virus in the pathogenesis of these changes. (H&E, ×10.)

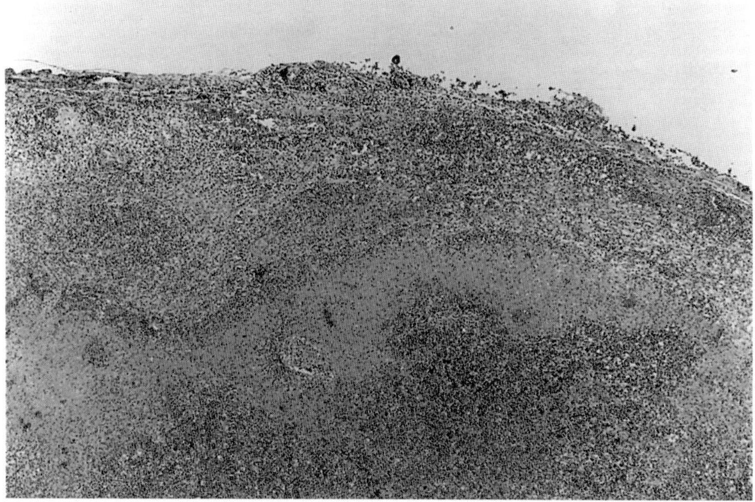

Fig. 9-2. This lymph node shows diffuse hyperplasia with an area of early confluent subcapsular necrosis. Rare residual follicles were seen elsewhere. Negligible spillover of cells beyond the capsule is noted in this field. Intralesional Epstein-Barr virus was demonstrated, and the process was interpreted as infectious mononucleosis. Atypical immunoblasts were not a feature of the proliferation. The vast majority of cells in this node were plasmacytic, and the process may actually be intermediate between typical infectious mononucleosis and plasma cell hyperplasia. (H&E, ×40.)

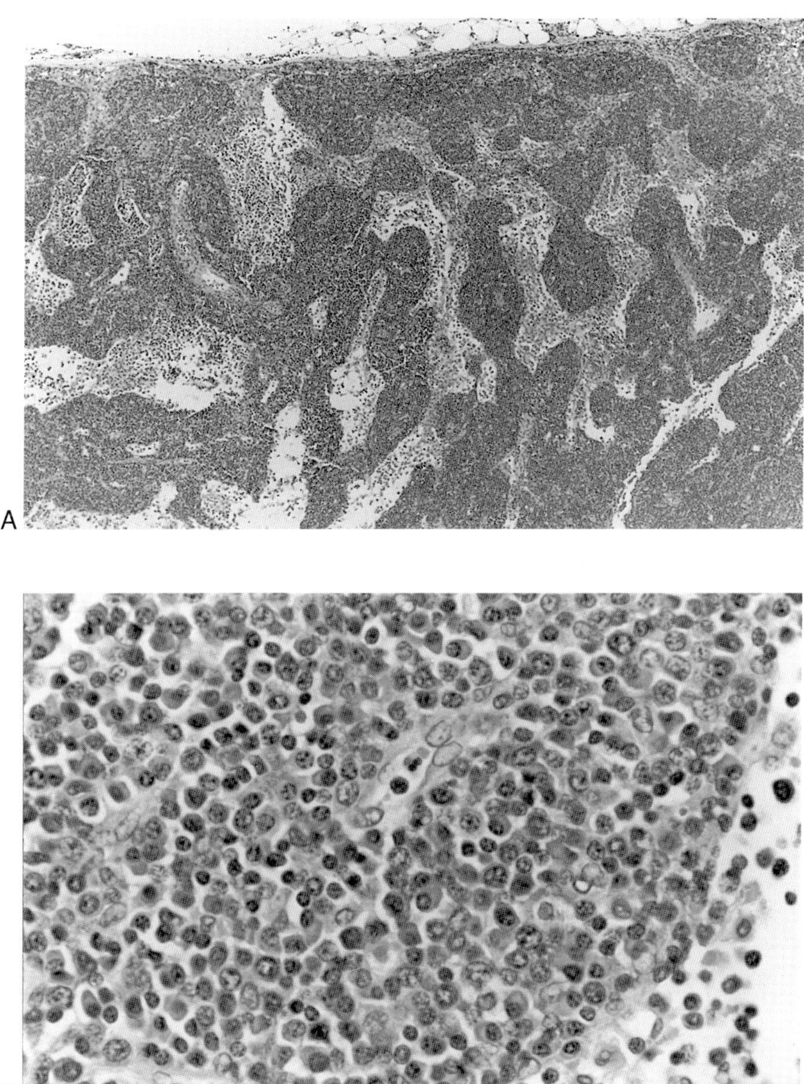

Fig. 9-3. **(A)** Plasma cell hyperplasia in lymph node. Cortex and medullary cords contain a diffuse proliferation of cells with no obvious follicle formation. Sinusoids are well demarcated. No significant extracapsular spread is noted. (H&E, ×10.) **(B)** A bland, uniform, predominantly plasmacellular population is present. The patient had concurrent gastrointestinal PTLD and disseminated cytomegalovirus infection. The tumors were resected, and the patient ultimately expired due to superimposed sepsis. No evidence of residual PTLD was seen at autopsy. (H&E, ×400.)

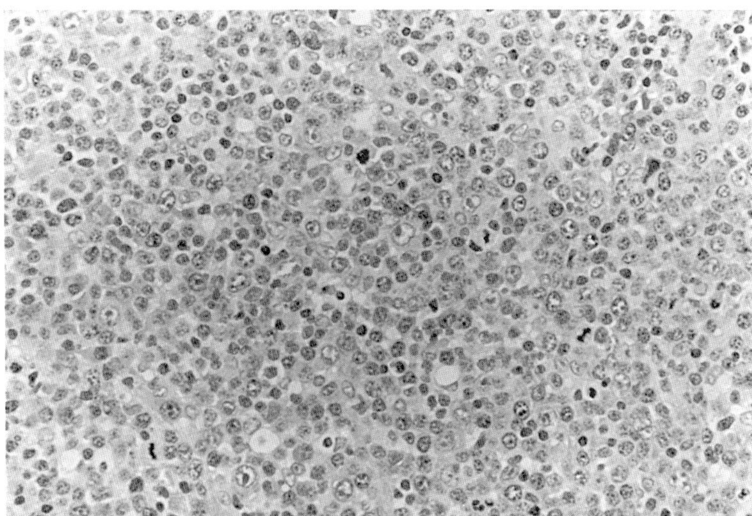

Fig. 9-4. Polymorphic diffuse B-cell hyperplasia. The heterogeneity of the mononuclear cells comprising this diffuse process is more marked than that seen in plasma cell hyperplasia. In addition to plasma cells, a follicular center cell component in the form of small round or angulated cells and larger centroblast-like cells can be seen. Immunophenotypic analysis also indicates the presence of a variable T-cell element. However, when clonal subpopulations are seen they are typically due to the B-cell population. (H&E, ×200.)

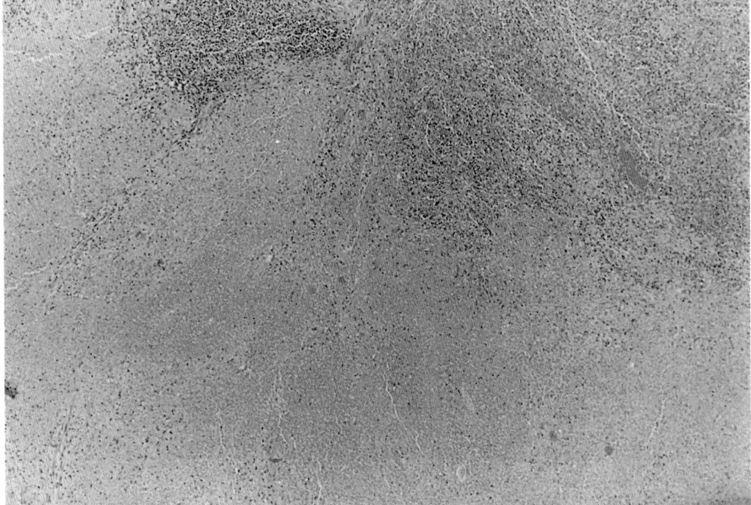

Fig. 9-5. Extensive necrosis in PTLD. The bulk of this lesion consists of necrotic material. Compare with Figure 9-2. In some cases it is possible to read through the necrosis to observe the amorphous ghosts of mononuclear cells in PTLD. Although this pattern cannot be recommended as sufficient for diagnosis, it may suggest this disorder when only small amounts of tissue are available. The possibility of extensive necrosis should reinforce prospective efforts to obtain adequate tissue samples from the surgeon.

nent plasmacytoid differentiation. The infiltrate may extend beyond the capsule into the adjacent tissue, but it is not associated with tissue destruction. In the pure form, only single-cell necrosis and no atypical lymphoid cells are seen.

Polymorphic B-cell lymphoma likewise grows in a diffuse fashion and displays marked heterogeneity in the appearance of its constituent lymphoid cells. One of its distinguishing features is the presence of more prominent necrosis that often assumes a characteristic swath-like or geographic configuration. Early areas of necrosis may contain confluent regions of nuclear pyknosis and/or apoptosis. In other cases necrosis may be the predominant feature of the specimen (Fig. 9-5). Such areas may contain residual nuclear debris, and close inspection reveals cell ghosts. A second distinguishing feature of polymorphic B-cell lymphoma is the presence of large atypical mononuclear cells, some of which may resemble Reed-Sternberg cells (atypical immunoblasts) (Fig. 9-6). These large cells contain irregular nuclei that may be bi- or multilobated and within which are found prominent nucleoli. The cells generally contain abundant cytoplasm. Except for these cells, true cellular anaplasia is not a feature of this condition.[2] In the pure form polymorphic B-cell lymphoma, both necrosis and atypical immunoblasts are seen. There is a tendency for atypical immunoblasts to be seen near or adjacent to necrotic zones. Finally, plasmacytoid differentiation is less prominent than in polymorphic diffuse B-cell hyperplasia.

The categorical distinction between polymorphic B-cell hyperplasia and lymphoma is not absolute, and individual cases may show features intermediate between the two.[35,36]

Additional lymphoid neoplasias in transplant recipients have histologic appearances similar to those found in nonimmunosuppressed populations.[2,4,7,9,35,37–48] The overwhelming majority are of non-Hodgkin's type. Virtually all are diffuse, high grade lesions. Within this group, immunoblastic lymphomas comprise the largest subtypes (Fig. 9-7). Some examples of small noncleaved cell lymphomas also exist (Fig. 9-8). Intermediate grade lesions are largely represented by diffuse large cell lymphomas. Rare cases of small lymphocytic and follicular large cell lymphomas may also occur. In our experience, these rare cases do not contain EBV. Examples of extramedullary plasmacytoma and multiple myeloma have been described, as have occasional cases of T-cell lymphoma (Fig. 9-9). Hodgkin's disease[41,49,50] and Hodgkin's-like lymphomas[51] (Fig. 9-10) have been described in small numbers of allograft recipients.

Cell Phenotype and Clonal Status

Phenotypic Studies of Cell-Associated Molecules

Immunophenotypic analysis of cell lineage markers has supported the primary role of B lymphocytes in the majority of these disorders.[35] The heterogeneity of the lesions is reflected in the fact that about 36 percent of cases are polyclonal by immunophenotypic studies, 29 percent are monoclonal, 20 percent are immunoglobulin negative but are positive for other B-cell antigens, and 15 percent contain both polyclonal and monoclonal lesions.[12,52] The B cells in PTLDs may express CD antigens 19, 20, 21, and 22. Within this group, CD21 is inconstantly expressed. The activated phenotype of many of these cells is also reflected in the presence of adhesion molecules LFA-1/CD11a, ICAM-1/CD54, and LFA-3/CD58, together with the activation marker CD23 in reported cases.[53] Variable numbers of T lymphocytes are also found within these tumors (Fig. 9-11). In most cases such cells represent small lymphocytes that are thought to be a reflection of the host response to the B-cell growth. To date, this hypothesis has not been tested. In occasional cases the PTLD may be of T cell origin.[9] CD8+ or CD4−8− phenotypes may be more frequent in these lesions.[12]

CD30+ B-cell lymphoproliferations with an anaplastic large cell morphology have been described in the posttransplant setting.[54] One case that was interpreted as Hodgkin's-like lymphoma contained large atypical cells with the

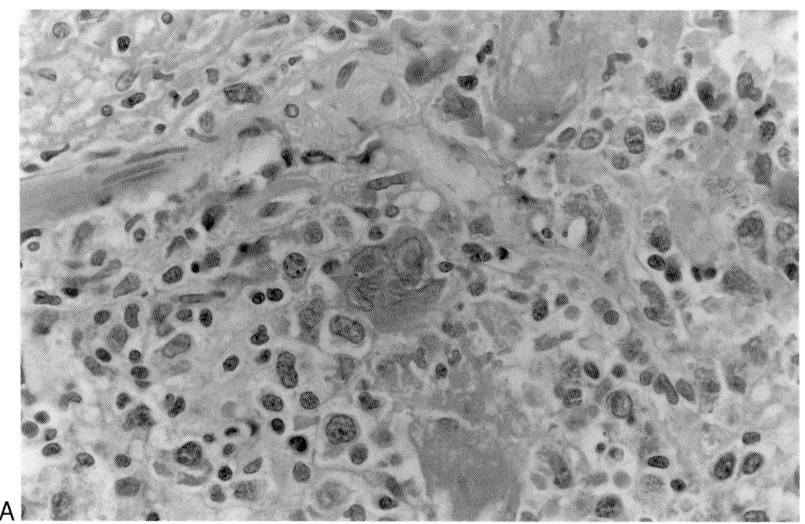

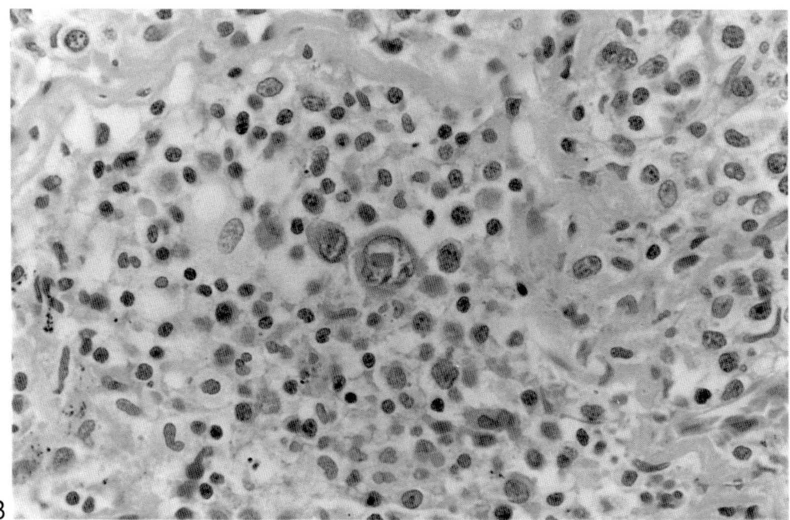

Fig. 9-6. Polymorphic B-cell lymphoma (polymorphic PTLD). **(A)** A large atypical blast with a multilobated nucleus is seen in a heterogeneous background of mononuclear cells. Two small areas of amorphous material at the top and bottom of the photomicrograph represent the edges of necrotic foci. (H&E, ×400.) **(B)** Separate field from same cases as A, showing more frequent small mononuclear cells and a bizarre immunoblast. (H&E, ×400.) *(Figure continues.)*

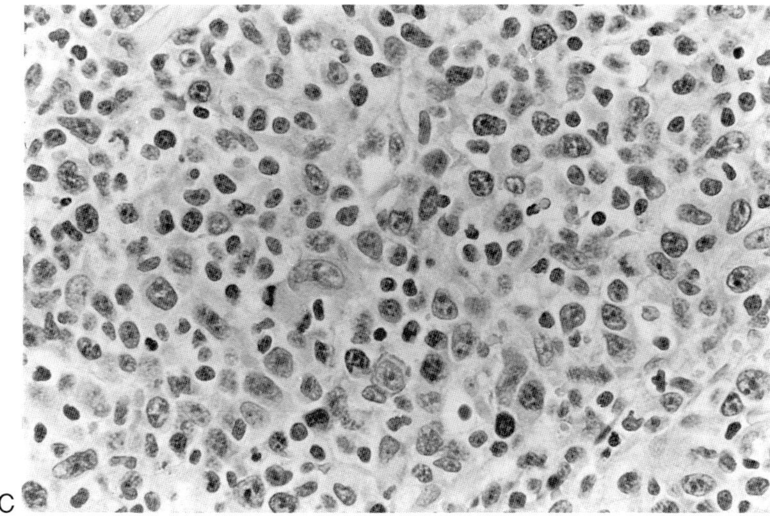

Fig. 9-6 *(Continued).* **(C)** Separate example of polymorphic B-cell lymphoma immunostained for EBV latent membrane protein (LMP) in a region removed from necrosis. The centroblast-like cell component is more prominent in this case. The LMP stain is seen in only rare cells in this case. This is unusual but serves to reinforce the point that the antibody may occasionally lead to a false negative conclusion regarding the presence of PTLD if only a small fragment of tissue is available. Avidin-biotin-peroxidase with hematoxylin counterstain. (×400.)

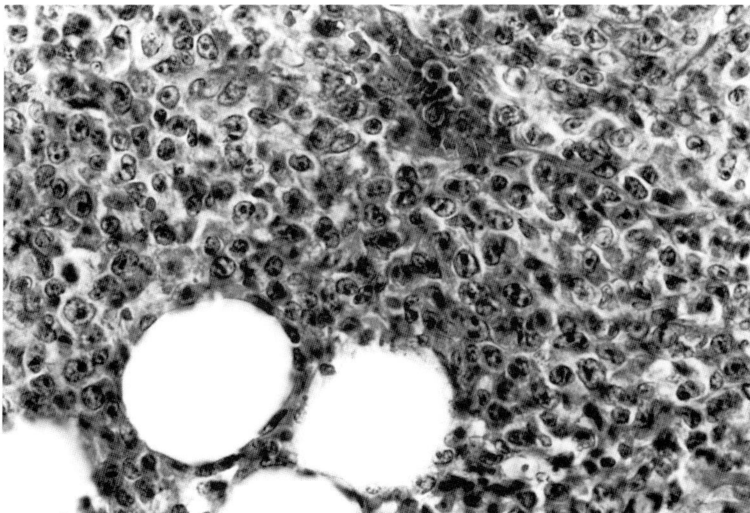

Fig. 9-7. Posttransplant lymphoma (monomorphic PTLD, large cell/immunoblastic). A uniform population of cells with vesicular, round to ovoid nuclei and small irregularities in the peripheral chromatin/nuclear membrane contours contain prominent, centrally placed nucleoli. The nuclei resemble those of immunoblasts, although the cytoplasm is somewhat sparse. The presence of fat reflects the extranodal location of this tumor. (H&E, ×400.)

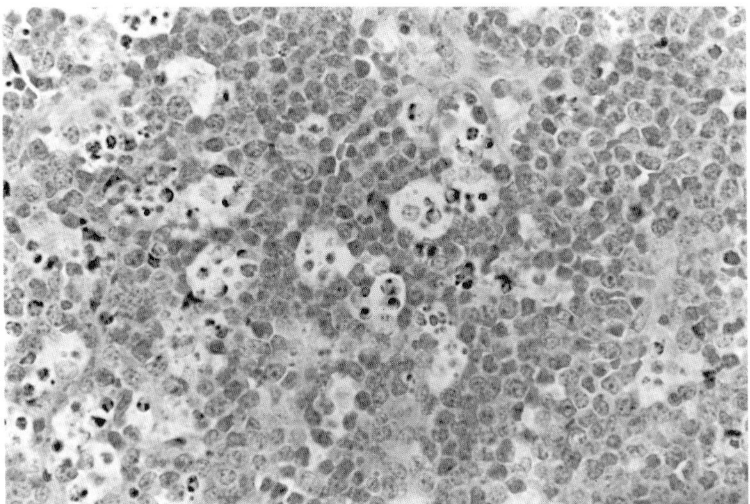

Fig. 9-8. Posttransplant lymphoma (monomorphic PTLD, small cell noncleaved). The monotonous cell population does not contain the prominent nuclei as seen in Fig. 9-7. Macrophages containing karyorrhectic nuclear debris are interspersed among the tumor cells. (H&E, ×200.)

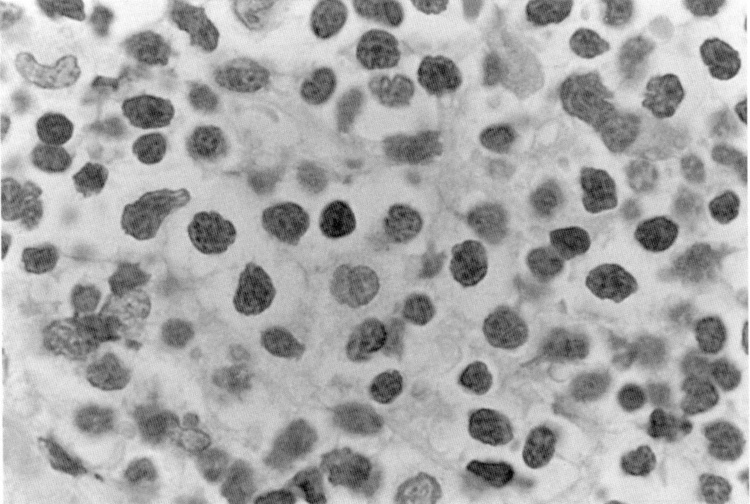

Fig. 9-9. Posttransplant T-cell lymphoma. The cells in this lesion contain small nucleoli and dense granular chromatin set in round nuclei with shallow invaginations. Some heterogeneity in the size of these otherwise uniform cells is observed. The interpretation of T-cell lymphoma was supported by flow cytometric analysis and by demonstration of clonal rearrangement of the T-cell receptor in the absence of immunoglobulin gene rearrangement. Clonal EBV was also present in this tumor. (H&E, ×1,000.)

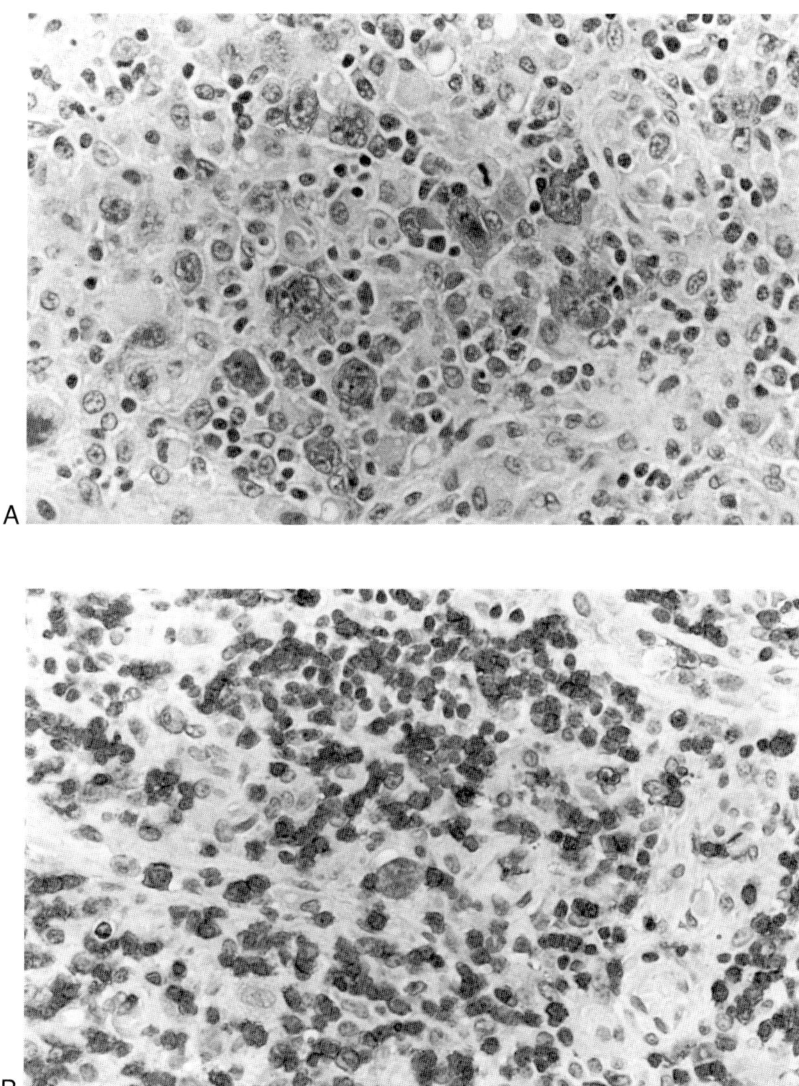

Fig. 9-10. Posttransplant lymphoproliferative disorder with features of Hodgkin's disease. **(A)** CD15+ atypical cells appear similar to the atypical immunoblasts observed in polymorphic B-cell lymphoma (compare with Fig. 9-6B,C). These cells are much more frequent in the present example. Some transformed cells are seen in the heterogeneous background, unlike the usual situation in typical Hodgkin's disease. (Avidin-biotin peroxidase with hematoxylin counterstain, ×300.) **(B)** T lymphocytes (CD3+) are a prominent subpopulation in this case. The atypical cell population was negative for this marker, as shown by a representative cell in the center of the photograph. Immunoglobulin gene rearrangement analysis showed a clonal subpopulation, whereas no evidence of T-cell receptor rearrangement was seen. The large atypical cells were positive for CD20 (not shown), and it is thought likely that these represent a B-cell-derived monoclonal population. (Avidin-biotin-peroxidase with hematoxylin counterstain, ×200.) *(Figure continues.)*

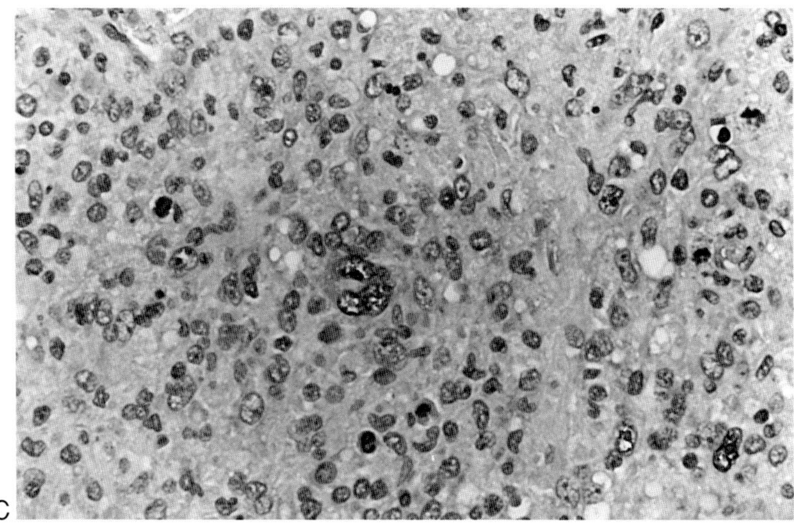

Fig. 9-10 *(Continued).* **(C)** Epstein-Barr virus was detected by EBER in situ hybridization and was localized primarily to the large cell population. (Biotin-streptavidin-peroxidase with hematoxylin counterstain, ×200.)

phenotype CD15+, LN1+, LN2+, CD30+, EMA−, LCA− (Fig. 9-10).[51]

Molecular Analysis of Clonal Composition

Immunoglobulin gene rearrangement analysis has also served to support the primary role of the B lymphocyte in the pathogenesis of PTLDs. The heterogeneity of these lesions extends to the molecular level. Hanto et al.[55] described both polyclonal and monoclonal tumors in their series. In the Pittsburgh series, approximately 32 percent of lesions were polyclonal and 68 percent contained a monoclonal component when immunoglobulin rearrangements were examined by Southern blot analysis.[5,56] Of those containing monoclonal elements, 18 percent showed only a minor clone in a polyclonal background, whereas the remainder showed a more substantial proportion of the tumor to contain clonally rearranged cells. It was noted that histologically monomorphic tumors (i.e., non-Hodgkin's lymphomas) were invariably monoclonal, but those with a polymorphic histology (polymorphic diffuse B-cell hyperplasia and polymorphic B-cell lymphoma showed divergent clonalities. In the series of Knowles et al.,[7] no evidence of immunoglobulin gene rearrangement was seen in 9 of 10 examples of plasmacytic hyperplasia, whereas the tenth case contained only a minor clonal component. Significant clonal rearrangement of immunoglobulin genes was seen in the remaining 17 cases, including all examples of polymorphic diffuse B-cell hyperplasia, polymorphic B-cell lymphoma, immunoblastic lymphoma, and multiple myeloma. Occasional cases with germline immunoglobulin genes are described[54,55] and represent 21 percent of a recent French series.[8]

Examination of concurrent noncontiguous PTLDs may disclose a variety of clonal alterations.[5,57] Some tumors may share identical rearrangements, signifying metastatic disease. In other examples, unique rearrangements within individual tumors points to multicentric clonal disease. In yet other instances more than one clone may be seen within an individual tumor. Such oligoclonal proliferations have been described in EBV-related tumors arising in other immunodeficiency states as well.[58]

Several examples of clinically recurrent PTLD have been examined for immunoglobulin gene rearrangements. The initial report of Hanto et al.[59] documented the clinical progression of

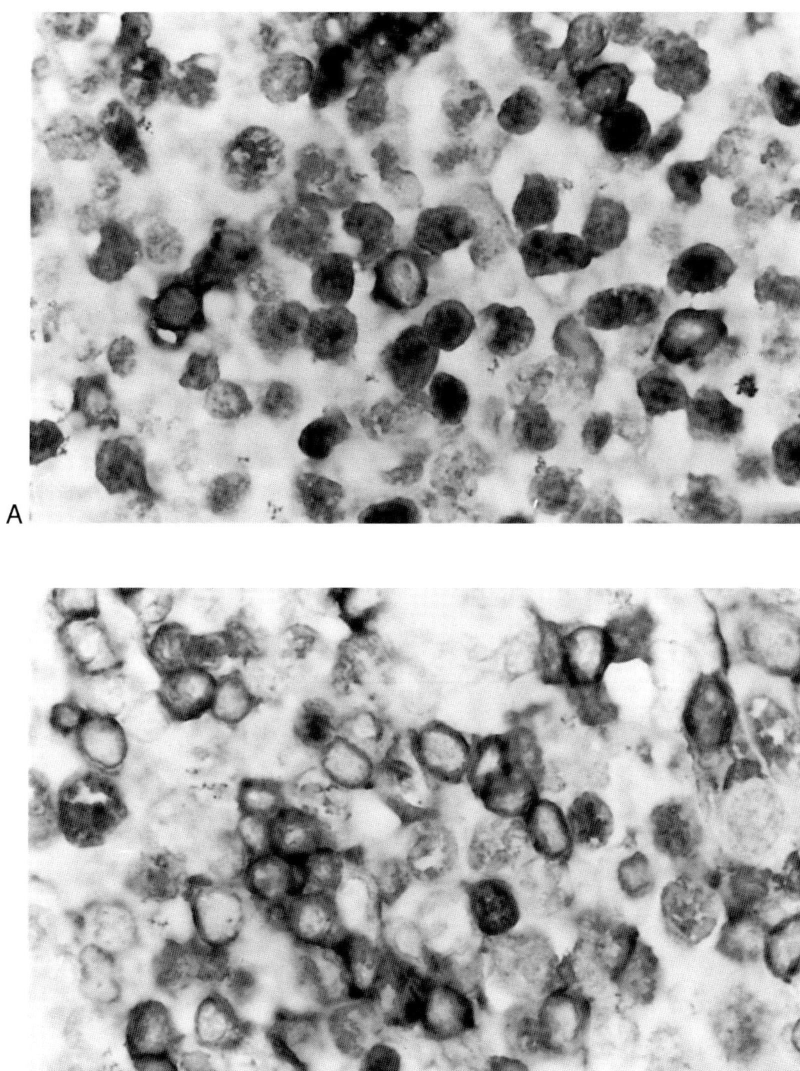

Fig. 9-11. T lymphocytes within PTLD. **(A)** CD3 + T cells are demonstrated by cell surface staining and EBER + cells present as cells with nuclear staining. Since no counterstain was used, nuclear is due to deposition of EBER-localized reaction product. The majority of cells are EBER positive and are negative for CD3. ×1,000. **(B)** The CD3 + and EBER + populations are usually mutually exclusive with PTLDs. Rare exceptions are noted, as in this example of a single CD3 + cell that also shows clear-cut evidence of EBER positivity. (×1,000.) (CD3 avidin-biotin-peroxidase developed with diaminobenzidine, EBER biotin-avidin-alkaline phosphatase developed with BCIP/INT; original procedure from L. Weiss, M.D., City of Hope, Duarte, CA.)

a polyclonal PTLD to a monoclonal tumor. The more recent study of Wu et al.[48] documented 11 transplant patients who developed recurrent EBV-associated lesions. Four of these patients had matched immunoglobulin gene rearrangement studies performed on primary and recurrent disease. One patient who progressed from a mononucleosis-like pattern to polymorphic PTLD showed no evidence of clonal rearrangement in the primary lesion but had a monoclonal component identified in the recurrence. Two of the four patients showed identical clonal rearrangements in both primary and recurrent tumors. Histologic examination in one case showed polymorphic PTLD in both examples. The second patient had a large cell lymphoma (monomorphic PTLD) in each instance. The fourth patient in this group demonstrated unique rearrangements in each lesion. In this case the first lesion was interpreted as a polymorphic PTLD, whereas the recurrence resembled Hodgkin's disease.[51]

Oncogenes and Tumor Suppressor Genes

Rearrangements of c-*myc* were observed in 3 of 40 specimens in one series.[5] Tumors containing this alteration were histologically monomorphic and invariably progressed. More recently, Knowles et al.[7] and Delecluse et al.[40] showed c-*myc* rearrangements in one example each of plasmacytoid immunoblastic lymphoma and plasmacytoid small cell lymphoma. In addition, the first of these tumors contained an N-*ras* mutation, as did both examples of multiple myeloma in this series.[7] Both cases of pleomorphic immunoblastic lymphoma showed *p53* mutations. No evidence of similar mutations was seen in any example of polymorphic PTLD or plasma cell hyperplasia.

Karyotypic Studies

Cytogenetic studies of PTLDs have only rarely been reported.[2,15,36,60–62] No consistent anomaly has been detected to date. Translocations or loss of material involving chromosome 6 and trisomy or duplication of chromosome 11 have been most frequently reported. Translocations between chromosomes 8 and 14, as seen in Burkitt's lymphoma, have been reported in only two cases,[15,40] although we are aware of several unreported examples. An increase in unrelated clonal or nonclonal karyotypic abnormalities has been reported in PTLD specimens.[36,60–62] This is similar to changes seen in angioimmunoblastic lymphadenopathy[12] and also serves to differentiate PTLD lesions from in vitro cultures of EBV-infected lymphoblastoid cell lines. In these latter examples, the karyotype is stable.

CLASSIFICATION SYSTEMS OF POSTTRANSPLANT LYMPHOID HYPERPLASIAS AND NEOPLASIAS

Prior to the 1980s, the term *reticulum cell sarcoma* was uniformly applied to abnormal lymphoproliferations occurring in transplant patients.[63,64] A study from the University of Minnesota sampled four histologically distinct categories of LPDs in this patient population[1,2] and introduced the concept that these lesions represented a range of disorders. Two then newly described conditions, namely, polymorphic diffuse B-cell hyperplasia and polymorphic B-cell lymphoma, were interpreted as hyperplastic and early neoplastic members of this syndrome (Table 9-1). This conclusion was later supported by clonal analysis in some cases. These two conditions were to be distinguished from nonspecific reactive hyperplasia at one end and immunoblastic sarcoma at the other end of this scale. However, the clinical relevance of the differentiation between polymorphic diffuse B-cell hyperplasia and polymorphic B-cell lymphoma was unclear at that time.[2]

Initial studies from the Stanford University heart transplant series suggested that all posttransplant lymphoid lesions were monoclonal as based on immunoglobulin gene rearrange-

Table 9-1. Classification Systems of Posttransplant Lymphoproliferations

Frizzera et al.[2]	Nalesnik et al.[4]	Knowles et al.[7]
(Reactive hyperplasia)[a]		
	(Infectious mononucleosis)	
	(Plasma cell hyperplasia)	Plasma cell hyperplasia
Polymorphic diffuse B-cell hyperplasia	Polymorphic posttransplant lymphoproliferative disorder	Polymorphic posttransplant lymphoproliferative disorder (polymorphic diffuse B-cell hyperplasia)
Polymorphic B cell lymphoma	Polymorphic posttransplant lymphoproliferative disorder	Polymorphic posttransplant lymphoproliferative disorder (polymorphic B-cell lymphoma)
	"Minimally polymorphic" posttransplant lymphoproliferative disorder	
Immunoblastic sarcoma	Monomorphic posttransplant lymphoproliferative disorder	Immunoblastic lymphoma, multiple myeloma

[a] Terms in parentheses were either not considered as a proven component of the PTLD process by the individual authors (reactive hyperplasia, plasma cell hyperplasia) or were considered a part of the spectrum but were not reported as a part of the original series (infectious mononucleosis).

ment analysis.[38] This observation was subsequently expanded when multiple concurrent lesions from individual patients were observed.[57] Unique clonal rearrangements within individual tumors raised the possibility that the lesions were actually multicentric growths.

An analysis of lymphoproliferations arising in the organ transplant population studied at the University of Pittsburgh showed a range of histologies similar to that described in the Minnesota series.[4] No clinical differences could be discerned between those patients diagnosed as having polymorphic B-cell hyperplasia and those diagnosed as having polymorphic B-cell lymphoma. Thus, these two categories were merged under the simplified heading of *polymorphic PTLD* (Table 9-1). A separate subgroup of patients had lesions histologically identical to non-Hodgkin's lymphomas. Although immunoblastic sarcomas were well represented within this group, other lesions resembled different forms of non-Hodgkin's lymphomas. The inclusive term of *monomorphic PTLD* was employed to distinguish such lesions from the polymorphic hyperplasia/lymphoma category. On the basis of this patient series it was concluded that polymorphic lesions as a group were more likely to respond to conservative therapy (whether or not a monoclonal component was detectable; see below) than were histologically monomorphic PTLDs. Despite this difference in behavior, the term *lymphoma* was not applied to any of these lesions at that time, since the relationship of these EBV-carrying lesions to true non-Hodgkin's lymphomas was unknown.

Two other types of lesions were observed in this study. The first was reactive diffuse plasmacytic hyperplasia and consisted of a diffuse proliferation of benign-appearing plasma cells with retention of underlying architecture. This was seen in conjunction with PTLD elsewhere in the patient. It was not known whether this itself was a virus-driven condition or if it represented a reaction to lymphoproliferative disease elsewhere.

The second type of lesion consisted of a diffuse invasive lymphoproliferation, also with a marked plasmacellular component. Polymorphism was present but was minimal in such cases due to this restricted cellular composition. It was suggested that such lesions might respond more favorably to therapy than purely "monomorphic" lesions.

Additional experience at other centers disclosed cases with features intermediate between those described from the above three series. The term *atypical lymphoid hyperplasia* was applied to lesions that occurred in the paracortex of lymph nodes or interstitium of tissues and were composed of a polymorphic mononuclear cell infiltrate without evidence of invasion or of destruction of underlying tissue.[36] Atypical polymorphic diffuse B-cell hyperplasia was a term applied to lesions intermediate between polymorphic diffuse B-cell hyperplasia and polymorphic B-cell lymphoma.[36] Lesions morphologically equivalent to infectious mononucleosis,[28] multiple myeloma,[37,43] or T-cell lymphoma[9] have since been described as manifestations of PTLD.

Knowles et al.[7] divided their series of 28 PTLDs into five histologic categories, namely, plasmacytic hyperplasia, polymorphic diffuse B-cell hyperplasia, polymorphic B-cell lymphoma, immunoblastic lymphoma, and multiple myeloma (Table 9-1). From this range they were able to construct three clinicopathologic groups. Plasmacytic hyperplasia presented an appearance similar to that defined above and constituted the first group of lesions. These investigators defined polymorphic diffuse B-cell hyperplasia and polymorphic B-cell lymphoma according to the original criteria[2] and concluded that there was no clinical difference between the behavior of these two types of lesions. They therefore grouped them as a second class and termed them *polymorphic PT-LPD*. Finally, immunoblastic lymphoma and multiple myeloma were representative of the third group of lesions. Immunoblastic lymphomas could consist of monomorphic collections of cytologically malignant cells or, in some cases, uniform-appearing lesions composed of plasmacytoid cells. Conversely, some cases showed a more heterogeneous or polymorphic population of malignant cells. Multiple myeloma was defined as consisting of a monomorphic population of cytologically atypical plasma cells.[7] These investigators did not observe other forms of non-Hodgkin's lymphomas in their series of adult cardiac transplant recipients.

THE EPSTEIN-BARR VIRUS AND PTLD

Prologue: Epstein-Barr Virus Infection and Host Response

EBV is a double-stranded DNA herpesvirus that preferentially infects B lymphocytes via an interaction between the viral envelope glycoprotein 350/220 and the B-cell surface protein CD21.[65,66] Primary infection occurs mainly by salivary exchange, and the oropharynx is a site of viral replication. Although normal[67] and abnormal[68] epithelial cells may support such replication, recent studies suggest that it is the lymphocytes in this area, and not the oropharyngeal epithelial cells, that serve as the reservoir for the virus and for the passage of virus between hosts.[69] Eradication of infection following bone marrow transplantation in some patients also suggests that the hematopoietic cell compartment is a major site of virus persistence.[70]

Upon B-cell receptor–virus ligand interaction, EBV is internalized and carried into the cell nucleus. The linear viral DNA forms a circular episome by fusion of terminal repeat segments at either end of the viral genome. This is associated with variable loss of some of the segments, such that individual viral particles may have different multiples of terminal repeats. The episomal form of virus corresponds to the latent, rather than the lytic or infectious, form of infection. Latent infection normally persists for the life of the host.[65,66]

In the case of latent infection, a small number of viral proteins may be produced. These include six EBNAs (Epstein-Barr nuclear antigens), as well as three proteins that localize primarily to the cell surface (latent membrane proteins, LMP-1, -2a, -2b). Several nontranslated RNAs are also produced in high copy number (EBERs, EBV early RNAs).[71]

In vitro studies indicate that expression of LMP-1 and EBNAs 2, 3A, 3C, and LP are essential for the transformation or immortalization of B lymphocytes.[72] The viral proteins interact to upregulate B-cell activation markers such as CD23 as well as adhesion markers (e.g., LFA-

1, LFA-3, ICAM-1) and vimentin.[73–79] Such infected cells may progress through the cell cycle and proliferate.

The viral episomes divide and distribute themselves randomly among the chromosomes during cell mitosis so as to produce more or less equal numbers of viral progeny within each of the daughter lymphocytes.[80] The daughter virus particles generally retain the same multiple of terminal repeat segments as found in the original virus particle. This phenomenon has been exploited to determine the ''clonal'' status of the virus within a PTLD (see below).

Cellular *bcl*-2 production is induced by viral LMP-1, and this serves to inhibit apoptosis.[81–83] The net sum of these effects is a rapid expansion of the B-cell compartment.

The above events are normally either subclinical in very young children or are associated with infectious mononucleosis in a slightly older population.[18] The B-cell stimulation triggers a host response that modulates and eventually controls this lymphoproliferation.[65] Natural killer cells (NK cells) increase in number early during typical EBV-related infectious mononucleosis.[84] These cells are soon eclipsed by the more numerous cytotoxic CD8+ T cells, which mediate their effects in a class I HLA-restricted manner.[85–89] Some studies indicate restricted T-cell receptor usage and increased numbers of $\gamma\delta$ T cells early in the response.[90–92] Variability in response to different viral epitopes has been demonstrated in an HLA-dependent manner in vitro.[80]

Despite a strong cellular immune response, patients with infectious mononucleosis can develop transient cutaneous anergy. This may be due to a combination of T-suppressor activity or direct interference with the T-cell receptor signal. Both processes have been demonstrated in vitro during acute EBV infection.[93,94]

This immunologic storm that comprises infectious mononucleosis is accompanied by a variety of alterations in cytokine levels. Elevations of interferon-γ, interleukin-2 (IL-2), and IL-1α have been described in infectious mononucleosis.[95] Andersson et al.[96] have observed a more prominent IL-2, interferon-γ, and tumor necrosis factor-β expression in infectious mononucleosis tonsils than in tonsils with recurrent tonsillitis. There is some evidence that IL-2 and possibly other cytokines may serve to prevent apoptosis in responding T cells.[97]

The serologic response to infectious mononucleosis has been well described.[18,66] IgM production against the viral capsid antigen is an indicator of primary infection. This is superseded by IgG production, which persists for the life of the host. Antigens of the early viral lytic cycle also induce antibody production. Antibodies to EBV nuclear antigens develop later in infection and usually persist for life.

The acute infection typically subsides after 1 to 3 months. The virus persists in latent form within B lymphocytes, and the bone marrow has been shown to function as a major virus reservoir.[98] Several forms of virus latency have been defined by in vitro studies.[99] These differ according to viral promoter usage as well as in the number and types of viral proteins produced. Different types of latency exist in vitro for lymphoblastoid cell lines, for Burkitt's lymphoma cells, and for EBV-infected Hodgkin's or Reed-Sternberg cells.[100] The in vivo phenotype of the latent infected B cell has also been an object of study. Recent studies suggest that this phenotype is more similar to the antigenically silent Burkitt's lymphoma cell than to the heavily activated lymphoblastoid cell line.[101] If this viewpoint is correct, then one may speculate that the lifelong persistence of antibodies and cytotoxic cells specific for EBV reflects an ongoing host response to sporadic, small-scale activation of infected B cells that are reexpressing the lymphoblastoid cell line and/or lytic phenotype. Such a scenario has not yet been proven, however.

In the transplant recipient, antirejection immunosuppression is thought to inhibit the specific T-cell cytotoxicity that serves to control EB viral infection.[3,102,103] A high incidence of lymphoproliferative disorders in patients who have received large doses of the anti-T-cell antibody OKT3[14] as well as the 24 percent frequency of PTLD in bone marrow recipients who receive T-cell-depleted allogeneic grafts[36] may be examples of this concept carried to somewhat extreme lengths. Interference with T-cell anti-EBV immunosurveillance as the sole reason for PTLD may be simplistic, however, since (1) not every patient who receives augmented immunosuppression develops PTLD, (2) some patients develop PTLD despite rigorous control of immunosuppression, and (3) some patients sustain primary posttransplant EBV infection with no clinical complications.

Detection of EBV—Methods and Application

Detection of EBV DNA in transplant-associated lymphoproliferations was initially performed using Southern blot hybridization analysis of DNA extracted from fresh tumor specimens.[104] More recently, the development of specific reagents for immunohistochemistry, in situ hybridization, and the polymerase chain reaction (PCR) made possible the detection of EBV from routinely processed paraffin-embedded tissue specimens.[105–109]

Molecular Detection of EBV

EBV is a double-stranded herpes virus 172 kb in length.[110] There are several internal repeat regions alternating with unique regions. At either end of the genome are a series of terminal repeats, which fuse when viral DNA circularizes.

Initial methods of detection focused on internal repeat sequences to demonstrate the viral genome in tumor tissues.[104] Since the internal repeat regions vary among individual viruses, analysis of these sequences has also been used to document transmission of virus via transplanted organs and to show that the subsequent lymphoproliferations derived from the transmitted as opposed to endogenous host virus.[111]

In 1986, Raab-Traub and Flynn[112] developed a novel probe to the viral genome. These investigators reasoned that by isolating a restriction fragment that contained the entire sequence of terminal repeats, it would be possible to determine the number of repeat segments for a given virus. It was presumed that a virus particle that was present in the cell prior to the proliferation of that cell would give rise to progeny with an identical number of terminal repeats in each virus particle. Therefore size fractionation and subsequent Southern hybridization of the reaction product would show a single sized restriction fragment corresponding to this event. In contrast, superinfection of an existing tumor by EBV would give rise to a panoply of different progeny virus particles, each family with its own particular number of terminal repeat fragments. Thus, this approach could not only indicate the presence of virus within tumor but could also determine the clonality of the virus in a manner analogous to determination of clonality of the cell itself. The two variables were generally found to correspond with rare exceptions. Furthermore, the approach gave insight into the latent versus lytic nature of the infection. Use of this probe has shown that latently infected cells comprise the predominant population of PTLDs. Lytic infection is typically seen in the context of specimens morphologically consistent with infectious mononucleosis. Some PTLDs may show a minor lytic component in addition to a predominant latent infection pattern.[5]

The sensitivity of the PCR allows detection of the virus in approximately in 1 in 10^6 cells.[113] However, its application is complicated by the fact that EBV infection persists for the life of the host.[66] Therefore, a baseline presence of virus can be expected that in itself may have no clinical significance. Furthermore, there is evidence to indicate that the host–virus equilibrium is shifted upward in favor of more virus in transplant patients.[114,115] Indeed, Marchevsky et al.[116] described several cases in which EBV was identified by PCR within an allograft lung, yet the patients responded to antirejection therapy. For this reason a negative PCR result may actually serve a more useful function by excluding the presence of virus in a given problematic case.[109]

This difficulty will likely be overcome to some degree by the more widespread use of quantitative PCR. Data at this point suggest that a rise in EBV DNA as detected by quantitative PCR from peripheral blood specimens may be predictive of subsequent PTLD.[117] Further data are needed to substantiate this, however.

In Situ Hybridization

Initial detection of EBV in situ utilized cloned probes directed against internal repeat segments of the virus. The sensitivity of this approach is such that a subset of PTLD cells exhibit a positive reaction. By using this approach Borisch-Chappuis et al.[118] showed two general patterns of EBV positivity that they likened to patterns detected in infectious mononucleosis or to Burkitt's lymphoma.

Randhawa et al.[119] utilized a ^{35}S-labeled *Bam*HI-W EBV internal repeat fragment DNA probe to study the distribution of the virus in 12 cases of disseminated and fatal PTLD. The estimated sensitivity of the probe was one viral genome per cell. As expected, they found the virus to be present within all sites of PTLD. Surprisingly, positive signals were also found in some hepatocytes and/or adrenal cortical epithelial cells in 5 of the 12 cases. Of interest, all five cases involved children.

A more commonly employed hybridization procedure to detect EBV in histologic specimens utilizes a probe against the early RNA of EBV (EBV early RNA, EBER).[71,120,121] This RNA has a considerable secondary structure that renders it somewhat resistant to the RNAses, which usually limit the ability of the pathologist to perform RNA hybridization studies on routinely processed tissues. Additionally, this RNA is produced in large amounts, reportedly up to 10^7 copies per cells. Thus, it can be detected by nonradioactive as well as radioactive means (Figs. 9-10C, 9-11). Utilization of this approach showed that EBV was actually present in the majority of cells of selected post-transplant lesions. Combination of this procedure with immunocytochemical stain showed that infiltrating T lymphocytes rarely contained the virus in these lesions (Fig. 9-11B).

One study utilized digoxigenin-labeled EBER probe to examine allograft liver biopsies for the presence of EBV.[122] Positive signals were found in 71 percent of patients who subsequently went on to develop PTLD. In contrast, EBER-positive cells were found in only 10 percent of patients who remained free of PTLD throughout the follow-up interval. Due to the retrospective nature of the study, however, the predictive value of EBER positivity in this setting remains undefined at present. Hubscher et al.[123] utilized ^{35}S-labeled EBER probe on liver biopsy and resection specimens and reported occasional positive cells in disorders other than EBV hepatitis or PTLD.

Late arising lesions with large polymorphic malignant appearing cells may differ from the usual PTLD, since the majority of the background cells are negative for virus whereas the large cells and scattered smaller cells do contain the virus (e.g., Fig. 9-10C). This situation is similar to that described for Hodgkin's disease that contains EBV.

Immunohistochemistry

Immunologic detection of EBV using human sera and later antibodies to EBNA-1 were pioneered by Henle et al.[124] and Henle and Henle.[125] The antigen–antibody system was particularly labile and thus not well suited for routine pathologic tissue specimens. The development of antibodies specific to individual EBV proteins has shown that PTLD cells express a viral phenotype similar to that seen in lymphoblastoid cell lines (i.e., a full expression of latent viral proteins).[126] From this conclusion it was surmised that growth of PTLD was likely contingent upon specific host immunodeficiency and not due to downregulation of viral proteins to evade host immunosurveillance.[98]

LMPs of EBV include three related proteins, LMP-1, LMP-2a, and LMP-2b. A commercially available cocktail of monoclonal antibodies raised against LMP-1 is reactive in paraffin-embedded specimens and produces a crisp surface and cytoplasmic stain of infected cells. The cytoplasmic positivity is a reflection of the rapid turnover of this protein, which plays an important role in cell transformation by the virus.[73,76,127] In our experience the stain is specific, but it is not as sensitive as EBER hybridization. However, the protein does appear to persist in areas of necrosis within the PTLD. Therefore, it may give presumptive evidence of viral presence in necrotic samples if care is taken to exclude background staining.

Commercially available monoclonal antibody to EBNA-2 has been designed to work in frozen sections. We have found that it is also applicable in paraffin tissues if an antigen retrieval technique, such as microwave pretreatment, is used. As of this time, we have been unsuccessful in applying any of the commercially available EBNA-1 antibodies to routinely processed paraffin sections, although they have been utilized for immunohistochemical staining by others.[128]

A commercially available monoclonal antibody directed against the virus protein encoded by the BZLF-1 segment of the genome exists. The target protein plays an important role in the transition of the virus from latency to a lytic state.[66,129] The antibody can be applied to both frozen and paraffin-embedded tissues, the latter requiring antigen retrieval for optimum results. Positive staining confirms the presence of EBV and suggests the presence of lytic as well as latent virus.[130] However, despite the presence of this protein in a number of PTLDs, other proteins indicative of late or productive stages of lytic infection (membrane glycoprotein, GHQ 140220) are not found.[130] Thus, an abortive entry into the lytic cycle may be common in these lesions. This question remains to be resolved. The possibility that this abortive lytic cycle exists may be a point in favor of the addition of antiviral drugs to therapeutic regimens,[55] although this point also remains unresolved.

SEPARATION OF PTLD CATEGORIES AND THEIR DIFFERENTIAL DIAGNOSIS FROM OTHER CONDITIONS

PTLDs are uncommon lesions, and current therapeutic strategies are based on the results of relatively small patient series. For this reason it is incumbent upon the histopathologist to apply precise criteria in delineating where to place a given specimen within the PTLD spectrum. This diagnosis should be supported whenever possible by phenotypic, clonal, and EBV analyses.

Infectious mononucleosis may be identified as such in uncomplicated cases by retention of follicles in the setting of nonuniform paracortical expansion. Transformed lymphocytes, including immunoblasts and plasma cells, exist in a background of small lymphocytes in these regions. Mitotic activity may be brisk, and in some cases aggregates of immunoblasts may occur. The overall process leads to distortion but not destruction of the underlying nodal architecture. Damage is restricted to single cell or small foci of necrosis. Reed-Sternberg-like cells may be seen in small numbers and may be found near these necrotic areas.

Many of the changes in infectious mononucleosis are shared by other forms of lymphadenitis, although the extent of changes are usually more prominent in EBV-related cases. Demonstration of the virus by any of the procedures mentioned above is extremely helpful in the differential diagnosis. In situ hybridization for EBER is more sensitive than immunohistochemical stain for LMP-1 or BZLF1 in detecting viral presence. Molecular studies may also be used to verify viral presence, although results of nonquantitative PCR need to be interpreted with caution. The presence of nonclonal cytogenetic abnormalities does not exclude the diagnosis of infectious mononucleosis, but clonal cytogenetic abnormalities would be inconsistent with the diagnosis.

Plasma cell hyperplasia may represent a variant of infectious mononucleosis in the immunosuppressed population. In plasma cell hyperplasia there is an exaggeration of the B-cell component as manifested by the predominance of plasma cells throughout. Plasma cell hyperplasia is a diffuse process in which virtually the entire node may resemble medullary cords. Cell anaplasia is not seen, and this helps to distinguish it from malignant plasmacellular proliferations. The extreme cellular heterogeneity of the polymorphic PTLDs is not a feature of this condition. Small foci of necrosis may be seen in plasma cell hyperplasia. These tend to resemble those observed in infectious mononucleosis (i.e., they are discrete foci, tend to be subcapsular, and comprise a minority of the surface area of the specimen). Spillover of plasma cell hyperplasia beyond the capsule is not a prominent finding. In aggregate, the features suggest that plasma cell hyperplasia represents a variant of infectious mononucleosis in which B-cell maturation is predominant but occurs in an orderly fashion. It is also likely that forms intermediate between plasma cell hyperplasia and polymorphic B-cell hyperplasia exist.

Plasma cell hyperplasia was originally described as an empirical finding that may or may not be related to an EBV-stimulated process.[4] A more recent classification places it within the context of PTLD, even though not all cases demonstrated EBV in that series.[7] The decision as to whether or not to include all such lesions within the PTLD family on the basis of histology alone remains problematic. We have observed one case of plasma cell hyperplasia coincident with a typical PTLD within the gut, although an exuberant (extranodal) plasma cell reaction that occurred in direct contiguity to the PTLD was the seat of a prominent cytomegalovirus infection. Despite occasional cases of this type, it is reasonable to include such lesions in lymph nodes as forms of PTLD, once other causes such as cytomegalovirus have been excluded.

According to present criteria, plasma cell hyperplasia is a reactive process within which minor B-cell clones may arise. This pathophysiology may be reflected by the presence of a minor band upon immunoglobulin gene rearrangement studies. Such minor clones are not routinely detectable by immunohistochemistry or flow cytometry. No karyotypic studies of these lesions have been reported.

Polymorphic B-cell hyperplasia contains a diffuse and heterogeneous population of lymphoid cells with tendencies toward plasma cell differentiation. Residual follicles are not seen in typical cases. The marked necrosis and atypical cells observed in polymorphic B-cell lymphoma are not seen in this condition in the pure state. However, these two conditions appear to be closely related, and intermediate forms may contain early foci of necrosis and/or rare atypical large immunoblast-like cells. The best approach in such cases is to note the existence of these features and to evaluate the lesion on the basis of the predominant pattern.

Polymorphic B-cell lymphoma is easily distinguished from other lesions in this spectrum when abundant necrosis and obvious Reed-Sternberg-like cells or atypical immunoblasts exist in a diffuse and invasive heterogeneous mononuclear background. Necrosis and Reed-Sternberg-like cells may also be seen in infectious mononucleosis, but they are usually less extensive in that condition.

Polymorphic immunoblastic lymphoma may also show significant heterogeneity of cell size with large bizarre cells and variable necrosis. In these cases anaplasia is a predominant feature and is not confined to the largest cell population. In some other cases frequent large bizarre cells may be seen in a less activated background, and the resemblance is more to Hodgkin's disease. In our experience these unusual tumors may also invade the node in a pattern akin to Hodgkin's disease. The phenotype of the large cells may be similar to Reed-Sternberg cells, and clonal analysis may reveal a small B-cell clone that presumably corresponds to these cells. Yet other cases may contain large cells with an appearance and phenotype of anaplastic large cell lymphoma.

A few comments are in order regarding issues that surround interpretation of EBV status in the context of PTLD. The original description of PTLD was based on a tumorous lesion that contained this virus. In the ensuing 15 years additional experience and technical advances have modified this position slightly. In particular, the ability to detect EBV in routinely processed paraffin sections has raised two important questions: (1) what is the significance of EBV positivity in inflammatory infiltrates that do not fulfill other criteria of PTLD, and (2) are EBV-negative lymphoid tumors to be classified in a manner identical to those that contain the virus?

In our opinion, the diagnosis of PTLD remains primarily a histologic one. Redefining the diagnosis on the basis of EBV-positive cells within inflammatory infiltrates in the absence of characteristic histology would amount to an unacceptable degree of drift in this principle. Such inflammatory lesions should be regarded as manifestations of latent or active EBV infection occurring in the immunosuppressed patient. Whereas entities such as EBV hepatitis and infectious mononucleosis represent histologically well-defined examples, we may expect that information obtained from this heavily biopsied patient population will expand our knowledge regarding the full range of pathologies associated with this ubiquitous virus.

A different problem occurs in the case of an EBV-negative lymphoma in a transplant patient. This is an uncommon situation in this population in contrast to the situation in the AIDS population. Is the use of the term PTLD justified in this instance, or is this an inappropriate designation for what may simply represent a sporadic malignant lymphoma? This issue is unresolved at present. Although our initial bias is to regard such lesions as garden-variety lymphoma, we have seen examples of regression in EBV-negative lymphoma in the course of a trial of reduced immunosuppression. At present we continue to include such lesions as members of the PTLD syndrome. Segregation and thorough pathologic and molecular workup of EBV-negative posttransplant lymphomas in published series will help to define the behavior of this category of tumors vis à vis their histologic counterparts in the nonimmunosuppressed population.

PTLD at Extranodal Sites

A significant number of PTLDs are multicentric. Extranodal disease is most frequently seen in the setting of coexistent node involvement, but it may also exist alone. The range of appearances of PTLDs at all sites is similar, although features may be modified somewhat by the parenchymal composition of the particular organ or site.

Liver

Liver involvement by PTLD starts in the portal regions (Fig. 9-12). Nodular infiltrates expand the portal tracts and may extend into the

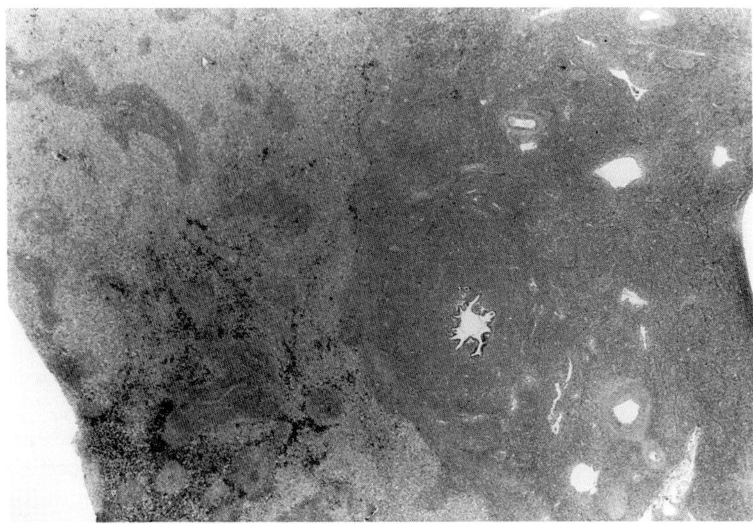

Fig. 9-12. Hepatic involvement by PTLD. Nodular portal infiltrates may coalesce to form larger tumors as in this case. In other cases, one or more tumors may occur as the only manifestation of this process in this organ. Note persistence of bile duct epithelium despite surrounding tumor. Mass effect of the infiltrate and cellular atypia favor the diagnosis of PTLD over EBV-associated hepatitis, but this distinction may be problematic at times.

periportal lobules.[23,131] Infiltration of vessels or bile ducts may occur, but the degree of bile duct infiltration is usually minimal given the intensity of the infiltrate. The infiltrate may show the heterogeneity typical of polymorphic PTLDs, or it may comprise a more uniform population. Diminished involvement of bile ducts (proportionate to rejection of similar cellular intensity) and atypia help to distinguish this from rejection. Nodularity of infiltrates and prominent atypia in some cases help to differentiate PTLD from EBV hepatitis.

Kidney

Early renal involvement by PTLD may track the perivascular region (Fig. 9-13). The infiltrate is usually dense and relatively circumscribed. Tubule infiltration may occur, but it is more common to see minimally involved tubules sitting amidst a lymphoid infiltrate. In other cases (or in other areas) tubular necrosis and disappearance may occur secondary to presumed ischemia. The lymphoid lesion may be heterogeneous or monotonous. Plasma cell differentiation is common.

The infiltrate may contain occasional eosinophils, although neutrophils are not a significant component (except adjacent to areas of necrosis). Thus, the infiltrate differs from that expected of a proportionately heavy rejection response. Long-term kidneys may contain periarterial aggregates of mature plasma cells. These are not infiltrative and should not be confused with PTLD. In our experience they have invariably been EBV negative.

We have recently seen a florid capsular repair reaction that histologically mimicked a lymphoproliferative disorder. Rare and occasional neutrophils were observed in this process, which was localized to the immediate subcapsular zone and occurred 2 weeks following transplant.

In resected allografts that contain lymphoproliferative disorders, involvement of the hilar fat may be seen.

Gastrointestinal Tract

The gastrointestinal tract may be involved at any site along its length.[132,133] The most frequent involvement appears at the site of the densest aggregate of lymphoid tissue (i.e., the ileocolic region). We have seen involvement of both native and allograft intestines in our series.

Native Gastrointestinal Tract

Involvement of the gastrointestinal tract by PTLD tends to occur in a multicentric fashion. The lesions arise in the submucosa and expand to induce ulceration with a heaped up border with subsequent infiltration and necrosis of the underlying muscularis propria (Fig. 9-14). Typical lesions do not infiltrate the mucosa substantially beyond the tumor site. Growth is rapid, and bowel perforation may occur within a few days of onset of symptoms.

Allograft Bowel

The onset of small bowel transplantation coincided with the introduction of in situ hybridization probes for EBV. Thus, the virus is most commonly detected within cells of a nonspecific inflammation within the lamina propria. Such inflammation may be extremely difficult to differentiate from early acute cellular rejection, and indeed it is possible that the two processes may coexist at this site. In any event, rapid transition from EBV-associated inflammation to rejection may occur in response to therapy. More fully developed cases of the PTLD within the allograft bowel resemble those seen within native bowel.

Central Nervous System

Similar to LPD at other sites, these lesions may present a polymorphic appearance or may resemble non-Hodgkin's lymphomas. The presence of atypical cells within cerebrospinal fluid may also be suggestive of this process within the central nervous system. Such an interpretation would need to be verified by the appropriate

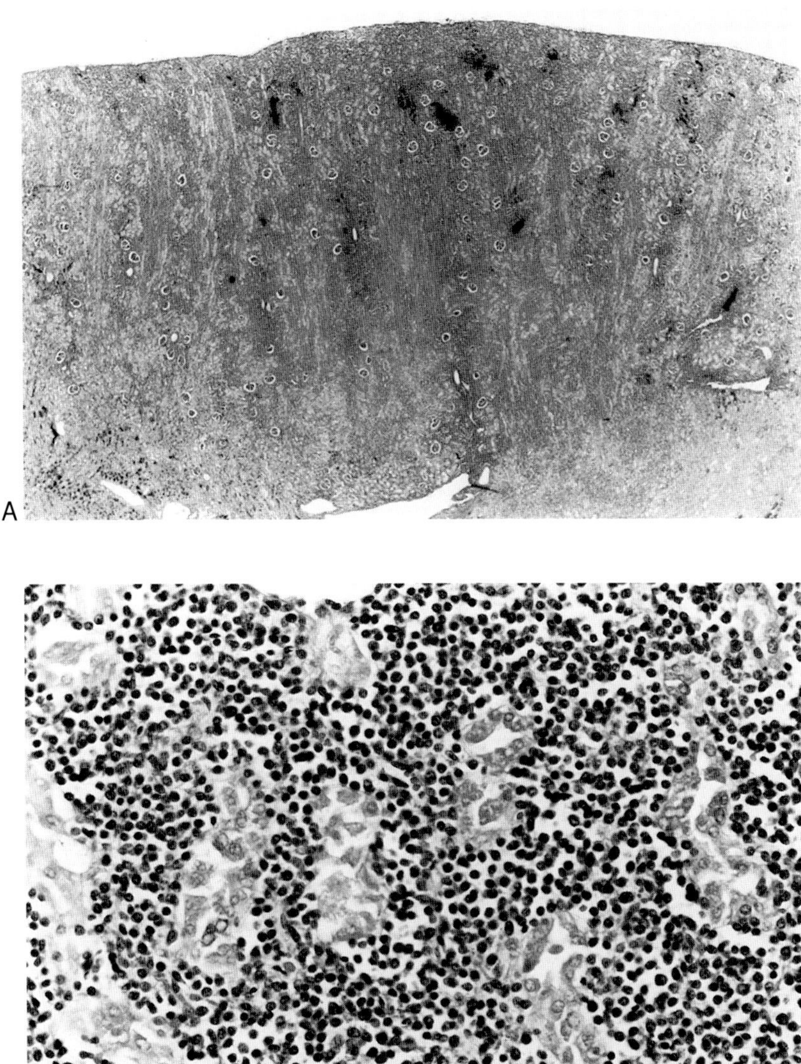

Fig. 9-13. Infiltrative PTLD involving allograft kidney. **(A)** A somewhat linear infiltrate alternates with areas of parenchyma less involved by the process. Glomeruli stand out in relief within the lesion. Darker areas represent foci of calcification. In some cases PTLD at this site presents as a mass lesion. However, even in an example such as this, a needle biopsy would tend to show an irregularly distributed process in contrast to the more uniform pattern of rejection. (H&E, ×10.) **(B)** The cells comprise a uniform population of lymphocytes and plasmacytoid forms without the ancillary cells expected in cellular rejection of an equivalent magnitude. Necrotic tubules are seen within the infiltrate. Tubulitis is present but is not an outstanding feature. (H&E, ×200.)

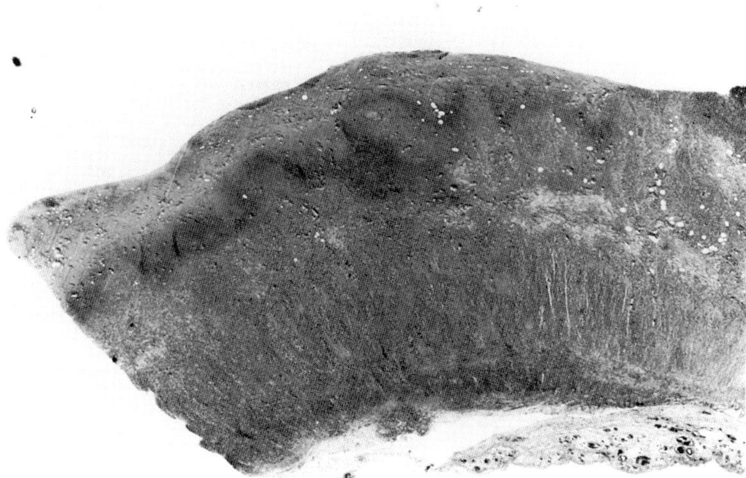

Fig. 9-14. Low power photomicrograph of intestinal PTLD. The upper portion consists of a fibrinoinflammatory exudate overlying the ulcerated bowel. These superficial areas frequently contain abundant bacteria. The tumor grows rapidly to infiltrate the entire bowel wall. In this example the muscularis propria is largely replaced by tumor. For this reason initial abdominal discomfort may rapidly progress to signs and symptoms of intestinal perforation. (H&E, ×10.)

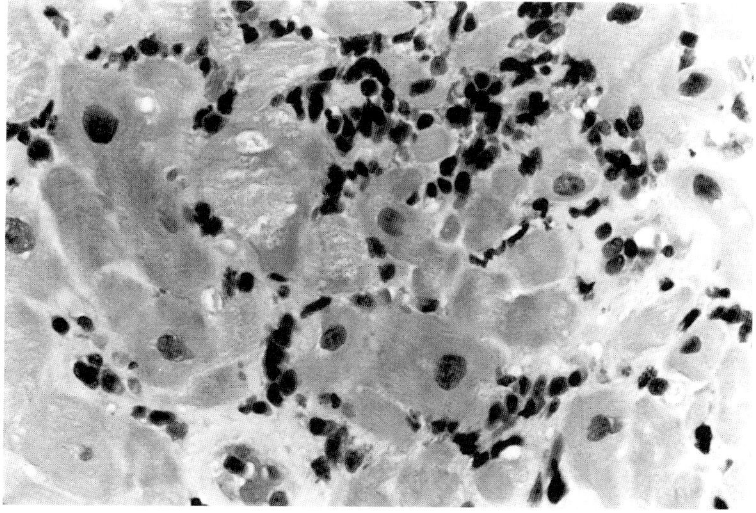

Fig. 9-15. Endomyocardial biopsy of allograft heart with PTLD. A uniform mononuclear infiltrate involves allograft myocardium. The cell nuclei are only slightly smaller than those of the adjacent myocytes. Some plasma cell differentiation is observable. Although the nuclei are larger than small lymphocytes, they still retain a hyperchromatic appearance. In some cases nuclear irregularities were seen. Occasional mitoses were also noted. None of the ancillary cells typical of an active rejection process (i.e., eosinophils and neutrophils) were present. The patient expired shortly thereafter with disseminated PTLD. (H&E, ×400.)

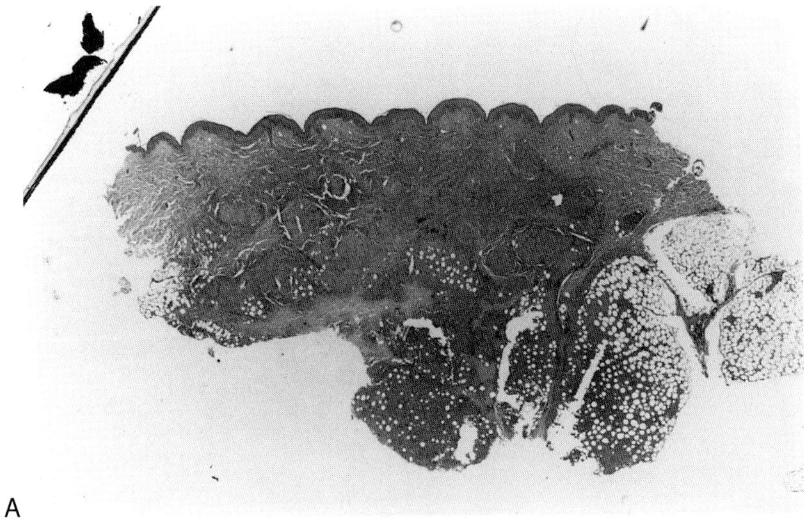

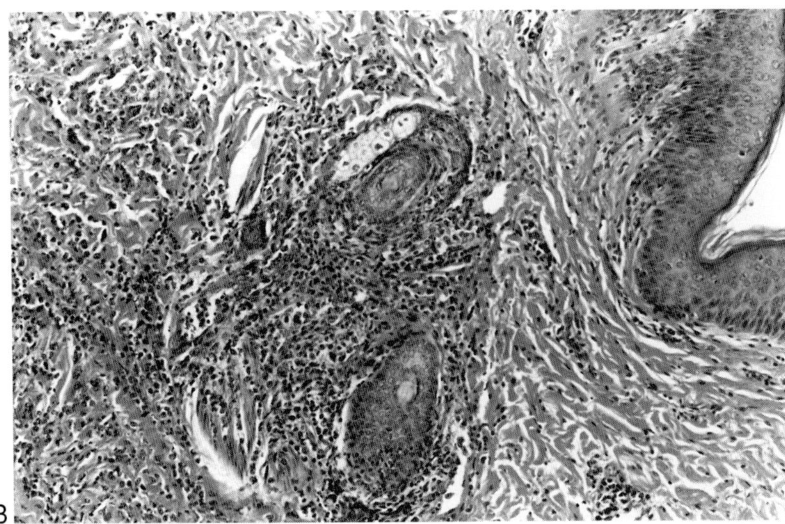

Fig. 9-16. Skin involvement by post-transplant lymphoproliferative disorder. **(A)** The distribution of the infiltrate does not diminish within the lower dermis and subcutaneous fat in this monomorphic PTLD. This pattern is typical of lymphomas involving this site. (H&E, ×10.) **(B)** Higher magnification shows preferential adnexal involvement. The upper dermis is largely spared in this example. (H&E, ×20.)

viral stains or isolation techniques, since other viral syndromes may also cause this appearance.[134]

Heart

The heart is rarely involved by EBV-associated lymphoproliferative disorders and then primarily in the setting of disseminated disease. Rarely, a diagnosis of lymphoproliferative disorder may be rendered on endomyocardial biopsy (Fig. 9-15).[135,136] The cells appear larger than those mediating rejection, and some atypia or plasmacytoid differentiation may be seen. In addition, aggregation of these cells may be seen in contrast to the usual mixed inflammation associated with rejection, in which eosinophils and neutrophils may also be found. A high level of suspicion must be maintained, since the diagnosis can be easily missed.

Lung

PTLD may grow as both infiltrative processes and tumor masses within the lung. Their relatively circumscribed nature leads to a growth pattern of one or more pulmonary nodules. A combination of interstitial and intraalveolar growth can occur. Vascular infiltration may be observed, and necrosis may be a prominent feature in our experience. A number of these lesions have a pronounced tendency for plasmacellular differentiation. Any of the lesions within the PTLD family may occur at this site. A uniform infiltrate with more than 25 percent B cells and over 30 percent large lymphoid cells favored PTLD in one study.[25] These authors recommended immunohistochemical staining for EBV LMP-1 as an even more useful criterion, however, since it was positive in all 11 study cases and negative in the same number of matched controls.

Skin

PTLD can occasionally present as ulcerations or nodules in the skin or underlying soft tissue (Fig. 9-16). In some cases, this has been related back to local inoculation of an immunosuppressive agent, whereas in other cases no associated lesion or procedure can be documented. Both inflammatory and neoplastic variants of lymphoproliferative disorder can be seen in the skin. Early lesions are associated with a tendency to involve skin adnexa. In more advanced cases, pandermal and subcutaneous involvement typical of lymphomas may be demonstrated.

CONCLUSION: PATHOGENETIC ASPECTS OF PTLDs

A number of authors have offered their opinions regarding the pathogenesis of PTLDs.[2,3,7,12,34,35,39,40,45,51–53,55,58,82,98,100,103,113,117,118,120,130,137–158] The following brief discussion incorporates a number of features from these and other authors in order to weave a coherent, if speculative, account of this disorder from the anatomic pathologist's standpoint. We offer this simply as one way to consider these tumors. Many of the individual points are unproven, although they are directly testable.

EBV infection of B lymphocytes in the setting of immunosuppression appears to be an important precondition for the majority of PTLDs. Exacerbation of either of these two variables (i.e., elevated levels of EBV or higher levels of immunosuppressive drugs) appears to be associated with an increased risk of the disorder. The different morphologies of PTLD may reflect different unrelated conditions, but it is logically appealing to view them as different aspects of a single underlying process. The EBV-stimulated B lymphocyte is normally brought under control by an immune response dominated by the cytotoxic T cell. The latter cell is a major target of antirejection therapy, and interference with the functions of this cell provides a mechanism by which explosive B-cell outgrowth may be possible. This process may be operative in cases of disseminated disease, in which widespread multiclonal or polyclonal lesions are often associated with other evidence of immunodeficiency (i.e., infections). In a more attenuated form, direct interference with T-cell function may be the major contributory factor to the increased incidence of LPDs in patients seronegative for EBV at the time of transplant. In these cases, the naive immune system must mount its primary antiviral response in the face of iatrogenic immunosuppression. In many cases, such lesions are amenable to modification of drug dose, antiviral therapy, and supportive care.

The appearances of infectious mononucleosis, plasma cell hyperplasia, and polymorphic PTLD (polymorphic diffuse B-cell hyperplasia and polymorphic B-cell lymphoma) may be a reflection of the intralesional dynamics between the virus-associated cell expansion and the efforts of the body to control it. T lymphocytes are likely most prominent in mononucleosis, although direct comparative quantitative studies among these conditions have not been reported. It is conceivable that a lesser degree of immune control may exist in polymorphic PTLD and may allow clonal competition among the stimulated B cells, thereby favoring outgrowth of small numbers of clones, or even a single clone. Such tumors often occur within the first year after transplant and may be more of a result of this disordered population-based proliferation than a result of true malignant transformation of individual cells. This viewpoint is supported by both the presence of clonal populations and the absence of oncogene changes in these lesions to date.

The heterogeneous cell appearance of polymorphic PTLD may also be a harbinger of the nature of the late-arising lesions. The overwhelming number of EBV-infected cells appear as transformed B cells in these lesions. Perhaps this is a reflection of the normal distribution of infection in other individuals who do not present with frank tumors at this time. Rare atypical immunoblasts are seen, and T lymphocytes, although they may occur in substantial numbers, are also only rarely infected by the virus. The proportions of infected cells in these lesions may crudely correspond to the relative frequencies of late tumors of the corresponding cell types.

The precise route by which such tumors arise remains undefined. Several studies suggest that the true latent infected B cell maintains a "silent" phenotype, unlike the case of in vitro infected cells. If this is true, then a source of B-cell stimulation might be required to activate expression of viral proteins. Alternatively, cell senescence itself might have a role in this process, since it is known that the virus has at its disposal the ability to save the cell from apoptosis via *bcl*-2 expression. If this is an important strategy of virus survival, it is possible that "illegitimate" rescue from apoptosis occurs, leading to proliferation of cells with cumulative accretion of random cytogenetic abnormalities. Such cells could provide a reservoir from which late-arising malignancies occur. Furthermore, the addition of mutations or rearrangements of specific oncogenes/antioncogenes may supplement these alterations and lead to true malignancies. It may be that the virus itself is no longer required at this point and is lost as clonal progression occurs within the tumor. In other cases, persistence of virus expression may provide targets for the immune system even in the presence of true immunity.

What are the implications of this to the surgical pathologist? At a minimum, it should reemphasize the importance of careful evaluation of these conditions. It is possible to provide an accurate diagnosis based on histology alone, supplemented with special stains to detect EBV and to ascertain the phenotype of the cell of interest. It is highly desirable to set aside material for molecular analysis of clonality and to provide fresh tissue for cytogenetic studies. In this manner, accurate statements can be made regarding the relationship between disease and response to therapy. The nature of these disorders remains such that one or several well-studied cases may provide a significant addition to our collective understanding of herpesvirus-associated lymphomagenesis.

ACKNOWLEDGMENTS

The generosity of Dr. Eduardo Yunis of Children's Hospital of Pittsburgh, PA, in providing material for a number of the photomicrographs is gratefully acknowledged. The assistance of Dr. Ronald Jaffe of Children's Hospital of Pittsburgh, PA, in providing the specimen for Figure 9-8 is also appreciated.

REFERENCES

1. Hanto DW, Frizzera G, Purtilo DT et al: Clinical spectrum of lymphoproliferative disorders in renal transplant recipients and evidence for the role of Epstein-Barr virus. Cancer Res 41:4253, 1981
2. Frizzera G, Hanto DW, Gajl-Peczalska KJ et al: Polymorphic diffuse B-cell hyperplasias and lymphomas in renal transplant recipients. Cancer Res 41:4262, 1981
3. Starzl TE, Nalesnik MA, Porter KA et al: Reversibility of lymphomas and lymphoprolifera-

tive lesions developing under cyclosporine–steroid therapy. Lancet i:584, 1984
4. Nalesnik MA, Jaffe R, Starzl TE et al: The pathology of post-transplant lymphoproliferative disorders occurring in the setting of cyclosporine A–prednisone immunosuppression. Am J Pathol 133:173, 1988
5. Locker J, Nalesnik M: Molecular genetic analysis of lymphoid tumors arising after organ transplantation. Am J Pathol 135:977, 1989
6. Chen JM, Barr ML, Chadburn A et al: Management of lymphoproliferative disorders after cardiac transplantation. Ann Thorac Surg 56:527, 1993
7. Knowles DM, Cesarman E, Chadburn A et al: Correlative morphologic and molecular genetic analysis demonstrates three distinct categories of posttransplantation lymphoproliferative disorders. Blood 85:552, 1995
8. Leblond V, Sutton L, Dorent R et al: Lymphoproliferative disorders after organ transplantation: a report of 24 cases observed in a single center. J Clin Oncol 13:961, 1995
9. van Gorp J, Doornewaard H, Verdonck LF et al: Posttransplant T-cell lymphoma. Report of three cases and a review of the literature. Cancer 73:3064, 1994
10. Penn I: Immunosuppression—a contributing factor in lymphoma formation. Clin Transplant 6:214, 1992
11. Penn I: The changing pattern of posttransplant malignancies. Transplant Proc 23:1101, 1991
12. Frizzera G: Atypical lymphoproliferative disorders. P. 459. In Knowles DM (ed): Neoplastic Hematopathology. Williams & Wilkins, Baltimore, 1992
13. Calne RY, Rolles K, White DJ et al: Cyclosporine A initially as the only immunosuppressant in 34 recipients of cadaveric organs: 32 kidneys, 2 pancreases, and 2 livers. Lancet 2:1033, 1979
14. Swinnen LJ, Costanzo-Nordin MK, Fisher SG et al: Increased incidence of lymphoproliferative disorder after immunosuppression with the monoclonal antibody OKT3 in cardiac transplant recipients. N Engl J Med 323:1723, 1990
15. Ho M, Jaffe R, Miller G et al: The frequency of Epstein-Barr virus infection and associated lymphoproliferative syndrome after transplantation and its manifestations in children. Transplantation 45:719, 1988
16. Ho M, Miller G, Atchison RW et al: Epstein-Barr virus infections and DNA hybridization studies in posttransplantation lymphoma and lymphoproliferative lesions: the role of primary infection. J Infect Dis 152:876, 1985
17. Malatack JJ, Gartner JC, Urbach AH et al: Orthotopic liver transplantation, Epstein-Barr virus, cyclosporine, and lymphoproliferative disease: a growing concern. J Pediatr 118:667, 1991
18. Cheeseman SH: Infectious mononucleosis. Semin Hematol 25:261, 1988
19. Emery RW, Lake KD, Brouwer RML et al: Letters. Reply to [Swinnen LJ, Costanzo-Nordin MK, Fisher SG et al: Increased incidence of lymphoproliferative disorder after immunosuppression with the monoclonal antibody OKT3 in cardiac transplant recipients. N Engl J Med 323:1723, 1990]. N Engl J Med 324:1437, 1991
20. Kheterpal S, Kirkby GR, Neuberger JM et al: Intraocular lymphoma after liver transplantation. Am J Ophthalmol 116:507, 1993
21. Palmer BF, Sagalowsky AI, Mcquitty DA et al: Lymphoproliferative disease presenting as obstructive uropathy after renal transplantation. J Urol 153:392, 1995
22. Markin RS, Linder J, Zuerlein K et al: Hepatitis in infectious mononucleosis. Gastroenterology 93:1210, 1987
23. Randhawa PS, Williams PA, Markin RS et al: Epstein-Barr virus associated syndromes in immunosuppressed liver transplant recipients: clinical profile and recognition on routine allograft biopsy. Am J Surg Pathol 14:538, 1990
24. Jin DC, Yoon YS, Yoon SA et al: Ten cases of malignancies in kidney allografts. Transplant Proc 26:1975, 1994
25. Rosendale B, Yousem SA: Discrimination of Epstein-Barr virus-related posttransplant lymphoproliferations from acute rejection in lung allograft recipients. Arch Pathol Lab Med 119:418, 1995
26. Cohen JI: Epstein-Barr virus lymphoproliferative disease associated with acquired immunodeficiency. Medicine 70:137, 1991
27. Martinez AJ, Ahdab-Barmada M: The neuropathology of liver transplantation: comparison of main complications in children and adults. Mod Pathol 6:25, 1993
28. Billiar TR, Hanto DW, Simmons RL: Inclusion of infectious mononucleosis in the spectrum of Epstein-Barr virus infections in transplant recipients. Transplantation 46:159, 1988
29. Salvador AH, Harrison EG, Kyle RA: Lym-

phadenopathy due to infectious mononucleosis: its confusion with malignant lymphoma. Cancer 27:1029, 1971

30. Gowing NFC: Infectious mononucleosis: histopathologic aspects. Pathol Annu 10:1, 1975
31. Childs CC, Parham DM, Berard CW: Infectious mononucleosis: the spectrum of morphologic changes simulating lymphoma in lymph nodes and tonsils. Am J Surg Pathol 11:122, 1987
32. Strickler JG, Fedeli F, Horwitz CA et al: Infectious mononucleosis in lymphoid tissue. Histopathology, in situ hybridization, and differential diagnosis. Arch Pathol Lab Med 117:269, 1993
33. Lukes RJ, Tindle BH, Parker JW: Reed-Sternberg-like cells in infectious mononucleosis [letter]. Lancet 2:1003, 1969
34. Reynolds DJ, Banks PM, Gulley ML: New characterization of infectious mononucleosis and a phenotypic comparison with Hodgkin's disease. Am J Pathol 146:379, 1995
35. Swerdlow SH: Post-transplant lymphoproliferative disorders: a morphologic, phenotypic and genotypic spectrum of disease. Histopathology 20:373, 1992
36. Shapiro RS, McClain K, Frizzera G et al: Epstein-Barr virus associated B cell lymphoproliferative disorders following bone marrow transplantation. Blood 71:1234, 1988
37. Chucrallah AE, Crow MK, Rice LE et al: Multiple myeloma after cardiac transplantation: an unusual form of posttransplant lymphoproliferative disorder. Hum Pathol 25:541, 1994
38. Cleary ML, Warnke R, Sklar J: Monoclonality of lymphoproliferative lesions in cardiac-transplant recipients. N Engl J Med 310:477, 1984
39. Craig FE, Gulley ML, Banks PM: Posttransplantation lymphoproliferative disorders. Am J Clin Pathol 99:265, 1993
40. Delecluse HJ, Rouault JP, French M et al: Posttransplant lymphoproliferative disorders with genetic abnormalities commonly found in malignant tumours. Br J Haematol 89:90, 1995
41. Doyle TJ, Kumarapuram K, Venkatachalam MD et al: Hodgkin's disease in renal transplant patients. Cancer 51:245, 1983
42. Griffith RC, Saha BK, Janney CV: Immunoblastic lymphoma of T-cell type in a chronically immunosuppressed renal transplant patient. Am J Clin Pathol 93:280, 1990
43. Joseph G, Barker RL, Yuan B et al: Posttransplantation plasma cell dyscrasias. Cancer 74: 1959, 1994
44. Medeiros LJ, Kingma DW, Martin AW et al: Epstein-Barr virus (EBV)-induced lymphoproliferative disorders (LPD) manifesting as plasmacytomas, abstracted. Lab Invest 68:96A, 1993
45. Nalesnik MA, Makowka L, Starzl TE: The diagnosis and treatment of posttransplant lymphoproliferative disorders. Curr Prob Surg 25:365, 1988
46. Oldhafer KJ, Bunzendahl H, Frei U et al: Primary Hodgkin's lymphoma: an unusual case of graft dysfunction after kidney transplantation. Am J Med 87:218, 1989
47. Spiro IJ, Yandell DW, Li C et al: Brief report: lymphoma of donor origin occurring in the porta hepatis of a transplanted liver. N Engl J Med 329:27, 1993
48. Wu TT, Swerdlow S, Locker J et al: Pathologic analysis of recurrent posttransplant lymphoproliferative disorders. Transplant Proc 27:1193, 1995
49. Sterling W, Wu L, Dowling E: Hodgkin's disease in a renal transplant recipient. Transplantation 17:315, 1974
50. Cerilli J, Rynosiewicz J, Rothermel W: Hodgkin's disease in human renal transplantation. Am J Surg 133:182, 1977
51. Nalesnik MA, Randhawa P, Demetris AJ, et al: Lymphoma resembling Hodgkin disease after posttransplant lymphoproliferative disorder (PTLD) in a liver transplant recipient. Cancer 72:2568, 1993
52. Ferry JA, Jacobson JO, Conti D et al: Lymphoproliferative disorders and hematologic malignancies following organ transplantation. Mod Pathol 2:583, 1989
53. Thomas JA, Hotchin NA, Allday MJ et al: Immunohistology of Epstein-Barr virus-associated antigens in B cell disorders from immunocompromised individuals. Transplantation 49:944, 1990
54. Borisch B, Gatter KC, Tobler A et al: Epstein-Barr virus-associated anaplastic large cell lymphoma in renal transplant patients. Am J Clin Pathol 98:312, 1992
55. Hanto DW, Frizzera G, Gajl-Peczalska KJ et al: Epstein-Barr virus, immunodeficiency, and B cell lymphoproliferation. Transplantation 39: 461, 1985
56. Nalesnik M, Locker J, Jaffe R et al: Experience with posttransplant lymphoproliferative disor-

ders in solid organ transplant patients. Clin Transplant 6:249, 1992

57. Cleary ML, Sklar J: Lymphoproliferative disorders in cardiac transplant recipients are multiclonal lymphomas. Lancet 2:489, 1984
58. Shearer WT, Ritz J, Finegold MJ et al: Epstein-Barr virus-associated B-cell proliferations of diverse clonal origins after bone marrow transplantation in a 12 year old patient with severe combined immunodeficiency. N Engl J Med 312:1151, 1985
59. Hanto DW, Frizzera G, Gajl-Peczalska K et al: Epstein-Barr virus-induced B-cell lymphoma after renal transplantation. Acyclovir therapy and transition from polyclonal and monoclonal B-cell proliferation. N Engl J Med 306:913, 1982
60. Cabanillas F, Pathak S, Zander A et al: Monosomy 21, partial duplication of chromosome 11, and structural abnormalities of chromosome 1q21 in a case of lymphoma developing in a transplant recipient: characteristic abnormalities of secondary lymphoma? Cancer Genet Cytogenet 24:7, 1987
61. Olopade OI, Anastasi J, Thangavelu M et al: Cytogenetic abnormalities in a secondary lymphoma complicating cardiac transplantation. Leukemia 3:303, 1989
62. Gollin SM, Cen H, Storto PD et al: Consistent nonclonal cytogenetic abnormalities in posttransplant lymphoproliferative disease, abstracted. Am J Hum Genet, suppl 3 47:A7, 1990
63. Deodhar SD, Kuklinca AG, Vidt DG et al: Development of reticulum cell sarcoma at the site of antilymphocyte globulin injection in a patient with renal transplant. N Engl J Med 280:1104, 1969
64. Cotton JR, Searls AG, Remmers AR et al: The appearance of reticulum cell sarcoma at the site of antilymphocyte globulin injection. Transplantation 16:154, 1973
65. Kieff E, Liebowitz D: Epstein-Barr virus and its replication. P. 1889. In Fields BN, Knipe DM, Chanock RM et al. (eds): Fields Virology. 2nd Ed. Lippincott-Raven, Philadelphia, 1990
66. Miller G: Epstein-Barr virus: biology, pathogenesis, and medical aspects. p. 1921. In Fields BN, Knipe DM, Chanock RM et al: (eds): Fields Virology. 2nd Ed. Lippincott-Raven, Philadelphia, 1990
67. Sixbey JW, Nedrud JG, Raab-Traub N et al: Epstein-Barr virus replication in oropharyngeal epithelial cells. N Engl J Med 310:1225, 1984
68. Greenspan JS, Greenspan D, Lennette E et al: Replication of Epstein-Barr virus within epithelial cells of oral ''hairy'' leukoplakia, an AIDS-associated lesion. N Engl J Med 313:1564, 1985
69. Anagnostopoulos I, Hummel M, Kreschel C et al: Morphology, immunophenotype, and distribution of latently and/or productively infected Epstein-Barr virus-infected cells in acute infectious mononucleosis: implications for the interindividual infection route of Epstein-Barr virus. Blood 85:744, 1995
70. Gratama JW, Oosterveer MAP, Zwaan FE et al: Eradication of Epstein-Barr virus by allogeneic bone marrow transplantation: implications for site of latency. Proc Natl Acad Sci USA 85: 8693, 1988
71. Glickman JN, Howe JG, Steitz JA: Structural analysis of EBER1 and EBER2 ribonucleoprotein particles present in Epstein-Barr virus-infected cells. J Virol 62:902, 1988
72. Kaye KM, Izumi KM, Kieff E: Epstein-Barr virus latent membrane protein-1 is essential for B-lymphocyte growth transformation. Proc Natl Acad Sci USA 90:9150, 1993
73. Kaye KM, Izumi KM, Mosialos G et al: The Epstein-Barr virus LMP1 cytoplasmic carboxy terminus is essential for B-lymphocyte transformation: fibroblast cocultivation complements a critical function within the terminal 155 residues. J Virol 69:675, 1995
74. Tong X, Wang F, Thut CJ et al: The Epstein-Barr virus nuclear protein 2 acidic domain can interact with TFIIB, TAF40, and RPA70 but not with TATA-binding protein. J Virol 69:585, 1995
75. Johannsen E, Koh E, Mosialos G et al: Epstein-Barr virus nuclear protein 2 transactivation of the latent membrane protein 1 promoter is mediated by j kappa and PU.1. J Virol 69:253, 1995
76. Wang F, Gregory C, Sample C et al: Epstein-Barr virus latent membrane protein (LMP1) and nuclear proteins 2 and 3C are effectors of phenotypic changes in B lymphocytes: EBNA-2 and LMP1 co-operatively induce CD23. J Virol 64: 2309, 1990
77. Wang F, Kikutani H, Tsang SF et al: Epstein-Barr nuclear protein 2 transactivates a cis-acting CD23 DNA element. J Virol 65:4101, 1991
78. Cohen JI, Wang F, Mannick J et al: Epstein-Barr virus nuclear protein 2 is a key determinant

of lymphocyte transformation. Proc Natl Acad Sci USA 86:9558, 1989
79. Birkenbach M, Liebowitz D, Wang F et al: Epstein-Barr virus latent infection membrane protein increases vimentin expression in human B-cell lines. J Virol 63:4079, 1989
80. Orlowski R, Polvino-Bodnar M, Hearing J et al: Inhibition of specific binding of EBNA 1 to DNA by murine monoclonal and certain human polyclonal antibodies. Virology 176:638, 1990
81. Rowe M, Pengpilon M, Huen DS et al: Upregulation of *bcl*-2 by the Epstein-Barr virus latent membrane protein LMP1: a B-cell-specific response that is delayed relative to NF-kappa B activation and to induction of cell surface markers. J Virol 68:5602, 1994
82. Henderson S, Rowe M, Gregory C et al: Induction of *bcl*-2 expression by Epstein-Barr virus latent membrane protein 1 protects infected B cells from programmed cell death. Cell 65:1107, 1991
83. Hickish T, Robertson D, Clarke P et al: Ultrastructural localization of BHRF1: an Epstein-Barr virus gene product which has homology with *bcl*-2. Cancer Res 54:2808, 1994
84. Zverkova AS, Faktorova EI: Large granule-containing lymphocytes in patients with infectious mononucleosis. Vrachebnoe Delo 6:72, 1991
85. Svedmyr E, Jondal M: Cytotoxic effector cells specific for B cell line transformed by Epstein-Barr virus and present in patients with infectious mononucleosis. Proc Natl Acad Sci USA 72: 1622, 1975
86. Lee SP, Thomas WA, Murray RJ et al: HLA A2.1-restricted cytotoxic T-cells recognizing a range of Epstein-Barr virus isolates through a defined epitope in latent membrane protein LMP2. J Virol 67:7428, 1993
87. Burrows SR, Sculley TB, Misko IS et al: An Epstein-Barr virus-specific cytotoxic T cell epitope in EBV nuclear antigen 3 (EBNA 3). J Exp Med 171:345, 1990
88. Gavioli R, De Campos-Lima PO, Kurilla MG et al: Recognition of the Epstein-Barr virus-encoded nuclear antigens EBNA-4 and EBNA-6 by HLA-A11-restricted cytotoxic T lymphocytes: implications for down-regulation of HLA-A11 in Burkitt lymphoma. Proc Natl Acad Sci USA 89:5862, 1992
89. Murray RJ, Kurilla MG, Brooks JM et al: Identification of target antigens for the human cytotoxic T cell response to Epstein-Barr virus (EBV): implications for the immune control of EBV-positive malignancies. J Exp Med 176: 157, 1992
90. Smith TJ, Terada N, Robinson CC et al: Acute infectious mononucleosis stimulates the selective expression/expansion of V beta 6.1-3 and V beta 7 T cells. Blood 81:1521, 1993
91. Strickler JG, Movahed LA, Gajl-Peczalska KJ et al: Oligoclonal T cell receptor gene rearrangements in blood lymphocytes of patients with acute Epstein-Barr virus-induced infectious mononucleosis. J Clin Invest 86:1358, 1990
92. Hassan J, Feighery C, Bresnihan B, et al: Elevated T cell receptor gamma delta + T cells in patients with infectious mononucleosis. Br J Haematol 77:255, 1991
93. Perez-Blas M, Regueiro JR, Ruiz-Contreras JR et al: T lymphocyte anergy during acute infectious mononucleosis is restricted to the clonotypic receptor activation pathway. Clin Exp Immunol 89:83, 1992
94. Tosato G, Magrath I, Koski I et al: Activation of suppressor T cells during Epstein-Barr-virus-induced infectious mononucleosis. N Engl J Med 301:1133, 1979
95. Linde A, Andersson B, Svenson S et al: Serum levels of lymphokines and soluble cellular receptors in primary Epstein-Barr virus infection and in patients with chronic fatigue syndrome. J Infect Dis 165:994, 1992
96. Andersson J, Abrams J, Bjork L et al: Concomitant in vivo production of 19 different cytokines in human tonsils. Immunology 83:16, 1994
97. Uehara T, Miyawaki T, Ohta K et al: Apoptotic cell death of primed CD45RO + T lymphocytes in Epstein-Barr virus-induced infectious mononucleosis. Blood 80:452, 1992
98. Gratama JW, Zutter MM, Minarovits J et al: Expression of Epstein-Barr virus-encoded growth-transformation-associated proteins in lymphoproliferations of bone-marrow transplant patients. Int J Cancer 47:188, 1991
99. Rowe M, Lear A, Croom-Carter D et al: Three pathways of Epstein-Barr virus gene activation from EBNA1-positive latency in B lymphocytes. J Virol 66:122, 1992
100. Klein G: Epstein-Barr virus strategy in normal and neoplastic B cells. Cell 77:791, 1994
101. Miyashita EM, Yang B, Lam KMC et al: A novel form of Epstein-Barr virus latency in normal B cells in vivo. Cell 80:593, 1995
102. Purtilo DT: Biology of disease. Defective im-

mune surveillance in viral carcinogenesis. Lab Invest 51:373, 1984

103. Purtilo DT, Tatsumi E, Manolov G et al: Epstein-Barr virus as an etiological agent in the pathogenesis of lymphoproliferative and aproliferative diseases in immune deficient patients. Int Rev Exp Pathol 27:113, 1985
104. Saemundsen AK, Purtilo DT, Sakamoto K et al: Documentation of Epstein-Barr virus infection in immunodeficient patients with life-threatening lymphoproliferative diseases by Epstein-Barr complementary RNA/DNA and viral DNA/DNA hybridization. Cancer Res 41:4237, 1981
105. Weiss LM, Movahed LA, Warnke RA et al: Detection of Epstein-Barr viral genomes in Reed-Sternberg cells of Hodgkin's disease. N Engl J Med 320:502, 1989
106. Hamilton-Dutoit SJ, Karkov J, Franzmann MB et al: AIDS-related central nervous system lymphoma. Demonstration of Epstein-Barr virus DNA by in situ hybridization. P. 110. In Racz P, Haase AT, Gluckman JC (eds): Modern Pathology of AIDS and Other Retroviral Infections. Basel, Karger, 1991
107. Hamilton-Dutoit SJ, Pallesen G: Demonstration of Epstein-Barr viral genomes in routine paraffin sections of lymphoproliferative and epithelial lesions by in situ hybridization. Prog Surgical Pathol XII:97, 1992
108. Barletta JM, Kingma DW, Ling Y et al: Rapid in situ hybridization for the diagnosis of latent Epstein-Barr virus infection. Mol Cell Probe 7: 105, 1993
109. Ambinder RF, Mann RB: Detection and characterization of Epstein-Barr virus in clinical specimens. Am J Pathol 145:239, 1994
110. Baer R, Bankier AT, Biggin AT et al: DNA sequence and expression of the B95-8 Epstein-Barr virus genome. Nature 310:207, 1984
111. Cen H, Breinig MC, Atchison RW et al: Epstein-Barr virus transmission via the donor organs in solid organ transplantation: polymerase chain reaction and restriction fragment length polymorphism analysis of IR2, IR3, and IR4. J Virol 65:976, 1991
112. Raab-Traub N, Flynn K: The structure of the termini of the Epstein-Barr virus as a marker of clonal cellular proliferation. Cell 47:883, 1986
113. Purtilo DT, Strobach RS, Okano M et al: Epstein-Barr virus-associated lymphoproliferative disorders. Lab Invest 67:5, 1992
114. Yao QY, Rickinson AB, Gaston JSH et al: In vitro analysis of the Epstein-Barr virus: host balance in long-term renal allograft recipients. Int J Cancer 35:43, 1985
115. Preiksaitis JK: Lymphoproliferative disorders in renal transplant recipients: virologic aspects. Clin Transplant 6:235, 1992
116. Marchevsky A, Hoffmann DG, Gedebou M et al: Detection of Epstein-Barr virus by polymerase chain reaction in transbronchial biopsies of lung transplant recipients: evidence of infection?, abstracted. Lab Invest 68:133A, 1993
117. Riddler SA, Breinig MC, Mcknight JLC: Increased levels of circulating Epstein-Barr virus (EBV)-infected lymphocytes and decreased EBV nuclear antigen antibody responses are associated with the development of posttransplant lymphoproliferative disease in solid-organ transplant recipients. Blood 84:972, 1994
118. Borisch-Chappuis B, Nezelof C, Muller H et al: Different Epstein-Barr virus expression in lymphomas from immunocompromised and immunocompetent patients. Am J Pathol 136:751, 1990
119. Randhawa PS, Jaffe R, Demetris AJ et al: The systemic distribution of Epstein-Barr virus genomes in fatal posttransplant lymphoproliferative disorders: an in-situ hybridization study. Am J Pathol 138:1027, 1991
120. Weiss LM, Movahed LA: In situ demonstration of Epstein-Barr viral genomes in viral-associated B cell lymphoproliferations. Am J Pathol 134:651, 1989
121. Wu T, Mann RB, Charache P et al: Detection of EBV gene expression in Reed-Sternberg cells of Hodgkin's disease. Int J Cancer 46:801, 1990
122. Randhawa PS, Jaffe R, Demetris AJ et al: Expression of Epstein-Barr virus-encoded small RNA (by the EBER-1 gene) in liver specimens from transplant recipients with post-transplantation lymphoproliferative disease. N Engl J Med 327:1710, 1992
123. Hubscher SG, Williams A, Davison SM et al: Epstein-Barr virus in inflammatory diseases of the liver and liver allografts: an in situ hybridization study. Hepatology 20:899, 1994
124. Henle W, Henle GE, Horwitz CA: Epstein-Barr specific diagnostic tests in infectious mononucleosis. Hum Pathol 5:551, 1974
125. Henle W, Henle G: Epstein-Barr virus-specific serology in immunologically compromised individuals. Cancer Res 41:4222, 1981

126. Young L, Alfieri C, Hennessy K et al: Expression of Epstein-Barr virus transformation-associated genes in tissues of patients with EBV lymphoproliferative disease. N Engl J Med 321: 1080, 1989
127. Cuomo L, Trivedi P, Wang F et al: Expression of the Epstein-Barr virus (EBV)-encoded membrane antigen (LMP) increases the stimulatory capacity of EBV-negative B lymphoma lines in allogeneic mixed lymphocyte cultures. Eur J Immunol 20:2293, 1990
128. Grasser FA, Murray PG, Kremmer E et al: Monoclonal antibodies directed against the Epstein-Barr virus-encoded nuclear antigen 1 (EBNA1): immunohistologic detection of EBNA1 in the malignant cells of Hodgkin's disease. Blood 84:3792, 1994
129. Zhang Q, Gutsch D, Kenney S: Functional and physical interaction between *p53* and BZLF1—implications for Epstein-Barr virus latency. Mol Cell Biol 14:1929, 1994
130. Rea D, Fourcade C, Leblond V et al: Patterns of Epstein-Barr virus latent and replicative gene expression in Epstein-Barr virus B cell lymphoproliferative disorders after organ transplantation. Transplantation 58:317, 1994
131. Markin RS: Manifestations of Epstein-Barr virus-associated disorders in liver. Liver 14:1, 1994
132. Guettier C, Hamilton-Dutoit S, Guillemain R et al: Primary gastrointestinal malignant lymphomas associated with Epstein-Barr virus after heart transplantation. Histopathology 20:21, 1992
133. Nalesnik MA: Involvement of the gastrointestinal tract by Epstein-Barr virus-associated posttransplant lymphoproliferative disorders. Am J Surg Pathol, suppl 14 1:92, 1990
134. Kappel TJ, Manivel JC, Goswitz JJ: Atypical lymphocytes in spinal fluid resembling posttransplant lymphoma in a cardiac transplant recipient. A case report. Acta Cytol 338:470, 1994
135. Eisen HJ, Hicks D, Kant JA et al: Diagnosis of posttransplantation lymphoproliferative disorder by endomyocardial biopsy in a cardiac allograft recipient. J Heart Lung Transplant 13:241, 1994
136. Fernandez-Gonzalez AL, Herreros-Gonzalez JM, Mindan JP: Value of endomyocardial biopsy in the diagnosis of lymphoproliferative disorder after heart transplantation. J Heart Lung Transplant 13:1146, 1994
137. Briggs JD, Hamilton DNH, Macsween RNM et al: Infectious mononucleosis, herpes simplex infection, and diffuse lymphoma in a renal transplant patient. Transplantation 25:227, 1978
138. Nagington J, Gray J: Cyclosporin A immunosuppression, Epstein-Barr antibody and lymphoma. Lancet II:536, 1980
139. Bird AG, McLachlan SM: Cyclosporin A and Epstein-Barr virus. Lancet 2:418, 1980
140. Hanto D, Sakamoto K, Purtilo DT et al: The Epstein-Barr virus in the pathogenesis of posttransplant lymphoproliferative disorders. Surgery 90:204, 1981
141. Hanto D, Gajl-Peczalska K, Frizzera G et al: Epstein-Barr (EBV) induced polyclonal and monoclonal B-cell lymphoproliferative diseases occurring after renal transplantation. Ann Surg 198:356, 1983
142. Purtilo DT: Opportunistic cancers in patients with immunodeficiency syndromes. Arch Pathol Lab Med 111:1123, 1987
143. Cleary ML, Nalesnik MA, Shearer WT et al: Clonal analysis of transplant associated lymphoproliferations based on the structure of the genomic termini of the Epstein-Barr virus. Blood 72: 349, 1988
144. Ioachim HL: The opportunistic tumors of immune deficiency. Adv Cancer Res 54:301, 1990
145. Purtilo DT, Falk K, Pirrucello SJ et al: SCID mouse model of Epstein-Barr virus-induced lymphomagenesis of immunodeficient humans. Int J Cancer 47:510, 1991
146. Thomas JA, Allday MJ, Crawford DH: Epstein-Barr virus-associated lymphoproliferative disorders in immunocompromised individuals. Adv Cancer Res 57:329, 1991
147. McCune JM: Epstein-Barr virus associated lymphoproliferative disease in mice and men. Lab Invest 65:377, 1991
148. Magrath IT, Rowe M, Filipovich AH et al: Advances in the understanding of EBV associated lymphoproliferative disorders. p. 243. In Ablashi DV, Huang AT, Pagano JS et al (eds): Epstein-Barr Virus and Human Diseases—1990. Humana Press, Clifton, NJ, 1991
149. Rowe M, Young LS, Crocker J et al: Epstein-Barr virus (EBV)-associated lymphoproliferative disease in the SCID mouse: implications for the pathogenesis of EBV-positive lymphomas in man. J Exp Med 173:147, 1991
150. Alfrey E, Friedman A, Grossman R et al: Two distinct patterns of post-transplantation lympho-

proliferative disorder (PTLD): early and late onset. Clin Transplant 6:246, 1992

151. Frizzera G: Atypical lymphoproliferative disorders: when of age? Virchows Arch A Pathol Anat Histol 422:261, 1993
152. Heslop HE, Brenner MK, Rooney C et al: Clinical protocol. Administration of neomycin resistance gene marked EBV specific cytotoxic T lymphocytes to recipients of mismatched-related or phenotypically similar unrelated donor marrow grafts. Hum Gene Ther 5:381, 1994
153. Nalesnik MA, Starzl TE: Epstein-Barr virus, infectious mononucleosis, and posttransplant lymphoproliferative disorders. Transplant Sci 4: 60, 1994
154. Crompton CH, Cheung RK, Donjon C et al: Epstein-Barr virus surveillance after renal transplantation. Transplantation 57:1182, 1994
155. Lones MA, Mishalani S, Shintaku IP et al: Changes in tonsils and adenoids in children with posttransplant lymphoproliferative disorder: report of three cases with early involvement of Waldeyer's ring. Hum Pathol 26:525, 1995
156. Martinez OM, Villanueva JC, Lawrence-Miyasaki L et al: Molecular markers of Epstein-Barr virus infection in the circulation of transplant recipients. Transplant Proc 27:1211, 1995
157. Hornef MW, Wagner HJ, Fricke L et al: Immunocytochemical detection of Epstein-Barr virus antigens in peripheral B lymphocytes after renal transplantation. Transplantation 59:138, 1995
158. Oudejans JJ, Jiwa M, van den Brule AJC et al: Detection of heterogneous Epstein-Barr virus gene expression patterns within individual posttransplantation lymphoproliferative disorders. Am J Pathol 147:923, 1995

10

Ki-1 (CD30) Positive Large Cell Lymphoma

Bjarni A. Agnarsson and Marshall E. Kadin

In 1985, Stein et al.[1] described a high grade non-Hodgkin's lymphoma resembling malignant histiocytosis. The histology of this lymphoma was characterized by cohesive large anaplastic cells with a distinctive distribution in lymph node sinuses that marked positively with the Hodgkin's disease related antibody Ki-1 (CD30). Since then numerous reports delineating the clinical and morphologic spectrum of this Ki-1 positive large cell lymphoma (Ki-1 + LCL) have been published.[2–10] In this chapter, we describe primarily the histology and immunocytochemistry of Ki-1 + LCL, with special emphasis on its differential diagnosis from other disorders with which it may be confused. Concerning the biology of Ki-1 + LCL, the reader is referred to a recent article reviewing the pathogenesis of this disorder.[11]

CLINICAL FEATURES

Ki-1 + LCL may represent 1 to 8 percent of all non-Hodgkin's lymphomas,[1,10] 6 to 15 percent of all large cell lymphomas,[9] and 6 to 10 percent of non-Hodgkin's lymphomas in children.[12,13] Males are in general more commonly affected than females, with a ratio of 2.2–1.4 : 1,[1–3,5–7,10] although in one study from Japan this ratio was reversed.[8] The age range extends from 4 months of age to 91 years,[6,7] but in most series a bimodal age pattern is noted.[3,5,7,9,10] The peak age incidence is thus in the second decade, with a smaller peak found after age 60. Patients with cutaneous Ki-1 + LCL, however, seem to have an older median age of 60 to 67 years.[14,15]

Constitutional symptoms are present at diagnosis in 20 to 50 percent of patients.[2,3,5–9] The most common presenting complaint is peripheral lymphadenopathy (cervical, axillary, inguinal), which is present in the majority of patients, although in some cases more centrally located nodes may be affected, for example, in the mediastinum and/or retroperitoneum. Extranodal disease is often present, either alone or in combination with lymphadenopathy. The most common extranodal site is the skin, which is involved in 10 to 20 percent of patients.[6,9] It is noteworthy that skin lesions, as well as lymphadenopathy, may regress temporarily.[2,3,5,14] Other not uncommon extranodal sites are bone (osteolytic lesions),[5–7,9,16] lung and pleura,[6,7,9] stomach or small bowel,[1,3,5,7,9] and spleen.[7] Rarely lesions may occur in the liver,[7] kidney,[5] soft tissues,[3] or esophagus.[17] In most series the percentage of cases with bone marrow infiltrates is under 15 percent[2–5,7–9] although Chott et al.[6] reported bone marrow involvement in 30 percent of their cases.

The majority of patients with Ki-1 + LCL present with advanced stage disease (stages III and IV).[7,12,13,18] Most patients treated with intensive chemotherapy achieve complete remission, but relapses, especially in adult patients, are relatively frequent. Patients often, however, achieve durable remissions following relapse.[19,20] In a study of adult patients, 65 percent of patients remained disease free after a median follow-up of 24 months,[18] and in a recent large study of pediatric patients 80.6 percent of patients were still in complete remission after a median follow-up time of 2.5 years.[12] In a study comparing adult patients with LCL who were Ki-1+ to patients with Ki-1− LCL, it was found that the Ki-1+ patients had significantly better long-term survival.[21] Similar studies of childhood LCL have either found no prognostic significance associated with Ki-1 expression[19] or significantly better survival in the Ki-1+ group, but only in advanced stage disease.[13] A recent Children's Cancer Group study of advanced stage LCL has not been able to confirm these results (unpublished data). Patients with primary cutaneous Ki-1+ LCL, without extracutaneous disease at presentation, have an excellent prognosis and may be treated with simple excision and/or local radiotherapy if the lesions are solitary and localized.[14,22]

The chromosomal translocation t(2;5)(p23; q35), which was previously associated with malignant histiocytosis, has been found to be typical of nodal Ki-1+ LCL.[23–25] It has been reported that the t(2;5) translocation may be lacking in Ki-1+ LCL patients who do not have typical anaplastic cytology and may correlate with a worse prognosis.[26] The t(2;5) can now be detected by reverse transcriptase polymerase chain reaction and immunohistochemically.[27,28] The use of these methods suggests that the t(2; 5) is not specific for Ki-1+ LCL.[29]

Ki-1+ LCL may be divided into primary and secondary forms. In a small subset of patients with Ki-1+ LCL it appears that the disease transforms from another previously diagnosed lymphoproliferative disorder (most frequently peripheral T-cell lymphoma, mycosis fungoides, lymphomatoid papulosis, Hodgkin's disease, or angioimmunoblastic lymphadenopathy),[10,22] underscoring the close clinical, pathologic, and sometimes clonal relationship that exists between these different disorders.[22,30,31] Patients with secondary Ki-1+ LCL appear to have a worse prognosis than patients who have primary disease.

HISTOLOGY

Lymph nodes

It has become apparent that the histology of Ki-1+ LCL is quite heterogenous. Most cases of Ki-1+ LCL may, however, be divided into two main types based on cytology. Thus approx-

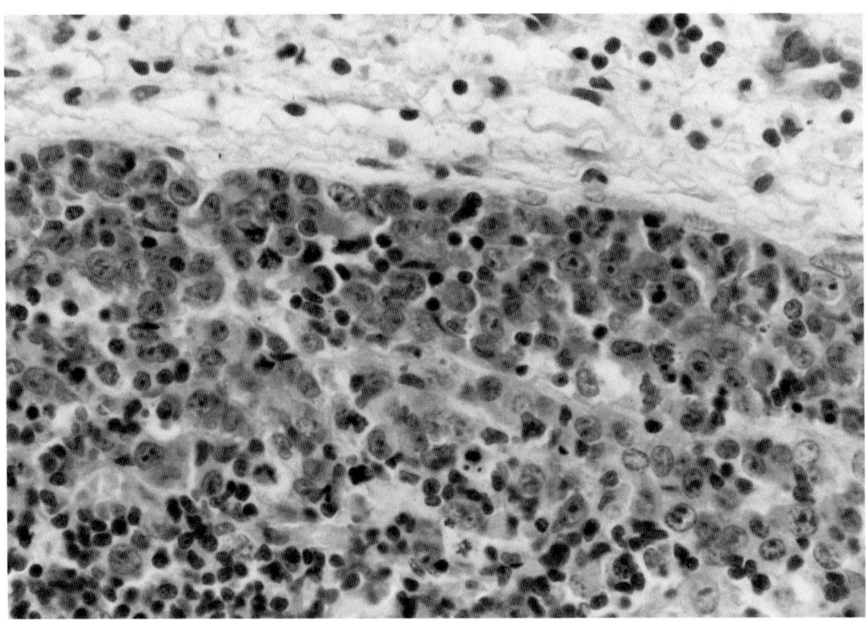

Fig. 10-1. Tumor cells infiltrating subcapsular sinus of lymph node.

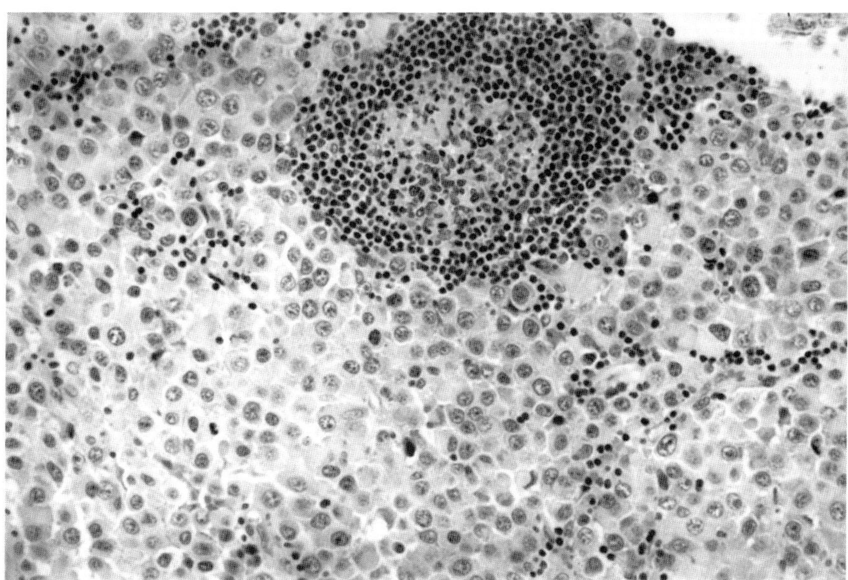

Fig. 10-2. Tumor cells surround, but spare, a B-cell follicle that contains a germinal center.

imately two-thirds of cases have an *anaplastic* appearance, while the remaining one-third appear *monomorphic*. First the defining histologic features that are common to both types are reviewed, and then the cytology of each type is discussed in detail.

The most distinctive histologic feature of Ki-1+ LCL is its distribution in lymph node sinuses (Fig. 10-1). although a dense paracortical infiltrate with sparing of B-cell follicles is also usually seen (Fig. 10-2). In some cases, however, the lymph node architecture is completely effaced. It is of interest to note that this preferential T-zone distribution may be seen in both Ki-1+ LCL of T and B-cell types. A helpful histologic feature of Ki-1+ LCL is the partial lymph node involvement seen in approximately 50 percent of cases, since this finding is unusual in other high grade non-Hodgkin's lymphomas. At low power examination tumor cells often appear cohesive, imparting a trabecular pattern to the involved areas, while in other areas the cells may appear dispersed. Capsular thickening with fibrous bands that divide the tissue into nodules may be seen (Fig. 10-3). More centrally fibrosis is often present in the form of delicate collagenous bands encircling small clusters of cells.

In both cytologic types mitoses are usually abundant. Necrosis is present in a minority of cases (less than 25 percent).[3,5,9,10] A starry-sky pattern may occasionally be present.[3] Frequently intermingled with the neoplastic cells are inflammatory cells. Most often these are small lymphocytes and histiocytes, but also frequently seen are plasma cells, neutrophils, and eosinophils.[2,3,5,6,8–10] These reactive cells may sometimes be very numerous. Erythrophagocytosis by tumor cells may be seen but is not a conspicuous feature of Ki-1+ LCL. Macrophages, however, may exhibit erythrophagocytosis, especially in the small cell variant and the variant with a high content of histiocytes (see below).

The cytologic appearance of Ki-1+ LCL is that of a high grade lymphoma. We believe, as mentioned above, that two subtypes of Ki-1+ LCL may be distinguished based on the cytologic appearance of the tumor cells. The more common type is the anaplastic type, which appears to be similar to the type II (basophilic cell) Ki-1+ LCL described by Chan et al.[5] and the type A Ki-1+ LCL of Chott et al.[6] This type is characterized by large round or oval pleomorphic cells in various stages of transformation. Nuclei are commonly eccentrically located and

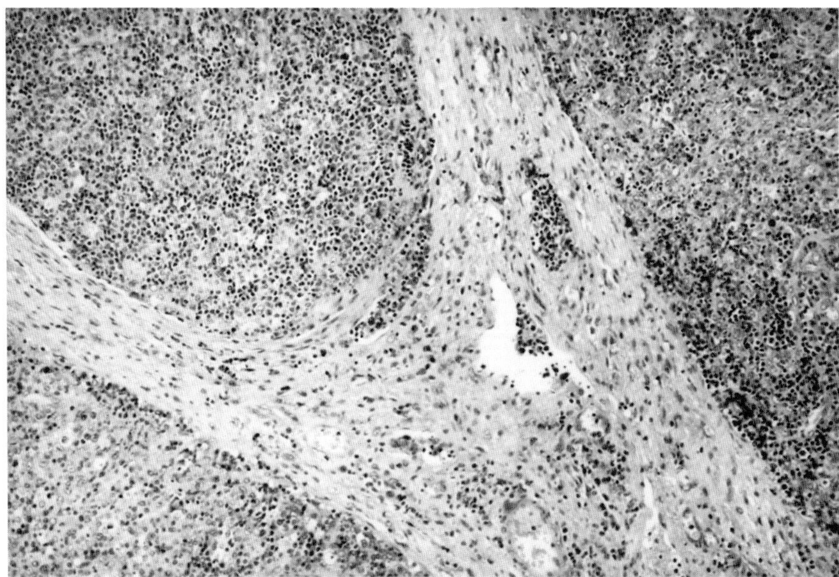

Fig. 10-3. Bands of collagen divide the tissue into nodules containing an admixture of tumor cells and lymphocytes.

lobated or horseshoe-like (Fig. 10-4), and multinucleated giant cells, sometimes with wreath-like (Fig. 10-5) or doughnut-shaped nuclei (Fig. 10-6), may be seen. Nucleoli are generally multiple and large and in some cases may be inclusion-like. These cells may be indistinguishable from classic (Fig. 10-7) or lacunar variants of Reed-Sternberg cells. Chromatin is generally coarse, and a paranuclear halo or hof is commonly present. The cytoplasm is usually abundant, amphophilic or basophilic, and may be finely vacuolated. Occasional cases are charac-

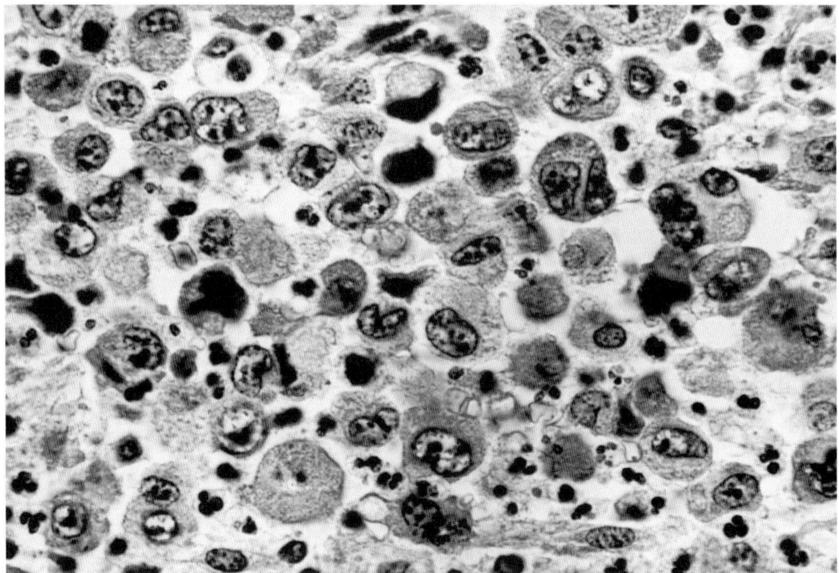

Fig. 10-4. Ki-1+ LCL with anaplastic cytology. Note admixture of neutrophils.

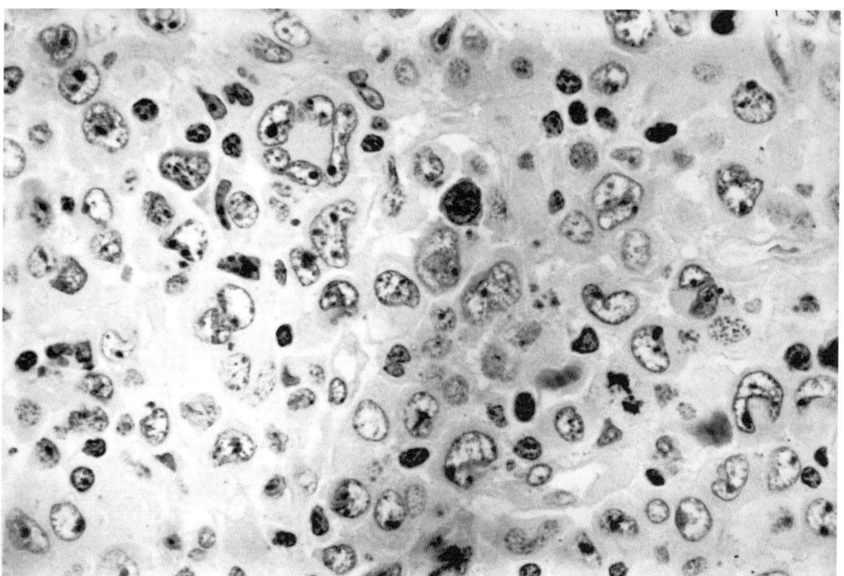

Fig. 10-5. Ki-1+ LCL with anaplastic cytology. Wreath-like cell and cells with lobated or reniform nuclei.

terized by cells with clear cytoplasm and distinct cell membranes (Fig. 10-8). Multilobated cells as described by Pinkus et al.[32] are not a feature of Ki-1+ LCL.

In contrast, the monomorphic type is characterized by a monotonous appearance of the tumor cells, which are fairly uniform in size and shape. Many of these cases may correspond to the type I (pale cell) Ki-1+ LCL of Chan et al.[5] or the type B described by Chott et al.[6] Nuclei are in general round or oval and centrally placed (Fig. 10-9). Nucleoli tend to be less prominent than in the anaplastic type, but may be multiple. Reed-Sternberg-like cells and/or multinucleated

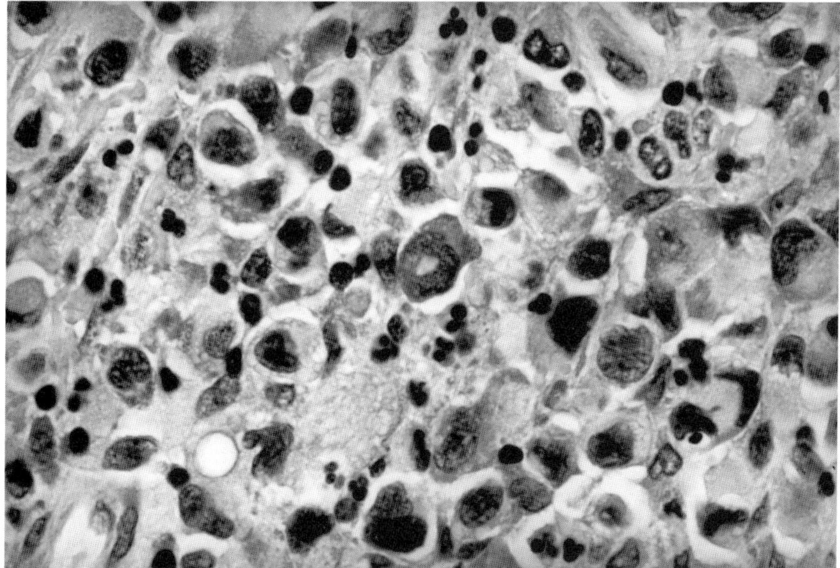

Fig. 10-6. Ki-1+ LCL with anaplastic cytology. "Doughnut" cell in center.

giant cells are rarely seen. A paranuclear clear area is not present. Cytologically these cases may appear similar to Ki-1− large cell lymphomas. Salient distinguishing features of the anaplastic and monomorphic types are presented in Table 10-1.

Ultrastructurally Ki-1+ LCL contains activated lymphocytes with reniform nuclei with dispersed chromatin and prominent nucleoli.[33,34] There is abundant organelle-poor cytoplasm containing polyribosomes and scattered lysosomes. Surface microvillous projections may be present.

In general the distinction between anaplastic and monomorphic types is straightforward, but in rare cases both anaplastic and monomorphic cytology may be seen in the same tissue and in some areas morphology that appears intermediate between anaplastic and monomorphic types may be seen (Fig. 10-10). Initial studies have indicated that patients with monomorphic cytology more often present at an advanced stage of disease and may have a worse prognosis than patients who have anaplastic cytology.[5,6,9,26] A recent clinical study of Romaguera et al.[21] of adult patients as well as a Children's Cancer Group study of pediatric patients with advanced stage disease (unpublished results) have not, however, shown significant differences in prognosis in Ki-1+ LCL according to histologic subtype. In both these studies, however, the numbers of patients were small, and the significance of differences in morphology in Ki-1+ LCL remains unclear.

Skin

Skin lesions are most often solitary nodules or tumors but may be multiple. The histologic appearance with the exception of a sinus pattern is similar to that seen in lymph nodes. Thus cohesive sheets of tumor cells, most often of the anaplastic type, are present in the dermis and often extend to the subcutis (Fig. 10-11).[14,15] Ulceration and pseudoepitheliomatous hyperplasia are common, but a Grenz zone or epidermotropism by tumor cells is not a usual feature of Ki-1+ LCL of the skin, although epidermotropism may rarely be seen (Fig. 10-12). Monomorphic cytology appears to be uncommon, although 7 of 47 patients with primary cutaneous CD30+ lymphoma of the skin described by Beljaards et al.[14] had "nonanaplastic" cytology. There was no difference in prognosis between patients with anaplastic and nonanaplastic cytology in this setting. The histology in skin and lymph nodes may be discordant. Thus in some patients there are anaplastic cells in the skin while monomorphic larger cells are found in the lymph nodes of the same patient (Figs. 10-13, 10-14).

Other Sites

Ki-1+ LCL in other extranodal sites is generally characterized by anaplastic cytology, often with extensive necrosis.[3,6,9] Involvement of bone marrow may be subtle (isolated large cells), neccesitating immunocytochemical methods for its identification,[5] or focal and diffuse.[6]

Table 10-1. Morphologic Characteristics of Anaplastic and Monomorphic Variants of Ki-1+ LCL

	Anaplastic	Monomorphic
Cell size	Large and pleomorphic	Monomorphic (large or small)
Nuclei	Round, oval, irregular, convoluted, lobated, wreath-like	Round, oval, vesicular
Nucleoli	Prominent, large (may be inclusion-like)	Inconspicuous, small
Reed-Sternberg-like cells	Common	Rare
Multinucleate giant cells	Common	Rare
Paranuclear hof	Yes	No
Site of nucleus	Eccentric	Central
Cytoplasm	Basophilic/amphophilic/clear	Basophilic/amphophilic

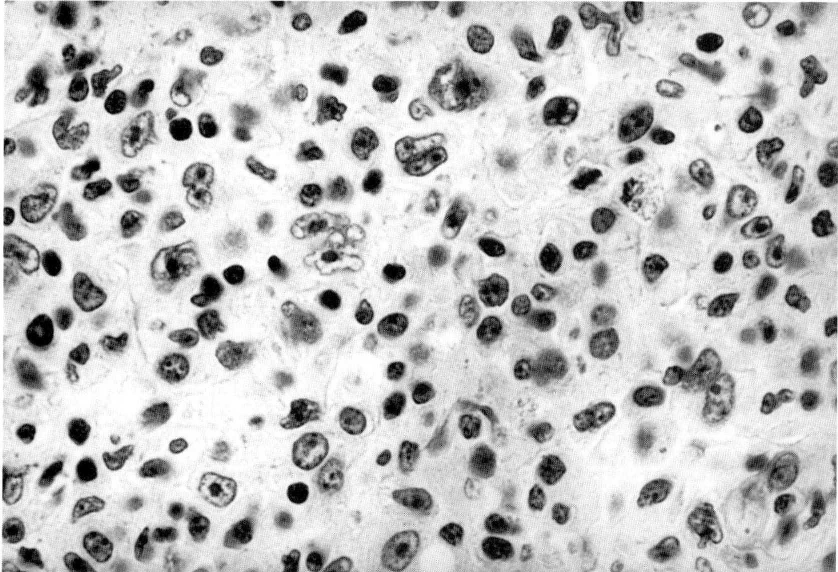

Fig. 10-7. Ki-1 + LCL with anaplastic cytology. Reed-Sternberg-like cell near center.

If close attention is paid to the characteristic histology decribed above, Ki-1 + LCL may usually be easily recognized. In a blinded study (unpublished results) involving 41 large cell lymphomas, we were able to identify morphologically 88 percent of the lymphomas, which turned out to be CD30 + . The cases that could not be identified were all of the monomorphic type and lacked a sinus pattern. A typical case of Ki-1 + LCL thus has a distinct sinus pattern with sparing of B-cell areas, but may have either anaplastic or monomorphic cytology. In con-

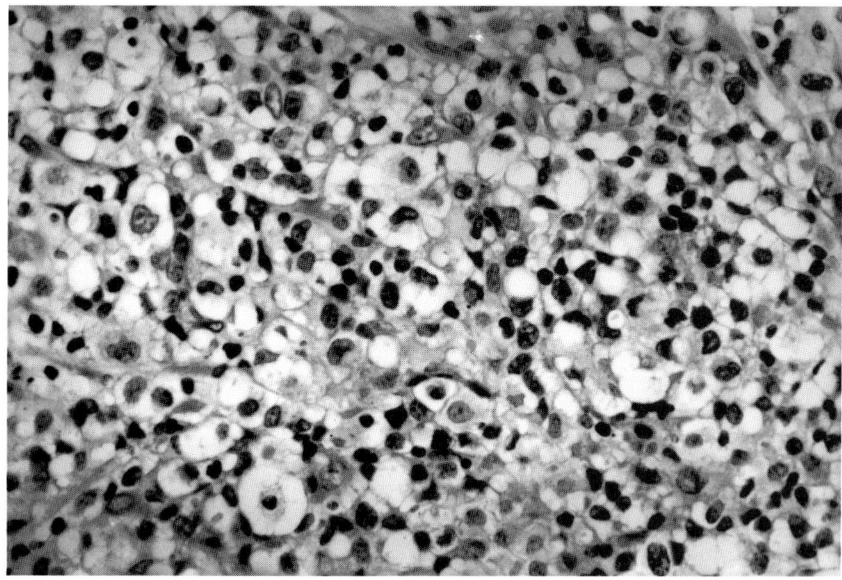

Fig. 10-8. Ki-1 + LCL with clear cell appearance.

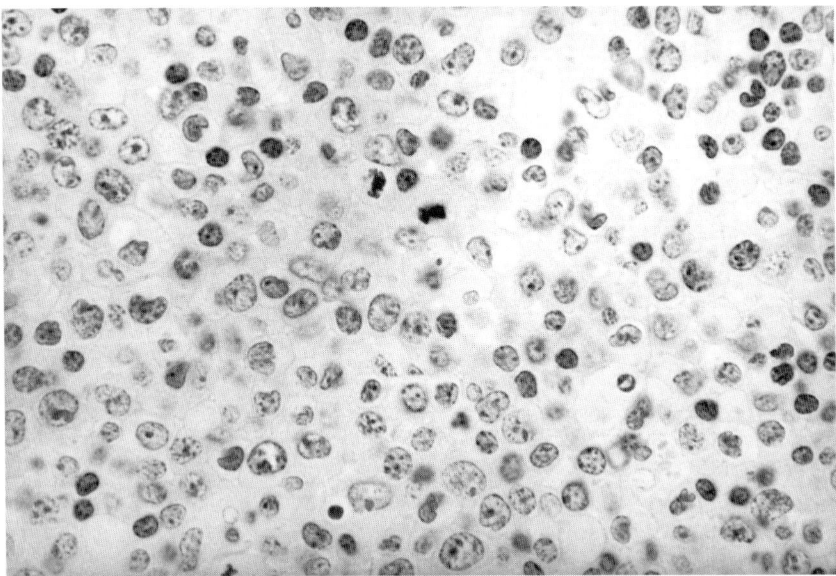

Fig. 10-9. Ki-1+ LCL with monomorphic cytology. Tumor cells are uniform in size and shape and have inconspicuous nucleoli.

trast, CD30− lymphomas almost never have a sinus pattern and seldom display anaplastic cytology.

Since Ki-1+ LCL is not included in most lymphoma classifications histologic subtyping may be problematic. Most cases with anaplastic cytology have been classified in the Working Formulation as high grade immunoblastic lymphomas, but in some cases with monomorphic cytology a diagnosis of diffuse large cell lymphoma or even diffuse mixed lymphoma may be more appropriate. In the recently updated Kiel classification this lymphoma has been termed *large cell anaplastic lymphoma* and is further

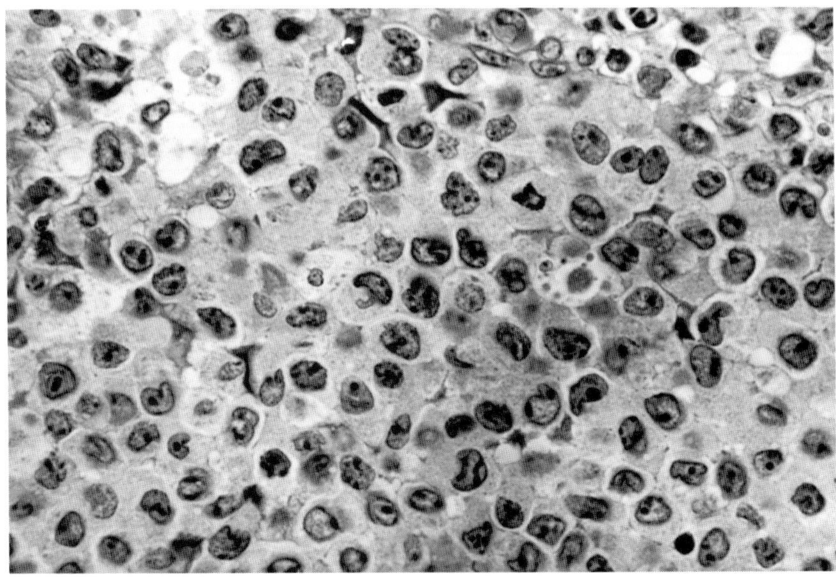

Fig. 10-10. Ki-1+ LCL with intermediate morphology.

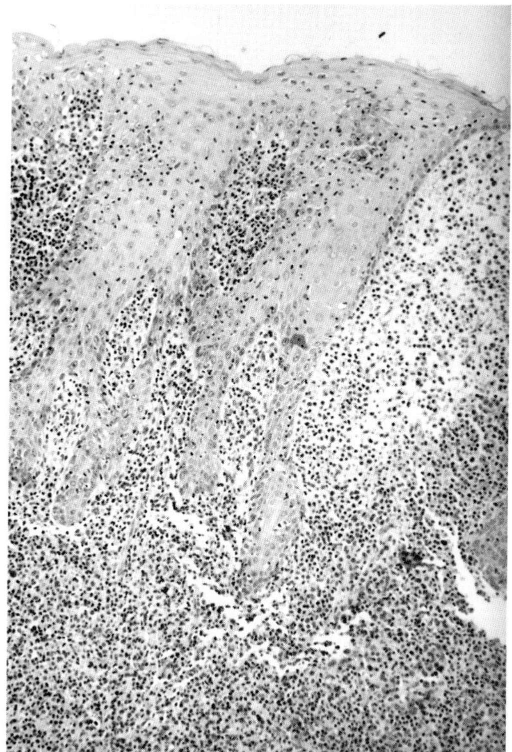

Fig. 10-11. Ki-1+ LCL of skin. In this case numerous lymphocytes are present in infiltrate and exhibit exocytosis, but tumor cell epidermotropism is not seen. Note epidermal hyperplasia.

categorized according to phenotype.[10] According to Lennert and Feller,[10] about a fourth of lymphomas expressing CD30 may be classified in previously recognized categories (B centroblastic; B or T immunoblastic; or T-pleomorphic, medium sized, and large cell lymphomas). Further studies are needed to elucidate the clinical significance of CD30 expression in these cases, especially since it is likely that their differentiation from cases of Ki-1+ LCL with monomorphic cytology can be difficult.

VARIANTS OF Ki-1+ LCL

Variant with a High Content of Reactive Histiocytes (Lymphohistiocytic T-cell Lymphoma)

In 1990, Pileri et al.[35] described 13 young patients who presented with systemic symptoms and peripheral lymphadenopathy. In this variant of Ki-1+ LCL the lymph node architecture is effaced and variant numbers of CD30+ anaplastic cells are present singly, in small clusters, or in sinuses intermingled with numerous benign reactive histiocytes. In these cases immunophenotyping of the large cells is important to distinguish this variant from malignant histiocytosis or hyperimmune reactions such as virus-associated hemophagocytic syndrome. The patients responded well to aggressive chemotherapy.

Sarcomatoid Variant

In 1990, Chan et al.[36] brought attention to a case of K1+ LCL presenting as a subcutaneous tumor of the lower extremity that mimicked a sarcoma both clinically and histologically. The histology of this lesion at the primary site and in a lymph node was characterized by spindle cells that had a storiform pattern with myxoid stroma reminiscent of malignant fibrous histiocytoma. The lymphoid nature of this case was confirmed by immunohistochemistry. A spindle cell component in otherwise typical Ki-1+ LCL has also been reported.[3]

Small Cell Variant

Kinney and associates[37] have recently described nine patients with a small cell predominant variant of Ki-1+ LCL. In these cases the predominant cell was a markedly irregular small lymphocyte often with a cerebriform appearance (Fig. 10-15). The large cells were present singly or in small clusters and could be found in sinuses or surrounding small vessels. The large cells and some small cells were CD30+. Two patients developed typical Ki-1+ LCL in later biopsies, and in four cases the t(2;5) translocation typical of Ki-1+ LCL was found. Thus, in spite of the unusual morphology, these cases appear to be part of the spectrum of Ki-1+ LCL. It is of interest to note that without immunologic staining it could be difficult to identify the CD30+ large atypical cells. It is possible that some of these cases are similar to the variant with a high content of histiocytes decribed above, since

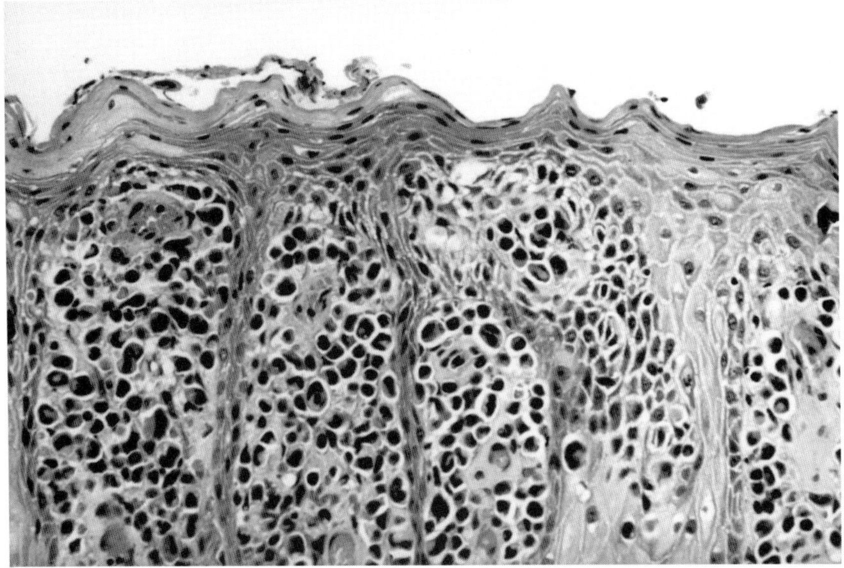

Fig. 10-12. Unusual occurrence of extensive tumor cell epidermotropism in Ki-1 + LCL of skin.

large numbers of histiocytes were present in two patients.

Hodgkin's-Like and Giant Cell-Rich Variants

European investigators have defined two additional types of Ki-1 + LCL with anaplastic cytology, namely, a Hodgkin's-like variant resembling Hodgkin's disease and a giant cell-rich subtype that frequently has a B-cell phenotype.[38] In the Hodgkin's-like variant, tumor cells have bizarre nuclei and are consistently large and cohesive. Neoplastic cells are mixed with reactive cells that always represent a minor population. Tumor cells frequently collect in nodules with surrounding sclerosis and capsular thickening, similar to nodular sclerosing Hodgkin's disease (Fig. 10-3). Clinically, the Hodgkin's-like variant is consistently associated with a mediastinal mass, often bulky; has a mean age of onset of 34 years versus 27 for the common type of Ki-1+ LCL; and more frequent occurrences of stage II disease.[39]

IMMUNOCYTOCHEMISTRY

By definition most or all of the tumor cells in Ki-1 + LCL are CD30 +, using either the original Ki-1 antibody on frozen material or the BerH2 antibody, which recognizes a formalin and paraffin resistant epitope of the Ki-1 antigen.[40] The neoplastic cells display strong membrane and frequently a dot-like paranuclear staining pattern. Formalin-fixed tissue should preferably be used to detect the CD30 antigen in archival material, since B5 fixation is not reliable for its detection. Although initial studies indicated that all or almost all cases of Ki-1 + LCL were CD45 +,[3,5,7,9] it has become increasingly apparent that slightly less than one-half to one-third of cases may be CD45 − in paraffin-embedded tissues.[6,41] The Hodgkin's disease related CD15 antibody is usually negative in Ki-1 + LCL,[3,6,8] although occasional positive cases have been described.[7,9]

Ki-1 + LCL appears to be primarily a neoplasm of activated lymphoid cells. Markers typical of activated cells, namely, HLA-DR (Ia), CD25 (IL-2 receptor), and T9 (transferrin receptor), are thus expressed in almost all cases.[1,3,5,6,8] These antibodies are, however, of little discriminatory value in the differential diagnosis of other lymphomas.

On frozen material approximately 60 to 70 percent of Ki-1 + LCL express a T-cell phenotype and about 10 to 20 percent a B-cell phenotype, and in approximately 20 percent of cases

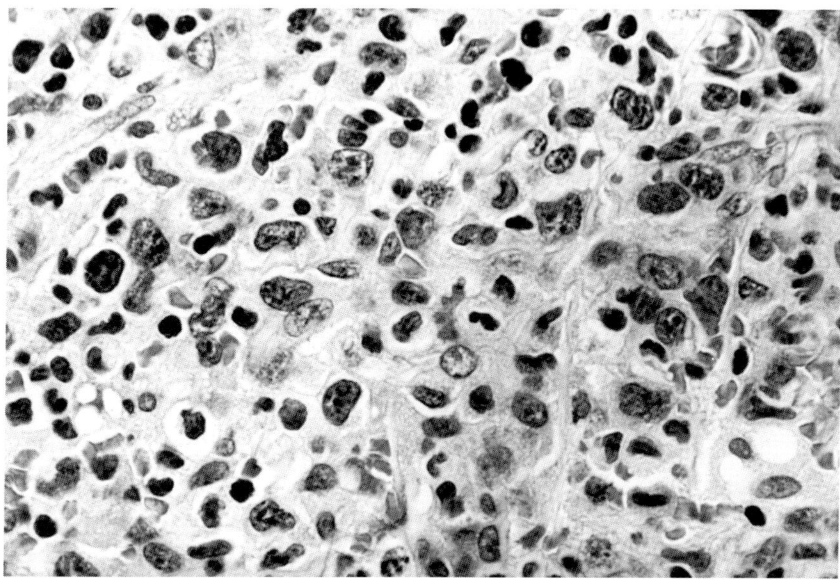

Fig. 10-13. Anaplastic tumor cell infiltrate in dermis of patient with Ki-1 + LCL.

neither a T- nor a B-cell phenotype is expressed.[1,3,5–10] In a few cases a mixed B- and T-cell phenotype has been described.[1,5] In paraffin-embedded tissues, lower frequencies of T- and B-cell expression are to be expected. The majority of the T-cell cases express a T-helper (CD4) phenotype (50 to 80 percent), while a T-suppressor phenotype (CD8) is infrequently found (0 to 15 percent). An aberrant T-cell phenotype in these cases is usually present. Thus expression of CD2 is found in the majority of cases (50 to 80 percent), while expression of the

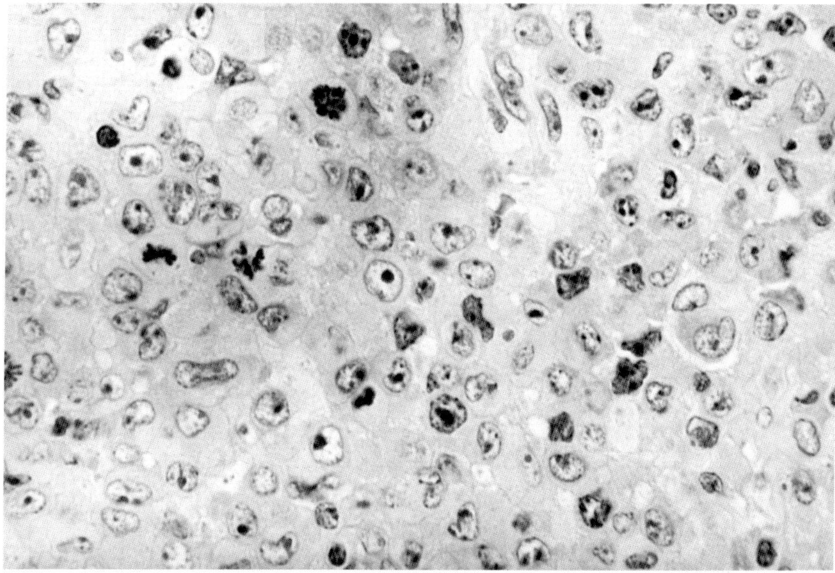

Fig. 10-14. Lymph node with monomorphic appearance from same patient as in Figure 10-13. Morphology is clearly discordant between different tumor sites.

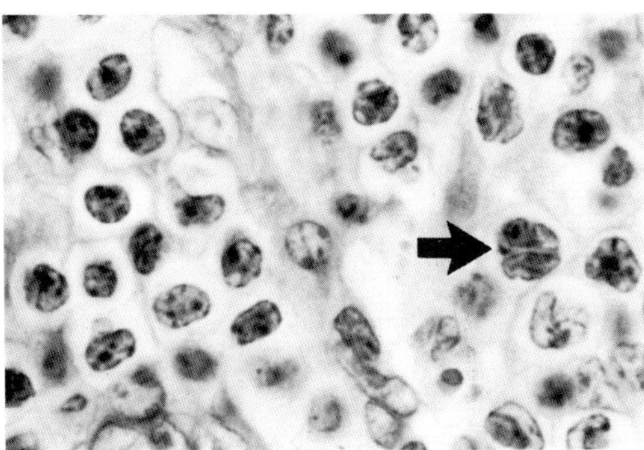

Fig. 10-15. Small cell predominant variant of Ki-1 + lymphoma containing tumor cell with ceribriform nucleus (*arrow*). (Adapted from Kinney et al.,[34] with permission.)

CD3, CD5, and CD7 antigens is variable, but relatively infrequent.[1,3,6,8,9] Most of the B-cell cases express both the CD20 and CD22 antigens. Although it is not possible to exclude a true histiocytic origin for some of the Ki-1 + LCLs that have a null cell phenotype, markers specific for histiocytes in general have been negative.[1-3,5,6] It should be emphasized that positive staining for α_1-antitrypsin and α_1-antichymotrypsin, which has been reported in some cases of Ki-1 + LCL,[1,9] is not specific for histiocytes and may be present in cells of lymphoid origin.[1]

Most investigators have found that epithelial membrane antigen (EMA) is expressed in a majority of cases (60 to 70 percent) and is therefore a useful marker of this lymphoma.[5-9,42] The typical phenotype of Ki-1 + LCL is thus CD30 +, CD45 +, CD15 −, EMA +, and T or B +, but the expression of these antigens (with the exception of CD30) in different cases is quite variable.

DIFFERENTIAL DIAGNOSIS

Malignant Histiocytosis

Many cases of Ki-1 + LCL have initially been diagnosed as malignant histiocytosis.[1,3,5,43] Malignant histiocytosis has been described as a rare systemic disorder that usually pursues a rapidly fatal course.[44,45] Atypical cells resembling histiocytes are found in lymph node sinuses, and phagocytosis by tumor cells is characteristic. When cases initially diagnosed as malignant histiocytosis have been reevaluated,[46,47] the majority of cases have been found to be CD30 + and have shown a T- or a B-cell lineage and lack macrophage-associated antigens. Thus most cases previously diagnosed as malignant histiocytosis are now classified as Ki-1 + LCL. Rare "null cell" Ki-1 + LCL may express macrophage-associated antigens and therefore be of true histiocytic origin.[41,48,49] Whether these cases should be termed *Ki-1 + LCL of histiocytic type* or *malignant histiocytosis expressing CD30 antigen* is a moot point. There are clearly more similarities than differences between Ki-1 + LCL and malignant histiocytosis, and a diagnosis of malignant histiocytosis should not be made without compelling immunohistochemical or ultrastructural evidence of histiocytic lineage.[43,47]

Hodgkin's Disease

CD30 expression is typical of Hodgkin's disease as well as Ki-1 + LCL. Ki-1 + LCL may have broad collagenous bands that define nodules containing tumor cells resembling lacunar variants of Reed-Sternberg cells (Fig. 10-3), intermingled with inflammatory cells, and may thus be confused with Hodgkin's disease,[1,3,7] especially the syncytial variant of nodular sclerosis described by Strickler et al.[50] Also, some patients with Hodgkin's disease develop secondary Ki-1 + LCL,[10] and in both disorders a bimodal age distribution is seen. Extranodal disease, however, is much less common in Hodgkin's disease than in Ki-1 + LCL. Sheets of tumor cells are more commonly seen in Ki-1 + LCL than in Hodgkin's disease, classical Reed-Sternberg cells are infrequently present in Ki-1 + LCL, and sinusoidal involvement is rare in Hodgkin's disease. Immunohistochemistry may be very useful in resolving difficult cases, since Ki-1 + LCL usually express CD45 and EMA,[51] but lack CD15, while the converse is true of Hodgkin's disease of the nodular sclerosis type.

T- and B-cell antigens also are more often detected on tumor cells in Ki-1 + LCL than Hodgkin's disease. Rare cases of Ki-1 + LCL may, however, be CD45 − and CD15 +, thus creating a possible diagnostic pitfall.[52]

Metastatic Carcinoma

Because of the frequent sinusoidal pattern of involvement and cohesive or trabecular pattern of the tumor cells as well as EMA positivity, Ki-1 + LCL is often confused with metastatic carcinoma.[3,5,7] Also, prominent perivascular cuffing of tumor cells in Ki-1 + LCL may result in a pseudoglandular appearance that may be confused with adenocarcinoma.[53] Close attention to the clinical history and the use of CD30, CD45, and cytokeratin markers should resolve most cases. Embryonal carcinomas and some pancreatic carcinomas have, however, been reported to be CD30 +,[38,54] and rare Ki-1 + LCLs may be cytokeratin positive and LCA negative.[55]

Regressing Atypical Histiocytosis

Regressing atypical histiocytosis was described as a cutaneous noduloulcerative proliferation of atypical histiocytes,[56] which initially was thought to be a self-limiting disorder. However, long-term follow-up has shown that recurrence is common and that dissemination may occur.[57] It has been shown that these lesions may be clonal lesions of T-cell lineage and may express the CD30 antigen.[2,14] We know of no significant differences between regressing atypical histiocytosis and primary cutaneous Ki-1 + LCL in terms of clinical presentation, histology, immunophenotype, genotype, and response to therapy and therefore believe that regressing atypical histiocytosis and cutaneous Ki-1 + LCL represent the same disorder.[3,14,15]

Sarcomas

Occasionally Ki-1 + LCL closely mimics a soft tissue sarcoma such as malignant fibrous histiocytoma, and the CD30 antigen may be expressed in various mesenchymal tumors, at least on frozen sections.[58] In these cases a high index of suspicion is needed for the tumor to be correctly diagnosed. In Ki-1 + LCLs simulating sarcomas, both CD45 and CD30 should be positive in the spindle cells.[36] Staining with vimentin is not useful in this differential diagnosis, since, as in most other lymphomas, this intermediate filament is usually expressed in Ki-1 + LCL.[55]

Melanoma

Ki-1 + LCL may simulate malignant melanoma due to the presence of single frequently ulcerated cutaneous tumors composed of cohesive sheets of anaplastic cells in the dermis. In contrast to Ki-1 + LCL, however, malignant melanoma is seldom seen in children and young adults. Unequivocal staining for CD30 and CD45 and negative staining for S100 protein and specific antimelanoma antibodies such as HMB-45 would support a diagnosis of Ki-1 + LCL, although weak cytoplasmic staining for CD30 may be seen in malignant melanomas[40] and S100 protein may be found in occasional tumor cells in Ki-1 + LCL.[8] The ultrastructural demonstration of premelanosomes is diagnostic of melanoma.[43]

Other Lymphomas

Two types of lymphoma deserve special mention due to their frequent intrasinusoidal pattern in lymph nodes.

In 1980, Osborne et al.[59] decribed a sinusoidal LCL in which the neoplastic cells were in part or entirely sinusoidal. Most cases were classified as immunoblastic sarcomas, often showing considerable nuclear pleomorphism. Only occasional tumor cells showed positive cytoplasmic staining for heavy and light chain immunoglobulins, which was not unequivocally monoclonal. The lack of monoclonal cytoplasmic staining for immunoglobulins may suggest a possible T-cell phenotype, and it is possible that some cases of sinusoidal LCL may in fact represent Ki-1+ LCL.

So-called microvillous lymphomas may be confused with Ki-1+ LCL because of their frequently prominent sinus growth pattern.[34] In contrast to Ki-1+ LCL, however, microvillous lymphomas do not express CD30 and EMA, usually have a B-cell phenotype, and possess numerous cytoplasmic processes that are rarely seen in Ki-1+ LCL. Some cases of sinusoidal LCL may correspond to microvillous lymphomas.

Cutaneous T-Cell Lymphoma

Cutaneous T-cell lymphoma may be confused with cutaneous Ki-1+ LCL[43] due to the common skin involvement in Ki-1+ LCL. Also, patients with cutaneous T-cell lymphoma may develop secondary Ki-1+ LCL.[10] Tumor nodules characteristic of cutaneous Ki-1+ LCL are, however, infrequently seen in cutaneous T-cell lymphoma in which multiple patches or plaques are usually present. Also, in contrast to Ki-1+ LCL, cutaneous T-cell lymphoma is seldom seen in children and young adults. Large CD30 cells may be found in cutaneous T-cell lymphoma, but these are in general not numerous.[60] Cutaneous T-cell lymphoma is characterized by epidermotropism of tumor cells and the presence of small to medium sized cerebriform cells. With the exception of the small cell variant,[37] cerebriform cells are seldom seen in Ki-1+ LCL, and tumor cell epidermotropism is usually lacking.

Lymphomatoid Papulosis

The most difficult differential diagnosis encountered in conjunction with cutaneous Ki-1+ LCL is its differentiation from lymphomatoid papulosis, type A. Lymphomatoid papulosis is a regressing but recurrent skin disorder in which 10 to 20 percent of patients later develop lymphoma[61–63] that may be Ki-1+ LCL.[10] The phenotype of lymphomatoid papulosis is identical to that of Ki-1+ LCL, including CD30 expression,[64] and both disorders appear to be clonal.[65,66] It is clear that the histology of type A lymphomatoid papulosis and Ki-1+ LCL may be very similar, if not identical, and it may thus be exceedingly difficult if not impossible to differentiate these two disorders both immunologically and histologically. Features favoring Ki-1+ LCL are single tumors, predominance of large cells, more extensive dermal involvement, and less prominent admixture of reactive cells

Table 10-2. Differential Diagnosis of Ki-1+ Large Cell Lymphoma

	Age	Clinical Features	Morphology
Ki-1+ large cell lymphoma	Bimodal	Peripheral lymphadenopathy, skin lesions, may be multiple	Sinus pattern in nodes, anaplastic/ monomorphic, sheets of cells
Hodgkin's disease	Bimodal	Lymphadenopathy, often in mediastinum, rarely extranodal	No sinus pattern, typical Reed-Sternberg cells, often single tumor cells
Carcinoma	Rare in children	Variable, lymphadenopathy	Sinus pattern in nodes, cohesive cells
Sarcoma	Rare in children	Soft tissue mass, lymphadenopathy rare	Spindle cells, myxoid stroma
Melanoma	Rare in children	Single skin lesion	Nests of tumor cells at D-E junction, melanin in cells
Cutaneous T-cell lymphoma	Rare in children	Cutaneous plaques and patches	Cerebriform cells, epidermotropism
Lymphomatoid papulosis	Mainly adults	Recurrent papules, no lymphadenopathy	Anaplastic cells, singly or in clusters, inflammatory cells

[a] Exceptions may occur (see text).

than is generally seen in lymphomatoid papulosis.[15] Because of the close similarities between Ki-1 + LCL and lymphomatoid papulosis it is probable that these conditions are part of a continuous spectrum and that lymphomatoid papulosis may represent a relatively benign form of Ki-1 + LCL.[5,22,43,67] Preliminary results indicate that lack of t(2;5) in cutaneous lesions of either lymphomatoid papulosis or Ki-1 + LCL may possibly be correlated with a favorable prognosis.[68] Key features of the differential diagnosis of Ki-1 + LCL are summarized in Table 10-2.

TERMINOLOGY

Of the lymphoma classifications in common use, only the recently updated Kiel classification includes Ki-1 + LCL. In that classification the term *large cell anaplastic lymphoma* is used. Since, however, there exists significant morphologic heterogeneity in this type of tumor, including a monomorphic or nonanaplastic variant, not all cases can be included by using that terminology. We therefore believe that the term *Ki-1 (or CD30) positive large cell lymphoma* is, at least at the present time, more appropriate. This term also emphasizes the combined morphologic and immunologic approach that we believe is neccessary for accurate diagnosis of this type of lymphoma. *Anaplastic large cell lymphoma, CD30 +, T- and null-cell types* are included as a specific entity in the recent Revised European-American Lymphoma (REAL) classification.[69] The B lineage Ki-1 + LCL, however, are included within the larger category of diffuse large cell B-cell lymphoma and are not recognized as a specific entity.

CONCLUSION

Ki-1 + LCL is a high grade non-Hodgkin's lymphoma characterized by either peripheral lymphadenopathy with frequent extranodal disease (most often skin lesions), infrequent bone marrow involvement, and chromosomal translocation t(2;5)(p23;q35) or by primary skin disease without extracutaneous disease. Nodal Ki + LCL is clinically a high grade lymphoma while primary cutaneous disease has an excellent prognosis. Ki-1 + LCL may be found in all age groups but is relatively frequent in children and young adults. Primary or secondary forms of Ki-1 + LCL are recognized.

The most distinctive histologic feature of Ki-1 + LCL is intrasinusoidal spread of the tumor cells, and most cases may be classified as anaplastic or monomorphic on the basis of cytology. Variants of Ki-1 + LCL are a Hodgkin's-related type; a giant cell-rich type; a histiocyte-rich type; a sarcomatoid type; and a small cell predominant type.

The characteristic phenotype of Ki-1 + LCL is CD30 + CD45 + CD15 − EMA +, but expression of these antigens (except CD30) is variable. Approximately 60 to 70 percent of cases are of T-cell type, 10 to 20 percent are B-cell type, and 20 percent are null cell type.

The main differential diagnoses of Ki-1 + LCL are Hodgkin's disease, metastatic carcinoma, soft tissue sarcoma, malignant melanoma, and certain other lymphomas including cutaneous T-cell lymphoma and lymphomatoid papulosis. Regressing atypical histiocytosis and most cases of malignant histiocytosis are now felt to represent Ki-1 + LCL. Lymphomatoid papulosis may represent a cutaneous form of Ki-1 + LCL with a favorable prognosis.

ACKNOWLEDGMENTS

This work was supported by NIH grant R01CA/54062 to Dr. Kadin and the Beth Israel Hospital Pathology Foundation.

REFERENCES

1. Stein H, Mason DY, Gerdes J et al.: The expression of the Hodgkin's disease associated antigen Ki-1 in reactive and neoplastic lymphoid tissue: evidence that Reed-Sternberg cells and histiocytic malignancies are derived from activated lymphoid cells. Blood 66:848, 1985

2. Kadin ME, Sako D, Berliner N et al: Childhood Ki-1 lymphoma presenting with skin lesions and peripheral lymphadenopathy. Blood 68:1042, 1986
3. Agnarsson BA, Kadin ME: Ki-1 positive large cell lymphoma. A morphologic and immunologic study of 19 cases. Am J Surg Pathol 12:264, 1988
4. Schnitzer B, Roth MS, Hyder DM, Ginsburg D.: Ki-1 lymphomas in children. Cancer 61:1213, 1988
5. Chan JKC, Ng CS, Hui PK et al: Anaplastic large cell Ki-1 lymphoma. Delineation of two morphological types. Histopathology 15:11, 1989
6. Chott A, Kaserer K, Augustin I et al: Ki-1-positive large cell lymphoma. A clinicopathologic study of 41 cases. Am J Surg Pathol 14:439, 1990
7. Greer JP, Kinney MC, Collins RD et al: Clinical features of 31 patients with Ki-1 anaplastic large-cell lymphoma. J Clin Oncol 9:539, 1991
8. Nakamura S, Takagi N, Kojima M et al: Clinicopathologic study of large cell anaplastic lymphoma (Ki-1-positive large cell lymphoma) among the Japanese. Cancer 68:118, 1991
9. Penny RJ, Blaustein JC, Longtine JA, Pinkus GS: Ki-1-positive large cell lymphomas, a heterogenous group of neoplasms. Morphologic, immunophenotypic, genotypic and clinical features of 24 cases. Cancer 68:362, 1991
10. Lennert K, Feller AC: Histopathology of Non-Hodgkin's Lymphomas (Based on the Updated Kiel Classification). 2nd Ed. Springer-Verlag, Berlin, 1992
11. Kadin ME, Kinney MC: Pathogenesis of Ki-1+ lymphomas. In Magrath IT (ed): The Non-Hodgkin's Lymphomas. 2nd Ed. Edward Arnold, London, 1995
12. Reiter A, Schrappe M, Tiemann M et al: A successful treatment strategy for Ki-1 anaplastic large cell lymphoma of childhood. A prospective analysis of 62 patients enrolled in three consecutive BFM group studies. J Clin Oncol 12:899, 1994
13. Sandlund JT, Pui C-H, Santana VM et al: Clinical features and treatment outcome for children with CD30-positive large cell non-Hodgkin lymphoma. J Clin Oncol 12:895, 1994
14. Beljaards RC, Kaudewitz P, Berti E et al: Primary cutaneous CD30-positive large cell lymphoma: definition of a new type of cutaneous lymphoma with a favorable prognosis. A European multicenter study of 47 patients. Cancer 71:2097, 1993
15. Krishnan J, Tomaszewski M-M, Kao GF: Primary cutaneous CD30-positive anaplastic large cell lymphoma. Report of 27 cases. J Cutan Pathol 20:193, 1993
16. Chan JKC, Ng C-S, Hui P-K et al: Anaplastic large cell Ki-1 lymphoma of bone. Cancer 68: 2186, 1991
17. Pearson JM, Borg-Grech A: Primary Ki-1 (CD30)-positive, large cell, anaplastic lymphoma of the esophagus. Cancer 68:418, 1991
18. Shulman LN, Frisard B, Antin JH et al: Primary Ki-1 anaplastic large cell lymphoma in adults: clinical characteristics and therapeutic outcome. J Clin Oncol 5:937, 1993
19. Vecchi V, Burnelli R, Pileri S et al: Anaplastic large cell lymphoma (Ki-1+/CD30+) in childhood. Med Pediatr Oncol 21:402, 1993
20. Salhany KE, Collins RD, Greer JP, Kinney MC: Long-term survival in Ki-1 lymphoma. Cancer 67:516, 1991
21. Romaguera JE, Manning JT, Tornos CS et al: Long term prognostic importance of primary Ki-1 (CD30) antigen expression and anaplastic morphology in adult patients with diffuse large-cell lymphoma. Ann Oncol 5:317, 1994
22. Kaudewitz P, Stein H, Dallenbech F: Primary and secondary cutaneous Ki-1+ (CD30+) anaplastic large-cell lymphomas. Morphologic, immunologic and clinical characteristics. Cancer 135: 355, 1989
23. Morgan R, Hecht BK, Sandberg AA, et al.: Chromosome 5q35 breakpoint in malignant histiocytosis. N Engl J Med 314:1322, 1986
24. Le Beau MM, Bitter MA, Larson RA et al: The t(2;5) (p23;q35): a recurring chromosomal abnormality in Ki-1 positive anaplastic large cell lymphoma. Leukemia 12:866, 1989
25. Mason DY, Bastard C, Rimokh R et al: CD30-positive large cell lymphomas (''Ki-1 lymphoma'') are associated with a chromosomal translocation involving 5q35. Br J Haematol 74: 161, 1990
26. Bitter MA, Franklin WA, Larson RA et al: Morphology in Ki-1 (CD30)-positive non-Hodgkin's lymphoma is correlated with clinical features and the presence of a unique chromosomal abnormality, t(2;5)(p23;q35). Am J Surg Pathol 14:305, 1990
27. Lopategui JR, Sun L-H, Chain JKC et al.: Low frequency association of the t(2;5)(p23;q35) chromosomal translocation with CD30+ lymphomas from American and Asian patients. A

reverse transcriptase-polymerase chain reaction study. Am J Pathol 146:323, 1995
28. Shiota M, Fujimoto J, Takenaga M et al.: Diagnosis of t(2;5)(p23;q35)-associated Ki-1 lymphoma with immunohistochemistry. Blood 84:3648, 1994
29. Downing J, Shurtleff S, Head D et al.: Molecular detection of t(2;5) of non-Hodgkin's lymphoma by reverse transcriptase polymerase chain reaction (RT-PCR). Lab Invest 72:109A, 1995
30. Davis T, Morton CM, Miller-Cassman R et al.: Hodgkin's disease, lymphomatoid papulosis and cutaneous T-cell lymphoma derived from a common T-cell clone. N Engl J Med 326:1115, 1992
31. Volkenandt M, Bertino JR, Shenoy BV et al: Molecular evidence for a clonal relationship between lymphomatoid papulosis and Ki-1 positive anaplastic large cell lymphoma. J Dermatol Sci 6: 121, 1993
32. Pinkus GS, Said JW, Hargreaves HK: Malignant lymphoma, T cell type: a distinct morphologic variant with large multilobated nuclei. Report of four cases. Am J Clin Pathol 72:540, 1979
33. Burns BF, Dardick I: Ki-1 positive non-Hodgkin's lymphomas. An immunophenotypic, ultrastructural, and morphometric study. Am J Clin Pathol 93:327, 1990
34. Kinney MC, Glick AD, Stein H, Collins RD: Comparison of anaplastic large cell Ki-1 lymphomas and microvillous lymphomas in their immunologic and ultrastructural features. Am J Surg Pathol 14:1047, 1990
35. Pileri S, Falini B, Delsol G et al: Lymphohistiocytic T-cell lymphoma (anaplastic large cell lymphoma CD30+/Ki-1+ with a high content of reactive histiocytes). Histopathology 16:383, 1990
36. Chan JKC, Buchanan R, Fletcher CDM: Sarcomatoid variant of anaplastic large-cell Ki-1 lymphoma. Am J Surg Pathol 14:983, 1990
37. Kinney MC, Collins RD, Greer JP et al: A small-cell-predominant variant of primary Ki-1 (CD30)+ T-cell lymphoma. Am J Surg Pathol 17:859, 1993
38. Stein H, Dallenbach F: Diffuse large cell lymphomas of B and T cell types. pp. 675–714. In Knowles DM (ed): Neoplastic Hematopathology, Williams & Wilkins, Baltimore, 1992
39. Pileri S, Bocchia M, Baroni CD et al: Anaplastic large cell lymphoma (CD30+/Ki-1+): results of a prospective clinico-pathologic study of 69 cases. Br J Haematol 86:513, 1994
40. Schwarting R, Gerdes J, Dürkop H et al.: BER-H2: a new anti-Ki-1 (CD30) monoclonal antibody directed at a formol-resistant epitope. Blood 74:1678, 1989
41. Falini B, Pileri S, Stein H et al.: Variable expression of leucocyte-common (CD45) antigen in CD30 (Ki-1)-positive anaplastic large-cell lymphoma: Implications for the differential diagnosis between lymphoid and nonlymphoid malignancies. Hum Pathol 21:624, 1990
42. Delsol G, al Saati T, Gatter KC et al.: Coexpression of epithelial membrane antigen (EMA), Ki-1, and interleukin-2 receptor by anaplastic large cell lymphomas. Diagnostic value in so-called malignant histiocytosis. Am J Pathol 130:59, 1988
43. Kinney MC, Greer JP, Glick AD et al.: Anaplastic large-cell Ki-1 malignant lymphomas. Recognition, biological and clinical implications. Pathol Annu 26:1, 1991
44. Byrne GE, Rappaport H: Malignant histiocytosis. GANN Monogr Cancer Res 15:145, 1973
45. Ducatmann BS, Wick MR, Morgan TW, et al.: Malignant histiocytosis. A clinical, histologic and immunohistochemical study of 20 cases. Hum Pathol 15:368, 1984
46. Cattoretti G, Villa A, Vezzoni P et al.: Malignant histiocytosis. A phenotypic and genotypic investigation. Am J Pathol 136:1009, 1990
47. Wilson MS, Weiss LM, Gatter KC et al.: Malignant histiocytosis. A reassessment of cases previously reported in 1975 based on paraffin section immunophenotyping studies. Cancer 66:530, 1990
48. Andreesen R, Bruggen W, Löhr GW, Bross KJ: Human macrophages can express the Hodgkin's cell-associated antigen Ki-1 (CD30). Am J Pathol 134:187, 1989
49. Carbone A, Gloghini A, De Re V et al.: Histopathologic, immunophenotypic, and genotypic analysis of Ki-1 anaplastic large cell lymphomas that express histiocyte-associated antigens. Cancer 66:2547, 1990
50. Strickler JG, Michie SA, Warnke RA, Dorfman RF: The "syncitial variant" of nodular sclerosing Hodgkin's disease. Am J Surg Pathol 10:470, 1986
51. Delsol G, Gatter KC, Stein H et al.: Human lymphoid cells express epithelial membrane antigen. Implications for the diagnosis of human neoplasms. Lancet 2:1124, 1984
52. Perkins PL, Ross CW, Schnitzer B: CD30 posi-

tive anaplastic large-cell lymphomas that express CD15 but lack CD45: a possible diagnostic pitfall. Arch Pathol Lab Med 116:1192, 1992
53. Sioutos N, Kadin ME: Perivascular Ki-1+ lesions. Int J Hematol 55:275, 1992
54. Pallesen G, Hamilton-Dutoit SJ: Ki-1 (CD 30) antigen is regularly expressed by tumor cells of embryonal carcinoma. Am J Pathol 133:446, 1988
55. Gustmann C, Altmannsberger M, Osborn M, et al.: Cytokeratin expression and vimentin content in large cell anaplastic lymphomas and other non-Hodgkin's lymphomas. Am J Pathol 138:1413, 1991
56. Flynn KJ, Dehner LP, Gajl-Peczalska KJ et al.: Regressing atypical histiocytosis: a cutaneous proliferation of atypical neoplastic histiocytes with unexpectedly indolent biologic behavior. Cancer 49:959, 1982
57. Headington JT, Roth MS, Schnitzer B: Regressing atypical histiocytosis: a review amd critical appraisal. Semin Diagn Pathol 4:28, 1987
58. Mechtersheimer G, Möller P: Expression of Ki-1 antigen (CD 30) in mesenchymal tumors. Cancer 66:1732, 1990
59. Osborne BM, Butler JJ, Mackay B: Sinusoidal large cell (''histiocytic'') lymphoma. Cancer 46: 2484, 1980
60. Van der Putte SCJ, Toonstra J, Van Wichen DF et al.: The expression of the Hodgkin's disease-associated antigen Ki-1 in cutaneous infiltrates. Acta Dermatol Venereol (Stockh) 68:202, 1988
61. Macauley WL: Lymphomatoid papulosis. A continuing self-healing eruption, clinically benign—histologically malignant. Arch Dermatol 97:23, 1968
62. Willemze R, Meijer CJLM, Van Vloten WA, Scheffer E: The clinical and histological spectrum of lymphomatoid papulosis. Br J Dermatol 107:131, 1982
63. Sanchez NP, Pittelkow MR, Muller SA et al.: The clinicopathologic spectrum of lymphomatoid papulosis: study of 31 cases. J Am Acad Dermatol 8:81, 1983
64. Kadin M, Nasu, Sako D, et al.: Lymphomatoid papulosis. A cutaneous proliferation of activated helper T-cells expressing Hodgkin's disease associated antigens. Am J Pathol 119:315, 1985
65. Weiss LM, Wood GS, Trela M et al.: Clonal T-cell populations in lymphomatoid papulosis: evidence of a lymphoproliferative origin for a clinically benign disease. N Engl J Med 315:475, 1986
66. Kadin ME, Vonderheid EC, Sako D et al.: Clonal composition of T cells in lymphomatoid papulosis. Am J Pathol 126:13, 1987
67. Kadin ME: The spectrum of Ki-1+ cutaneous lymphomas. Curr Probl Dermatol 19:132, 1990
68. Kadin ME: Ki-1+ (anaplastic) large-cell lymphoma: maturation of a clinicopathologic entity with prospects of effective therapy. J Clin Oncol 12:884, 1994
69. Harris NL, Jaffe E, Stein H et al: A revised European-American classification of lymphoid neoplasms: a proposal from the International Lymphoma Study Group. Blood 84:1361, 1994

11

Histiocytic and Dendritic Cell Proliferations

Karen L. Chang and Lawrence M. Weiss

NORMAL HISTIOCYTES AND DENDRITIC CELLS

Normal histiocytes derive from the bone marrow stem cells (granulocyte-macrophage colony-forming units), have a high content of lysosomal enzymes, and are capable of phagocytosis.[1,2] Fixed tissue histiocytes, also called *macrophages*, populate virtually all organs and include the Kupffer cells of the liver, lung alveolar macrophages, and tingible-body macrophages of lymph node germinal centers. Circulating, or freely mobile, histiocytes are localized to the lymph node, tonsil, and splenic sinuses. Morphologically, all histiocytes generally have bland medium sized nuclei and a moderate to marked amount of cytoplasm, depending on their functional state. Ultrastructural studies show that the histiocyte cytoplasm contains numerous lysosomes, vacuoles, and mitochondria.[3] Histiocytes also contain a well-developed Golgi apparatus and cytoskeletal system. There are residual bodies in their cytoplasm, which often shows numerous folds and microvillous projections. Cytochemically, the cells are reactive for nonspecific esterase, acid phosphatase, lysozyme, α_1-antitrypsin, and α_1-chymotrypsin.[1] Immunologically, histiocytes/macrophages have been shown to express class II major histocompatibility (MHC) molecules as well as CD45, CD68 and a variety of other antigens, depending on their functional state.[1,4,5]

Dendritic cells are bone marrow-derived cells present in small numbers in almost all tissues.[6,7] Unlike histiocytes and macrophages, which have phagocytic properties, dendritic cells do not function as phagocytic elements, but as antigen-presenting cells.[7–12] Cells of this series include Langerhans cells, follicular dendritic (dendritic reticulum) cells, interdigitating dendritic (interdigitating reticulum) cells, and indeterminate cells. These cells all have a dendritic morphology and contain low levels of lysosomal enzymes. Most of the cells of this class have ATPase activity and do not have peroxidase activity.[1] They strongly express class II histocompatibility proteins and HLA-DR antigen, and they have receptor sites for the Fc portion of the IgG molecule and the third component of complement.[1,11] CD45 staining has also been reported.[1] The cell surface glycoprotein HB15, a new member of the immunoglobulin superfamily, has been found to be uniquely expressed on Langerhans cells and interdigitating dendritic cells.[13]

The Langerhans cell is the most extensively studied dendritic cell and is usually found in epithelia.[1,14] It is most commonly present in the upper part of the squamous layer of epidermis and helps to form a meshwork throughout the epidermis. It recognizes and presents antigen to immunocompetent T-lineage lymphocytes. Ultrastructural studies reveal small vesicles, multivesicular bodies, lysosomes, and a characteristic organelle termed the *Birbeck granule*.[15] The latter is a racket- or rod-shaped structure of about 200 to 400 nm in length and about 33 nm in width with an osmiophilic core and a double outer sheath. The Langerhans cell lacks microvilli, desmosomes, tonofilaments, and melanosomes. The Langerhans cell also has low nonspecific esterase activity, 5′ nucleotidase,

ATPase, small amounts of acid phosphatase, and small amounts of placental alkaline phosphatase.[16–18] The cell also expresses S100 antigen, CD1, CD4, CD11, and CD14, variably expresses CD15 and CD21, and does not usually exhibit CD35.[12,19]

The interdigitating dendritic cell is the antigen-presenting cell of the lymph node paracortex. It has similar morphology and immunophenotype to Langerhans cells.[20] However, unlike the Langerhans cell, it lacks Birbeck granules, contains an organelle of undetermined function (the tubulovesicular system), and expresses only variable amounts of CD1.[21,22] The cell also expresses S100 protein, CD4, CD15, and CD11c, variable amounts of CD14, and many macrophage-associated antigens. It lacks complement receptors.

The follicular dendritic cell is the antigen-processing cell of the germinal center and surrounding mantle zone and is a multinucleated cell with long, slender cytoplasmic processes that form a network with other follicular dendritic cells via desmosomal attachments.[23] Because this cell retains antigens on its surface, it is capable of providing a sustained reaction to that antigen, a potentially important feature in immune memory.[24] It expresses CD4, CD21, and CD35 and variable amounts of S100, CD11, and CD14, in addition to a cell-specific antigen recognized by monoclonal antibodies R4/23, Ki-M4, and BU-10.[23,25–29] Unlike the Langerhans cell, it does not express CD1. The follicular dendritic cell also shows activity for nonspecific esterase and acid phosphatase.[16,17]

Indeterminate cells are dendritic cells of the skin that are morphologically and antigenically similar to Langerhans cells with the one exception that Birbeck granules are not identified.[30] These cells are present in both the epidermis and dermis.

HISTIOCYTIC AND DENDRITIC CELL PROLIFERATIONS

Table 11-1 lists the histiocytic and dendritic cell proliferations discussed in this chapter. For the sake of parsimony, the following diseases that show histiocytic proliferations are omitted from discussion: storage disorders in which histiocytic accumulation of metabolic byproducts is a secondary phenomenon, the majority of cutaneous histiocytic disorders (such as juvenile xanthogranuloma), acute and chronic monocytic leukemias, and the majority of inflammatory/infectious disorders (such as tuberculosis or sarcoidosis).

Table 11-1. Classification of Histiocytic and Dendritic Cell Proliferations

I.	Benign histiocytic proliferations
	Sinus hyperplasia
	Sinus histiocytosis with massive lymphadenopathy
	Infection-associated hemophagocytic syndrome
	Familial hemophagocytic lymphohistiocytosis
	Malignant lymphoma with benign erythrophagocytosis
	Erythrophagocytic Tγlymphoma
II.	Benign dendritic proliferations
	Dermatopathic lymphadenopathy
III.	Borderline and malignant dendritic proliferations
	Langerhans cell histiocytosis
	Dendritic and indeterminate cell neoplasms
IV.	Malignant histiocytic proliferations
	True histiocytic lymphoma and malignant histiocytosis
	Malignant histiocytosis associated with mediastinal germ cell tumor
	Intravascular histiocytosis
	Histiocytic medullary reticulosis
	Regressing atypical histiocytosis

BENIGN HISTIOCYTIC PROLIFERATIONS

Sinus Hyperplasia

Sinus hyperplasia or sinus histiocytosis is an extremely common finding in lymph nodes.[31,32] In many instances, the cause of the hyperplasia is unknown. It may be prominent in lymph nodes draining the extremities and the mesenteric region and in lymph nodes draining sites of malignant neoplasms or of prosthesis placement. Histologic features include dilated subcapsular and trabecular lymph node sinuses, filled with uniform-sized histiocytes with cytologically bland nuclei and abundant cytoplasm. Erythrophagocytosing histiocytes may be seen, particularly in the axillary lymph nodes of patients with breast cancer who otherwise show no signs of systemic hemophagocytic syndrome.[33]

A rare signet ring variant of sinus histiocytosis has been reported, again most commonly in the axillary lymph nodes recovered from a radical mastectomy specimen.[34,35] In this rare variant, the sinusoidal histiocytes contain clear cytoplasmic vacuoles that displace the nuclei to the periphery. The vacuoles do not stain for mucin, but may contain lipid. Unlike the cells of metastatic signet ring cell carcinoma, the cells of signet ring variant of sinus histiocytosis show no nuclear atypia.

Sinus Histiocytosis with Massive Lymphadenopathy

Sinus histiocytosis with massive lymphadenopathy (SHML) is a rare idiopathic proliferative histiocytic disorder first described in the 1960s.[36–38] Approximately 90 percent of patients present with cervical lymph node enlargement. Extranodal sites are involved in approximately 40 percent of cases. The eponym ''Rosai-Dorfman disease'' may be applied to SHML, particularly in cases of extranodal disease.

Afflicted patients are usually in their first or second decade of life, with a median age of 20 years. However, the disease affects all age groups, from neonates presenting with congenital disease to the elderly.[39] The male to female ratio is approximately 3:2. Men of African descent are only slightly more commonly affected than Caucasian men. A small percentage of patients are Asian or other races. Worldwide, the incidence of SHML is greatest in the United States, Western Europe, and Africa. Interestingly, two pairs of identical twins were reported to develop SHML within a 5 year interval.[39,40]

SHML usually presents as isolated, massive bilateral, and painless cervical lymphadenopathy. Other lymph node groups may also be involved, including axillary, inguinal, para-aortic, and mediastinal, with or without concomitant cervical disease. Rarely is a single lymph node involved. Fever, weight loss, malaise, joint symptoms, and night sweats may accompany the adenopathy, but hepatosplenomegaly is rare. Extranodal sites of disease include the upper respiratory tract, bone, soft tissues of the eyelid and orbit, and, less often, skin and subcutaneous tissue.[39,41,42] Other rarely involved extranodal sites include the gastrointestinal and genitourinary tracts and the thyroid. The bone marrow and spleen seem to be spared.[39]

Patients with SHML may have a mild normochromic, normocytic anemia or hypochromic, microcytic anemia; a minority of patients have red cell autoantibodies, which may manifest as severe hemolytic anemia. Leukocytosis with relative lymphopenia and relative granulocytosis may also be present; a reversal in the CD4/CD8 ratio is often found. A moderate polyclonal hypergammaglobulinemia is often present, as is hypoalbuminemia. The erythrocyte sedimentation rate is typically elevated. A minority of patients may test positive for rheumatoid factor or have a positive lupus erythematosus cell preparation test, but whether these represent false positive results is not yet clear. Elevated antibody titers to Epstein-Barr virus (EBV) and measles virus have been observed in some patients, and some cases have been associated with EBV or herpesvirus 6.[43,44] However, specific etiology has not been documented. No consistent lymphocyte, granulocyte, or histiocyte abnormalities have been found, and lipid studies are normal.

Gross examination of involved lymph nodes shows marked enlargement with a yellowish-white cut surface. The histologic features include a very fibrotic lymph node capsule; in contrast to Hodgkin's disease, the fibrosis does not extend into the lymph node parenchyma. A striking feature in most cases is massive dilatation of the sinuses, resulting in partial or complete architectural effacement (Fig. 11-1A). Numerous histiocytes with highly characteristic features fill and distend the lymphatic sinuses (Fig. 11-1B). These unique histiocytes have an intermediate sized nucleus with a vesicular chromatin pattern and one to several nucleoli. The nu-

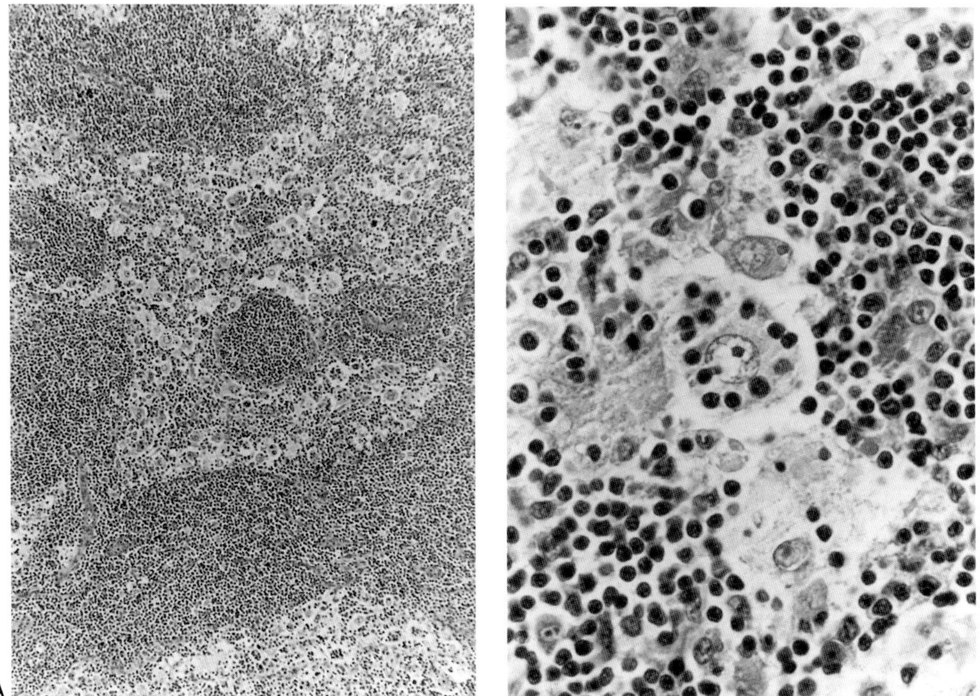

Fig. 11-1. Sinus histiocytosis with massive lymphadenopathy. **(A)** The sinusoidal pattern of involvement is distinctive. **(B)** The characteristic cells have medium sized nuclei with one or several prominent nucleoli. There is abundant cytoplasm. Lymphophagocytosis is seen. Plasma cells are easily found.

clear membrane is delicate but distinct. Cytologic atypia is usually not seen, but may be present in rare cases. The voluminous cytoplasm, amphophilic to eosinophilic in hematoxylin and eosin stains, contains intact lymphocytes (termed *lymphophagocytosis* or *emperipolesis*) and, less often, may contain plasma cells, neutrophils, and red blood cells. Sometimes, the cytoplasm of the characteristic cells may appear foamy. The sinuses and intrasinusal tissues are often filled with mature plasma cells. Eosinophils are not seen. Germinal centers are usually present, but generally are not a prominent feature. The histologic findings of SHML in extranodal sites are similar to that seen in lymph nodes, even to the extent of having dilated sinuses in some cases. However, fibrosis is greater, and the number and prominence of the characteristic cells is usually less than in nodal disease.

The proliferating cells of SHML appear to share properties of histiocytes and dendritic cells. Ultrastructural studies show histiocytic features: numerous complex filopodia and the presence of lipid vacuoles and varying numbers of lysosomes in the cytoplasm. Birbeck granules are absent, as are viral particles or other evidence of infection. Histochemical studies demonstrate the presence of neutral fat and periodic acid-Schiff positive, diastase-resistant material in the cytoplasm. Cytochemical stains show that the cells contain acid phosphatase, α-naphthyl-acetate, and α-butyrate esterase, providing additional evidence for a histiocytic differentiation.[45,46]

Paraffin section immunohistochemical studies show that the cells of SHML express S100 protein, lysozyme, α_1-antitrypsin, α_1-antichymotrypsin, CD68, CD14, CD15, as well as the macrophage-specific markers HAM56 (panmacrophage) and Mac-387 (associated with early inflammation).[47] CD30 reactivity is present in approximately 50 percent of cases.[47] Frozen section immunoperoxidase studies show that the histiocytes of SHML express numerous macrophage and macrophage-associated antigens, including several antigens not found on interdigitating dendritic cells. The cells of SHML do not usually express the CD1 antigen found on Langerhans cells and also lack expression of R4/23, a monoclonal antibody with high specificity for follicular dendritic cells.[46] Gene rearrangement studies show a germline configuration for both the immunoglobulin heavy chain gene and the β- and T-cell receptor gene.[46] The evidence to date suggests a relationship between the cells of SHML and cells of the histiocytic lineage. However, the strong S100 reactivity of the cells of SHML implies only a tenuous relation to normal sinus histiocytes, which are negative for S100 protein, and in fact may suggest some relationship to dendritic cells. Recently, the histiocytes of SHML involving lymph nodes were shown by molecular methods to be polyclonal.[47a]

The conditions that may be confused with SHML in lymph nodes include reactive sinus hyperplasia, in which the sinuses are usually less expanded than in SHML. More importantly, the histiocytes of reactive sinus hyperplasia do not usually express S100 and differ cytologically from the characteristic cells of SHML. Langerhans cell histiocytosis (histiocytosis X) has a similar low power appearance to SHML, but the cytologic characteristics of Langerhans cells and the presence of eosinophils in Langerhans cell histiocytosis helps to distinguish between the two diseases. Furthermore, CD1 expression, the presence of Birbeck granules, and lack of emperipolesis in Langerhans cell histiocytosis differs from CD1-negative SHML. Close examination of the cytologic features of the proliferating cells and differing immunohistochemical profiles also help distinguish SHML from sinusoidal involvement by metastatic carcinoma, malignant melanoma, and sinusoidal malignant lymphoma (Fig. 11-2).

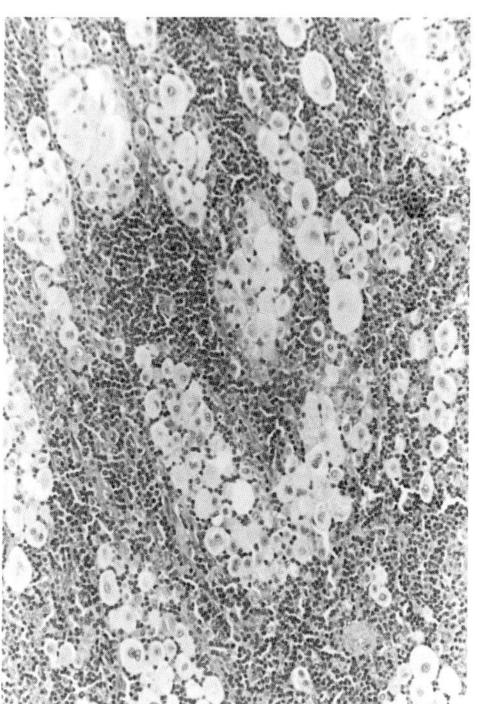

Fig. 11-2. Metastatic melanoma. The sinusoidal infiltration of balloon-cell variant melanoma cells closely mimics the low power appearance of sinus histiocytosis with massive lymphadenopathy.

In general, therapy is both unnecessary and ineffective. The majority of patients with SHML undergo spontaneous remission, with disease manifestations gradually subsiding over several months to years.[39,48] Extranodal disease appears to regress before nodal disease. Another large group of patients may have persistent but stable disease and do not require therapy. Some patients require surgery beyond the initial biopsy for cosmetic reasons or to alleviate obstruction. Chemotherapy has been administered to patients whose extensive disease compromises organ function, with response rates inferior to those seen in most other hematolymphoid neoplasms. Radiation therapy has also been given to some patients with extensive disease; again, the response rates are inferior to those seen in the majority of malignant lymphomas. A small number of patients with SHML have died, either directly of disease or with SHML significantly contributing to their death.[39,40,48,49] Patients with an aggressive clinical course tend to have involvement of a larger number of node groups and a larger number of extranodal sites. Many of these patients also have evidence of immunologic abnormalities.

Infection-Associated Hemophagocytic Syndrome

Infection-associated hemophagocytic syndrome (IAHS) is a non-neoplastic, systemic proliferation of benign-appearing histiocytes. The disease was originally described to be associated with viral infections, particularly cytomegalovirus and and other herpesviruses.[50] The list of agents associated with the induction of a hemophagocytic syndrome has expanded beyond viruses to include almost any infectious agent, including gram-positive and gram-negative bacteria, mycobacteria, fungi, rickettsia, and leishmaniasis.[51–60] IAHS is most likely a manifestation of an impaired immune response to an infectious process.[54] Many, but not all, patients have a documented primary or iatrogenic (e.g., organ-transplant-related) immunodeficiency.[61] Patients who develop IAHS and do not have an obvious immunodeficiency may have a subtle immunologic deficit, possibly specific for particular types of infectious agents.[52,57]

IAHS has been reported in children without evidence of an underlying disease and in patients of all ages with a history of immunosuppression.[59] Affected patients usually present with evidence of multisystem involvement, including fever and other constitutional symptoms, and often have hepatosplenomegaly, generalized lymphadenopathy, a skin rash, and bilateral pulmonary infiltrates.[51–53,62–63] Similar symptoms, accompanied by morphologic changes nearly identical to those seen in IAHS, have been induced in juvenile rhesus monkeys treated with interleukin-3.[64] A prodromal period of several weeks of a viral-like illness may precede development of more severe symptomatology. Laboratory evaluation usually reveals pancytopenia, liver function abnormalities, and abnormal coagulation parameters that are more severe than expected on the basis of abnormal liver function alone. A rapidly progressive variant of IAHS has been described in Taiwan and other parts of the Orient. This clinically agressive form affects infants and toddlers and is EBV associated.[65–67]

The pathologic features vary with the time that biopsies are performed. Early in the disease, lymph nodes may exhibit a marked immunoblastic proliferation with only partial lymph node effacement. The number of histiocytes is low. Later in the disease, one observes lymphoid depletion and possibly massive sinusoidal infiltration by benign-appearing histiocytes (Fig. 11-3A). The histiocytes have no cytologic atypia and may show prominent platelet phagocytosis and hemophagocytosis (Fig. 11-3B). Germinal centers may be present but generally are not prominent. Other hematolymphoid organs may also show striking findings. Early in the disease, the bone marrow may be hypercellular with few infiltrating histiocytes. Erythrophagocytosis is best seen in the aspirate smears. Later in the disease, the bone marrow is hypocellular with decreased numbers in the erythroid and granulocytic series, but with relatively normal or slightly increased numbers of megakaryocytes. Moderate to marked histiocytic hyperplasia is always present. The histiocytes appear benign and often show prominent phagocytosis. Granulomas and necrotic areas may be observed. Platelets and erythrophagocytosis generally predominate, but phagocytosis of other cellular debris may also be seen. Histiocytic hyperplasia may also be seen in the spleen, where the red pulp is preferentially involved. Histiocytic hyperplasia involving the liver generally affects both the sinusoidal and portal areas.

Similarities in clinical presentation may render IAHS difficult to distinguish from other hematolymphoid malignancies that involve the lymph node sinuses and that secondarily induce benign hemophagocytosis. The cytologically benign histiocytes of IAHS can generally be distinguished from the atypical proliferating cells of hematolymphoid malignancies involving lymph node sinuses. For cases in which this distinction may be difficult (because of inadequate sample size), repeat biopsies may help resolve the problem.[68] T-cell lymphomas, and a minority of other lymphomas, may induce a florid hyperplasia of morphologically benign hemophagocytizing lymphocytes, possibly resulting in confusion with IAHS.[57,58,69–74] Identification of the malignant cells of the lymphoma will help separate the IAHS from the malignancy.

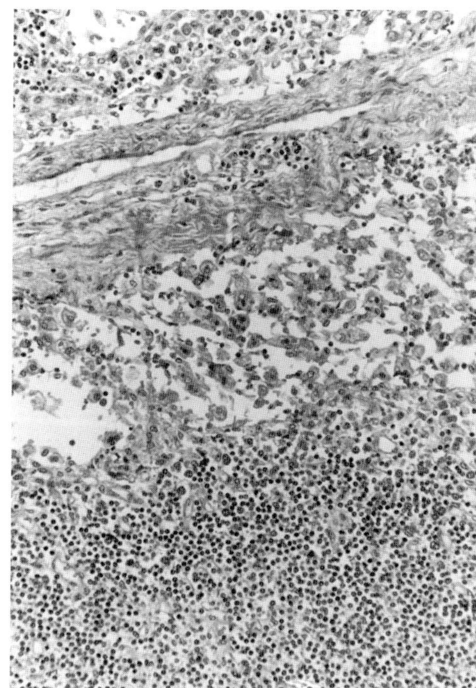

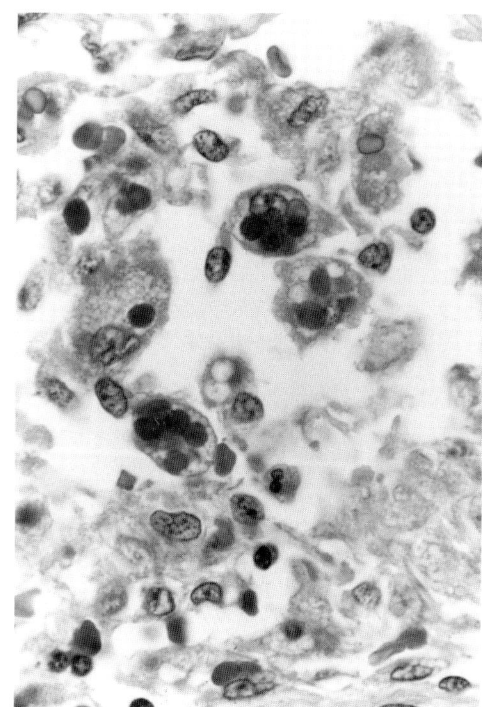

Fig. 11-3. Infection-associated hemophagocytic syndrome. **(A)** The sinuses are dilated with numerous histiocytes. **(B)** Abundant histiocytes showing erythrophagocytosis are present.

Patients with IAHS may recover within a period of months from this benign, self-limiting condition.[75,76] However, many affected patients will die during the acute disease episode due to multisystem failure or later due to infectious complications exacerbated by their underlying immunodeficiency.[61,65] Death from nontraumatic splenic rupture has been reported.[77] EBV-associated hemophagocytic syndrome is often fatal.[65–67] Reports of immunosuppressive therapy used in cases in which the diagnosis of IAHS was mistaken for other histiocytic malignancies, such as malignant histiocytosis, show that the use of immunosuppressive agents has been deleterious.

Familial Hemophagocytic Lymphohistiocytosis

Familial hemophagocytic lymphohistiocytosis is an extremely rare and usually fatal disease of early childhood that is characterized by marked lymphohistiocytic infiltration in multiple organs.[59,78] Synonyms include *familial hemophagocytic reticulosis, generalized lymphohistiocytosis of infancy,* and *familial lymphohistiocytic syndrome*. The typical patient is less than 1 year old (two-thirds of patients are less than 3 months old)[79,80] and has intermittent fevers, pallor, and failure to thrive. Males are affected slightly more than females, and the disease occurs in all ethnic groups. About three-fourths of cases are familial, with an autosomal recessive mode of inheritance.[81] Common physical findings at presentation include hepatosplenomegaly, pulmonary effusions, and a maculopapular skin rash. Two siblings were reported to have disseminated T-cell lymphoma at the time of diagnosis of FHLH.[82] Laboratory findings include pancytopenia, a severe hypofibrinogenemia without abnormalities of other clotting facts, hyperlipidemia, and hyperbilirubinemia.

The lymph nodes and bone marrow are the most frequently involved sites, followed by involvement of the spleen, liver, and central nervous system.[82] The affected lymph nodes are cell poor and are partially to completely effaced by sinusoidal infiltrates of benign-appearing histiocytes, lymphocytes, and, often, plasma cells. The histiocytosis is quite pronounced and is accompanied by striking erythrophagocytosis. Lymphophagocytosis and phagocytosis of other cellular debris may also be observed. The bone marrow is hypercellular and contains large numbers of hemophagocytic histiocytes, accompanied by relative erythroid hyperplasia and myeloid hypoplasia. A hemophagocytic histiocytosis may also be present in the red pulp of involved spleens and the sinusoids of involved livers. The latter can be seen particularly well by fine-needle aspiration of the liver.[83] Diffuse infiltration of the leptomeninges and perivascular spaces by the characteristic histiocytes is observed in the white matter of involved brains. The thymus shows severe lymphoid depletion.

The proliferating cells show histochemical evidence of acid phosphatase, nonspecific esterase, and lysozyme.[80] Immunophenotypic analysis of the histiocytic cells shows expression of CD14 and HLA-DR, with variable expression of CD15.[81,84] Both of these observations support histiocytic derivation. Evidence against a dendritic cell lineage for these proliferating cells is the lack of S100 protein, CD1 antigen, and Birbeck granules.

Familial hemophagocytic lymphohistiocytosis may be clinically and pathologically difficult to distinguish from IAHS. In fact, some investigators hypothesize that they represent the same disease, with familial hemophagocytic lymphohistiocytosis presenting as IAHS in individuals with familial immunodeficiencies. Cellular and humoral immunity are defective in this disorder.[53,85–87] Cytogenetic abnormalities, including the presence of double minute chromosomes and occasional loss of chromosomes 7 and 12, were found in unstimulated peripheral blood cells of one patient. These karyotypic findings have been associated with dyserythropoietic and leukemic states and suggest a primary proliferative disorder.[88]

In the majority of cases, familial hemophagocytic lymphohistiocytosis is rapidly fatal, with death due to sepsis, bleeding, or a lymphocytic meningitis accompanied by refractory seizure. Survival of several months to years has been reported. To date, there is no proven effective therapy for familial hemophagocytic lymphohistiocytosis, although bone marrow transplantation has been attempted, with mixed results.[81,89]

Malignant Lymphoma with Benign Erythrophagocytosis

Malignant lymphoma with benign erythrophagocytosis refers to a mixed process that combines features of both lymphoma and a reactive histiocytic disorder.[69,70,90] The lymphoma is usually of T-cell lineage, and the lymphoma cells are well demarcated from a proliferation of benign histiocytes that display prominent erythrophagocytosis.[57,58] The histiocytic proliferation is similar to that seen in IAHS, but is not associated with a systemic infection.

Malignant lymphoma with benign erythrophagocytosis has primarily two different clinical presentations. Patients with known lymphoma may develop a syndrome mimicking IAHS.[57,69,92–94] In these patients, lymphoma is often disseminated and usually shows T-cell lineage or ''activated killer cell'' phenotype.[58] In one study, approximately one-third of such patients had active infections, mostly of viral origin.[58] Morphologically, clusters or sheets of malignant cells are physically separate from a marked proliferation of cytologically benign histiocytes that show erythrophagocytosis as well as phagocytosis of leukocytes and platelets. This latter process is most evident in lymph node sinuses, bone marrow, splenic red pulp, and hepatic sinusoids.[95,96] The occurrence of erthyrophagocytosis is usually a terminal event in a patient with advanced stage lymphoma.[58]

In the second predominant clinical presentation, the hemophagocytic syndrome occurs in the absence of any previously diagnosed disease.[62,70] In this setting, benign hemophagocytizing histiocytes are intimately interspersed with the malignant lymphoma cells. This lymphoma often involves the bone marrow, spleen, and liver. Paraffin and frozen section immunophenotyping studies usually demonstrate a T-cell lineage. The prognosis is extremely poor in most patients.

The prominent phagocytosis by the benign histiocytes of malignant lymphoma with benign erythrophagocytosis may be mediated by production of a lymphokine by the neoplastic cells.[91] In support of this hypothesis, a factor that augments the phagocytosis of IgG-coated ox red blood cells by the human monocyte/macrophage line U9437 has been identified in two patients with this disease.[95]

Hemophagocytosis is also a feature of a unique subtype of acute myelomonocytic leukemia associated with the cytogenetic abnormality t(8 : 16)(p11 : 13) and its variants.[97,98]

Erythrophagocytic Tγ Lymphoma

Erythrophagocytic Tγ lymphoma is an exceedingly rare neoplasm reported in 1981.[99] Its clinical and pathologic features resemble those of malignant histiocytosis, as defined in the early 1980s. Immunologic studies show that the malignant cells of erythrophagocytic Tγ lymphoma belong to a subpopulation of T lymphocytes known as Tγ cells. In current nomenclature, this entity most likely represents hepatosplenic T-cell lymphoma, with associated hemophagocytosis.[100,101]

BENIGN DENDRITIC PROLIFERATIONS: DERMATOPATHIC LYMPHADENOPATHY

Dermatopathic lymphadenopathy, initially termed *lipomelanosis reticularis of Pautrier*, refers to the reactive condition seen in lymph nodes that drain areas near disruption of the skin integrity.[102,103] Patients usually have some form of chronic dermatosis, but typically have a generalized exfoliative dermatitis with pruritus. The skin disorders may be benign, such as psoriasis, or malignant, such as mycosis fungoides. Rarely, changes of dermatopathic lymphadenopathy may be seen in the absence of skin disease.

Grossly, the lymph node is enlarged and fleshy and may have a streaky melanotic pigment in the periphery of the lymph node. Histologically, the overall lymph node architecture is preserved. Varying degrees of paracortical expansion are comprised of a population of dendritic cells and histiocytes, often admixed with immunoblasts, eosinophils, plasma cells, and a variable number of small lymphocytes with nuclear atypia (Fig. 11-4). The histiocyte cytoplasm may contain phagocytosed melanin and neutral fat. Reactive follicular hyperplasia is typically present. The lymph node sinuses are usually intact. The numerous dendritic cells, which include interdigitating dendritic cells and Langerhans cells, express the S100 antigen.

Dermatopathic lymphadenopathy involving

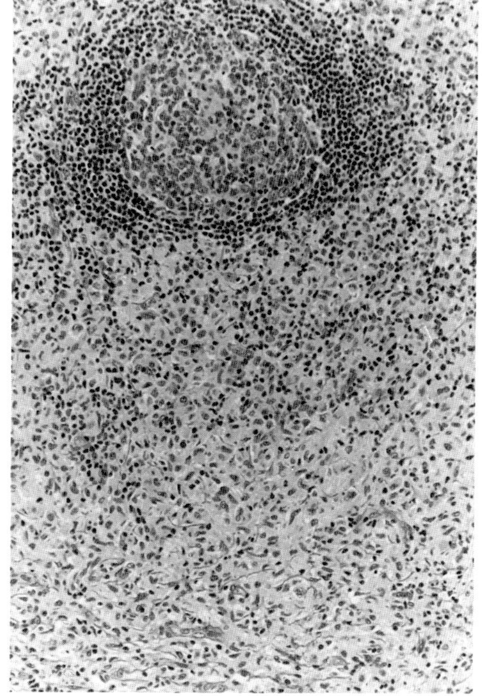

Fig. 11-4. Dermatopathic lymphadenitis. The paracortex of the lymph node is expanded by a collection of histiocytes, interdigitating cells, and Langerhans cells.

the lymph node may be confused with Langerhans cell histiocytosis, Hodgkin's disease, and monocytic leukemia. However, the paracortical location and bland morphology of the proliferating cells of dermatopathic lymphadenopathy are not features of the other disorders. Differentiating dermatopathic lymphadenopathy from mycosis fungoides involving the lymph node may be extremely difficult. Patients whose lymph nodes show dermatopathic changes may have skin lesions for which mycosis fungoides is a clinical consideration. Conversely, the lymph nodes of patients with mycosis fungoides may have dermatopathic changes with or without involvement by mycosis fungoides. As described above, the sinuses of lymph nodes with dermatopathic lymphadenopathy may contain individual or clusters of atypical lymphocytes. Thus, in order to establish definitively a diagnosis of mycosis fungoides involving the lymph node, one must see nearly complete effacement of the normal lymph node architecture by cells with malignant cytologic features. Immunohistochemical studies are not very useful in distinguishing between the two entities.[104] However, molecular evidence of a β T-cell receptor gene rearrangement provides evidence for mycosis fungoides.[105]

BORDERLINE AND MALIGNANT DENDRITIC PROLIFERATIONS

Langerhans Cell Histiocytosis

Langerhans cell histiocytosis (LCH), also known as *histiocytosis X* and *Langerhans cell granulomatosis,* encompasses many different clinical manifestations of a clonal proliferation of Langerhans cells. Historically, the disease comprises three main and sometimes overlapping clinical syndromes: unifocal disease (solitary eosinophilic granuloma), multifocal unisystem disease (including cases of Hand-Schüller-Christian syndrome), and multifocal multisystem disease (including cases of Letterer-Siwe syndrome.[106]

Langerhans cell histiocytosis is an extremely rare disease that affects approximately 1 in 2 million people.[107] Males are affected twice as often as females. Patients of Northern European descent are more frequently afflicted than patients of Hispanic heritage, and the disease has rarely been described in patients of African ancestry.[108,109] The age at presentation varies with the clinical syndrome, but the disease occurs primarily in the pediatric population. Unifocal disease is found predominantly in older children and young adults under the age of 30.[108,110] The age of presentation with multifocal unisystem disease is approximately 2 to 5 years. The median age of presentation with multifocal multisystem disease is less than 3 years.[110] Solitary lung involvement usually occurs in young adult males between 20 and 40 years.[111,112] However, all of the clinical syndromes have been reported in all age groups.[112] Early reports describe sibships and kindreds who had what appears to be Letterer-Siwe disease. Although many of the earlier reports were actually describing non-LCH reticulohistiocytic disorders, rare well-documented cases of LCH have appeared in families.[113,114]

The etiology of the disease is unknown. One group reported evidence of human herpesvirus 6 in lesions of LCH.[115] However, another group did not confirm this finding and in fact found no molecular evidence of seven other viruses, including EBV, in 50 cases of LCH.[116] Isolated LCH of the lung seems to be more common in active cigarette smokers than in nonsmokers; otherwise LCH has no known and consistent association with environmental factors.[112,117] Cigarette smoking may also be implicated in the high prevalence of pulmonary and extrapulmonary malignancies in patients with pulmonary LCH.[118] The alveolar macrophages of patients with pulmonary LCH have been shown to produce increased amounts of platelet-derived growth factor, which may lead to increased fibroblast replication and collagen production in LCH lesions.[119]

The most common site of presentation of unifocal unisystem disease is the bone, particularly the skull, femur, rib, mandible, vertebral body, or pelvis.[120–122] Pain and tender swelling are common symptoms, and the radiograph shows a sharply demarcated lytic lesion. Patients with isolated lymph node involvement (usually cervical or inguinal region) are typically afebrile and may have painful lymphadenopathy.[123] Patients with isolated lung involvement usually present with cough, dyspnea, chest pain, fever, hemoptysis, or weight loss. The chest radiograph varies from a diffuse pattern to a ''honeycomb lung'' appearance.[124] Some investigators suggest that isolated lung involvement by LCH may represent a peculiar reactive process and not a true neoplasm.[124,125] Other reported sites of isolated disease include lymph node, thymus, soft tissue, vulva, and spinal cord.[126,129]

Multifocal unisystem disease accounts for approximately 15 to 40 pencent of all cases of LCH.[109] Physical examination at presentation may reveal bony defects with exophthalmos (usually due to tumor infiltration of the orbital cavity and the orbital bones)[130] and loss of teeth (due to mandibular involvement and gum infiltration). The bones most often affected in this variant are the flat bones of the skull, ribs, pelvis, and scapula and, less frequently, long bones and the anterior portion of the vertebral bodies of the lumbrosacral vertebral bones.[131] Rarely, bones of the wrists, hands, knees, feet, or cervical vertebrae may be involved. Purulent external otitis media is common, due to involvement of the temporal bone. Diabetes insipidus affects 25 to 40 percent of patients who present with systemic disease and involvement of the skull.[121,132] The diabetes insipidus may worsen in patients with LCH who are pregnant.[133] Lymphadenopathy and skin rashes due to LCH have been reported to regress transiently during pregnancy.[134] Hypothalamic infiltration and pancreatic and thyroid tumor involvement may result in hyperprolactinemia and hypogonadism.[135]

Multifocal multisystem disease is the rarest (10 percent of all cases) and most severe form of LCH and generally involves the skin, lymph nodes, lung, and liver.[109] Symptoms include anorexia, failure to thrive, and pulmonary symptoms, such as cough, tachypnea, and pneumothorax. Chronic otitis media, lymphadenopathy, and hepatosplenomegaly are also common. Skin involvement usually manifests as a generalized erythematous or eczematoid rash affecting the scalp, ear canals, abdomen, intertriginous areas, and face.[136] Ulcerated and denuded skin may serve as a port of entry for microorganisms and may lead to sepsis. Laboratory abnormalities include anemia in the absence of iron deficiency or significant infection, leukopenia, neutropenia, or thrombocytopenia.

Langerhans cell histiocytosis may be diagnosed in lymph nodes draining the site of disease, in multisystem disease, in isolated disease (as a primary site), or, rarely, adjacent to a focus of malignant lymphoma. In general, the microscopic features do not allow distinction between the disseminated and localized forms of LCH. However, in lymph nodes that drain a site of bone (osteolymphatic) or skin (dermatolymphatic) disease, the affected lymph nodes are generally small and show focal LCH involvement of the sinuses. Lymph nodes may be slightly enlarged in those cases with superimposed dermatopathic changes, which are generally present in the paracortical areas. In the lymph node involvement of multisystem disease or of unifocal unisystem disease, the lymph node architecture is almost always intact. Partial or even complete effacement of architecture may be observed in advanced cases. In these cases, the Langerhans cell proliferation is seen in the sinusoids and often causes marked sinus distention, with extension into the perinodal tissues.

Despite the variation in the histologic appearance of LCH lesions, one always sees a sinusoidal proliferation of Langerhans cells in the appropriate cellular milieu (Fig. 11-5A). Langerhans cells are mononuclear cells, approximately 12 to 15 μm in diameter, with a moderate amount of eosinophilic cytoplasm. The nucleus of the Langerhans cell is characteristically folded, grooved, or lobulated and generally has small to inconspicuous nucleoli (Figure 11-5B). The nuclei appear cytologically benign, although slight cytologic atypia may be observed. The nuclear membrane is thin, and the chromatin is finely dispersed. Mitotic activity varies widely from lesion to lesion and ranges from 0 to 25 mitotic figures per 10 high power fields, with a

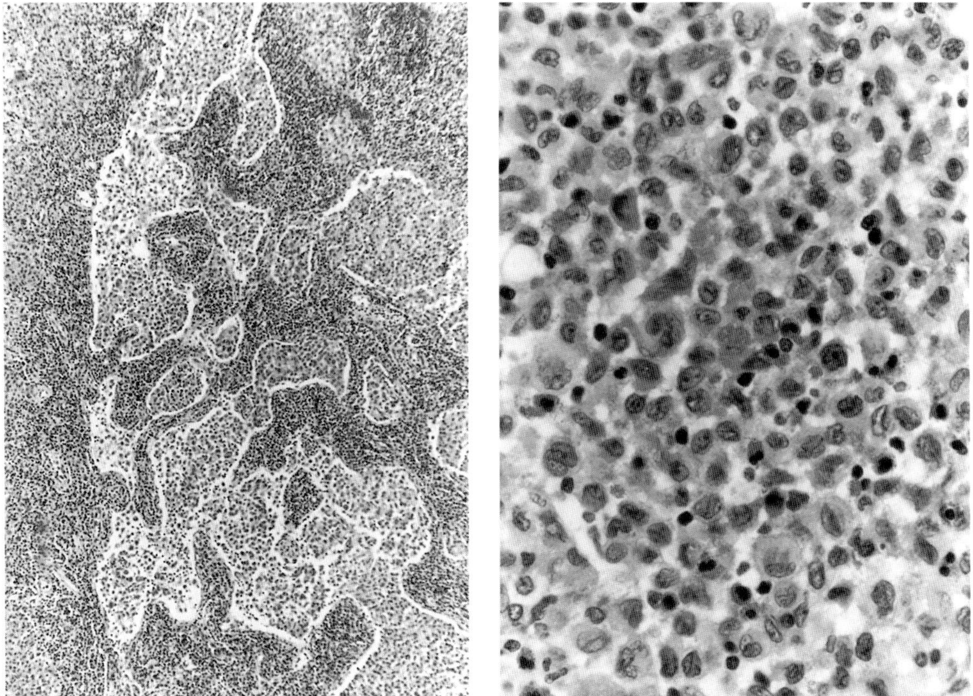

Fig. 11-5. Langerhans cell histiocytosis. **(A)** The lymph node sinuses are markedly distended. **(B)** A mixture of Langerhans cells, eosinophils, macrophages, lymphocytes, and giant cells is present. The Langerhans cells have the characteristic nuclear grooving and folding.

median of 2.[137] The typical cells of LCH are accompanied by varying numbers of reactive cells, including eosinophils, mononuclear and multinucleated histiocytes, neutrophils, and small lymphocytes; plasma cells are rare or absent. Clusters of eosinophils are typically accompanied by necrosis, forming so-called eosinophilic microabscesses. Areas of necrosis, eosinophils, and multinucleated histiocytes are typically more prevalent in bone lesions than in skin, lung, or lymph node specimens.[138] Early lesions usually contain large numbers of Langerhans cells and eosinophils.[138,139] As lesions age, they tend to have more histiocytes and fewer eosinophils. In very late lesions, fibrosis is markedly increased and the cellular composition may predominantly be foamy histiocytes, lymphocytes, and plasma cells, with only rare Langerhans cells.

The presence of a focus of LCH adjacent to a malignant lymphoma is rarely observed and may be seen in conjunction with either non-Hodgkin's lymphoma, Hodgkin's disease (Fig. 11-6), or leukemia (most typically acute nonlymphocytic leukemia).[123,140,141] In cases associated with non-Hodgkin's lymphoma, the LCH lesion is usually small, located adjacent to the lymphoma, and is not located in the sinusoids. The malignant lymphoma and LCH lesions are usually concurrent, but rarely LCH has subsequently developed at other sites in these patients.[141,142] In contrast, in cases of LCH associated with leukemia, the LCH typically precedes the diagnosis of malignancy.[141] LCH has also been described in association with a variety of solid tumors. One case of LCH with concurrence of viral-associated hemophagocytic syndrome has been reported.[143]

Neoplastic Langerhans cells have virtually the same ultrastructural features as their benign counterparts.[144] The cells have irregular plasma

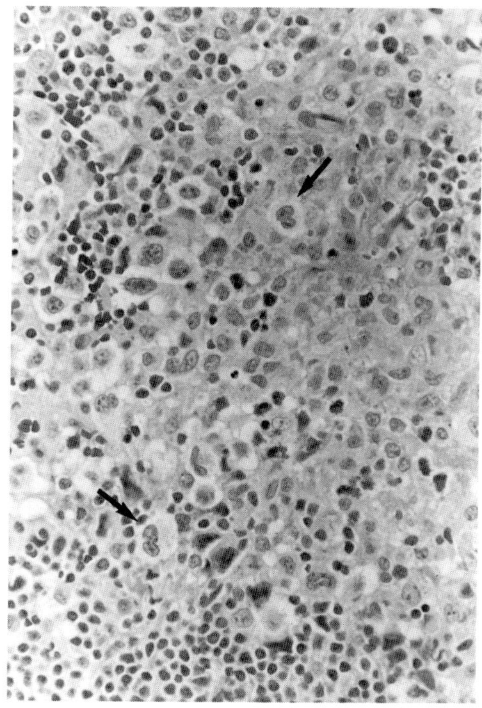

Fig. 11-6. Langerhans cell histiocytosis with Hodgkin's disease. Scattered lacunar cells (*arrows*) are interspersed in the proliferation of Langerhans cells.

membranes and lack cell junctions. The nuclei are irregularly shaped, and the cytoplasm contains a variable number of lysosomes. Birbeck granules, identical to those seen in benign Langerhans cells, can be identified in almost every neoplasm, but the percentage of cells containing the pathognomonic granules varies from case to case.[138,145,146] Some studies have reported a strong increase in the number of Birbeck granules in the cells of pulmonary LCH lesions compared with the bronchiolar Langerhans cells of normal people.[112]

The enzyme histochemical profile of the Langerhans cells of LCH also parallels that of benign Langerhans cells, although the neoplastic Langerhans cells may show greater cell-to-cell variation.[16] Similar to histiocytes and other dendritic cells, the neoplastic Langerhans cells exhibit activity for α-naphthyl acetate esterase (with variable inhibition by sodium fluoride), α-naphthyl butyrate esterase, acid phosphatase (not tartrate resistant), and adenosine triphosphatase.[16] The abnormal cells do not have 5′-nucleotidase, peroxidase, chloroacetate esterase, or β-glucuronidase. Compared with Langerhans cells from healthy patients, neoplastic Langerhans cells have decreased functional activity, as measured by allogeneic mixed cell reaction.[147]

Immunohistochemistry studies show an overlap between the antibody profiles of the Langerhans cells of neoplastic and reactive disorders. Paraffin section immunohistochemical studies of LCH show that neoplastic Langerhans cells virtually always express S100 protein and express vimentin, CD74, the Fc receptor, and HLA-DR in greater than 80 percent of cases.[19,148] Peanut agglutinin lectin also stains the proliferating cells of most cases.[142] Within a given LCH tumor, a variable fraction of neoplastic cells express CD68 and antiplacental alkaline phosphatase in a granular cytoplasmic pattern of variable intensity.[18,149] CD45 staining may also be observed after involved tissues have been subjected to heat-induced epitope retrieval methods.[150] The neoplastic Langerhans cells generally lack expression of CD45RA, CDw75, α_1-antitrypsin, epithelial membrane antigen, and CD15. However, CD15 reactivity may be observed after removal of sialic acid residues.[151] A minority of cells may also show immunoreactivity with lysozyme and α_1-antichymotrypsin.[149] Using paraffin or frozen section immunohistochemistry, Langerhans cells stain for CD1,[152] which is of great diagnostic utility as other histiocytic and dendritic cells lack this marker. Indeed, CD1 expression is limited to reactive and neoplastic Langerhans cells, immature thymocytes, and T-lineage lymphoblastic neoplasms. Neoplastic Langerhans cells also express CD4, CD11b (C3bi), CD11c, CD14, CD16, CD25, CDw32, CD71 (transferrin receptor), and HLA-A, -B, -C and -DR and do not express most B- and T-cell lineage markers.[147,153,154] Similar to paraffin section immunohistochemistry, the Langerhans cells in frozen section immunohistochemistry stain for CD45 and do not stain with antibodies to CD45RA or CD45RO.[16] The Langerhans cells of LCH, but not of reactive conditions, may show cytoplasmic CD2 and CD3.[19] Recently, the cells of LCH were shown to express adhesion molecules similar to those of cultured Langerhans cells and monocyte/macrophages.[155] The histiocytes, foamy histiocytes, and multinucleated cells often found in the lesions of LCH mark as ordinary non-neoplastic histiocytes and do not possess the antigenic characteristics of Langerhans cells.

By studying the patterns of X-chromosome inactivation in the X-linked human androgen receptor gene, researchers have demonstrated that LCH is a monoclonal proliferation.[156,157] These studies have included neoplastic tissues from female patients with unifocal, multifocal unisystem, or multifocal multisystem LCH. Molecular hybridization studies show a germline configuration for the immunoglobulin heavy chain and α, β, and γ T-cell receptor genes.[157,158] The cytogenetics of LCH has not yet been elucidated.

Rare cases of LCH may contain Langerhans cells with unequivocally malignant cytologic features and have been called *malignant histiocytosis X* or *malignant LCH*.[159] Reported cases show a male preponderance, a predilection for multisystem involvement, and a rapidly progressive clinical course.[159–161] Whether this phenomenon represents a distinct clinicopathologic entity or merely a variant of typical LCH is a subject of debate. Cases with malignant cytologic features that pursue a benign clinical course have also been described.[159]

The differential diagnosis of LCH is quite varied and depends on the site of involvement. Nodal involvement by LCH should be distinguished from other diseases that show a sinusoidal pattern of involvement, including reactive sinusoidal hyperplasia, SHML, metastatic neoplasms, and sinusoidal malignant lymphoma. The histiocytes of reactive sinusoidal hyperplasia do not have the distinctive cleaved nuclei that characterize the Langerhans cells of LCH; also the easily identified accompanying eosinophils of LCH are not usually present in benign sinusoidal hyperplasia. The proliferating cells of SHML also lack the folded nuclei of LCH and instead have round nuclei with a vesicular chromatin pattern and more prominent nucleoli. The larger quantity of cytoplasm, the phagocytosed cells and debris, the presence of abundant numbers of plasma cells, and the absence of eosinophils also help separate SHML from LCH, which generally lacks these morphologic features. Attention to the malignant morphologic features seen in metastatic malignancies and sinusoidal malignant lymphoma should help to avoid confusion with LCH. Dermatopathic lymphadenopathy may contain large numbers of Langerhans cells in the paracortical region and not the sinuses, as is the case in LCH. In dermatopathic lymphadenopathy, the proliferating cells are accompanied by numerous melanin-containing histiocytes and interdigitating reticulum cells.[162]

The multifaceted clinical presentations of LCH demand a unique approach to the therapy of each patient. Most clinicians advocate minimal therapy, unless critical structures are involved. Patients with unifocal unisystem or multifocal unisystem disease are generally treated with surgical curettage or resection, if possible.[163] Radiation therapy is generally reserved for residual disease, disease that recurs following curettage, lesions that increase in size, or in a critical site such as the orbit, mandible, or vertebral column. Radiation therapy is mandatory in patients who develop diabetes insipidus. Chemotherapy is usually reserved for multisystem disease. Both combination chemotherapy and single agent chemotherapy regimens have been employed.[164] Immunotherapy with thymic extracts and bone marrow transplantation remain experimental modalities.[163]

The clinical course of the disease is most greatly influenced by the number of affected organs at presentation, especially if involvement is accompanied by organ dysfunction.[18,165,166] The overall survival rate is greater than 95 percent in patients with unifocal unisystem disease, decreases to 75 percent when two organs are affected, and continues to decrease as the number of affected organs increases. The rate of progression of disease may also vary widely. In general, less than 10 percent of patients with unifocal unisystem disease undergo dissemination of disease. However, a unifocal unisystem lesion may rapidly progress to multisystem involvement, while cases of multisystem involvement have been rarely reported to undergo spontaneous regression.[167] Death, when it occurs, generally results from intercurrent infection or as a consequence of extensive marrow involvement.

Whether the patient's age also affects the clinical course and prognosis of LCH is a controversial observation. Some investigators believe that an age under 2 years and elderly ages are adverse prognostic variables,[165,168] while others believe that age has no effect independent of the pattern of organ involvement. Evaluation of histologic features does not generally help determine prognosis. Nuclear atypia and mitotic rate do not correlate with clinical outcome,[137] although nuclear atypia may be more prevalent in lesions from patients with multisystem involvement. The presence of eosinophils or lymphocytes was significantly associated with a more favorable outcome in one study.[149] Proliferating cell nuclear antigen staining of the tumor cells also may correlate with the clinical course.[136] Favorable response to initial chemotherapy has been shown to be associated with improved survival and overall disease control.[165,168]

Dendritic and Indeterminate Cell Neoplasms

These rare tumors exhibit differentiation consistent with follicular dendritic cell, interdigitating dendritic cell, or indeterminate cell lineage.

Follicular Dendritic Cell Sarcoma

The follicular dendritic sarcoma, also known as *follicular dendritic cell tumor* and *dendritic reticulum cell tumor/sarcoma,* is a neoplasm with similar morphologic and immunologic features to non-neoplastic dendritic reticulum cells, which normally reside in germinal centers.

This tumor is extremely rare and occurs with nearly equal sex predilection predominantly in adults.[25,169–175] Painless cervical lymphadenopathy is typical, although axillary presentation has also been reported. Subsequent enlargement of other lymph node sites has been reported, without biopsy confirmation of recurrent malignancy. Extranodal sites of occurrence include the soft palate, tonsil, small intestine, and retroperitoneal soft tissue.[173,175] One case has been reported as a complication of the hyaline-vascular type of Castleman's disease.[172]

The lymph node architecture may be partially effaced, with a sharp boundary between the neoplasm and residual lymphoid tissue. Complete replacement of the lymph node by the neoplastic process may also be seen. One generally sees a proliferation of oval to spindled cells that forms fascicles, nests, or a storiform pattern. Occasionally, a whorled growth pattern is observed, similar to the pattern commonly seen in meningiomas (Fig. 11-7A). The individual neoplastic cells are uniform and possess oval nuclei with a relatively bland, vesicular chromatin pattern (Fig. 11-7B). Pseudonuclear inclusions may be present, and nucleoli are not prominent. Multinucleated malignant cells may be seen. The mitotic rate is low. The cytoplasm is pale to slightly eosinophilic, and the cytoplasmic borders are not distinct. Small lymphocytes are usually found within the lesion, either as single cells or clusters, within perivascular spaces. Occasionally, germinal centers are seen between fascicles of the tumor. Necrosis is not a feature of this tumor.

Ultrastructurally, one sees spindled cells with long, slender cytoplasmic processes connected with each other through numerous desmosomes (mostly of the macula adherens type). Lysosomes are usually few in number. Other organelles, such as tonofilaments, Birbeck granules, dense-core secretory granules, basal lamina, and melanosomes, are usually not seen.

Enzyme histochemical studies have been reported for one case of follicular dendritic cell sarcoma. The tumor cells were reactive for acid phosphatase (almost completely inhibited by tartrate), nonspecific esterase (completely inhibited

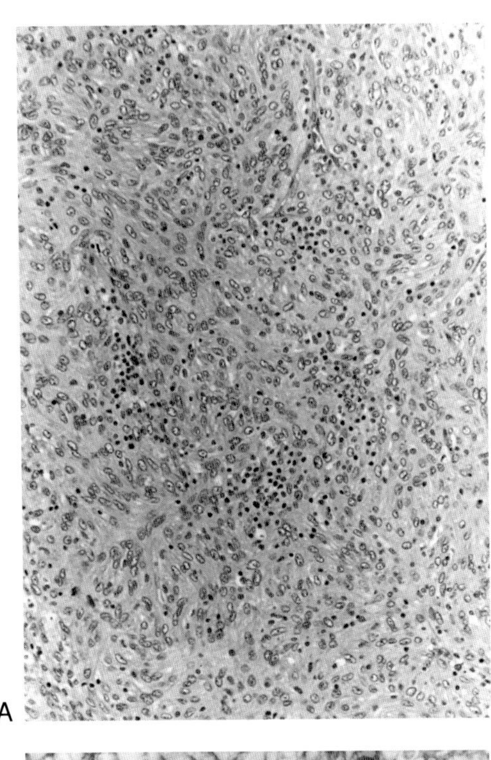

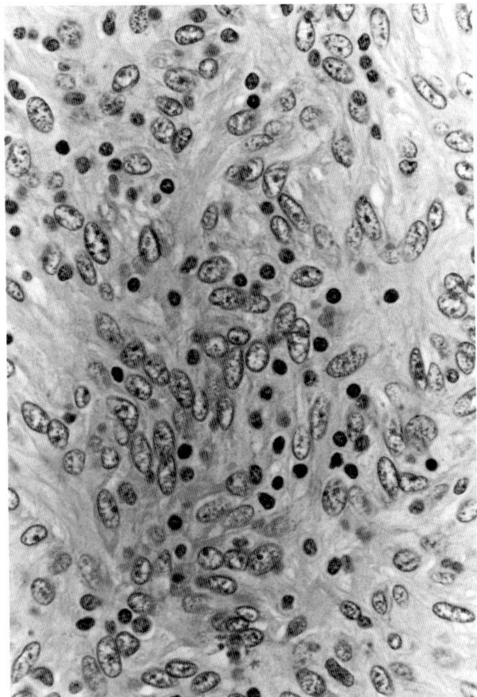

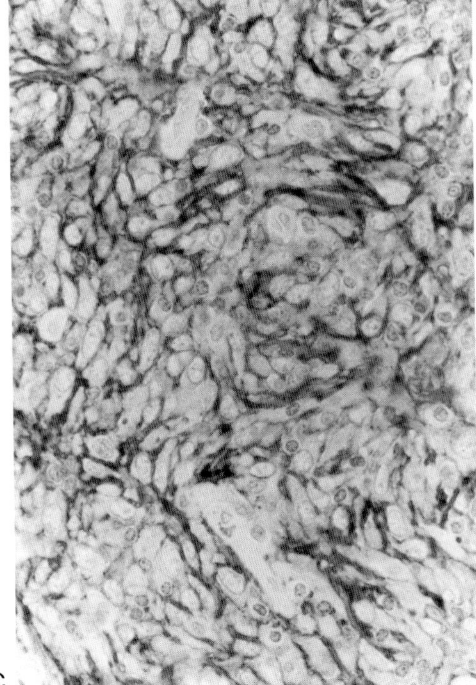

Fig. 11-7. Follicular dendritic cell sarcoma. **(A)** The spindled tumor cells exhibit a whorled growth pattern. **(B)** Tumor cells with bland nuclear features are intermixed with lymphocytes; **(C)** Antibody to CD21 highlights the dendritic meshwork of the tumor.

by fluoride), alkaline phosphatase, and 5′-nucleotidase.[25]

The immunophenotype of a follicular dendritic cell sarcoma closely parallels that of normal follicular dendritic cells. In paraffin sections, the neoplastic cells usually show equivocal or no staining for CD45 and may or may not express S100 protein.[25,169,170,175] The neoplastic cells almost always stain for CD35 (C3b complement receptor) and CD68, and the cells also almost always stain with monoclonal antibodies specific for dendritic reticulum cells, such as Ki-M4 and R4/23 (Fig. 11-7C).[25] Two extranodal cases showed aberrant epithelial membrane antigen staining.[175] In frozen sections, the cells stain for multiple macrophage markers, CD35 and CD21 (C3d receptor), HLA-DR, and the lymphocyte adhesion markers CD11a and CD18. The cells may also express one or more B-cell lineage markers, similar to normal follicular dendritic cells. CD1, which is expressed in Langerhans cells and immature T cells, is always negative, as are specific T-cell lineage antigens, keratin, desmin, or the melanocyte-associated antigen HMB-45.

Molecular study of two cases showed a germline configuration for both the immunoglobulin heavy chain gene and the β- and T-cell receptor gene.[170]

The differential diagnosis includes all spindled lesions that may occur in the lymph node. Nonhematopoietic malignancies may be excluded from the differential diagnosis by noting the malignant cytologic characteristics of such entities. Immunohistochemical studies may be necessary. Also in the differential diagnosis is the palisaded myofibroblastoma, also known as intranodal hemorrhagic spindle cell tumor with amianthoid fibers. This entity almost always occurs in an inguinal lymph node and is less cellular than follicular dendritic cell sarcoma. The former entity also lacks staining with dendritic reticulum cell markers. Lymphoma only very rarely appears spindled; immunohistochemical studies are very useful for identification of these cases. Thymoma and follicular dendritic cell sarcoma share morphologic features, such as the presence of numerous lymphocytes in perivascular spaces. The keratin immunohistochemical stain is useful, as thymomas are keratin positive and follicular dendritic cell sarcomas are not. Different immunohistochemical profiles separate follicular dendritic cell sarcoma, interdigitating dendritic cell sarcoma, and indeterminate cell tumor from one another. All three tumors have immunohistochemical staining patterns similar to those of their normal cell counterparts. In addition, ultrastructural studies of follicular dendritic cell sarcomas show well-formed desmosomes, which are not seen in the other dendritic neoplasms. The clinical relevance of these distinctions has yet to be shown conclusively.

Because most cases of follicular dendritic cell sarcoma present with localized disease, local excision is usually adequate. Chemotherapy or radiotherapy appears to offer no survival advantages over initial or repeat surgical excision.[170] Local recurrence may occur and may be at multiple sites. Recurrence appears to be independent of the type of therapy received. The one reported death due to this neoplasm followed several local recurrences.

Interdigitating Dendritic Cell Sarcoma

An interdigitating dendritic cell sarcoma is a neoplasm with lineage consistent with non-neoplastic interdigitating dendritic cells, which normally reside in the paracortical areas of a lymph node. It is also known as interdigitating dendritic cell tumor and interdigitating reticulum cell tumor/sarcoma.

The literature contains reports of approximately two dozen cases of this extremely rare tumor.[170,176–188] Four cases originally reported as follicular dendritic cell sarcoma are now considered more likely to be interdigitating dendritic cell sarcoma.[176] Well-documented cases report occurrence in teen-aged children and adults of both sexes. Solitary lymph node involvement at presentation is common, although presentation in extranodal sites such as the small intestine have been reported. A previous history of malignant lymphoma has been reported in two patients.[186] Systemic symptoms such as fatigue, fever, and night sweats may be present. Approximately one-half of cases present with disseminated disease, with involvement of numerous organs, including spleen, bone marrow, skin, liver, kidney, and lung.

The histologic features of interdigitating dendritic cell sarcoma are quite varied and may overlap with those of both malignant lymphoma and the follicular dendritic cell sarcoma. By light microscopy, some cases may appear identical to cases of follicular dendritic cell sarcoma. The neoplastic cells may have large round nuclei, with focal spindling (Fig. 11-8). Delicate nuclear folds and rare intranuclear cytoplasmic invaginations have been reported. Occasional nuclear grooves were described in another case. Some cases resemble pleomorphic large cell lymphoma with convoluted nuclei. One reported case showed a spindled neoplasm in the initial biopsy and a more pleomorphic and less spindled neoplasm in a recurrence.[170]

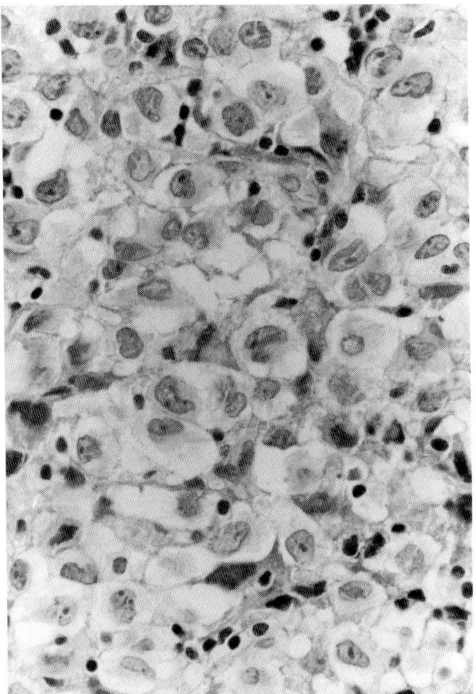

Fig. 11-8. Interdigitating dendritic cell sarcoma. The tumor cells grow in sheets. Occasional nuclear grooves are seen.

Ultrastructural features of the neoplastic cells and normal interdigitating cells are similar.[179,181,182,187] The neoplastic cells have elongated and complex cell processes, but, unlike follicular dendritic cell sarcomas, well-formed desmosomes are not present. Basal lamina, tonofilaments, Birbeck granules, dense-core secretory granules, and melanosomes are usually not seen.

The majority of studied cases express positivity for adenosine triphosphatase, α-naphthyl esterase, acid phosphatase, and 5′-nucleotidase.[175,177,179,181,182] No reaction is seen with alkaline phosphatase, peroxidase, β-glucuronidase, and chloroacetate esterase.

The diagnosis of interdigitating dendritic cell sarcoma rests on immunohistochemical studies. The neoplastic cells have an immunophenotype similar to normal interdigitating dendritic cells. In paraffin sections, the cells stain with antibodies to CD45, S100, and CD68.[170] In frozen sections, the cells stain for multiple macrophage markers and the lymphocyte adhesion markers CD11a and CD18. One generally sees no expression of CD1, complement receptor antigens, B-cell lineage antigens, specific T-cell lineage antigens, specific follicular dendritic cell antigens, keratin, desmin, or the melanocyte antigen HMB-45.

In the rare cases analyzed by molecular methods, germline configurations for both the immunoglobulin heavy chain gene and the β T-cell receptor gene have been found.[182]

The differential diagnosis of interdigitating dendritic cell sarcoma overlaps with the differential diagnosis for follicular dendritic cell sarcoma. Absence of desmosomes on ultrastructural examination and the absence of reactivity with monoclonal antibodies against complement receptors and the KiM4 and R4/23 antigens distinguishes interdigitating dendritic cell sarcoma from follicular dendritic cell sarcoma, which contains desmosomes and are reactive to those antibodies.

Patients with interdigitating dendritic cell sarcoma have been treated with local excision, usually with adjuvant radiotherapy and/or chemotherapy. One patient underwent bone marrow transplantation. Local recurrence may also occur. Approximately one-half of patients die of their disease, generally within 1 year of diagnosis. Prognosis appears to have no good correlation with any clinical, histologic, or treatment variables.

Indeterminate Cell Tumors (Precursor Langerhans Cell Histiocytosis)

An indeterminate cell tumor is a neoplasm that shows differentiation toward indeterminate cells, which are normal cells that are morphologically and immunologically similar to Langerhans cells, but without the characteristic Birbeck granules.[189,190]

Only rare cases of indeterminate cell tumors exist in the literature.[190–196] One case was originally reported as an interdigitating reticulum cell sarcoma.[196] The large majority of indeterminate cell tumors have been reported in adults. Patients typically present with one or multiple skin nodules, although one patient presented with lymph node involvement and others presented with disseminated disease in multiple organs. Three patients had an antecedent history of B-cell neoplasms (one with chronic lymphocytic leukemia, two with low grade follicular lymphoma), with the time intervals between diagnoses ranging from 4 months to 9 years. One patient had synchronous development of chronic lymphocytic leukemia. Another patient had previously diagnosed mast cell leukemia.

Indeterminate cell tumors morphologically appear very similar to LCH. In rare cases of lymph node involvement, the neoplastic process partially replaces the node and may invade angiolymphatic spaces. The tumor cells, which are arranged in a vaguely storiform pattern, have medium to large oval nuclei that may have irregular nuclear outlines, prominent eosinophilic nucleoli, and abundant clear to pink cytoplasm (Fig. 11-9). In the skin, the proliferating histiocytes also appear virtually identical to those seen in LCH and may show atypical cytologic features similar to those described in the malignant variant of LCH. The cytoplasm is abundant and

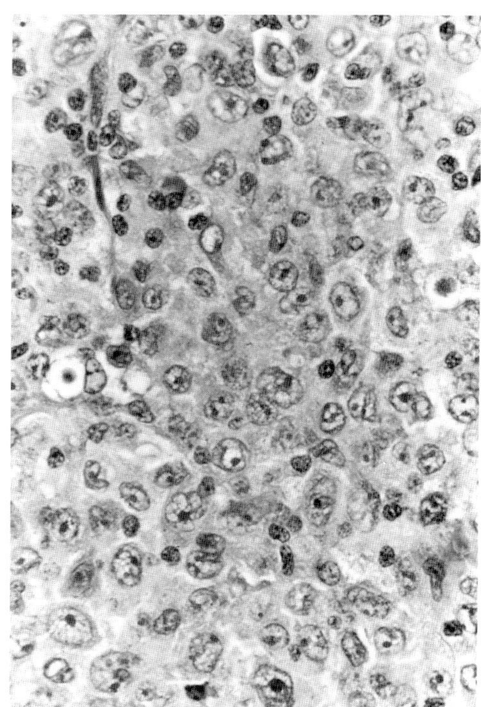

Fig. 11-9. Indeterminate cell tumor. The tumor cells have large vesicular nuclei. The diagnosis requires comprehensive immunologic study, because the morphologic features are not distinctive.

pale to eosinophilic. Multinucleated and foam cells may be present.

The ultrastructural characteristics of cells of an indeterminate cell tumor are nearly identical to those of Langerhans cells, with the important exception that Birbeck granules cannot be seen.

The neoplastic cells show cytochemical activity for adenosine triphosphatase, acid phosphatase (not tartrate resistant), and nonspecific esterase and lack alkaline phosphatase, 5′-nucleotidase, peroxidase, chloroacetate esterase, β-glucuronidase, and dipeptidyl-amino peptidase reactivity. This cytochemical profile parallels that of normal Langerhans cells and indeterminate cells.[195]

Immunohistochemically, one sees identical staining patterns to that of normal Langerhans cells and indeterminate cells. The neoplastic cells stain for S100 protein, CD1, CD45, macrophage markers, and lack of reactivity for specific

B- and T-cell-associated antigens.[189] To date, no published case has been studied by molecular techniques.

Ultrastructural and immunohistochemical studies are necessary to establish a diagnosis of indeterminate cell tumor. Absence of Birbeck granules may be the feature that distinguishes an indeterminate cell tumor from an LCH lesion. Indeterminate cell tumor CD1 expression is the most helpful antibody to differentiate indeterminate cell tumor from follicular and interdigitating dendritic cell tumors, which lack this antigen.

Most of the reported patients have been treated with chemotherapy, with varying results. One patient who presented with an isolated skin lesion was in remission after excisional biopsy alone. The clinical course appears variable. One patient who presented with systemic disease subsequently died of tumor, while another patient developed acute monocytic leukemia. One patient with multiple skin lesions had a progressive course terminating in death. One patient with a skin lesion developed metastasis to a regional lymph node. All other reported patients were free of disease at last follow-up.

MALIGNANT HISTIOCYTIC PROLIFERATIONS

True Histiocytic Lymphoma and Malignant Histiocytosis

Malignant histiocytosis (MH) and true histiocytic lymphoma (THL) are rare neoplasms in which the malignant cells demonstrate differentiation along histiocytic lineage. In lymph nodes, the term MH generally applies when the malignant cells are mostly confined to the sinusoids, and the term THL is usually reserved for cases in which the malignant proliferation effaces the existing lymph node architecture. We prefer to apply the term THL for all these neoplasms because the term MH has been greatly abused in the past.

Historically, the term MH was applied to a variety of different malignancies because of their morphologic and cytochemical similarities to histiocytes. In the past decade, several groups have reported that the majority of cases of MH studied in earlier reports were actually lymphoid in origin.[197–200] In the 1970s, Isaacson and colleagues[201,202] described cases of primary small intestinal neoplasms that were called *MH of the small intestine* because they were thought to arise from the histiocytic cells of the small bowel; they presented with systemic involvement and were associated with celiac disease. Nearly a decade later, the same investigators, as well as others, demonstrated by immunophenotypic and genotypic studies that these tumors were in fact T-cell lymphomas.[203,204] Fifteen cases reported as MH in 1975, on the basis of morphology, were re-evaluated by paraffin section immunohistochemistry 14 years later.[205] Eight cases were reclassified as CD30-positive anaplastic large cell lymphoma (including six T-lineage and two null phenotype), three cases were reclassified as T-cell lymphoma, two cases were reclassified as B-cell lymphoma, one case was reclassified as lymphoma of uncertain lineage, and one case was reclassified as most consistent with the infection-associated viral hemophagocytic syndrome. None of the 15 cases had malignant cells that expressed CD68. Another study found that tumors classified in the past as MH in children were more likely to be CD30-positive anaplastic large cell lymphoma of T-cell lineage.[197] An additional retrospective study of nine patients initially diagnosed with MH yielded only one patient to be reclassified as a possible histiocytic malignancy after an evaluation with immunohistochemical antibodies.[206]

With the emergence of more sophisticated study techniques, criteria for the diagnosis of THL have expanded to require immunohistochemical evidence of histiocytic lineage, accompanied by absence of specific T- and B-lineage markers and molecular evidence of a germline configuration for the T-cell receptor and immunoglobulin genes. Other more recently reported cases of putative THL are excluded from this strict definition of THL because of the presence of immunohistochemical evidence of T lineage,[207] CD30 expression,[197,208–210] gene rearrangements of the T-cell receptor, or heavy or light chain immunoglobulins.[208,210,211]

Using the strict immunologic and molecular criteria delineated previously, only rare cases of bona fide MH/THL have been reported.[210,212–215] The true incidence of this neoplasm is not known. However, two recent studies suggest that THL accounts for approximately 0.5 percent of all hematolymphoid neoplasms.[213,216,217] The etiology of the disease is not known.

The clinical features of the neoplasms are not well defined because most of the large clinicopathologic studies of THL were based on cases diagnosed almost solely on histologic features, because they were published prior to the availability of more recent methodologies, such as modern immunohistochemistry and molecular pathology.[218,219] In addition to lacking current technologies, these studies did not always distinguish between lymphoid malignancies that contained numerous reactive histiocytes and neoplasms in which the histiocytes themselves were considered the malignant cells. The recent more vigorous studies show that THL occurs in all age groups, although adults are more commonly affected than children. There is no gender predilection. Common sites of involvement at presentation include lymph node and skin; involvement of spleen, small intestine, lung, and bone marrow has also been reported.[220] Patients generally present with fever, fatigue, and weakness and may have weight loss, lymphadenopathy, skin lesions, or splenomegaly. Laboratory tests are generally normal, with rare reports of leukopenia and thrombocytopenia.

Involved lymph nodes may be partially (patchy, paracortical, or sinusoidal) or completely replaced by the malignant process. Typically, the neoplasm is composed of a proliferation of cytologically malignant cells that resemble histiocytes. The malignant cells vary in size and have abundant eosinophilic cytoplasm (occasionally foamy or vacuolated) and a large, eccentrically placed, bean-shaped nucleus with a prominent irregular nucleolus (Fig. 11-10). The nucleus may appear grooved. Multinucleated tumor cells with bizarre nuclei and multiple nucleoli, and hemophagocytosis by tumor cells, may also be present. Mitotic activity is usually high. In some cases of THL, the constituent cells may show only a slight degree of nuclear enlargement and irregular distribution of chromatin. In these instances, mitotic figures are rare or absent. In summary, no morphologic features help to distinguish the cells of THL from other malignant cells; thus, immunophenotypic and molecular studies are essential.

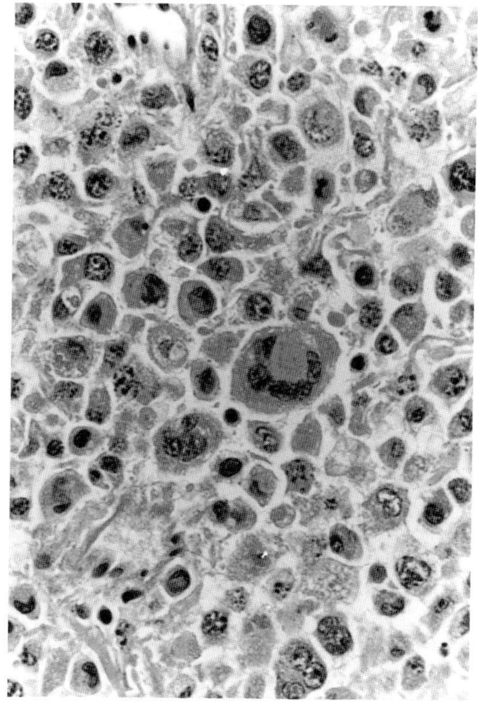

Fig. 11-10. True histiocytic lymphoma. The tumor cells have pleomorphic nuclei and abundant eosinophilic cytoplasm. (Courtesy of John K. C. Chan, M.D., Hong Kong.)

Virtually all cytochemical and ultrastructural studies of THL were performed on tissues designated MH or THL based solely on morphology. A recent study shows that the tumor cells lack neutrophilic elastase, myeloperoxidase, and chloroacetate esterase.[213]

By paraffin section immunohistochemistry, the tumor cells of THL should express CD68.[210,213,220] Also, they may stain with CD15, CD43, CD45, CD45RO, or lysozyme.[214,215] Some investigators advocate the presence of two or more monocyte/macrophage-lineage antibodies as minimum positive evidence for histiocytic lineage. The malignant cells generally lack S100 and CD30 antigens, and the tumor cells also should not stain with any of the antikeratin antibodies or HMB45. Frozen section immunohistochemical studies should show reactivity of the MH/THL cells with CD45, HLA-DR, CD14, CD11c, CD13, CD33, and CD68.[210] CD33 and CD35 expression has been reported in rare cases. Cytoplasmic (and not membrane) expression of CD4 has been reported in the majority of cases of THL. In contrast to the membrane CD4 expression of helper T cells, cytoplasmic CD4 expression has been demonstrated in cells of monocyte/macrophage lineage.[221] In addition to confirming the histiocytic lineage of a neoplasm, immunohistochemistry should be used to exclude the diagnosis of non-Hodgkin's lymphomas or nonhematolymphoid neoplasms from the list of diagnostic possibilities.

Paraffin and frozen section immunophenotyping studies may not clearly favor a histiocyte or lymphocyte lineage. Thus, one may need to resort to gene rearrangement studies. Theoretically, cases of THL should have germline configuration for T-cell receptor and immunoglobulin genes. In the recent past, many cases that had morphologic features of malignant histiocytes and that showed immunohistochemical evidence of histiocytic lineage in the absence of staining with B- or T-cell markers, were reported to have clonal T-cell receptor or immunoglobulin gene rearrangements.[177,200,210,222,223] In these instances, clonal rearrangements of the T-cell receptor genes appeared to be equally as common as clonal immunoglobulin gene rearrangements.[223] Many investigators favor the possibility that cases with some phenotypic evidence of histiocytic differentiation should still be regarded as histiocyte derived, regardless of the presence of T-cell receptor or immunoglobulin gene rearrangements.[210] However, as stated above, the authors think that until more data are available in this confused area, one would be prudent to limit making the diagnosis of THL to cases in which the phenotypic evidence clearly supports a histiocytic lineage, accompanied by absence of specific T- and B-lineage markers and a germline configuration for the T-cell receptor and immunoglobulin genes.[224–227]

The 5q35 breakpoint abnormality, a common finding in cases of anaplastic large cell lymphoma, was reported in the earlier literature in cases of MH/THL.[228–230] However, the cases used for study were assessed by morphology only and were most likely misdiagnosed cases of anaplastic large cell lymphoma. A high incidence of 17p13 chromosomal abnormalities in cases of MH was reported in 1988.[231] This finding has not been confirmed in cases of THL diagnosed by the rigorous criteria set forth above.

Entities that may be clinically and histologically confused with THL include anaplastic large cell lymphoma (often of T-lineage and expressing CD30), B-cell sinusoidal large cell lymphoma, anaplastic carcinomas exhibiting hemophagocytosis, malignant lymphomas associated with benign erythrophagocytosis, follicular dendritic cell neoplasms, hepatosplenic T-cell lymphoma, infection-associated hemophagocytic syndrome, storage disease such as Gaucher's disease and Niemann-Pick disease, and familial hemophagocytic lymphohistiocytosis. By adhering to the strict histologic, phenotypic, and molecular criteria outlined above, along with clinical presentation, one may separate THL from the other malignancies listed above.[58,91,232,233]

Most patients have been treated with multiagent chemotherapy, with poor results. The majority of patients die of their disease in a short time, ranging from weeks to 3 years after their diagnosis.[213,215] Rare patients with resectable disease, treated with surgery alone, have been reported to be free of disease, with follow-up times ranging from 13 to 92 months. One patient was reported to be alive with disease, having had her third recurrence 120 months following initial diagnosis. One patient underwent bone marrow transplantation 7 months after diagnosis and had recurrence of disease 2 months following transplant.

Malignant Histiocytosis Associated with Mediastinal Germ Cell Tumor

A relatively frequent association between hematologic malignancies and mediastinal germ cell tumors has been reported.[234,235] The majority of the reports describe nonseminomatous mediastinal germ cell tumors occurring predominantly in young men, in conjunction with hematologic disorders.[234–237] Approximately one-half of the hematologic malignancies have been characterized as MH, usually associated with a malignant teratoma, with or without yolk sac tumor differentiation. The rest of the hematologic disorders include acute nonlymphocytic leukemia and, less often, acute lymphoblastic leukemia and myeloproliferative disorders. Other unexplained hematologic abnormalities, such as refractory thrombocytopenia, have been described.[235] The hematopoietic malignancies have been hypothesized to be a consequence of multipotential differentiation of malignant germ cells, since teratocarcinoma cells are capable of differentiation along hematopoietic lines under the proper in vitro conditions.[234] The cases reported as MH have generally not been rigorously investigated to confirm their histiocytic nature.

Intravascular Histiocytosis

Intravascular lymphomatosis is a rare entity that is characterized by a proliferation of lymphoma cells within blood vessels.[238] The malignancy generally involves the blood vessels of the central nervous system and the skin but in the terminal stages of the disease may involve the lymph nodes, bone marrow, spleen, and liver. A rare variant of intravascular lymphomatosis is intravascular histiocytosis in which the proliferation of cells are morphologically and immunologically consistent with histiocyte origin.[239]

Histiocytic Medullary Reticulosis

Histiocytic medullary reticulosis was the term used by Scott and Robb-Smith[240] in 1939 for a clinicopathologic entity characterized by fever, weight loss, skin rash, hepatosplenomegaly, lymphadenopathy, and anemia with leukopenia. They described a systemic proliferation of histiocytes that showed erythrophagocytosis associated with Reed-Sternberg-like cells.[240] In 1990, Falini and colleagues[70] reported eight cases diagnosed by Professor Robb-Smith by morphology alone during the period from 1949 to 1965 and restudied with the addition of modern techniques. Their retrospective analysis suggested that the entity known as *histiocytic medullary reticulosis* included a myriad of current entities, including anaplastic large cell lymphoma, THL, T-cell lymphoma with hemophagocytic syndrome, disseminated LCH, Lennert's lymphoma, Hodgkin's disease, viral-associated hemophagocytic syndrome, and hyperimmune reaction. The term *histiocytic medullary reticulosis* should be confined to discussions of historical relevance and not be used as a designation for current diseases.

Regressing Atypical Histiocytosis

Regressing atypical histiocytosis is a cutaneous proliferation of cells that histologically resemble histiocytes. The disorder shares many clinical, morphologic, immunologic, and genotypic features with lymphomatoid papulosis and cutaneous CD30-positive anaplastic large cell lymphoma (Fig. 11-11). Several groups have suggested that these three entities most likely represent a spectrum of one disease entity, with the histologic and clinical characteristics determined by either the degree of biologic aggressiveness of the individual neoplasm or the strength of the host immune defenses.[241–243] Clonal rearrangements of the β T-cell receptor gene have been found in regressing atypical histiocytosis and lymphomatoid papulosis.[243] Thus, regressing atypical histiocytosis may be more appropriately regarded as a lymphoproliferative

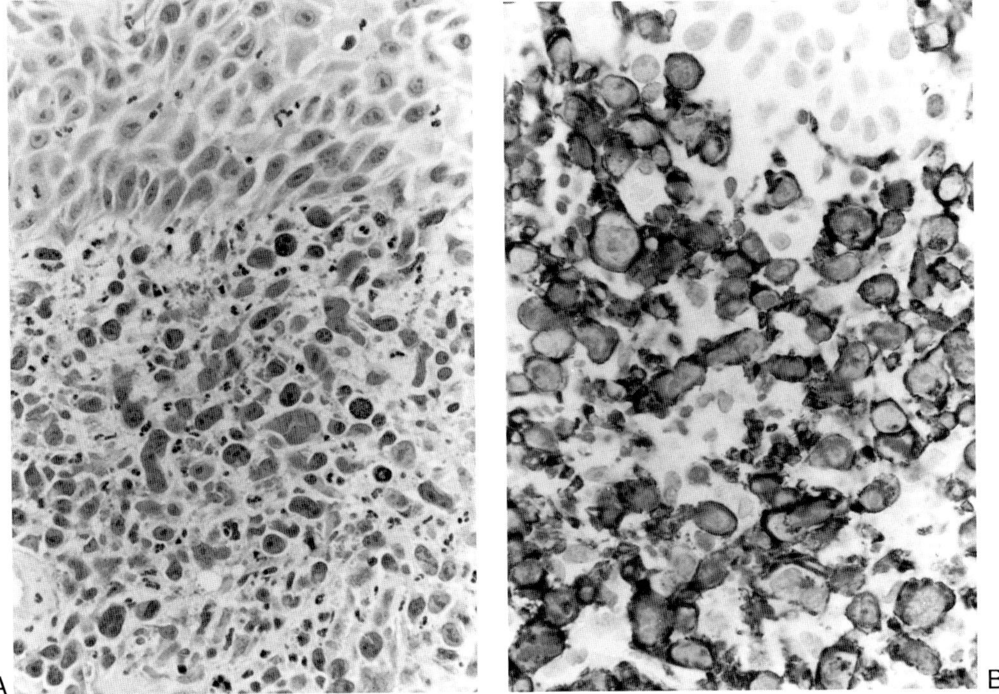

Fig. 11-11. Anaplastic large cell lymphoma of skin. **(A)** The large tumor cells under the epidermis superficially resemble histiocytes, hence its old name "regressing atypical histiocytosis." **(B)** The CD30 positivity and clinicopathologic picture are those of anaplastic large cell lymphoma.

disorder of T lymphocytes rather than a true histiocytic lesion.[242,243] Many investigators advocate abandonment of the term *regressing atypical histiocytosis* because of its pathobiologic and clinical overlap with lymphomatoid papulosis and because of its descriptive inaccuracy.[244]

REFERENCES

1. Foucar K, Foucar E: The mononuclear phagocyte and immunoregulatory effector (M-PIRE) system: evolving concepts. Semin Diagn Pathol 7:4, 1990
2. Cline MJ: Histiocytes and histiocytosis. Blood 84:2840, 1994
3. Clark SC, Kamen R: The human hematopoietic colony stimulating factors. Science 236:1229, 1987
4. Franklin WA, Mason DY, Pulford K et al: Immunohistological analysis of human mononuclear phagocytes and dendritic cells by using monoclonal antibodies. Lab Invest 54:322, 1986
5. Roholl PJM, Kleyne J, Prins MEF et al: Immunologic marker analysis of normal and malignant histiocytes. A comparative study of monoclonal antibodies for diagnostic purposes. Am J Clin Pathol 89:187, 1988
6. Steinman R: The dendritic cell system and its role in immunogenicity. Annu Rev Immunol 9: 271, 1991
7. Reid CDL, Fryer PR, Clifford C et al: Identification of hematopoietic progenitors of macrophages and dendritic Langerhans cells (DL-CFU) in human bone marrow and peripheral blood. Blood 76:1139, 1990
8. Nossal GJV, Abbot A, Mitchell J, Lummus Z: Antigens in immunity. XV. Ultrastructural features of antigen capture in primary and secondary follicles. J Exp Med 127:277, 1968
9. Gerdes J, Stein H, Mason DY, Ziegler A: Human dendritic reticulum cells of lymphoid follicles: their antigenic profile and their identification as multinucleated giant cells. Virchows Arch [Cell Pathol] 42:161, 1983
10. Reis e Sousa C, Stahl PD, Austyn JM: Phagocy-

tosis of antigens by Langerhans cells in vitro. J Exp Med 178:509, 1993
11. Caux C, Dezutter-Dambuyant C, Schmitt D, Bachereau J: GM-CSF and TNF-α cooperate in the generation of dendritic Langerhans cells. Nature 360:258, 1992
12. Thomas R, Davis LS, Lipsky PE: Isolation and characterization of human peripheral blood dendritic cells. J Immunol 150:821, 1993
13. Zhou L-J, Schwarting R, Smith HM, Tedder TF: A novel cell-surface molecule expressed by human interdigitating reticulum cells, Langerhans cells, and activated lymphocytes is a new member of the immunoglobulin superfamily. J Immunol 149:735, 1992
14. Murphy GF, Messadi D, Fonferko I, Hancock WW: Phenotypic transformation of macrophages to Langerhans cells in the skin. Am J Pathol 123:401, 1986
15. Birbeck NS, Breathnach AS, Everall JD: An electron microscopic study of basal melanocytes and high-level clear cell (Langerhans' cell) in vitiligo. J Invest Dermatol 37:51, 1961
16. Beckstead JH, Wood GS, Turner RR: Histiocytosis X cells and Langerhans cells: enzyme histochemical and immunologic similarities. Hum Pathol 15:826, 1984
17. Wood GS, Turner RR, Shiurba RA et al: In situ immunophenotypic definition of subsets that exhibit specific morphologic and microenvironmental characteristics. Am J Pathol 119:73, 1985
18. Hage C, Willman CL, Favara BE, Isaacson PG: Langerhans' cell histiocytosis (histiocytosis X): immunophenotype and growth fraction. Hum Pathol 24:840, 1993
19. O'Doherty U, Steinman RM, Peng M et al: Dendritic cells freshly isolated from human blood express CD4 and mature into typical immunostimulatory dendritic cells after culture in monocyte-conditioned medium. J Exp Med 178:1067, 1993
20. Hoefsmit EChM, Cuyvestijn AM, Kamperdijk EW A: Relation between Langerhans cells, veiled cells, and *interdigitation* cells. Immunobiology 161:255, 1982
21. Lennert K: Malignant lymphomas, other than Hodgkin's disease. In: Handbuch der speziellen pathologischen Anatomie und Histologies 1/3/ B. Springer-Verlag, Berlin, 1978
22. van der Valk P, van der Loo EM, Jansen J et al: Analysis of lymphoid and dendritic cells in human lymph node, tonsil and spleen. A study using monoclonal and heterologous antibodies. Virchows Arch [Cell Pathol] 45:169, 1984
23. Orscheschek K, Merz H, Schlegelberger B, Feller AC: An immortalized cell line with features of human follicular dendritic cells. Antigen and cytokine expression analysis. Eur J Immunol 24:2682, 1994
24. Donaldson SL, Kosco MH, Szakal AK, Tew JB: Localization of antibody-forming cells in draining lymphoid organs during long-term maintenance of the antibody response. J Leuk Biol 40: 147, 1986
25. Pallesen G, Myhre-Jensen O: Immunophenotypic analysis of neoplastic cells in follicular dendritic cell sarcoma. Leukemia 1:549, 1987
26. Schriever F, Freedman AS, Freeman G et al: Follicular dendritic cells display a unique antigenic phenotype. J Exp Med 169:2043, 1989
27. Petrasch S, Perez-Alvarez C, Schmitz J et al: Antigenic phenotyping of human follicular dendritic cells isolated from non-malignant and malignant lymphatic tissue. Eur J Immunol 20: 1013, 1990
28. Naiem N, Gerdes J, Abdulaziz A et al: Production of a monoclonal antibody reactive with human dendritic cells and its use in the immunohistological analysis of lymphoid tissue. J Clin Pathol 36:167, 1983
29. Parwaresch MR, Radzun HJ, Hansmann M-L, Peters K-P: Monoclonal antibody Ki-M4 specifically recognizes human dendritic cells (follicular dendritic cells) and their possible precursors in blood. Blood 62:585, 1983
30. Murphy GF, Bhan AK, Harrist TJ, Mihm MC: In situ identification of T6-positive cells in normal human dermis by immunoelectron microscopy. Br J Dermatol 108:423, 1983
31. Black MM, Speer FD: Sinus histiocytosis of lymph node in cancer. Surg Gynecol Obstet 106: 163, 1958
32. Albores-Saavedra J, Vuitch F, Delgado R et al: Sinus histiocytosis of pelvic lymph nodes after hip replacement. A histiocytic proliferation induced by cobalt-chromium and titanium. Am J Surg Pathol 18:83, 1994
33. Listinsky CM: Common reactive erythrophagocytosis in axillary lymph nodes. Hum Pathol 89: 189, 1988
34. Gould E, Perez J, Albores-Saavedra J, Legaspi A: Signet ring cell sinus histiocytosis: a previously unrecognized histologic condition mim-

icking metastatic adenocarcinoma in lymph node. Am J Clin Pathol ;92:509, 1989
35. Frost AR, Shek YH, Lack EE: "Signet ring" sinus histiocytosis mimicking metastatic adenocarcinoma: report of two cases with immunohistochemical and ultrastructural study. Mod Pathol 5:497, 1992
36. Destombes P: Adenites avec surcharge lipidique, de l'enfant ou de l'adulte jeune, observees aux antilles et au mali. Quatre observations. Bull Soc Pathol Exot Filiales 58:1169, 1965
37. Rosai J, Dorfman RF: Sinus histiocytosis with massive lymphadenopathy: a newly recognized benign clinicopathological entity. Arch Pathol 87:63, 1969
38. Rosai J, Dorfman RF: Sinus histiocytosis with massive lymphadenopathy: a pseudolymphomatous benign disorder. Analysis of 34 cases. Cancer 30:1174, 1972
39. Foucar E, Rosai J, Dorfman RF: Sinus histiocytosis with massive lymphadenopathy (Rosai-Dorfman disease): review of the entity. Semin Diagn Pathol 7:19, 1990
40. Foucar E, Rosai J, Dorfman RF, Eyman JM: Immunological abnormalities and their significance in sinus histiocytosis with massive lymphadenopathy. Am J Clin Pathol 82:515, 1984
41. Montgomery EA, Meis JM, Frizzera G: Rosai-Dorfman disease of soft tissue. Am J Surg Pathol 16:122, 1992
42. Leighton SEJ, Gallimore AP: Extranodal sinus histiocytosis with massive lymphadenopathy affecting the subglottis and trachea. Histopathology 24:393, 1994
43. Levine PH, Jahan N, Murari P et al: Detection of human herpesvirus 6 in tissues involved by sinus histiocytosis with massive lymphadenopathy (Rosai-Dorfman disease). J Infect Dis 166: 292, 1992
44. Tsang WYW, Yip TTC, Chan JKC: The Rosai-Dorfman disease histiocytes are not infected by Epstein-Barr virus. Histopathology 25:88, 1994
45. Ngendahayo P, Roels H, Quatacker J et al: Sinus histiocytosis with massive lymphadenopathy in Rwanda: report of eight cases with immunohistochemical and ultrastructural studies. Histopathology 7:49, 1983
46. Bonetti F, Chilosi M, Menestrinia F et al: Immunohistological analysis of Rosai-Dorfman histiocytosis—a disease of S100+CD1− histiocytes. Virchows Arch [A] 411:129, 1987
47. Eisen RN, Buckley PJ, Rosai J: Immunophenotypic characterization of sinus histiocytosis with massive lymphadenopathy (Rosai-Dorfman disease). Semin Diagn Pathol 7:74, 1990
47a. Marmaduke DP, Rosai J, Warnke R et al: Molecular assessment of clonality in sinus histiocytosis with massive lymphadenopathy (SHML): a reactive disorder of polyclonal histiocytes. Mod Pathol 9:677A, 1996
48. Komp DM: The treatment of sinus histiocytosis with massive lymphadenopathy (Rosai-Dorfman disease). Semin Diagn Pathol 7:83, 1990
49. Foucar E, Rosai J, Dorfman RF: Sinus histiocytosis with massive lymphadenopathy. An analysis of 14 deaths occurring in a patient registry. Cancer 54:1834, 1984
50. Risdall RJ, McKenna RW, Nesbit ME et al: Virus-associated hemophagocytic syndrome. A benign histiocytic proliferation distinct from malignant histiocytosis. Cancer 44:993, 1979
51. Risdall RJ, Brunning RD, Hernandez JI, Gordon DH: Bacteria-associated hemophagocytic syndrome. Cancer 54:2968, 1984
52. McKenna RW, Risdall RJ, Brunning RD: Virus associated hemophagocytic syndrome. Hum Pathol 12:395, 1981
53. Gupta P, Hurley RW, Helseth PH et al: Pancytopenia due to hemophagocytic syndrome as the presenting manifestation of babesiosis. Am J Hematol 50:60, 1995
54. Marty AM, Dumler JS, Imes G et al: Ehrlichiosis mimicking thrombotic thrombocytopenic purpura. Case report and pathological correlation. Hum Pathol 26:920, 1995
55. Eliopoulos G, Vaiopoulos G, Kittas C, Fessas P: Tuberculosis associated hemophagocytic syndrome complicated with severe bone marrow failure and disseminated intravascular coagulation. Nouv Rev Fr Hematol 34:273, 1992
56. Gaffey MJ, Frierson HF Jr, Medeiros LJ, Weiss LM: The relationship of Epstein-Barr virus to infection-related (sporadic) and familial hemophagocytic syndrome and secondary (lymphoma-related) hemophagocytosis: an in situ hybridization study. Hum Pathol 24:657, 1993
57. Wong KF, Chan JK: Reactive hemophagocytic syndrome—a clinicopathologic study of 40 patients in an Oriental population. Am J Med 93: 177, 1992
58. Chang C-S, Wang C-H, Su I-J et al: Hematophagic histiocytosis: a clinicopathologic analysis of 23 cases with special reference to the association

with peripheral T-cell lymphoma. J Formos Med Assoc 93:421, 1994

59. Favara BE: Hemophagocytic lymphohistiocytosis: a hemophagocytic syndrome. Semin Diagn Pathol 9:63, 1992
60. Imashuku S, Hibi S: Cytokines in haemophagocytic syndrome. Br J Haematol 77:438, 1991
61. Rostaing L, Fillola G, Baron E et al: Course of hemophagocytic histiocytic syndrome in renal transplants. Transplantation 60:506, 1995
62. King PD, Diaz-Arias AA, Birkby WF, Loy TS: Reactive hemophagocytic syndrome simulating acute hepatitis. A case due to hepatic peripheral T-cell lymphoma. J Clin Gastroenterol 19:235, 1994
63. Smith KJ, Skelton HG, Yeager J et al: Cutaneous histopathologic, immunohistochemical, and clinical manifestations in patients with hemophagocytic syndrome. Arch Dermatol 128: 193, 1992
64. van Gils FC, Mulder AH, van den Bos C et al: Acute side effects of homologous interleukin-3 in rhesus monkeys. Am J Pathol 143:1621, 1993
65. Chen R-L, Su I-J, Lin K-H et al: Fulminant childhood hemophagocytic syndrome mimicking histiocytic medullary reticulosis. An atypical form of Epstein-Barr virus infection. Am J Clin Pathol 96:171, 1991
66. Kikuta H, Sakiyama T, Matsumoto S et al: Fatal Epstein-Barr virus-associated hemophagocytic syndrome. Blood 82:3259, 1993
67. Kikuta H: Epstein-Barr virus-associated hemophagocytic syndrome. Leuk Lymphoma 16:425, 1995
68. Weiss LM, Azzi R, Dorfman RF, Warnke RA: Sinusoidal hematolymphoid malignancy (''malignant histiocytosis'') presenting as atypical sinusoidal proliferation. A study of nine cases. Cancer 58:1681, 1986
69. Jaffe ES, Costa J, Fauci AS et al: Malignant lymphoma and erythrophagocytosis simulating malignant histiocytosis. Am J Med 75:741, 1983
70. Falini B, Pileri S, De Solas I et al: Peripheral T-cell lymphoma associated with hemophagocytic syndrome. Blood 75:434, 1990
71. Chubachi A, Imai H, Nishimura S et al: Nasal T-cell lymphoma associated with hemophagocytic syndrome. Immunohistochemical and genotypic studies. Arch Pathol Lab Med 116:1209, 1992
72. Craig FE, Clare CN, Sklar JL, Banks PM: T-cell lymphoma and the virus-associated hemophagocytic syndrome. Am J Clin Pathol 97:189, 1992
73. Gonzalez CL, Medeiros LJ, Braziel RM, Jaffe ES: T-cell lymphoma involving subcutaneous tissue. Am J Surg Pathol 15:17, 1991
74. Hathirat P, Chuansumrit A, Nitiyanant P et al: Histiocytoses in children: analysis of 120 cases and the bone marrow findings in infection-induced hemophagocytic syndrome vs. malignant histiocytosis. J Med Assoc Thai 76:72, 1993
75. Wu CS, Chang KY, Dunn P, Lo TH: Acute hepatitis A with coexistent hepatitis C virus infection presenting as a virus-associated hemophagocytic syndrome: a case report. Am J Gastroenterol 90:1002, 1995
76. Komatsuda A, Chubachi A, Miura AB: Virus-associated hemophagocytic syndrome due to measles accompanied by acute respiratory failure. Intern Med 34:203, 1995
77. Bell MD, Wright RK: Fatal virus-associated hemophagocytic syndrome in a young adult producing nontraumatic splenic rupture. J Forensic Sci 37:1407, 1992
78. Farquhar JW, Claireaux AF: Familial hemophagocytic reticulosis. Arch Dis Child 27:519, 1952
79. Stark B, Hershko C, Rosen N et al: Familial hemophagocytic lymphohistiocytosis (FHLH) in Israel. Cancer 54:2109, 1984
80. Janka GE: Familial hemophagocytic lymphohistiocytosis: review. Eur J Pediatr 140:221, 1983
81. Mache CJ, Slavc I, Schmid C et al: Familial hemophagocytic lymphohistiocytosis associated with disseminated T-cell lymphoma: a report of two siblings. Ann Hematol 69:85, 1994
82. Soffer D, Okon E, Rosen N et al: Familial hemophagocytic lymphohistiocytosis in Israel. II. Pathologic findings. Cancer 54:2423, 1984
83. Silverman JF, Singh HK, Joshi VV et al: Cytomorphology of familial hemophagocytic syndrome. Diagn Cytopathol 9:404, 1993
84. Wieczorek R, Greco A, McCarthy K et al: Familial erythrophagocytic lymphohistiocytosis: immunophenotypic, immunohistochemical and ultrastructural demonstration of the relation to sinus histiocytes. Hum Pathol 17:55, 1986
85. Fullerton P, Ekert H, Hosking C, Tauro GP: Hemophagocytic reticulosis. A case report with investigations of immune and white cell function. Cancer 36:441, 1975
86. Ladisch S, Holiman B, Poplack DG, Blaese RM:

Immunodeficiency in familial erythrophagocytic lymphohistiocytosis. Lancet 1:581, 1978
87. Granert C, Elinder G, Ost A, Henter JI: Kala-azar in a one-year-old Swedish child. Diagnostic difficulties because of active hemophagocytosis. Acta Paediatr 82:794, 1993
88. Kletzel M, Gollin SM, Gloster ES et al: Chromosome abnormalities in familial hemophagocytic lymphohistiocytosis. Cancer 57:2153, 1986
89. Ahmed T, Mehta R, Patel P et al: Bone marrow transplantation for familial hemophagocytic lymphohistiocytosis. Anticancer Res 9:1567, 1989
90. Boyd AW, Ellis DW, Kannourakis G et al: Activated killer cell lymphoma: an erythrophagocytic syndrome simulating histiocytic medullary reticulosis. Pathology 20:265, 1988
91. Ohshima K, Kikuchi M, Mizuno S et al: Hepatosinusoidal leukaemia/lymphoma consisting of Epstein-Barr virus-containing natural killer cell leukaemia/lymphoma and T-cell lymphoma; mimicking malignant histiocytosis. Hematol Oncol 13:83, 1995
92. Chan YF, Lee KC, Llewellyn H: Subcutaneous T-cell lymphoma presenting as panniculitis in children: report of 2 cases. Pediatr Pathol 14: 595, 1994
93. Cheng AL, Su IJ, Chen YC et al: Characteristic clinicopathologic features of Epstein-Barr virus-associated peripheral T-cell lymphoma. Cancer 72:909, 1993
94. Kaplan MA, Jacobson JO, Ferry JA, Harris NL: T-cell lymphoma of the vulva in a renal allograft recipient with associated hemophagocytosis. Am J Surg Pathol 17:842, 1993
95. Simrell CF, Margolick JB, Crabtree GR et al: Lymphokine-induced phagocytosis in angiocentric immunoproliferative lesions (AIL) and malignant lymphoma arising in AIL. Blood 65: 1469, 1985
96. Takeshita M, Kikuchi M, Ohshima K et al: Bone marrow findings in malignant histiocytosis and/ or malignant lymphoma with concurrent hemophagocytic syndrome Leuk Lymphoma 12:79, 1993
97. Juneja JS, Elder FFB, Rakaraman S: Acute monoblastic leukemia with a single chromosomal rearrangement involving breakpoints on chromosomes 8 and 16, 46,XX,t(8;16)(p11p13). Acta Haematol 78:1, 1987
98. Stark B, Resnitzky P, Jeison M et al: A distinct subtype of M4;M5 acute myeloblastic leukemia (AML) associated with t(8;16)(p11:NOp13), in a patient with the variant t(8;16)(p11:NOq-13)—case report and review of the literature. Leuk Res 19:367, 1995
99. Kadin ME, Kamoun M, Lamberg J: Erythrophagocytic T-γ lymphoma. A clinicopathologic entity resembling malignant histiocytosis. N Engl J Med 304:648, 1981
100. Farcet K, Gaulard P, Marolleau JP et al: Hepatosplenic T-cell lymphoma: sinusal/sinusoidal localization of malignant cells expressing the T-cell receptor $\gamma\delta$. Blood 75:2213, 1990
101. Wong KF, Chan JK, Matutes E et al: Hepatosplenic $\gamma\delta$ T-cell lymphoma: a distinctive aggressive lymphoma type. Am J Surg Pathol 6:718, 1995
102. Dorfman RF, Warnke R: Lymphadenopathy simulating the malignant lymphomas. Hum Pathol 5:519, 1974
103. Gould E, Porto R, Albores-Saavedra J, Ibe MJ: Dermatopathic lymphadenitis. The spectrum and significance of its morphologic features. Arch Pathol Lab Med 112:1145, 1988
104. Weiss LM, Warnke RA, Wood GS: Immunophenotypic differences between dermatopathic lymphadenopathy and lymph node involvement in mycosis fungoides. Am J Pathol 120:179, 1985
105. Weiss LM, Hu E, Wood GS et al: Clonal rearrangements of the T-cell receptor gene in mycosis fungoides and dermatopathic lymphadenopathy. N Engl J Med 284:539, 1985
106. Lichtenstein L: Histiocytosis X: integration of eosinophilic granuloma of bone, Letterer-Siwe disease and Schuller-Christian disease as related manifestations of a single nosologic entity. Arch Pathol 56:84, 1953
107. Berry DH, Becton DL: Natural history of histiocytosis X. Hematol Oncol Clin North Am 1:23, 1987
108. Mickelson MR, Bonfiglio M: Eosinophilic granuloma and its variations. Orthop Clin North Am 8:933, 1977
109. Winkelmann RK: The skin in histiocytosis X. Mayo Clin Proc 44:535, 1969
110. Alessi DM, Maceri D: Histiocytosis X of the head and neck in a pediatric population. Arch Otolaryngol Head Neck Surg 118:945, 1992
111. Tazi A, Bonay M, Grandsaigne M et al: Surface phenotype of Langerhans cells and lymphocytes in granulomatous lesions from patients with pul-

monary histiocytosis X. Am Rev Respir Dis 147:1531, 1993

112. Colby TV, Lombard C: Histiocytosis X in the lung. Hum Pathol 14:847, 1983
113. Katz AM, Rosenthal SD, Jakubovic HR et al: Langerhans cell histiocytosis in monozygotic twins. J Am Acad Dermatol 24:32, 1991
114. Hanapiah F, Yaacob H, Ghani KS, Hussin AS: Histiocytosis X: evidence for a genetic etiology. J Nihon Univ Sch Dent 35:171, 1993
115. Leahy MA, Knejei SM, Friedmanash M et al: Human herpesvirus 6 is present in lesions of Langerhans cell histiocytosis. J Invest Dermatol 101:642, 1993
116. McClain K, Jin H, Gresik V, Favara B: Langerhans cell histiocytosis—lack of viral etiology. Am J Hematol 47;16, 1994
117. Friedman PJ, Liebow AA, Sokoloff J: Eosinophilic granuloma of lung. Clinical aspects of primary pulmonary histiocytosis in the adult. Medicine 60:385, 1981
118. Tomashefski JF, Khiyami A, Kleinerman J: Neoplasms associated with pulmonary eosinophilic granuloma. Arch Pathol Lab Med 115: 499, 1991
119. Uebelhoer M, Bewig B, Kreipe H et al: Modulation of fibroblast activity in histiocytosis X by platelet-derived growth factor. Chest 107:701, 1995
120. Writing Group of the Histiocyte Society: Histiocytosis syndromes in children. Lancet i:208, 1987
121. Hartman KS: Histiocytosis X: a review of 114 cases with oral involvement. Oral Surg 49:38, 1980
122. Wester SM, Beabout JW, Unni KK, Dahlin DC: Langerhans' cell granulomatosis (histiocytosis X) of bone in adults. Am J Surg Pathol 6:413, 1982
123. Motoi M, Helbron D, Kaiserling E, Lennert K: Eosinophilic granuloma of lymph nodes—a variant of histiocytosis X. Histopathology 4: 585, 1980
124. Travis WD, Borok Z, Roum JH et al: Pulmonary Langerhans' cell granulomatosis (histiocytosis X). A clinicopathologic study of 48 cases. Am J Surg Pathol 17:971, 1993
125. Soler P, Kambouchner M, Valeyre D, Hance AJ: Pulmonary Langerhans' cell granulomatosis. Annu Rev Med 43:105, 1992
126. Siegal GP, Dehner LP, Rosai J: Histiocytosis X (Langerhans' cell granulomatosis) of the thymus: clinicopathologic study of four childhood cases. Am J Surg Pathol 9:117, 1985
127. Williams JW, Dorfman RF: Lymphadenopathy as the initial manifestation of histiocytosis X. Am J Surg Pathol 3:405, 1979
128. Savell V, Hanna R, Benda JA, Argenyi ZB: Histiocytosis X of the vulva with a confusing clinical and pathologic presentation. A case report. J Reprod Med 40:323, 1995
129. Hamilton B, Connolly ES, Mitchell WT Jr: Isolated intramedullary histiocytosis-X of the cervical spinal cord. Case report. J Neurosurg 83: 716, 1995
130. Erly WK, Carmody RF, Dryden RM: Orbital histiocytosis X. Am J Neuroradiol 16:1258, 1995
131. Enriquez P, Dahlin DC, Hayles AB, Henderson ED: Histiocytosis X: a clinical study. Mayo Clin Proc 42:88, 1967
132. Greenberger JS, Crocker AC, Vawter G et al: Results of treatment of 127 patients with systemic histiocytosis (Letterer-Siwe syndrome, Schuller-Christian syndrome and multifocal eosinophilic granuloma). Medicine 60:311, 1981
133. DiMaggio LA, Lippes HA, Lee RV: Histiocytosis X and pregnancy. Obstet Gynecol 85: 806, 1995
134. Scherbaum WA, Seif FJ: Spontaneous transient remission of disseminated histiocytosis X during pregnancy. J Cancer Res Clin Oncol 121: 57, 1995
135. Braunstein GD, Kohler PO: Endocrine manifestations of histiocytosis. Am J Pediatr Hematol Oncol 3:67, 1981
136. Helm KF, Lookingbill DP, Marks JG Jr: A clinical and pathologic study of histiocytosis X in adults. J Am Acad Dermatol 1993 29:166, 1993
137. Risdall RJ, Dehner LP, Duray P et al: Histiocytosis X (Langerhans' cell histiocytosis). Prognostic role of histopathology. Arch Pathol Lab Med 107:59, 1983
138. Nezelof C, Frileux-Herbet F, Cronier-Sachot J: Disseminated histiocytosis X. Analysis of prognostic factors based on a retrospective study of 50 cases. Cancer 44:1824, 1979
139. Favara BE, Jaffe R: Pathology of Langerhans cell histiocytosis. Hematol Oncol Clin North Am 1:75, 1987
140. Burns BF, Colby TV, Dorfman RD: Langerhans' cell granulomatosis (histiocytosis X) associated with malignant lymphomas. Am J Surg Pathol 7:529, 1983

141. Egeler RA, Neglia JP, Puccetti DM et al: Association of Langerhans cell histiocytosis with malignant neoplasms. Cancer 71:865, 1993
142. Neumann MP, Frizzera G: The coexistence of Langerhans' cell granulomatosis and malignant lymphoma may take different forms: report of seven cases with a review of the literature. Hum Pathol 17:1060, 1986
143. Hesseling PB, Wessels G, Egeler RM, Rossouw DJ: Simultaneous occurrence of viral-associated hemophagocytic syndrome and Langerhans cell histiocytosis: a case report. Pediatr Hematol Oncol 12:135, 1995
144. Favara BE: Langerhans cell histiocytosis: pathobiology and pathogenesis. Semin Oncol 18: 3, 1991
145. Fartasch M, Vigneswaran N, Diepger TL, Hornstein OP: Immunohistochemical and ultrastructural study of histiocytosis X and non-X histiocytoses. J Am Acad Dermatol 23:885, 1990
146. Mierau GW, Favara BE, Brenman JM: Electron microscopy in histiocytosis X. Ultrastr of Pathol 3:137, 1982
147. Yu RC, Morris JF, Pritchard J, Chu TC: Defective alloantigen-presenting capacity of "Langerhans cell histiocytosis cells." Arch Dis Child 67:1370, 1992
148. Azumi N, Sheibani K, Swartz WG et al: Antigenic phenotype of Langerhans cell histiocytosis: an immunohistochemical study demonstrating the value of LN-2, LN-3 and vimentin. Hum Pathol 19:1376, 1988
149. Ruco LP, Pulford KAF, Mason D et al: Expression of macrophage-associated antigens in tissues involved by Langerhans′ cell histiocytosis (histiocytosis X). Am J Clin Pathol 92:273, 1989
150. Battifora H, Alsabeh R, Jenkins KA, Gown A: Epitope retrieval (unmasking) in immunohistochemistry. Adv Pathol Lab Med 8:101, 1995
151. Santamaria M, Llamas L, Ree HI et al: Expression of sialylated Leu-M1 antigen in histiocytosis X. Am J Clin Pathol 89:211, 1988
152. Krenacs L, Tiszlavicz L, Krenacs T, Boumsell L: Immunohistochemical detection of CD1a antigen in formalin-fixed and paraffin-embedded tissue sections with monoclonal antibody O10. J Pathol 171:99, 1993
153. Ornvold K, Ralfkiaer E, Carstensen H: Immunohistochemical study of the abnormal cells in Langerhans cell histiocytosis (histiocytosis X). Virchows Arch [A] 416:403, 1990
154. Ruco LP, Remotti D, Monardo F et al: Letterer-Siwe disease: immunohistochemical evidence for a proliferative disorder involving immature cells of Langerhans′ lineage. Virchows Arch [A] 413:239, 1988
155. Ruco LP, Stoppacciaro A, Vitolo D et al: Expression of adhesion molecules in Langerhans′ cell histiocytosis. Histopathology 23:29, 1993
156. Willman CL, Busque L, Griffith BB et al: Langerhans′-cell histiocytosis (histiocytosis X)—a clonal proliferative disease. N Engl J Med 331:154, 1994
157. Yu RC, Chu C, Buluwela L, Chu AC: Clonal proliferation of Langerhans cells in Langerhans cell histiocytosis. Lancet 343:767, 1994
158. Yu RC, Chu AC: Lack of T-cell receptor gene rearrangements in cells involved in Langerhans cell histiocytosis. Cancer 75:1162, 1995
159. Ben-Ezra J, Bailey A, Azumi N et al: Malignant histiocytosis X—a distinct clinicopathologic entity. Cancer 68:1050, 1991
160. Wood C, Wood GS, Deneau DG et al: Malignant histiocytosis X. Report of a rapidly fatal case in an elderly man. Cancer 54:347, 1984
161. Delabie J, De Wolf-Peeters C, De Vos R et al: True histiocytic neoplasm of Langerhans′ cell type. J Pathol 163:217, 1991
162. Weiss LM, Beckstead JH, Warnke RA, Wood GS: Leu-6-expressing cells in lymph nodes: dendritic cells phenotypically similar to interdigitating cells. Hum Pathol 17:179, 1986
163. Ceci A, de Terlizzi M, Colella R et al: Langerhans cell histiocytosis in childhood: results from the Italian Cooperative AIEOP-CNR-H.X '83 study. Med Pediatr Oncol 21:259, 1993
164. Yu LC, Shenoy S, Ward K, Warrier RP: Successful treatment of multisystem Langerhans cell histiocytosis (histiocytosis X) with etoposide. Am J Pediatr Hematol Oncol 16:275, 1994
165. Komp DM, Herson J, Starling KA et al: A staging system for histiocytosis X: a Southwest Oncology Group Study. Cancer 147:798, 1981
166. Lahey ME: Prognostic factors in histiocytosis X. Am J Pediatr Hematol Oncol 3:57, 1981
167. Broadbent V, Pritchard J, Davies EG et al: Spontaneous remission of multi-system histiocytosis X. Lancet i:253, 1984
168. Bartholdy N, Thommesen P: Histiocytosis X. VIII. Prognostic significance of skull lesions. Acta Radiol Oncol 22:125, 1983
169. Monda L, Warnke R, Rosai J: A primary lymph

node malignancy with features suggestive of dendritic reticulum cell differentiation. A report of 4 cases. Am J Pathol 122:562, 1986

170. Weiss LM, Berry GJ, Dorfman RF et al: Spindle cell neoplasms of lymph nodes of probable reticulum cell lineage. True reticulum cell sarcoma? Am J Surg Pathol 14:405, 1990
171. Hollowood K, Pease C, Mackay AM, Fletcher CDM: Sarcomatoid tumors of lymph nodes showing follicular dendritic cell differentiation. J Pathol 163:205, 1991
172. Chan JKC, Tsang WYW, Ng CS: Follicular dendritic cell tumor and vascular neoplasm complicating hyaline-vascular Castleman's disease. Am J Surg Pathol 18:517, 1994
173. Chan JKC, Tsang WYW, Ng CS et al: Follicular dendritic cell tumors of the oral cavity. Am J Surg Pathol 148, 1994
174. Stricker JG, Parkin JL, Schmidt CM: Primary skin malignancy with features suggestive of dendritic reticulum cell differentiation. Ultrastruct Pathol 14:273, 1990
175. Hollowood K, Stamp G, Zouvani I, Fletcher CDM: Extranodal follicular dendritic cell sarcoma of the gastrointestinal tract. Morphologic, immunohistochemical and ultrastructural analysis of two cases. Am J Clin Pathol 103:90, 1995
176. van der Valk P, Ruiter DJ, den Ottolander GJ et al: Dendritic reticulum cell sarcoma? Four cases of a lymphoma probably derived from dendritic reticulum cells of the follicular compartment. Histopathology 6:269, 1982
177. Turner RR, Wood GS, Beckstead JH et al: Histiocytic malignancies. Morphologic, immunologic and enzymatic heterogeneity. Am J Surg Pathol 8:485, 1984
178. Salisbury JR, Ramsay AD, Isaacson PG: Histiocytic lymphoma: a report of a case with an unusual phenotype. J Pathol 146:99, 1985
179. van den Oord JJ, de Wolf-Peeters C, de Vos R et al: Sarcoma arising from interdigitating reticulum cells: report of a case studied with light and electron microscopy, and enzyme- and immunohistochemistry. Histopathology 10:509, 1986
180. Hui PK, Feller AC, Kaiserling E et al: Skin tumor of T accessory cells (interdigitating reticulum cells) with high content of T lymphocytes. Am J Dermatopathol 9:129, 1987
181. Nakamura S, Hara K, Suchi T et al: Interdigitating cell sarcoma. A morphologic, immunohistologic, and enzyme-histochemical study. Cancer 61:562, 1988
182. Rabkin MS, Kjeldsberg CR, Hammond ME et al: Clinical, ultrastructural, immunohistochemical and DNA content analysis of lymphomas having features of interdigitating reticulum cells. Cancer 61:1594, 1988
183. Hammer SP, Rudolph RH, Bockus DE, Remington FI: Interdigitating reticulum cell sarcoma with unusual features. Ultrastruct Pathol 15:631, 1991
184. Yamakawa M, Matsuda M, Imai Y et al: Lymph node interdigitating cell sarcoma, a case report. Am J Clin Pathol 97:139, 1992
185. Miettinen M, Fletcher CDM, Lasota J: True histiocytic lymphoma of small intestine. Analysis of two S-100 protein-positive cases with features of interdigitating reticulum cell sarcoma. Am J Clin Pathol 100:285, 1993
186. Rousselet M-C, François S, Croué A et al: A lymph node interdigitating reticulum cell sarcoma. Arch Pathol Lab Med 118:183, 1994
187. Feltkamp CA, van Heerde P, Feltkamp-Vroom TM, Koudstaal J: A malignant tumor arising from interdigitating cells; light microscopical, ultrastructural, immuno- and enzyme-histochemical characteristics. Virchows Arch [Pathol Anat] 393:183, 1981
188. Vasef MA, Zaatari GS, Chan WC et al: Dendritic cell tumors assoicated with low-grade B-cell malignancies. Report of three cases. Am J Clin Pathol 104:696, 1995
189. Murphy GS, Bhan AK, Harrist TJ, Mihm MC Jr: In situ identification for T6-positive cells in normal human dermis by immunoelectron microscopy. Br J Dermatol 108:423, 1983
190. Segal GH, Mesa MV, Fishleder AJ et al: Precursor Langerhans cell histiocytosis. An unusual histiocytic proliferation in a patient with persistent non-Hodgkin lymphoma and terminal acute monocytic leukemia. Cancer 70:547, 1992
191. Kolde G, Bröcker E-B: Multiple skin tumors of indeterminate cells in an adult. J Am Acad Dermatol 15:591, 1986
192. Berti E, Gianotti R, Alessi E: Unusual cutaneous histiocytosis expressing an intermediate immunophenotype between Langerhans′ cells and dermal macrophages. Arch Dermatol 124:1250, 1988
193. Wood GS, Haber RS: Novel histiocytoses considered in the context of histiocyte subset differentiation. Arch Dermatol 129:210, 1992

194. Wood GS, Hu C-H, Beckstead JH et al: The indeterminate cell proliferative disorder: report of a case manifesting as an unusual cutaneous histiocytosis. J Dermatol Surg Oncol 11:1111, 1985
195. Bonetti F, Knowles DM, Chilosi M et al: A distinctive cutaneous malignant neoplasm expressing the Langerhans cell phenotype. Synchronous occurrence with B-chronic lymphocytic leukemia. Cancer 55:2417, 1985
196. Chan WC, Zaatari G: Lymph node interdigitating cell sarcoma. Am J Clin Pathol 85:739, 1986
197. Srichaikul T, Sonalkul D, Meejungwal P et al: Pleomorphic large cell hemato-lymphoma (the so-called malignant histiocytosis): clinicopathological and immunophenotypic studies in 35 cases. J Med Assoc Thai 77:588, 1994
198. Su IJ, Hsu YH, Lin MT et al: Epstein-Barr virus-containing T-cell lymphoma presents with hemophagocytic syndrome mimicking malignant histiocytosis. Cancer 72:2019, 1993
199. Ornvold K, Carstensen H, Junge J et al: Tumours classified as "malignant histiocytosis" in children are T-cell neoplasms. APMIS 100: 558, 1992
200. Weiss LM, Trela MJ, Cleary ML et al: Frequent immunoglobulin and T-cell receptor gene rearrangements in "histiocytic" neoplasms. Am J Pathol 121:369, 1985
201. Isaacson P, Wright DH: Malignant histiocytosis of the intestine. Its relationship to malabsorption and ulcerative jejunitis. Hum Pathol 9:661, 1978
202. Hodges JR, Isaacson P, Smith CL, Sworn MJ: Malignant histiocytosis of the intestine. Dig Dis Sci 24:631, 1979
203. Isaacson P, Wright D, Jones DE: Malignant lymphoma of true histiocytic (monocyte/macrophage) origin. Cancer 51:80, 1983
204. Salter DM, Krajewski AS, Dewar AE: Immunophenotype analysis of malignant histiocytosis of the intestine. J Clin Pathol 39:8, 1986
205. Wilson MS, Weiss LM, Gatter KC et al: Malignant histiocytosis. A reassessment of cases previously reported in 1975 based on paraffin section immunophenotyping studies. Cancer 66: 530, 1990
206. Egeler RM, Schmitz L, Sonneveld P et al: Malignant histiocytosis: a reassessment of cases formerly classified as histiocytic neoplasms and review of the literature. Med Pediatr Oncol 25: 1, 1995
207. Oka K, Mori N, Yatabe Y, Kojima M: Malignant histiocytosis. A report of three cases. Arch Pathol Lab Med 116:1228, 1992
208. Cattoretti G, Villa A, Vezzoni P et al: Malignant histiocytosis. A phenotypic and genotypic investigation. Am J Pathol 136;1009, 1990
209. Hsu SM, Ho YS, Hsu PL: Lymphomas of true histiocytic origin. Expression of different phenotype in so-called true histiocytic lymphoma and malignant histiocytosis. Am J Pathol 138: 1389, 1991
210. Hanson CA, Jaszcz W, Kersey JH et al: True histiocytic lymphoma: histopathologic, immunophenotypic and genotypic analysis. Br J Haematol 73:187, 1989
211. van der Kwast TH, van Dongen JJM, Michiels JJ et al: T-lymphoblastic lymphoma terminating as malignant histiocytosis with rearrangement of immunoglobulin heavy chain gene. Leukemia 5:78, 1991
212. Franchino C, Reich C, Distenfeld A et al: A clinicopathologically distinctive primary splenic histiocytic neoplasm. Demonstration of its histiocytic derivation by immunophenotypic and molecular genetic analysis. Am J Surg Pathol 12:398, 1988
213. Ralfkiaer E, Delsol G, O'Connor NTJ et al: Malignant lymphomas of true histiocytic origin. A clinical, histological, immunophenotypic and genotypic study. J Pathol 160:9, 1990
214. Milchgrub S, Kamel OW, Wiley E et al: Malignant histiocytic neoplasms of the small intestine. Am J Surg Pathol 16:11, 1992
215. Kamel OW, Gocke CD, Kell DL et al: True histiocytic lymphoma: a study of 12 cases based on current definition. Leuk Lymphoma 18:81, 1995
216. Aozasa K, Ohsawa M, Saeki K et al: Histiocytic neoplasias: immunohistochemical evaluation of their frequencies among malignant lymphoma and related conditions in Japan. J Surg Oncol 47:215, 1991
217. Bryne GE, Rappaport H: Malignant histiocytosis. P. 145. In Adazaki K, Rappaport H, Berard CW et al (eds): Malignant Disease of the Hematopoietic System. Gann Monograph on Cancer Research 15. University of Tokyo Press, Tokyo, 1973
218. Warnke RA, Kim H, Dorfman RF: Malignant histiocytosis ("histiocytic medullary reticulosis"). I. Clinicopathologic study of 29 cases. Cancer 34:215, 1975
219. Risdall RJ, Sibley RK, McKenna RW et al: Ma-

lignant histiocytosis. A light - and electron - microscopic and histochemical study. Am J Surg Pathol 4:439, 1980

220. Arai E, Su WPD, Roche PC, Li C-Y: Cutaneous histiocytic malignancy. Immunohistochemical re-examination of cases previously diagnosed as cutaneous ''histiocytic lymphoma'' and ''malignant histiocytosis.'' J Cutan Pathol :20:115, 1993
221. Wood GS, Warner NL, Warnke RA: Anti-Leu3/ T4 antibodies react with cells of monocyte/ macrophage and Langerhans lineage. J Immunol 131:212, 1983
222. Isaacson PG, Spencer J, Connolly CH et al: Malignant histiocytosis of the intestine: a T-cell lymphoma. Lancet 1:688, 1985
223. Levine EG, Hanson CA, Jaszcz W, Peterson BA: True histiocytic lymphoma. Semin Oncol 18:39, 1991
224. Weiss LM, Crabtree GS, Rouse RV, Warnke RA: Morphologic and immunologic characterization of 50 peripheral T cell lymphomas. Am J Pathol 118:316, 1985
225. Picker LJ, Weiss LM, Medeiros LJ et al: Immunophenotypic criteria for the diagnosis of non-Hodgkin's lymphoma. Am J Pathol 128:181, 1987
226. Weiss LM, Picker LJ, Grogan TM et al: Absence of beta and gamma T cell receptor gene rearrangements in a subset of peripheral T cell lymphomas. Am J Pathol 130:436, 1988
227. Weiss LM, Picker LJ, Copenhaver CM et al: Large-cell hematolymphoid neoplasms of uncertain lineage. Hum Pathol 19:967, 1988
228. Morgan R, Hecht BK, Sandberg AA et al: Chromosome 5q35 breakpoint in malignant histiocytosis. N Engl J Med 314:1322, 1986
229. Benz-Lemoine E, Brizard A, Huret J-L et al: Malignant histiocytosis: a specific t(2;5)(;23; q35) translocation? Review of the literature. Blood 72:1045, 1988
230. Nezelof C: The 5q35bp chromosomal abnormality characterizes certain CD30 positive anaplastic large cell lymphoma offering a new definition of malignant histiocytosis in childhood. Nouv Rev Fr Hematol 35:463, 1993
231. Abe R, Akaike T, Yokoyama A et al: High incidence of 17p13 chromosomal abnormalities in malignant histiocytosis. Cancer 65:2689, 1990
232. Okada Y, Nakanishi I, Nomura H et al: Angiotropic B-cell lymphoma with hemophagocytic syndrome. Pathol Res Pract 190:718, 1994
233. Bucksy P, Favara B, Feller AC et al: Malignant histiocytosis and large cell anaplastic (Ki-1) lymphoma in childhood: guidelines for differential diagnosis—report of the Histiocyte Society. Med Pediatr Oncol 22:200, 1994
234. DeMent SH: Association between mediastinal germ cell tumors and hematologic malignancies: an update. Hum Pathol 21:699, 1990
235. Nichols CR, Roth BJ, Heerema N et al: Hematologic neoplasia associated with primary mediastinal germ-cell tumors. N Engl J Med 322:1425, 1990
236. Koo CH, Reifel J, Kogut N et al: True histiocytic malignancy associated with a malignant teratoma in a patient with 46XY gonadal dysgenesis. Am J Surg Pathol 16:175, 1992
237. Takahashi S, Asamoto M, Nakazawa T et al: Robb-Smith type malignant histiocytosis associated with a mediastinal germ cell tumor. Jpn J Clin Oncol 24:327, 1994
234. Cudennec CA, Johnson GR: Presence of multipotential hemopoietic cells in teratocarcinoma cultures. J Embryol Exp Morphol 61:51, 1981
238. Domizio P, Hall PA, Cotter F et al: Angiotropic large cell lymphoma: morphological, immunohistochemical and genotypic studies with analysis of previous reports. Hematol Oncol 7:195, 1989
239. O'Grady JT, Shahidullah H, Doherty VR, Al-Nafussi A: Intravascular histiocytosis. Histopathology 24:265, 1994
240. Scott RB, Robb-Smith AHT: Histiocytic medullary reticulosis. Lancet 2:194, 1939
241. Headington JT, Roth MS, Ginsburg D et al: T cell receptor gene rearrangements in regressing atypical histiocytosis. Arch Dermatol 123:1183, 1987
242. Weiss LM, Wood GS, Trela MJ et al: Clonal T cell populations in lymphomatoid papulosis: evidence for a lymphoproliferative etiology in a clinically benign disease. N Engl J Med 315: 475, 1986
243. Kadin ME, Vonderheid EC, Sako D et al: Clonal composition of T cells in lymphomatoid papulosis. Am J Pathol 126:13, 1987
244. Willemze R, Beljaards RC: Spectrum of primary cutaneous CD30 (Ki-1)-positive lymphoproliferative disorders. J Am Acad Dermatol 28:973, 1993

Index

Page numbers followed by f *indicate figures; those followed by* t *indicate tables.*